Cardiac Anesthesia

CLINICAL CARDIOLOGY MONOGRAPHS

SERIES CONSULTANTS: J. Willis Hurst, M.D., and Dean T. Mason, M.D.

Atheroslerosis: Its Pediatric Aspects edited by William B. Strong

Advances in Heart Disease, Volume 2 edited by Dean T. Mason

Infective Endocarditis edited by Shahbudin H. Rahimtoola

Hyperlipidemia: Diagnosis and Therapy edited by Basil M. Rifkind and Robert I. Levy

Cardiac Arrhythmias: Electrophysiologic Basis for Clinical Interpretation edited by Yoshio Watanabe and Leonard S. Dreifus

Advances in Heart Disease, Volume 1 edited by Dean T. Mason

Echocardiography: A Teaching Atlas by Joel M. Felner and Robert C. Schlant

Advances in Electrocardiography, Volume 2 edited by Robert C. Schlant and J. Willis Hurst

Clinical Cardiovascular Physiology edited by Herbert J. Levine

The Acute Coronary Attack by J. F. Pantridge, A.A.J. Adgey, J.S. Geddes, and S.W. Webb

The Peripheral Circulations edited by Robert Zelis

Rheumatic Fever and Streptococcal Infection by Gene H. Stollerman

Shock in Myocardial Infarction edited by Rolf M. Gunnar, Henry S. Loeb, and Shahbudin H. Rahimtoola

Noninvasive Cardiology edited by Arnold M. Weissler

Advances in Cardiovascular Surgery edited by John W. Kirklin

Cardiac Pacing edited by Philip Samet

Myocardial Diseases edited by Noble O. Fowler

Advances in Electrocardiography, Volume 1 edited by Robert C. Schlant and J. Willis Hurst

Cardiac Anesthesia

Edited by

Joel A. Kaplan, M.D.

Associate Professor, Department of Anesthesiology
Director, Division of Cardiothoracic Anesthesia
Emory University School of Medicine
Atlanta, Georgia

GRUNE & STRATTON
A Subsidiary of Harcourt Brace Jovanovich, Publishers
New York   London   Toronto   Sydney   San Francisco

Library of Congress Cataloging in Publication Data
Main entry under title:

Cardiac anesthesia.

Includes bibliographical references and index.
1. Anesthesia in cardiology. I. Kaplan, Joel A.
[DNLM: 1. Anesthesia. 2. Heart—Drug effects.
3. Heart surgery. WG169 C267]
RD598.C34   617'.967'412   78-21566
ISBN 8-8089-1125-2

Grune & Stratton, Inc.
111 Fifth Avenue
New York, New York 10003

Distributed in the United Kingdom by
Academic Press, Inc. (London) Ltd.
24/28 Oval Road, London NW 1

Library of Congress Catalog Number 78-21566
International Standard Book Number 0-8089-1125-2

Printed in the United States of America

This book is dedicated to the memory of Robert D. Dripps, M.D., mentor, teacher, friend. His inspiration, guidance, knowledge, and expertise were invaluable to me.

Contents

Foreword

J. Willis Hurst, M.D.
Charles R. Hatcher, Jr., M.D.
John E. Steinhaus, M.D.

Preface

Contributors

Part I: Pharmacology and Monitoring

1 Pharmacology—Anesthetic Drugs
  Carl C. Hug, Jr., M.D., Ph.D.   *3*

2 Pharmacology—Cardiac Drugs
  Carl C. Hug, Jr., M.D., Ph.D., and Joel A. Kaplan, M.D.   *39*

3 Hemodynamic Monitoring
  Joel A. Kaplan, M.D.   *71*

4 Electrocardiographic Monitoring
  Joel A. Kaplan, M.D.   *117*

Part II: Disease Entities and Anesthesia

5 Preoperative Management
  Lawrence M. Abrams, M.D., and Donn A. Chambers, M.D.   *169*

6 Anesthesia for the Patient with Acquired Valvular Heart Disease
  Donn A. Chambers, M.D.   *197*

7 Anesthesia for Coronary Revascularization
  John L. Waller, M.D., Joel A. Kaplan, M.D., and Ellis L. Jones, M.D.   *241*

8 Anesthesia for Treatment of Congenital Heart Defects
  James W. Bland, M.D., and Willis H. Williams, M.D.   *281*

9 Pacemakers
  James R. Zaidan, M.D.   *347*

10 Thoracic Aneurysms
  Ronald W. Dunbar, M.D.   *369*

11   Anesthesia for Noncardiac Surgery in Patients with
     Cardiac Disease
     Joel A. Kaplan, M.D., and Ronald W. Dunbar, M.D.   *377*

Part III: Support of the Circulation
12   Cardiopulmonary Bypass
     Donald C. Finlayson, M.D., and Joel A. Kaplan, M.D.   *393*
13   Assisted Circulation
     Joel A. Kaplan, M.D., and Joseph M. Craver, M.D.   *441*

Part IV: Postoperative Care of the Patient
14   Postoperative Intensive Care
     Donald C. Finlayson, M.D.   *473*
15   Pericardial Diseases
     Joel A. Kaplan, M.D.   *491*
16   Cardiopulmonary Resuscitation
     John T. Bonner, M.D.   *501*

Index   **509**

Foreword

A Cardiologist's View of Cardiac Anesthesia

There was a time when pain was considered to be decreed by God. Accordingly, the people of that era believed that anyone who tried to alleviate pain was interfering with God's plans. By the early part of the nineteenth century, the United States Congress offered to award $100,000 to anyone who discovered an agent that would relieve pain.

Dr. Crawford W. Long, a country physician practicing in Jefferson, Georgia, removed a tumor from the neck of James Venable on March 30, 1842. The patient felt no pain because Dr. Long used ether anesthesia. Long did not publish his discovery. Dr. William Morton, a Boston dentist, demonstrated ether anesthesia on October 16, 1846, in the "Ether Dome" at the Massachusetts General Hospital. Claims and counterclaims were heard from all quarters as to who was the first to use ether anesthesia. The conflict made it possible for Congress to withhold the $100,000 that had been offered for the discovery of an anesthetic agent. Accordingly, this interesting method of stimulating research did not gain popularity. (I have never understood why the political geniuses of the period did not give Long and Morton $50,000 each.) This conflict is one reason investigators publish so quickly today. They want their views and discoveries documented in scientific journals.

One hundred years passed after ether anesthesia was first used before anesthesiology was well established. The fledgling discipline had the usual problems associated with achieving "identity," but by 1942 the specialty of anesthesiology was accepted. At that point in time, it was the anesthesiologist who knew the most about all the drugs that relieved pain. It was the anesthesiologist who knew the most about hypoxia and how to prevent it. It was the anesthesiologist who knew the most about the acute problems of the heart and circulation, such as shock, cardiac arrhythmias, acute heart failure, fluid balance, and resuscitation. It was the anesthesiologist who knew the most about pulmonary physiology and blood gases. By then, the anesthesiologist was assuming the responsibility of the safe conduct of the patient through a surgical procedure. By then, some anesthesiologists followed their patients for three days following surgery and were often the first to recognize postoperative complications.

Now, in 1978, the anesthesiologist is a highly skilled clinical pharmacologist, cardiologist, pulmonary expert, and intensivist. The field has contributed to and benefited from many of the recent advances in medicine. The field itself has now become subdivided into specialities. This book is testimony to this fact. This specialization has produced remarkable improvement in patient care. For example, both my surgical and medical colleagues give credit to our cardiac anesthesiologists for lowering the operative mortality for coronary bypass surgery at Emory University Hospital from 2–5 percent to 0.2–1.2 percent.

The modern cardiac anesthesiologist is highly skilled in:

- The preoperative evaluation of a patient. He may discover carotid artery disease that has not been identified earlier. This may lead the decison-making team to alter their plan of management for the patient. He may discover that the patient has been taking aspirin, and because of aspirin's effect on platelet function, this may alter the date of surgery. The medical consultant knows better than to recommend that a patient be given a certain anesthetic agent. The smart medical consultant is so smart that he or she chooses the anesthesiologist rather than the agent and never writes trite statements on the patient's record, such as "Please avoid hypotension and hypoxia." The latter statement is currently referred to as a cardiac insult rather than a cardiac consult!
- The use of technical procedures. The anesthesiologist may insert a Swan-Ganz catheter and perform other procedures, requiring entrance into a vein or artery, better than anyone else. The anesthesiologist can insert an endotracheal tube with great skill. He can also employ cardiopulmonary resuscitation (CPR) better than anyone else. In many hospitals, such as ours, the anesthesiologists take the leadership in teaching CPR.
- The monitoring of vital signs and functions of the heart and lungs. He can interpret the meaning of blood gases, the wedge pressure, the pulmonary diastolic pressure, the electrocardiogram, and so forth.
- The treatment of cardiac arrhythmias, shock, heart failure, pulmonary dysfunction, and the like.
- The use of drugs such as propranolol, nitroprusside, intravenous nitroglycerin, dopamine, norepinephrine, epinephrine, isoproterenol, metaraminol, dobutamine, glucagon, digitalis, atropine, morphine, and so on. In fact, the cardiac anesthesiologist has discovered new applications of certain drugs that are now used in situations unrelated to cardiac surgery.
- The use of numerous anesthetic agents.
- The immediate postoperative care of the patient. The postcardiac surgical intensive care unit is extremely important to the care of the postoperative patient. The cardiac surgical nurses are extremely talented and devoted to the cause. The cardiac surgeon, medical cardiologist, pulmonary expert, respiratory therapist, and hematologist all contribute to the care of the patient. It is now evident that the anesthesiologist plays a very important role in the intensive care unit. Many anesthesiologists have become "intensivists." An "intensivist" is skilled in the care of the patients who require intensive observation and treatment. Accordingly, at Emory University Hospital, the

anesthesiologist who administered the anesthesia continues to contribute to the follow-up care of the patient in the postoperative intensive care unit. The anesthesiologist is able to add the information he has regarding the experience he had with the patient during surgery. He assists in the management of hypotension, hypertension, arrhythmias, and so forth and assists in the ventilation of the patient, including determining when the endotracheal tube can be removed. It is necessary to carefully define the duties of the professional people involved in this care of the patient in the unit. Once this is done the patient care improves.

This book speaks for itself. It is what our anesthesiologists do at Emory University Hospital. The titles of the chapters indicate the scope of expertise exhibited by modern cardiac anesthesiologists. This cardiologist views the modern cardiac anesthesiologist with awe. I am grateful to them for what they do for our patients and for all they have taught me.

J. Willis Hurst, M.D.
Professor of Medicine (Cardiology)
Chairman of the Department of Medicine
Emory University School of Medicine
Atlanta, Georgia

A Cardiac Surgeon's View of Cardiac Anesthesia

Today, thousands of open heart surgical procedures are performed annually throughout the United States. In many hospitals such as our own, open heart procedures are among the most frequently performed operations and are considered entirely routine. Such widespread acceptance of the surgical treatment of congenital and acquired heart disease is based largely upon the remarkable benefits obtained at low risk. A major factor, if not *the* major factor, in the current remarkably low operative mortality for open heart surgery has been the emergence of the cardiac anesthesiologist.

Only a few years ago, critically ill cardiac patients were considered temporarily or permanently inoperable by competent anesthesiologists applying traditional modes of evaluation. Today, the frontiers of cardiac surgery have been expanded to include almost any patient, regardless of condition, and our anesthesiology colleagues have joined in these heroic efforts with enthusiasm to the mutual benefit of all concerned. Functioning as an integral member of the "open heart team," cardiac anesthesiologists are frequently involved in cardiac patient care long before the patient reaches the operating theater. Proper drug therapy alone or in concert with mechanical assistance to the failing circulation may permit diagnostic studies and surgery in desperate clinical situations. In less tenuous circumstances, the cardiac anesthesiologist joins with the cardiologists and cardiac surgeons in the critical effort of placing the patient in the operating room at the proper time in relation to a threatening disease process. Once surgery is undertaken, the cardiac anesthesiologist provides the impressive expertise necessary to induce anesthesia without significant cardiovascular depression—a formidable task requiring a thorough knowledge of monitoring devices and a complete understanding of modern cardiac pharmacology and physiology. Again, with surgery completed and extracorporeal circulation discontinued, the cardiac anesthesiologist assumes a primary role in adjusting anesthetic agents and cardiac drugs to provide maximum safe cardiac output. Finally, cardiac anesthesiologists participate actively in patient care in the cardiac surgical intensive care unit until patients are extubated and stable. Dr. Joel Kaplan, director of Cardiac Anesthesia at Emory University Hospital, is a cardiac anesthesiologist of the first rank. Dr. Kaplan and his associates in cardiac anesthesiology have made remarkable contributions to the care of cardiac patients in our institution and, at the same time, have conducted exciting basic and clinical research. As teachers of cardiac pharmacology and physiology to students and house staff, this group of cardiac anesthesiologists has been invaluable.

This timely book is based on the extensive experience of Dr. Kaplan and his associates. The chapters on the pharmacology of cardiac and anesthetic drugs are definitive for the practicing anesthesiologist. Anesthesia for the spectrum of cardiac diseases is amply covered in the chapters on coronary, valvular, and congenital heart disease. The discussion of cardiopulmonary bypass and assisted circulation will be of value to the anesthesiologist of limited experience who wishes to expand his role into the cardiac area. The chapter entitled "Anesthesia for Noncardiac Surgery in Patients with Cardiac Disease," should be required reading for all medical practitioners administering general anesthesia.

I believe that this work will be extremely well received by numerous segments of the medical profession. I congratulate Dr. Kaplan upon his factual information, his grasp of difficult problems, and his informative writing style. It has been my pleasure to work side by side with our cardiac anesthesiologists; and I have watched with pride their development, culminating in this book.

Charles R. Hatcher, Jr., M.D.
Professor of Surgery
Chief of the Division of Thoracic
    and Cardiovascular Surgery
Emory University School of Medicine
Director of Emory University Clinic
Atlanta, Georgia

An Anesthesiologist's View of Cardiac Anesthesia

As research in the medical sciences has continued to grow and the clinical applications of these findings are made, our medical knowledge base has expanded, creating new medical specialties and new subspecialties within established medical disciplines. Cardiac anesthesia has become a division within anesthesiology because of the need to synthesize the medical knowledge found within the cardiovascular areas of physiology and pharmacology, together with the clinical knowledge of heart disease basic to the cardiologist. This information must be combined and coordinated with the anesthesia knowledge and the special techniques of the anesthesiologist in order to provide safe anesthesia care for the increasing number of patients who have cardiac surgery for severe heart disease. Changes in cardiac rhythm and myocardial contractility produced by drugs, acid-base abnormalities, and hypoxemia, as well as the maintenance of adequate blood supply to all elements of the heart, pose special problems during anesthesia for cardiac surgery. The above factors are superimposed on a cardiovascular system that is already seriously altered by the patient's disease. Concurrently, the surgical procedure may require interruption of the heart's function and usual blood supply, as well as surgical invasion of coronary vessels, myocardium, or valves.

Although this book is devoted to the special problems of cardiac anesthesia, the information provided is exceedingly valuable to all anesthesiologists, since the maintenance of cardiovascular function is probably the most challenging problem facing the anesthesiologist giving general anesthesia for other kinds of surgery, especially with seriously ill patients. Not only does the usual surgical schedule contain a significant number of patients who are suffering from a variety of heart and vascular diseases in addition to the surgical disease for which the operation is planned, but practically all anesthetic drugs have the potential for causing serious cardiovascular changes such as myocardial depression, increased cardiac irritability, vasodilatation, or vasoconstriction. Furthermore, the autonomic drugs administered exogenously or released endogenously cause significant and serious circulatory alterations. Even the opiates and muscle relaxants, which cause relatively minor changes in cardiac function, can induce significant cardiovascular effects, including rate and vasomotor changes. Circulatory effects produced by anesthesia and surgery must be managed in patients who may have various degrees of fluid and electrolyte imbalance. Respiratory changes that cause disturbances of oxygen and carbon dioxide tensions may also produce serious alterations of the circulation. Consequently, the highly specialized area of cardiac anesthesia provides much information for the anesthesiologist predominately involved in other types of surgery. This book, valuable to both the general as well as the specialized anesthesiologist, brings together a segment of anesthetic technique and theory not readily available from other sources.

John E. Steinhaus, M.D.
Professor and Chairman, Department of
    Anesthesiology
Emory University School of Medicine
Atlanta, Georgia

Preface

This book was written for the purpose of improving anesthesia care for patients with cardiac disease. The text reflects the experience of the cardiac anesthesia group at Emory University School of Medicine. It is intended to present methods, materials, philosophy, attitudes, and fundamentals to enable those who use it to provide safe, individualized anesthetic care.

The focus of this book ranges from the preoperative visit by the anesthesiologist, through premedication, induction, and maintenance of anesthesia, circulatory, and respiratory support during surgery, to postoperative care of the patient in the intensive care unit. The book is organized into four parts, consisting of sixteen chapters and hundreds of illustrations. The four major areas covered are (1) pharmacology and monitoring, (2) disease entities and anesthesia, (3) mechanical support of the circulation, and (4) postoperative care of the patient. Throughout, the emphasis is on using sophisticated measurement techniques to determine proper therapeutic interventions and results. All aspects of patient care are presented in the belief that preoperative and postoperative management of the patient is as important as intraoperative management.

The material in the book is intended as an overview of the highly specialized field of cardiac anesthesia. Many medical disciplines have contributed to the development of this field. Therefore, this work may serve as a source book for use by anesthesia residents, cardiac anesthesia fellows, anesthesiologists interested in the field of cardiac anesthesia, cardiologists, cardiac surgeons, and, in particular, any practitioner interested in providing the best possible care for the cardiac patient undergoing any type of surgery.

I gratefully acknowledge the help of my fellow cardiac anesthesiologists at Emory for the expertly written chapters they contributed to this book. In addition, I would like to thank my colleagues in surgery and cardiology who have supplied valuable information and illustrations to me, as well as those authors from whose works I have borrowed pertinent illustrative material.

Further thanks must be expressed to Grover Hogan for his excellent graphic work on my behalf and to Joe Jackson and Marianne Stang for their photographic expertise.

In particular, my sincerest thanks to Lola Righton and Marianne Stang for the hours of overtime they spent preparing this manuscript for publication. Without their tireless efforts, it would never have been ready on time. Thanks also to the others who helped in its preparation—Cindy Lewis, Elaine Hall, Valeria Maier, and Elizabeth Lindley.

Above all, my deepest appreciation goes to my wife, Norma, for all the hours she spent inserting commas, correcting grammar, and undangling participles.

Joel A. Kaplan, M.D.

Contributors

LAWRENCE M. ABRAMS, M.D., Assistant Professor of Anesthesiology, Baylor College of Medicine, Houston, Texas.

JAMES W. BLAND, JR., M.D., Associate Professor of Anesthesia and Pediatrics, Director of Pediatric Cardiovascular Anesthesia, Emory University School of Medicine, and Medical Director, Intensive Care Unit, Henrietta Egleston Hospital for Children, Inc., Atlanta, Georgia.

JOHN T. BONNER, M.D., Assistant Professor of Anesthesiology, Allied Health and Surgery, Emory University School of Medicine, Atlanta, Georgia.

DONN A. CHAMBERS, M.D., Assistant Professor of Anesthesiology, Emory University School of Medicine, Atlanta, Georgia.

JOSEPH M. CRAVER, M.D., Assistant Professor of Surgery (Thoracic), Emory University School of Medicine, Atlanta, Georgia.

RONALD W. DUNBAR, M.D., Professor of Anesthesiology, Emory University School of Medicine, Atlanta, Georgia.

DONALD C. FINLAYSON, M.D., F.R.C.P. (C), Professor of Anesthesiology, Emory University School of Medicine, Atlanta, Georgia.

CARL C. HUG, JR., M.D., Ph.D., Associate Professor of Anesthesiology and Pharmacology, and Associate Director, Division of Cardiothoracic Anesthesia, Emory University School of Medicine, Atlanta, Georgia.

ELLIS L. JONES, M.D., Associate Professor of Surgery (Thoracic), Emory University School of Medicine, Atlanta, Georgia.

JOEL A. KAPLAN, M.D., Associate Professor of Anesthesiology, and Director, Division of Cardiothoracic Anesthesia, Emory University School of Medicine, Atlanta, Georgia.

JOHN L. WALLER, M.D., Assistant Professor of Anesthesiology, Emory University School of Medicine, Atlanta, Georgia.

WILLIS H. WILLIAMS, M.D., Associate Professor of Surgery (Cardiovascular), Emory University School of Medicine, and Chief of Surgery, Henrietta Egleston Hospital for Children, Inc., Atlanta, Georgia.

JAMES R. ZAIDAN, M.D., Assistant Professor of Anesthesiology, Emory University School of Medicine, Atlanta, Georgia.

Cardiac Anesthesia

PART I

Pharmacology and Monitoring

Carl C. Hug Jr., M.D., Ph.D

1

Pharmacology—Anesthetic Drugs

INTRODUCTION

The classic triad of anesthetic objectives includes analgesia, unconsciousness, and skeletal muscle relaxation. Traditionally, a single general anesthetic drug (e.g., diethyl ether) was administered to achieve all of these objectives. Although still appropriate under certain circumstances, the practice of using a single anesthetic drug has generally been abandoned for several reasons:

1. The use of other drugs to supplement general anesthetics allows a satisfactory state of anesthesia to be achieved while limiting the dose and toxicity of the general anesthetic drug.
2. The selective use of drugs for their specific effects on individual organ systems permits the anesthesiologist to tailor the anesthetic more nearly to the condition of the patient and the needs of the surgeon. Volatile general anesthetics have the advantage of being readily controlled in terms of overall depth of general anesthesia, but they have the potential disadvantage of widespread effects on all organ systems that cannot be controlled independently.
3. The critically ill patient often cannot tolerate general anesthesia of even a moderate depth. Such a patient, however, may be ef-

fectively and safely anesthetized by combinations of drugs that produce a light level of anesthesia, a satisfactory degree of muscular relaxation, and minimal changes in the function of vital organs.

4. A fourth objective of general anesthesia has been recognized with the increasing use of light levels of anesthesia, namely the control of reflex activity, especially of sympathetic responses to noxious stimulation. These responses are usually suppressed by moderate to deep levels of anesthesia with potent inhalational agents but remain reactive with the light levels of anesthesia produced by nitrous oxide supplemented with muscle relaxants and other drugs. Excessive reflex sympathetic activity can impose an intolerable burden on the cardiovascular system as the demands for oxygen delivery to tissues increase dramatically.

Many patients undergoing cardiac surgery are critically ill in the immediate preanesthetic period and, as a result of anesthesia and surgery, acquire additional instability of vital organ function in the intraoperative and postoperative periods. Survival of such patients demands careful attention to all aspects of their anesthetic management, including the proper choice and use of anesthetic drugs.

This chapter discusses the clinical phar-

3

macology of anesthetic drugs of particular interest to the anesthesiologist engaged in the care of patients with cardiac disease. It is worth noting that anesthesia for cardiovascular disease, especially for cardiac surgery, has led the way in the development of anesthetic practices suited to critically ill patients undergoing all types of surgery.

CONSIDERATIONS IN THE CHOICE OF ANESTHETIC DRUGS FOR PATIENTS UNDERGOING CARDIAC SURGERY

The Patient

All the usual concerns of anesthesiologists for their patients (e.g., previous anesthetic complications, pulmonary disease, current drug therapy) are relevant to the patient scheduled for cardiac surgery, and in addition there are special concerns. One of the most important is the nature of the cardiac disease, particularly the functional status of the left ventricle. For example, a patient with poor left ventricular function as a result of chronic valvular heart disease may be very sensitive to the myocardial depressant effects of volatile anesthetic drugs such as halothane. On the other hand, a patient with coronary arterial occlusive disease and good left ventricular contractility may benefit from the use of halothane, which can depress contractility and limit myocardial oxygen demand in the face of a fixed oxygen supply. The basis for assessing left ventricular function is discussed elsewhere in this book.

Additional concerns about patients with cardiac disease include the following:

1. Dependence on sympathetic tone (e.g., compensation of congestive heart failure, circulatory hypovolemia)
2. Disturbances of rate and rhythm (e.g., predisposition to complete heart block)
3. Existence of hypertension (i.e., increased oxygen demand, pressure-sensitive dysrhythmias)
4. Pulmonary disease, which may impair oxygenation and also increases the work of breathing and the demand for oxygen, especially in the postoperative period
5. Current drug therapy (e.g., potential interactions with anesthetic drugs, loss of control of hypertension by discontinuation of the therapy in the preoperative period)

All these factors, and others as well (see individual chapters on various cardiac diseases), influence the choice of anesthetic drugs, may at least alter the manner in which they are used, and may determine the precision with which their effects need to be monitored.

The Surgery

The type of surgery, as well as the practices of the particular surgeon, influences the choice and use of anesthetic drugs. The approach to the operative site determines the intensity of noxious stimulation intraoperatively and the degree of discomfort and impairment of ventilatory effort likely in the postoperative period. If cardiopulmonary bypass is to be used, dosage requirements for intravenous anesthetic drugs may be altered by hemodilution, hypothermia, and changes in carbon dioxide tension. The quality of myocardial preservation and the care with which the heart is manipulated can influence the toleration of myocardial depressant drugs.

The Choice of Drugs

Factors such as those noted above should be taken into consideration when developing an anesthetic plan. Rather than merely representing contraindications to the choice of particular drugs, however, these factors indicate the need for skill in the use of any and all of the numerous anesthetic drugs available to the anesthesiologist. With precise monitoring of drug effects and thorough understanding of their pharmacologic basis, especially dose–response relationships, the competent anesthesiologist can safely employ drugs that are relatively contraindicated in order to achieve the anesthetic objectives for the patient and surgeon.

GENERAL PHARMACOLOGY

The emphasis of the following discussions of individual drugs and groups of drugs is on the anesthetic and cardiovascular effects relative to their use in cardiac surgery. The reader is referred to textbooks and other publications of anesthesiology and pharmacology for discussions of the important actions of these drugs on other organ systems, which are of no lesser concern in the anesthetic management of the cardiac patient than of any other type of patient.

Although generalizations are a necessary part of the accumulation and application of knowledge, two important qualifications must be borne in mind when considering pharmacology: (1) dose–response relationships and (2) the nature of the experimental subjects.

Dose–response relationships cannot be overemphasized in their importance, especially when dealing with critically ill patients with very limited reserves for homeostasis and toleration of stress. Given the wide range of variability in the responses of even healthy subjects to drugs, the average doses stated in brochures and textbooks may be totally inappropriate for the critically ill patient. It therefore seems wise to adjust the dosage of each drug to the responses of each patient by gradually increasing the dosage until either the desired effect is achieved or an adverse reaction is observed. In this manner, even very potent drugs with widespread effects such as the general anesthetics can be used to advantage to achieve one or more anesthetic objectives.

Experimental design, especially the nature of the experimental subject, influences the ultimate applicability of pharmacologic data to clinical medicine. Well-controlled studies in healthy volunteers are useful in identifying and quantitating the actions of the drug per se, as free as possible from the influence of extraneous variables. Information obtained in such studies of anesthetic drugs is directly applicable in anesthetizing essentially healthy patients. Its relevance to the critically ill patient is more limited, however, because the actions of anesthetic drugs are strongly influenced both qualitatively and quantitatively by disease processes, chronic drug therapy, intensity of surgical stimulation,

Table 1-1
Dose–Effect Relationships for
Nitrous Oxide in Healthy Subjects

20%	Analgesia equivalent to 15 mg morphine[1]
40%	Inability to cooperate
60%	Amnesia nearly complete
80%	Unconsciousness
100%	Lack of movement to surgical stimulation ("MAC")[2]

etc. Unfortunately, the many variables imposed by the patient's condition and the circumstances of anesthesia and surgery make it extremely difficult to gather meaningful data under clinical conditions. The difficulties can be reduced somewhat by the sophisticated techniques for monitoring vital functions during anesthesia and surgery.

INHALATIONAL ANESTHETICS

Nitrous Oxide (N₂O)

ANESTHETIC EFFECTS

Nitrous oxide, an odorless gas, is a weak general anesthetic under normal ambient conditions. Its lack of potency limits the effects it can produce under safe conditions, including the maintenance of a satisfactory supply of oxygen to the patient. In patients with impaired lung function, the requirement for oxygen supplementation of the inspired gas mixture is greater, and the maximum permissible concentrations of nitrous oxide are reduced accordingly.

The *dose*-effect relationships of nitrous oxide in essentially, healthy individuals are shown in Table 1-1.[1,2] The concentrations shown are for ambient conditions at sea level and are rounded off for easier memorization. Although less conventional, it would be more precise to state the dose in terms of partial pressures.* It should be noted that the *dose* refers to the percentages of nitrous oxide achieved in alveolar gas, which may differ considerably from the gas mixture delivered by the anesthesia machine, especially if there are leaks in the breathing circuit. Obviously, nitrous oxide concentrations above 80 percent cannot be used safely under ambient conditions because they infringe on the minimum requirements for oxygen in the inspired gas mixture.

Despite its limited potency, nitrous oxide is still the most widely used anesthetic and in fact, is often the primary anesthetic administered along with other drugs chosen to supplement its deficiencies. Skeletal muscle relaxants are the

* It is the partial pressure of anesthetic gases that determines the intensity of their effects. At a standard atmospheric pressure of 760 torr, a 20 percent concentration of gas would exert a partial pressure of 152 torr.

most frequently used supplements because nitrous oxide contains no relaxant properties.

The use of a nitrous oxide–muscle relaxant combination for general anesthesia is difficult because a totally paralyzed patient is not necessarily unconscious, although his lack of motor responses make him appear to be well anesthetized. Caution is indicated in evaluating the depth of anesthesia in a paralyzed patient, and if there is any uncertainty, it is customary to supplement nitrous oxide with one or more drugs, including low concentrations of the potent inhalational anesthetics (e.g., halothane, enflurane), narcotic analgesics, barbiturates, and minor or major tranquilizers. The pharmacology of these supplements and their interactions with nitrous oxide are discussed below.

CARDIOVASCULAR ACTIONS

In terms of the cardiovascular system, there is only one well-controlled study detailing the effects of nitrous oxide alone in normal volunteers. Eisele and Smith demonstrated that substituting 40 percent nitrous oxide in oxygen for a 40 percent nitrogen-in-oxygen mixture produced a 15 to 20 percent reduction in cardiac output as a result of decreases in both heart rate and contractility.[3] This was matched by a 20 percent increase in systemic vascular resistance, so the net effect on systemic blood pressure was nil. Modest increases in circulating catecholamines, primarily norepinephrine, were noted in these volunteers during nitrous oxide inhalation. Studies in animals suggest that the rise in vascular resistance results from increased sympathetic nervous system activity owing to an action of nitrous oxide on suprapontine areas of the brain.[4,5] Increased peripheral resistance and the associated rise in arterial blood pressure may activate baroreceptors and lead to a reflex inhibition of cardiac functions. Nitrous oxide also has a direct depressant effect on the heart.[6]

In essentially healthy individuals, the changes induced in cardiovascular function by nitrous oxide are small. In patients with compromised cardiac function, the myocardial depressant effects of nitrous oxide can be detrimental and may require discontinuation of its administration in some cases. Eisele et al. also studied the effects of substituting 40 percent nitrous oxide for 40 percent nitrogen in oxygen on cardiovascular function at the end of cardiac catheterization and coronary angiography in patients complaining of angina.[7] In 9 patients with angiographically demonstrable obstructions of the coronary arteries and evidence of impaired left ventricular function, nitrous oxide further depressed left ventricular function, as indicated by a 14 percent decrease in pressure development (dP/dt), 21 percent increase in end-diastolic pressure, and a 5 percent decrease in systemic blood pressure. In 4 patients without objective evidence of coronary artery disease, smaller and statistically insignificant changes in these hemodynamic variables were found.

It is our practice to reduce the inspired concentration or, more frequently, to stop the administration of nitrous oxide to cardiac patients exhibiting undesirable degrees of hypotension and reduced cardiac output. Usually, a trend toward more normal blood pressure is evident within a minute or two. It is not certain whether this recovery is due to elimination of cardiac depression by nitrous oxide or to a reduced level of anesthesia with increased sympathetic activity from the noxious stimulation of surgery.

The weak sympathetic stimulation and cardiovascular effects of nitrous oxide are still evident when it is combined with other anesthetic drugs in healthy volunteers (Table 1–2).[8–12] The effects of adding nitrous oxide to other drugs have been more variable in surgical patients, however.[13–16] The variability probably reflects the modest potency of nitrous oxide, especially in the face of preanesthetic medication, alterations of ventilation, surgical stimulation, and disease-related factors influencing cardiovascular functions. The net effect on cardiovascular functions of the combinations of nitrous oxide with other anesthetic drugs in patients is generally small and reflects three actions of nitrous oxide:

1. To the extent that nitrous oxide reduces the dose of the other drugs, it limits the cardiovascular effects of these other drugs. For example, 50 percent nitrous oxide reduces the required anesthetic concentration of potent volatile anesthetics by approximately 50 percent,[17] and it is anticipated that the dose-related depression of the cardiovascular system by the potent anesthetics would be similarly reduced.

2. Even in the presence of a stable dose of general anesthetic drug, the addition of nitrous oxide tends to raise blood pressure

Table 1-2

Cardiovascular Changes After Adding Nitrous Oxide
to General Anesthesia in Volunteers

Hemodynamic Variable	Baseline Anesthetic			
	None[3]	Morphine[8]	Halothane[9-11]	Enflurane[12]
Blood pressure	—	—	↑	—
Heart rate	↓	↓	—	↓
Cardiac output	↓	↓	—	↑
Vascular resistance	↑	↑	↑	—
Venous pressure	↑	↑	↑	—

primarily by increasing systemic vascular resistance. These effects are small in degree in healthy volunteers and may be overshadowed completely in the presence of disease and debilitation.

3. The direct cardiac depressant action of nitrous oxide may be masked by cardiac depression induced by the more potent volatile anesthetics, but it is evident in subjects under the influence of narcotic analgesics that do not impair cardiac function. This effect and the accompanying hypotension can limit or even preclude the use of nitrous oxide in critically ill patients.

Nitrous oxide can affect cardiovascular function indirectly through actions on the other organ systems. To the extent that the administration of nitrous oxide depresses spontaneous ventilation, carbon dioxide will accumulate and alter cardiovascular function by its effects on the activity of the sympathetic nervous system and on vascular smooth muscle.[18] If its concentration in the inspired gas mixture reduces the concentration of oxygen below that required for optimal oxygenation of the blood, the resulting hypoxemia can alter cardiovascular functions.[19] Hypoxemia also occurs as a result of "diffusion hypoxia" in the first 5 to 10 minutes following abrupt discontinuation of nitrous oxide administration *if* the patient is allowed to breathe room air instead of 100 percent oxygen.[20] In combination with narcotic analgesics, nitrous oxide potentiates the development of truncal rigidity, and positive pressure ventilation in the face of poor thoracic compliance can impair venous return and cardiac output.[21] The ability of nitrous oxide to enter and to expand air-filled spaces can lead to exacerbation of an existing pneumothorax and to enlargement of air emboli.[22,23]

The latter effect on air-filled spaces is particularly important in the patient undergoing cardiac surgery because of the frequency of the occurrence of pneumothorax and air emboli as a consequence of surgery. As long as the thoracic cavity is adequately vented and positive pressure ventilation is maintained, a pneumothorax presents no problem for the patient. Air emboli present a definite risk of morbidity and mortality, especially when they occur in the cerebral, coronary, or pulmonary circulations. Nitrous oxide diffuses extremely rapidly into air emboli and will expand them in proportion to its inspired concentration. That is, the volume of an expansile air space will increase by 1.5, 2, 4, or 5 times when the inspired concentration of nitrous oxide is 33, 50, 75, or 80 percent, respectively. Small, clinically insignificant emboli can enlarge and produce major obstructions to blood flow within a few minutes after the start of nitrous oxide administration.[22]

Important features of nitrous oxide pharmacology include a rapid onset and offset of action, the absence of arrhythmogenic actions, and no significant alterations in the responses to cardiovascular drugs.

Halothane

ANESTHETIC EFFECTS

The prototype of currently used volatile anesthetics is halothane (Fluothane). It is a complete anesthetic in that all the objectives of anesthesia can be achieved with sufficiently high concentrations of this agent alone.[24] Halothane is rarely used as the sole anesthetic, however, because of its potential toxicity, which includes a dose-dependent depression of the cardiovascular system and the potential for delayed toxicity involving the liver.[25,26] It is a customary practice for all types of surgery to reduce the dose requirements for halothane by the use of preanesthetic medication, nitrous oxide, and muscle relaxants.[27] It often becomes a moot point as to whether halothane is the primary or a supplemental anesthetic drug in such combinations. There is no question, however, that low concentrations (0.15 to 0.5 percent) of halothane can produce unconsciousness, especially in debilitated patients and in combination with nitrous oxide; can potentiate the relaxant effects of nondepolarizing neuromuscular blocking agents;[28] and can suppress sympathetic responses to noxious stimulation.[29] The last effect is particularly useful to the anesthesiologist who is trying to prevent episodes of tachycardia and hypertension in order to minimize the work and oxygen demand of the heart.[30]

CARDIOVASCULAR ACTIONS

Halothane is a fully potent depressant of the cardiovascular system in that it can produce dose-dependent depression through the stage of cardiac arrest and peripheral vascular collapse.[31] The mechanisms of this cardiovascular depression are complex and involve direct actions on cardiac and vascular smooth muscle as well as indirect effects mediated by depression of activity at several levels of the sympathetic nervous system. Studies by many different investigators have demonstrated that halothane decreases sympathetic activity emanating from the central nervous system through depressant effects on medullary vasomotor centers and possibly on the input to those centers from peripheral receptors and from higher brain centers.[32-36] In addition, halothane has been shown to depress transmission through sympathetic autonomic ganglia and to the adrenal medulla.[37-39] Direct effects on autonomic nerve terminals have not been demonstrated,[40] and there is no reason to believe nor any evidence to support the notion that halothane may act on adrenergic receptors. The net result of all the actions of halothane is a reduction in the output of catecholamines from adrenergic nerve terminals and the adrenal medulla.

Direct depressant effects of halothane on myocardial and vascular smooth muscle have been demonstrated with isolated tissues in vitro.[41,42] In addition, direct depression of cardiac function by halothane has been observed in the dog heart-lung preparation and in humans during cardiopulmonary bypass.[43,44]

Eger et al. described the overall effects of halothane on the cardiovascular system of human volunteers maintained at normal body temperature, ventilated to maintain normocarbia, and given no other drugs.[45] Concentrations of halothane were varied systematically between 1 and 2.5 percent in end-tidal gas. There was a dose-dependent fall in cardiac output (up to 50 percent control at 2 percent halothane) reflecting equivalent reductions in stroke volume and cardiac contractility (as measured by the I-J wave of the ballistocardiogram). Heart rate did not change, right atrial pressure increased, and mean systemic arterial blood pressure fell in parallel with the decline in cardiac output. Compared to awake controls, systemic vascular resistance was only slightly lower (10 percent) during the first hour of anesthesia, and did not vary with the concentration of halothane. An interesting but unexplained finding of this study was the gradual decrease in systemic vascular resistance and improvement in cardiac output between the first and fifth hour of halothane anesthesia. Other conditions were imposed on the experimental subjects in this interval and may have contributed to the absolute change in the values measured. The dose-related depression of cardiac function was still evident after 5 hours, however. These systematic observations of volunteers by Eger et al. are essentially in agreement with the findings of other groups of investigators for human volunteers and surgical patients.[46-49] Of course, variations in experimental technique, the presence of other drugs, hypercarbia during spontaneous ventilation under anesthesia, surgical stimulation, and a whole host of other factors may modify, at least quantitatively, the cardiovascular responses to halothane.[50-53]

The negative inotropic effects of halothane may be beneficial under certain conditions. In the patient with coronary artery occlusive disease and a fixed coronary blood flow, halothane anesthesia may reduce or at least limit the increases in myocardial work and oxygen demand during anesthesia and surgery. Marked reductions in mean arterial blood pressure could reduce coronary blood flow and myocardial oxygen supply, however. Two studies in dogs suggest that in the absence of ventricular failure, halothane may shift the myocardial oxygen supply/demand relationship in a favorable direction. Grover et al. demonstrated little or no decrease in coronary blood flow in dogs given 0.5 to 2.0 percent halothane; coronary flow was reduced by approximately 25 percent when the mean arterial pressure fell by almost 50 percent in response to the administration of 2.5 percent halothane.[54] Bland and Lowenstein found that 0.75 percent halothane superimposed on chloralose-urethane anesthesia in dogs limited the severity of myocardial ischemia created by temporary coronary artery occlusion, even though there was a slight degree of systemic arterial hypotension.[55] Although comparable data have not been reported for humans, halothane has been successfully used as a primary anesthetic (0.5 to 1 percent) or as an anesthetic supplement (0.15 to 0.5 percent) for patients undergoing myocardial revascularization operations. The incidence of hypotension has been no greater than that with other anesthetic drugs, but fewer and less severe episodes of hypertension and tachycardia have been encountered.[56]

The negative inotropic effect of halothane precludes its use in patients with congestive heart failure. In patients with compensated failure and borderline levels of cardiac function, the use of halothane as a primary anesthetic is contraindicated, but precisely controlled low levels (0.15 to 0.5 percent) may be used to advantage for purposes of anesthesia without seriously impairing cardiovascular function. It is important to monitor such patients very carefully for signs of cardiac failure and to be prepared to discontinue halothane administration entirely if necessary. The potential for individual variation and the dose–response relationships must be kept constantly in mind if halothane is to be used safely and effectively in any patient, but especially in those with cardiac disease.

The reduction of systemic vascular resistance, although variable and not clearly related to dose in the normal subject,[45–57] nevertheless is predictable and dose-related in the patient during cardiopulmonary bypass.[44] Administration of 0.25 to 1.5 percent concentrations by a vaporizer interposed in the oxygen line to the pump oxygenator is used to control hypertension during bypass. The reduction of vascular resistance by halothane allows a blood flow comparable to that expected for a normal person of similar size and facilitates adequate perfusion of all tissues.

The clinical indications and contraindications for the use of halothane with its potential for cardiovascular depression are discussed in greater detail in the chapters dealing with the anesthetic management of patients with coronary artery, valvular, and congenital heart diseases.

MANAGEMENT OF HYPOTENSION

In the usual clinical setting, reversal of excessive cardiovascular depression by halothane involves a progressive series of steps:

1. Hyperventilation with 100 percent oxygen to facilitate the pulmonary excretion of halothane and to produce maximal oxygenation of blood in the presence of reduced cardiac output.
2. Augmentation of the return of venous blood to the heart by alteration of the patient's position and the infusion of intravenous fluids.
3. Administration of atropine or another anticholinergic drug to eliminate bradycardia mediated by the vagus nerves.
4. Antagonism of halothane's depression of myocardial contractility by intravenous injection of calcium or a noncatecholamine sympathomimetic agent (e.g., ephedrine*)[58]
5. Intravenous injection of antiarrhythmic drugs to correct dysrhythmias that are interfering with cardiac output and maintenance of blood pressure.
6. Cardiac massage, as indicated by the usual criteria of ineffective circulation.

CARDIAC DYSRHYTHMIAS

In addition to depression of myocardial contractility, halothane can interfere with cardiac output by altering cardiac rhythm. The most common types of dysrhythmia are bigeminy, nodal rhythms, and nodal and ventricular premature contractions. All types of dysrhythmia have been observed under halothane anesthesia, including ventricular fibrillation.[60–62]

---

* Because the magnitude of the vascular effects of halothane is less than the magnitude of cardiac depression, it is better to administer a mixed inotropic-vasopressor drug than one that acts primarily on vascular smooth muscle (e.g., methoxamine or phenylephrine). Increased peripheral resistance in the face of myocardial depression will, in fact, further reduce cardiac output.[59]

One mechanism of halothane-induced dysrhythmias is the sensitization of the myocardium to the actions of catecholamines.[*][63–67] The underlying cellular or membranal changes responsible for the sensitization by halothane are unknown. No relationship between the concentration of halothane and the degree of sensitization has, in fact, been defined. It may be that the interaction of multiple factors is so complex that it is difficult, if not impossible, to define a clear-cut dose–response relationship for halothane. Consider the following facts:

1. Halothane decreases activity of the sympathetic nervous system and reduces the output of catecholamines by adrenergic nerve endings and the adrenal medulla.[39]
2. Halothane sensitizes myocardial cells to the action of catecholamines.
3. Halothane does not appear to affect vagal nervous activity consistently, although atropine-reversible bradycardia occurs in patients anesthetized with halothane.
4. Deeper levels of halothane anesthesia depress pacemaker activity and conduction in the heart.
5. Relatively deep levels of halothane anesthesia have been successfully used in patients with elevated circulating levels of catecholamines from a pheochromocytoma.[68]

It may be that light-to-moderate levels of halothane anesthesia sensitize the heart, while deeper levels can reduce its responsiveness to catecholamines. Under any circumstances, avoidance of the combination of halothane and catecholamines is desirable. If the combination is necessary, then it is recommended that the total dose of subcutaneous or submucosal epinephrine be limited to 1–1.5 μg/kg per 10 minutes, not to exceed 4 μg/kg every hour.[65,67]

The use of isoproterenol intravenously or by endotracheal instillation for the treatment of bronchospasm during halothane anesthesia has not been thoroughly evaluated,[69] but the possibility of producing cardiac dysrhythmias war-

rants extreme caution.[70] Isoproterenol is the one catecholamine that does not produce hypertension, and the incidence of dysrhythmias may be less in the absence of hypertension and the associated baroreceptor-induced vagal stimulation of the heart. Certainly, strong vagal stimulation, which tends to inhibit normal pacemakers, predisposes to the development of ectopic beats from ventricular cells whose automaticity is increased by a catecholamine. Likewise, the use of aminophylline to relieve bronchospasm in patients anesthetized with halothane has not been evaluated, but the occurrence of dysrhythmias has been reported.[70]

Therapy of Dysrhythmias. The treatment of cardiac dysrhythmias under halothane general anesthesia also involves a sequence of steps:

1. Correct any inadequacy in ventilation of the patient. Hypercarbia and hypoxia can contribute to the development and persistence of dysrhythmias by reflex activation of the sympathetic nervous system.
2. Make a judgment: Are the arrhythmias related to an anesthetic level that is too light or too deep? If the answer is uncertain, it is better to discontinue or at least to reduce the dose of halothane. It is important, however, to know that premature beats, bigeminy, and nodal rhythms are common, especially in healthy patients under light levels of halothane anesthesia, and can be controlled by deepening the anesthetic level. Increasing the depth of anesthesia may be especially useful in preventing other major complications of light anesthesia (e.g., bronchospasm in an asthmatic patient).
3. Treat bradycardia with incremental intravenous doses of atropine (0.2–0.4 mg), up to a total of 2 mg for an adult. Alternatively, an indirect-acting sympathomimetic (e.g., ephedrine, mephentermine) may be used to elicit a positive chronotropic response and to correct bradycardia (which allows ectopic pacemaker activity to become manifest).
4. Use antiarrhythmic drugs to treat persistent dysrhythmias interfering with cardiac output. Lidocaine in bolus doses of 1 mg/kg administered intravenously one to three times is effective in controlling nodal and ventricular premature beats and tachycardia. Propranolol administered intravenously in increments of 0.25 mg, up to a total of 3–

---

* Sensitization is measured as the reduction in the concentration or dose of catecholamine (i.e., epinephrine, norepinephrine, isoproterenol, dopamine) required to elicit a dysrhythmia of any type in the presence compared to that in the absence of the sensitizing agent. The incidence and severity of dysrhythmias are proportional to the dose of catecholamine.

5 mg, is effective in treating atrial tachycardia. The use of other antiarrhythmic drugs is discussed in other chapters of this book. Note, however, that it is necessary to wait at least 1 to 3 minutes after the intravenous injection to see how effective it will be; otherwise, toxicity from overdoses of the antiarrhythmic drugs is likely.

5. Sample blood for detection of abnormalities of blood gases and electrolytes that may produce a return of the dysrhythmia.

HALOTHANE–DRUG INTERACTIONS

In addition to halothane–catecholamine interactions, there are other important drug interactions to be considered in the anesthetic management of any type of patient. Of particular interest to the cardiac anesthesiologist are those related to sympathomimetic blocking drugs. Two concerns are registered about such interactions: (1) the continued presence of adrenergic blocking drugs may render the patient taking them unusually sensitive to the cardiovascular depressant actions of halothane, and (2) in the event of excessive cardiovascular depression by halothane, the persistence of adrenergic receptor blockade will interfere with therapy involving sympathomimetic drugs.

With the accumulation of clinical experience, it is now possible to state some guidelines for the management of these interactions. First, if there is not a clear therapeutic indication for the use of adrenergic blockers, they should be discontinued well in advance of elective surgery so that potential drug interactions with any anesthetic will be obviated. In cases where the indication for the adrenergic blocking drug is definite (e.g., for hypertension, angina pectoris, dysrhythmias), it is usually best to continue the chronic therapy up to the night before surgery in order to prevent exacerbation of the disease and its consequences in the perioperative period.[71–74] In some cases, it may be possible and desirable to reduce the maintenance dose to some degree, especially if the patient is at bed rest in the hospital. As a general rule, the dose reduction should be done decrementally as tolerated by the patient. If evidence of exacerbation of the disease symptoms appears, the dose should immediately be restored to the previously satisfactory level.

When the drug is continued, the risks of potential detrimental interactions can be minimized by taking certain precautions:

1. Reduce the need for sympathetic tone during general anesthesia by maintaining an adequate circulating blood volume and avoiding orthostatic stress.
2. Perform a gradual induction of anesthesia with halothane to minimize the risk of an overdose.
3. Be prepared to reduce the concentration of halothane and, if necessary, to substitute another anesthetic regimen.
4. Premedicate the patient appropriately and, if necessary, administer additional doses of narcotic analgesics and minor tranquilizers in order to reduce the concentration of halothane required for induction and maintenance of anesthesia.
5. If excessive hypotension occurs despite these precautions, be prepared to treat it in light of the pharmacology of the adrenergic blocker and halothane.

Propranolol. In practice, the above precautions have proven to be worthwhile in managing the cardiovascular interactions of halothane and propranolol. On the basis of studies of these drugs in dogs by Roberts et al.,[75–77] their interactions on cardiac function can be described as additive, predictable, and reversible by the elimination of halothane. Should the myocardial depression become excessive, therapeutic measures may include calcium, which is an inotropic drug that can antagonize the depressant effects of halothane and bypass the blockade of β-adrenergic receptors by propranolol.[58] Glucagon is another cardiac stimulant that bypasses β-adrenergic receptors.[78] Since propranolol is a competitive inhibitor of β-adrenergic receptors, larger than usual doses of isoproterenol should overcome the inhibition. Isoproterenol, however, may be contraindicated in the presence of halothane, which sensitizes the myocardium to the arrhythmogenic actions of catecholamines.[69,70]

We strongly believe that with the proper indications for its use, chronic therapy with propranolol should be continued in moderate doses (up to 320 mg daily) up to the time of surgery.[79–82] Not only will this minimize the occurrence of complications of the patient's disease in the preoperative period, but cardiovascular stability may actually be improved by the persistence of propranolol actions during anesthesia. The lower heart rate is favorable for minimizing myocardial oxygen demand, and the incidence and severity of episodes of tachycardia, dysrhythmias, and hypertension are probably less in patients maintained on propranolol up to the time of surgery than in similar patients not taking the drug.[82]

Of course, in the patient with poor left ventricular function and borderline compensation of congestive heart failure, halothane would be contraindicated whether or not the patient was receiving propranolol chronically.

Antihypertensive Drugs. The interactions of halothane with the more commonly used antihypertensive agents, such as thiazide-related diuretics, α-methyldopa, reserpine, clonidine, guanethidine, and hydralazine, have not been fully characterized, but they also have not proved to be a source of difficulty clinically. First, the preoperative control of chronic hypertension minimizes the development of hypotension as a result of halothane-induced vasodilation which unmasks the relative hypovolemia associated with a contracted intravascular space accompanying uncontrolled hypertension. Second, all of these antihypertensive drugs leave the α-adrenergic receptors on vascular smooth muscle responsive to vasopressors, which may ultimately be needed to treat undesirable degrees of halothane-induced hypotension that do not respond to the initial steps of the sequence outlined above.

Cardiac Glycosides. No detrimental interactions between halothane and the cardiac glycosides have been reported. Potentially, depression of atrioventricular (AV) nodal conduction by halothane could add to that of digitalis, but it should be readily reversible with atropine in the absence of digitalis toxicity. It terms of contractility, it has been demonstrated in dogs that digoxin can antagonize or reverse the depressant effects of halothane.[83] This finding suggests that it is beneficial to continue therapy with digitalis glycosides through the perioperative period, omitting only the morning dose on the day of surgery. In terms of the arrhythmogenic potential of the cardiac glycosides, Morrow has shown that halothane increases the dose of ouabain required to induce ventricular fibrillation in dogs.[84]

Enflurane

ANESTHETIC EFFECTS

Enflurane (Ethrane) is qualitatively identical to halothane in its anesthetic properties, except that high concentrations of enflurane, especially under conditions of hyperventilation, tend to produce electroencephalographic patterns and occasionally gross body movements suggestive of seizures.[85] There are only very minor quantitative differences between enflurane and halothane. Compared to halothane, enflurane is less potent (MAC* = 1.7 versus 0.8 percent) but is equivalent in efficacy as a general anesthetic.[86] Enflurane produces somewhat greater muscular relaxation than does halothane at equivalent anesthetic depths and may potentiate nondepolarizing relaxants to a greater degree.[87] The initial uptake of enflurane is slightly faster than that of halothane, and in accordance with its lesser affinity for lipids, its uptake by body fat is less and it is eliminated slightly more rapidly from the body than is halothane.[88] Lesser proportions of the absorbed dose of enflurane undergo biotransformation, and so far the incidence of postanesthetic hepatitis appears to be lower for enflurane than for halothane.[89] The release of fluoride ions by metabolism of enflurane is much less than that for methoxyflurane, and the incidence of renal toxicity would be expected to be correspondingly very low.[90,91]

CARDIOVASCULAR EFFECTS

The hemodynamic alterations induced by enflurane are also qualitatively identical and quantitatively similar to those described for halothane, although the newer anesthetic has been studied less intensively. A dose-dependent degree of hypotension reflects primarily a decreased stroke volume as a result of depression of myocardial contractility. Heart rate tends to increase, and systemic vascular resistance decreases slightly.[92–94] The changes result from reduced sympathetic nervous system activity

---

* Minimum alveolar concentration.[23]

and from a direct depressant action on the myocardial contractile elements.[95-97] As with halothane, the absolute values for cardiac output increase and those for systemic vascular resistance decrease over a 5-hour period of enflurane anesthesia; however, the pattern of dose-dependent depression remains the same.[92] Although the spontaneous outflow of impulses over sympathetic nerves is decreased and the output of catecholamines from the adrenal medulla and adrenergic nerves is reduced,[95,96,98] the remaining sympathetic activity can be further reduced by baroreceptor stimulation and can be increased in response to hypercarbia.[93,95]

The interaction of nitrous oxide with enflurane on cardiovascular function appears to be somewhat different than the interaction of nitrous oxide and halothane. In volunteers receiving no other medication and being ventilated artificially to maintain normocarbia, the addition of 70 percent nitrous oxide to a stable level of enflurane anesthesia produced minimal changes in cardiovascular variables.[12] When nitrous oxide-enflurane anesthesia in volunteers was compared to enflurane alone at the same anesthetic depth, there was less depression of cardiac contractility, heart rate increased less, and there was a tendency for blood pressure to decrease less with nitrous oxide present in the anesthetic mixture. The important point of difference between enflurane and halothane interactions with nitrous oxide in volunteers is the lack of a sympathomimetic response to the introduction of nitrous oxide in the presence of enflurane,[12] whereas, definite sympathomimetic signs are evident in the cardiovascular system and elsewhere when nitrous oxide is added to halothane.[10] In surgical patients receiving preanesthetic medication and encountering the common, uncontrolled clinical variables (e.g., surgical stimulation, hypothermia), the incremental addition of nitrous oxide produced progressive decreases in cardiac output and arterial blood pressure with a slight increase or no change in systemic vascular resistance.[16] It appears that nitrous oxide offers relatively little protection against the cardiovascular depressant effects of enflurane.[12,92]

Myocardial blood flow decreases in parallel with the decreased myocardial work and oxygen demand, so that no oxygen deficit is encountered.[97] In the face of a fixed coronary blood supply, the reduced oxygen demand is a desirable consequence of myocardial depression as long as there is no significant fall in coronary artery perfusion pressure.

The incidence of dysrhythmias under enflurane anesthesia is claimed to be less than that with halothane. Atlee et al. have observed that enflurane depresses atrioventricular conduction, as does halothane; but in contrast to halothane, enflurane does not increase the conduction time in His-Purkinje or ventricular fibers.[99] Perhaps this limits the chances of developing impulse reentry patterns and the associated dysrhythmias. Enflurane sensitization of the heart to the actions of catecholamines is less in degree than that of halothane.[67,100,101] Because of the gross alteration of the epinephrine dose–response curve in the presence of enflurane, it is not possible to specify precise limits on the use of catecholamines with this anesthetic. Generally, the incidence of dysrhythmias is low with epinephrine doses of less than 3.4 μg/kg, and when they occur, the dysrhythmias are less severe than those encountered with halothane.[101]

The interactions of enflurane with other drugs are likely to be similar to those described for halothane, but few actual studies have been reported. Horan et al. studied the interactions of enflurane and propranolol in dogs and compared them to those of halothane and propranolol.[102] Following the administration of propranolol, the hemodynamic changes induced by enflurane were much greater than those produced by equivalent anesthetic concentrations of halothane. The marked degree of hypotension resulted from impaired cardiac contractility and decreased cardiac output. The changes in heart rate and peripheral vascular resistance were insignificant. Additional stress on the cardiovascular system in the form of blood loss was tolerated poorly in the presence of enflurane and propranolol. The similarity of the cardiovascular responses to enflurane in dogs and humans suggests that, until the interaction is studied in humans, the concentrations of enflurane should be limited in patients receiving propranolol chronically. At least, the responses of such patients to enflurane should be closely monitored and the dose increased very gradually. We have noted that some hypotensive episodes are not corrected simply by reducing or discontinuing the administration of enflurane, and the administration of ephedrine has been necessary to restore blood pressure to acceptable levels.

Methoxyflurane

Methoxyflurane (Penthane) differs in several important ways from halothane. It is 4.6 times more potent as an anesthetic and has good analgesic properties in subanesthetic concentrations.[103,104] The onset of anesthesia is slow and the recovery prolonged owing to its very high solubility in body tissues. As much as 50 percent of an administered dose undergoes biotransformation with the release of fluoride ions.[105] The latter accumulate progressively as the depth and duration of anesthesia increase, and fluoride ions are responsible for the development of renal toxicity and failure.[106] In fact, the potential for impairment of renal function has led to the discontinuation of the use of methoxyflurane by many anesthesiologists.

The cardiovascular effects of methoxyflurane are characterized by a dose-related degree of hypotension. Reports of methoxyflurane anesthesia in human subjects have variously attributed the hypotension to decreases in cardiac output or systemic vascular resistance.[107,110] When cardiac output has declined, it was the result of a decreased stroke volume; heart rate increased slightly in all studies. It is clear from the study of dogs by Merin and Borgstedt that methoxyflurane impairs left ventricular function.[111] The lack of a consistent pattern of hemodynamic changes in humans may reflect the minimal effects of methoxyflurane on reflex activity of the sympathetic nervous system, as demonstrated in cats by Skovsted and Price.[112,113] Thus, hypotension can reduce baroreceptor activity and result in compensatory sympathetic stimulation to the heart and vasculature. In this regard, light levels of methoxyflurane may differ from those of halothane. Certainly overdoses of methoxyflurane can produce profound cardiovascular depression.

Methoxyflurane sensitizes the heart to catecholamines to a lesser degree than does halothane. Its interactions with β-adrenergic receptor blocking drugs in the dog can be characterized as potentiative, somewhat unpredictable, and not always reversible by discontinuation of methoxyflurane administration.[114] No studies of methoxyflurane–propranolol interactions have been made in humans.

It appears that low concentrations of methoxyflurane could be useful in providing light anesthesia, good analgesia, and minimal hemodynamic changes in patients with cardiac disease. Its potential renal toxicity has markedly reduced the clinical use of this anesthetic, however.

INTRAVENOUS DRUGS

Ultrashort-acting Barbiturates

The anesthetic properties of thiopental (Pentothal) and other ultrashort-acting barbiturates are discussed in standard textbooks of anesthesiology and pharmacology and need not be extensively reviewed here. There are a few basic points worth emphasizing, however, because a complete understanding of these properties is crucial to the interpretation of studies of the cardiovascular effects of these drugs as well as important for their effective use in patients with cardiac disease.

The depth of anesthesia and the intensity of cardiovascular actions of thiopental (and other ultrashort-acting barbiturates) are dose-related.[115–118] (These actions, in fact, are probably proportional to the concentration of thiopental in the circulating plasma, although not all investigators have been able to demonstrate such a relationship.)[119] Large intravenous bolus doses (4–5 mg/kg) used for rapid induction of anesthesia likely produce high plasma levels and intense, often excessive, effects that are usually short-lived. If additional large doses are administered to maintain anesthesia, widely fluctuating plasma levels and degrees of effect will be observed within a very short span of time. It is not often appreciated that the desired depth of anesthesia can be achieved, albeit more gradually, and maintained without such large fluctuations by the intermittent administration of small doses (0.3–1 mg/kg) or by continuous intravenous infusion (0.25–0.5 mg/kg/min) of thiopental.

Failure to recognize the above facts in designing experimental protocols and in the clinical application of intravenous barbiturates has led to confusion about the cardiovascular actions of these drugs and to absolute avoidance of their use in certain clinical situations where, in fact, their proper use may prove beneficial, even in terms of the cardiovascular system.

CARDIOVASCULAR EFFECTS

A detailed review of the hemodynamic effects of ultrashort-acting barbiturates was made by Conway and Ellis in 1969.[120] Very little new information has been added since that time except for the results of newer techniques of measuring cardiovascular function, and these have confirmed earlier observations.[121,122]

Although cardiovascular depression manifested by hypotension is a well-known response to intravenous barbiturates, the basic mechanisms are still in doubt. It has been clearly demonstrated in isolated hearts as well as in intact animals that myocardial contractility is impaired by these drugs.[118] This action has not been adequately substantiated in humans because other hemodynamic changes induced by the intravenous barbiturates complicate the interpretation of the indirect methods available for the study of human subjects. For example, a rise in central venous pressure resulting from myocardial depression may be masked by decreased venous blood return as a consequence of increased venous capacitance. Also, reductions in cardiac output (approximating 25 percent after moderate doses of ultrashort-acting barbiturates and approaching 50 percent with deep levels of anesthesia) can result from decreased stroke volume owing to reduced filling pressures, to myocardial depression, or to both.[120]

There is evidence that the intravenous barbiturates increase the capacitance of venous vessels and lead to peripheral pooling of blood.[123,124] This effect results, at least in part, from an action of the barbiturates within the central nervous system to reduce sympathetic tone.[125] Thus, it is likely that the decreased cardiac output measured in volunteers and patients results from (1) direct depressant action on myocardial contractility, (2) decreased ventricular filling pressures due to venous pooling of blood, and (3) decreased sympathetic outflow from the central nervous system. The latter effect is transient, as the depressant actions of the barbiturates are overcome by reflex sympathetic stimulation in response to hypotension.

The degree of hypotension is reduced by compensatory increases in heart rate (33 percent) and peripheral vascular resistance (32 percent).[120,126] It appears that a gradual induction of anesthesia by intermittent small doses or a slow infusion rate (50 mg/min in adults) allows suffi-

cient time for these reflex mechanisms to compensate for the myocardial depression and completely prevent hypotension.[116] On the other hand, very rapid injection of large doses has led to rapid decreases in systemic vascular resistance and profound hypotension, especially if barostatic reflexes were already impaired by other drugs.[127,128]

In patients without heart disease, the administration of an anesthetic dose of thiopental (4 mg/kg) produced hypotension and a compensatory tachycardia (32 percent) that was associated with a proportionally greater increase in myocardial oxygen consumption (55 percent), matched by an equivalent increase in coronary blood flow (55 percent). The increase in coronary blood flow resulted from coronary arterial vasodilatation (36 percent decrease in resistance) at a time when the mean systemic blood pressure was slightly decreased (9 percent) and the left ventricular end-diastolic pressure (LVEDP) was unchanged. The decrease in blood pressure reflected a 16 percent drop in cardiac index and a 9 percent increase in systemic vascular resistance.[126] It appears that the increases in myocardial oxygen demand occurred as a result of the compensatory tachycardia and in spite of an apparent depression of contractility. The increase in oxygen demand was matched by the increase in coronary blood flow in these patients without cardiac disease.

If these observations can be projected to patients with cardiac disease, then the following guidelines would be reasonable for the use of thiopental. Anesthetizing doses should not be used in patients with poor ventricular function because of the further impairment likely to be induced by thiopental. It is possible that small doses (0.5–1 mg/kg) may be tolerated satisfactorily, but diazepam, which produces little or no cardiac depression, would appear to be a safer choice for anesthetic supplementation in such patients.

In patients with coronary artery atherosclerosis and good left ventricular function, thiopental may be used to advantage *under certain circumstances*. Provided that reflex tachycardia is prevented (e.g., by residual propranolol from chronic use in the preoperative period), thiopental will decrease oxygen demand by its negative inotropic effect. Furthermore, it can blunt sympathetic stimulation of the heart by providing a pleasant induction and a rapid deepening of anesthesia as needed to counteract the noxious stimulation of tracheal intubation and surgery. It can be used in small, intermittent doses to maintain sleep while permitting a fairly prompt recovery of responsiveness.

Diazepam

Benzodiazepine derivatives, of which diazepam (Valium) is one, are qualitatively similar in their pharmacologic actions.[129] Although they are classified as minor tranquilizers, they resemble phenobarbital in their spectrum of central nervous system depression. That is, small doses are sedative and reduce anxiety. Larger doses can induce sleep and anesthesia. Anticonvulsant effects are evident in subanesthetic doses. The dose–response relationships for the benzodiazepines and for phenobarbital are such that both have a large margin of safety, and treatment of overdoses involves support of pulmonary and cardiovascular function. One significant difference between phenobarbital and the benzodiazepines is that the latter is much more expensive. No information is available concerning the use of phenobarbital as an anesthetic supplement for cardiac surgery, however.

Diazepam is the benzodiazepine most widely used by anesthesiologists because it is commercially available for both oral and parenteral administration and can be used for preanesthetic medication as well as for the induction and maintenance of general anesthesia, usually in combination with other drugs.[130–134] It has an amnesic action that is potentiated by scopolamine.[135] The doses required for these purposes produce relatively mild degrees of ventilatory and cardiovascular depression in most people, usually equivalent to that observed during natural sleep.[136] Diazepam elevates the seizure threshold to local anesthetic drugs and can be used to reduce the CNS side effects associated with regional anesthesia and the therapy of cardiac dysrhythmias.[137] One report suggests that diazepam itself has antiarrhythmic actions that add to those of lidocaine.[138]

Premedication with diazepam is better accomplished with oral administration than with intramuscular injection. Intramuscular injection is painful because of the vehicle in which diazepam is dissolved. Absorption of diazepam from parenteral injection sites is slow, erratic, and incomplete.[139] Diazepam's effects are predictable in onset and intensity after an oral dose.[140] We customarily prescribe a 0.1–0.2 mg/kg dose to be taken with 1 or 2 ounces of water 90 to 120 minutes before induction of anesthesia.

Because of the irritating properties of injectable diazepam and the association of phlebitis with its intravenous administration,[141] certain precautions are recommended. The drug should be injected directly into a large vein or if necessary into a rapidly flowing stream of intravenous fluids. It will be noted that a cloudy suspension forms in the intravenous tubing. The discomfort but not the inflammatory reaction can be minimized by injecting 10–40 mg (1–2 ml of a 1 to 2 percent solution) of lidocaine into the intravenous line a few minutes before administering diazepam.[142] Diazepam should not be mixed directly with any other drug.

Although intravenous injection of even large doses of diazepam (0.5–1.5 mg/kg) have generally produced only very mild degrees of ventilatory and cardiovascular depression[136,143] (see below), an occasional patient will become apneic with much smaller doses and episodes of severe hypotension have been noted in isolated case reports. The basis of these reactions is not known, but their possibility warrants careful titration of dosage (e.g., 2.5 or 5-mg increments) to the desired intensity of effect, especially in severely ill or debilitated patients.

When administered intravenously, diazepam has a rapid onset of action. Single, moderate doses appear to be short-lasting as a result of redistribution of diazepam from the brain to other body tissues that accumulate it. The ultimate elimination of the drug from the body is very slow [half-life $t_{\frac{1}{2}} = 20$ to 50 hours] and occurs primarily through biotransformation. An intermediate metabolite, desmethyldiazepam, is pharmacologically active and is transformed more slowly than is diazepam. Both diazepam and the N-demethylated metabolite accumulate with repeated doses, and recovery is prolonged accordingly.[144] A week or more is required for elimination of these compounds from plasma following discontinuation of chronic oral therapy.[129]

The interactions of diazepam with other drugs used in anesthesia are largely predictable from knowledge of its pharmacology. Diazepam adds to the depressant actions of other drugs (e.g., the dose of thiopental required for induction of anesthesia is reduced by diazepam).[145] It raises the seizure threshold for local anesthetics. Its interactions with general anesthetics and neuromuscular blocking drugs have not been evaluated, and the sites and mechanisms of muscular relaxation have not been definitely identified. No clinically important induction of microsomal drug-metabolizing enzymes occurs with diazepam or with other benzodiazepines.[129]

CARDIOVASCULAR EFFECTS

Because of its generally benign actions on the cardiovascular system, diazepam has become popular in the anesthetic management of critically ill patients, especially those with cardiac disease. Certainly the incidence and severity of cardiovascular complications with diazepam are much less than those associated with the ultrashort-acting barbiturates administered to an equivalent end point of CNS depression.[146]

The effects of diazepam on the hemodynamics of volunteers and essentially fit patients are characterized by small average reductions (5 to 20 percent) in arterial blood pressure.[136,143,147,148] A definite dose–response relationship has not been described in any single study of human subjects, and in fact, similar degrees of hypotension have been reported in studies using either low (0.1–0.2 mg/kg) or high (0.5–1.5 mg/kg) total doses of diazepam administered intravenously, usually in small increments. Other measures of cardiovascular function have shown comparably small changes. The only finding consistent among the four studies is a decrease in cardiac output, reflecting a reduction in stroke volume. This is associated with a fall in left ventricular diastolic pressure, a trend toward increased systemic vascular resistance, and in some cases, a very slight increase in heart rate. The decline in stroke volume is likely to result from a lower ventricular filling pressure rather than from impairment of the myocardial contractile mechanism. Direct measures of myocardial contractility in animals have shown transient decreases,*[149] no change,[150] or augmentation after diazepam.[151] One preliminary report of measures made in patients just before cardiopulmonary bypass showed no change in either LVEDP or the maximal short-

---

* The authors produced similar transient depression of ventricular performance with comparable volumes of commercially supplied diazepam or the vehicle alone.

ening velocity after 0.2 or 0.4 mg/kg doses of diazepam.[152] (These patients had received morphine, scopolamine, and pancuronium for anesthesia.)

Small doses of diazepam (0.1 mg/kg) administered during cardiac catheterization procedures are reported to have beneficial effects on myocardial function. Increased total coronary blood flow has been measured after administration of diazepam to humans and animals.[153,154] Proportionally larger increases were found in patients with coronary artery disease than in those with a normal coronary vasculature.[153] The significance of these observations for patients with coronary atherosclerosis is not yet clear because an increase in total coronary blood flow does not mean increased flow to potentially ischemic areas and, in fact, could be associated with reduced flow to those areas (i.e., coronary steal). Of greater importance perhaps are the observations indicating that diazepam reduces myocardial oxygen demand. In patients with elevated left ventricular end-diastolic pressures, a small dose of diazepam reduced the LVEDP by one-third,[148] and the usual increase in LVEDP following injection of the radiopaque dye was blunted.[155] Other studies have shown a decrease in left ventricular stroke work as well as an actual reduction in myocardial oxygen consumption.[136,148,155]

The sites and mechanisms underlying the myocardial effects of diazepam are not defined. To the extent that anxiety and the associated sympathetic activity contributes to myocardial stimulation, diazepam may reduce the stimulation by relieving anxiety. Diazepam appears to have no direct sympatholytic action, and it does not cause orthostatic hypotension.[156] Speculation has been offered that diazepam may activate postganglionic mechanisms to produce vasodilation, since its actions can be demonstrated in the isolated canine heart and are blocked by trimethapan, a ganglionic blocking drug.[157] No dilation of aortocoronary saphenous vein grafts occurs with diazepam.[158]

OTHER BENZODIAZEPINES

Chlordiazepoxide (Librium) is the only other benzodiazepine commercially available for parenteral injection in the United States and is not widely used by anesthesiologists. Newer benzodiazepine derivatives for oral administration have become available and are being used for sedation and sleep in the preoperative and postoperative periods. Oxazepam (Serax) offers a slightly shorter duration of action than diazepam because it is more readily inactivated by conjugation with glucuronic acid.[136] A derivative of oxazepam, lorazepam (Ativan) is available in the United States for oral administration and in other countries for both oral and parenteral use. It produces more amnesia than diazepam, but it may actually be less useful for anesthetic purposes because of its delayed onset and more prolonged duration of action after intravenous injection.[159,160]

Droperidol

Droperidol (Inapsine), also known as dehydrobenzperidol, is classified chemically as a butyrophenone and pharmacologically as a major tranquilizer with actions similar to chlorpromazine and other phenothiazines. Like other major tranquilizers, droperidol can reduce the anxiety and agitation accompanying psychoses, but it is less effective against acute situational anxiety such as that arising in the preoperative period. In this regard, as well as in the overall spectrum of its pharmacologic actions, droperidol is quite different from diazepam and the minor tranquilizers. Droperidol's actions on the central nervous and cardiovascular systems are of particular interest to the anesthesiologist.

Like chlorpromazine, droperidol induces the neuroleptic state characterized by an outwardly calm appearance with suppression of affect and slowing of motor function. The subject may sleep but is rather easily aroused and can follow simple commands.[161] In some patients given droperidol alone for premedication, considerable anxiety and inner discomfort have been masked by the outward manifestations of the neuroleptic state and have led to later recall of the unpleasantness of the experience as well as to erratic behavior under the influence of droperidol (e.g., unwarranted demands by the patient to cancel the surgery).[162–164] Because the degree of sedation and relief of anxiety is variable, it is recommended that droperidol be combined with other drugs for preanesthetic medication. In most instances, droperidol is combined with a narcotic analgesic, and the combination of their actions results in satisfactory and dependable sedation without interfering with the ability of the patient to cooperate when aroused.

Other actions of droperidol in the CNS include its antiemetic effect (particularly useful when combined with narcotic analgesics), suppression of temperature-regulating mechanisms (of value in reducing shivering with deliberate hypothermia), and reduction of total body oxygen consumption (25 percent decrease after a 10-mg dose in adults). The most distressing side effects result from extrapyramidal reactions manifested in a variety of ways (e.g., restlessness and agitation, torticollis, dysphagia, uncontrolled movements of all types, parkinsonian crises). Droperidol alone or in combination with narcotic analgesics does not produce amnesia, nor does it have an anticonvulsant action. Droperidol is neither an analgesic nor a significant depressant of respiration, and it probably does not potentiate these effects of the narcotic analgesics. Nevertheless, droperidol's relatively long duration of action ($t_\frac{1}{2}$ = 2 to 3 hours) and potential for interactions with other drugs should be considered when prescribing sedative and analgesic drugs in the postoperative period.[165]

CARDIOVASCULAR EFFECTS

Like chlorpromazine, droperidol can produce hypotension as a result of its actions within the central nervous system and its blockade of α-adrenergic receptors in vascular smooth muscle.[166–168] The relative contributions of the central and peripheral actions of droperidol to any particular episode of hypotension is usually uncertain. The hypotension can be effectively treated by the usual measures, including the use of sympathomimetic drugs.

Despite its potential for inducing hypotension, droperidol has shown surprisingly small and inconsistent effects on the hemodynamics of adult volunteers and patients given intravenous doses of 5–20 mg.* For example, Ferrari et al. administered droperidol intravenously in three 5-mg doses at intervals of 13 minutes to 5 volunteers receiving no other drugs.[169] Measurements were made 10 minutes after each dose.

---

* Because of its long duration of action, many anesthesiologists limit the total dose of droperidol to 10 mg in the average-sized adult and use other drugs to deepen the level of anesthesia.

The first dose was followed by a 24 to 31 percent decrease in peripheral vascular resistance, a 28 to 47 percent increase in cardiac output, and no change in arterial blood pressure. The second dose produced a very slight further change in resistance and output, but the third dose was followed by a return of peripheral resistance and cardiac output to control levels. Heart rate did not change significantly at any time during the course of the study. In another study of 5 volunteers, Graves et al. injected a single intravenous dose of droperidol (0.22 mg/kg, mean dose 17.5 mg) and made measurements 15 minutes later.[170] No statistically significant changes were found, although there was a trend toward decreased vascular resistance (10 percent) and a fall in central venous pressure (19 percent). Measurements repeated 60 minutes after droperidol injection again showed no significant changes, but the average peripheral resistance was now 10 percent higher than control and was associated with a 10 percent increase in $Paco_2$. Heart rate, stroke volume, and arterial blood pressure were approximately 10 percent less than the predrug level. Finally, MacDonald et al. administered 10 mg of droperidol intravenously over 10 minutes and made measurements over the succeeding hour in 4 patients with mitral valvular disease.[171] Both systemic and pulmonary vascular resistance decreased during the infusion and were accompanied by proportionate reductions in systemic and pulmonary arterial blood pressures. Following completion of the infusion, the resistances returned to the predrug levels in 20 to 30 minutes in 3 of the 4 patients. There were no consistent changes in cardiac output throughout the study.

Comparably small, transient, and somewhat inconsistent changes in hemodynamic measures have been observed when droperidol has been administered in the presence of other drugs including morphine,[133,172] fentanyl,[173,174] nitrous oxide,[175] and enflurane.[176] The practical implications of these findings are as follows: (1) hypotension may develop following intravenous injection of droperidol; (2) the hypotension probably results from a transient decrease in peripheral vascular resistance; (3) the hypotension is minimized when compensatory increases in cardiac output occur; and (4) the magnitude of change is generally too small and variable to consider droperidol as an effective therapy for the treatment of hypertension. Nevertheless, there have been suggestions that droperidol be used to minimize the development of hypertension during anesthesia involving ketamine or one of the narcotic analgesics.[177]

Another action of droperidol of interest to anesthesiologists is its antiarrhythmic effect.[178,179] It has been demonstrated in both animals and humans that the threshold for epinephrine-induced dysrhythmias is increased in the myocardium sensitized by halothane, cyclopropane, or chloroform. Droperidol has also prevented arrhythmias induced by coronary artery occlusion and by ouabain toxicity, although the last point is controversial. The mechanism of the antiarrhythmic action is uncertain, but two factors may be contributory. Droperidol has local anesthetic properties and may stabilize excitable membranes of myocardial cells. It may also reduce pressure-sensitive dysrhythmias by decreasing arterial blood pressure, especially the hypertensive response to epinephrine.

Narcotic Analgesics

Morphine is the oldest and still most widely used narcotic analgesic for anesthetic purposes. It is also the most thoroughly studied drug in this class. Other narcotic analgesics resemble morphine very closely; their major differences are in terms of potency and duration of action (Table 1-3).[180]

"ANESTHETIC" EFFECTS

Contrary to the anesthetics that produce a dose-related, generalized depression of the central nervous system, narcotic analgesics are quite selective in their actions. Profound analgesia and apnea can be achieved without rendering a healthy subject unconscious, providing that his ventilation is maintained mechanically to avoid hypoxia and hypercarbia. No amnesia or skeletal muscular relaxation results, and only certain reflexes are obtunded. Therefore, it is incorrect to refer to this group of drugs as "anesthetics" (anymore than one would refer to muscle relaxants or any other group of drugs with a limited spectrum of depressant effects as anesthetics).

In regard to patients with cardiac disease, it is worth distinguishing those who are able to maintain a satisfactory cardiac output and es-

Table 1-3

Comparison of Narcotic Analgesics

Duration*	Narcotic Analgesic	Equivalent Dose* (mg)
4 to 6 hours	Morphine	10
	Hydromorphone (Dilaudid)	1.5
	Oxymorphone (Numorphan)	1–1.5
2 to 4 hours	Meperidine (Demerol)	80–100
	Anileridine (Leritine)	25–30
1 to 2 hours	Fentanyl (Sublimaze)	0.1–0.15
	Alphaprodine (Nisentil)	40–60

* Based on subcutaneous injection.[180]

sentially normal function of body organs from patients who are severely ill from cardiac or other disease. For reasons still largely unknown, the severely ill person is usually very susceptible to the depressant effects of drugs of all types. In such patients, the narcotic analgesics alone can usually produce unconsciousness, whereas the more healthy subject may sleep only lightly under the influence of very large doses of morphine and its congeners.[181] It is most important to remember that the latter patients may be aroused by the noxious stimulation of surgery and that signs of arousal may not be evident if they are totally paralyzed by muscle relaxant drugs. For any individual patient, arousability is a function of the degree of drug-induced CNS depression versus the intensity of stimulus. In order to reduce the risk of the patient being aware and later recalling events occurring during surgery, it is a common practice to supplement a narcotic analgesic with other depressant drugs that can produce amnesia and unconsciousness. Such supplements also reduce the total dose requirements for the narcotic analgesics. For example, 1.5–3 mg/kg* doses of morphine may be required to induce sleep when it is used alone, whereas 0.3–0.5 mg/kg doses will often suffice when combined with diazepam (0.2–0.3 mg/kg).

It is usually necessary to supplement narcotic analgesics with muscle relaxants for anesthetic purposes. In addition to the relaxant

requirements imposed by tracheal intubation and surgical procedures, the narcotic analgesics are known to produce muscular rigidity, especially if they are administered rapidly in high doses and combined with nitrous oxide.[21,182,183] The rigidity occurs mainly in muscles of the body trunk and can severely impede positive pressure ventilation because of the marked decrease in thoracic compliance. (This also has implications for cardiovascular function; see below.) The rigidity can be relieved by small doses of either succinylcholine (0.1–0.3 mg/kg)† or one of the nondepolarizing relaxants. It can also be relieved or prevented by moderately deep levels of general anesthesia, a fact that suggests that the rigidity arises from a central action of the narcotic analgesics.[21]

The dose-related depression of ventilation and airway reflexes (i.e., cough) by narcotic analgesics can be used to advantage in minimizing diaphragmatic movement disruptive to the surgical procedure and in facilitating controlled ventilation during and after the operation. Changes in respiratory variables (e.g., $F_{I_{O_2}}$, hypercarbia, positive pressure ventilation) can influence cardiovascular functions and may be responsible for some of the hemodynamic alterations attributed to morphine.[184] These variables need to be controlled in order to identify the primary cardiovascular effects of morphine.

CARDIOVASCULAR EFFECTS

The introduction of "morphine anesthesia" by Lowenstein et al. was based on their obser-

* All doses are for intravenous administration unless other routes are specified in the text. These doses are given for induction of anesthesia and do not include those for premedication.

† The rigidity recurs when the relaxant effect of succinylcholine diminishes.

vations of minimal hemodynamic changes in critically ill patients receiving morphine in an intensive-care setting.[185] They demonstrated that even large doses (1 mg/kg) administered intravenously produced no significant changes in cardiovascular variables in subjects without cardiopulmonary disease and that there was a slight improvement in the hemodynamic status of patients with aortic valvular disease. The potential for cardiovascular stability and satisfactory anesthesia in critically ill patient has made morphine a popular drug for the anesthetic management of these patients during all types of surgery. However, certain precautions must be taken to maintain hemodynamic stability during the induction and maintenance of anesthesia with morphine.

Hypotension can occur during and following the administration of even relatively small doses of morphine. Three different mechanisms can contribute to a hypotensive response: (1) bradycardia, (2) histamine release, and (3) depression of the sympathetic nervous system.

Bradycardia results from increased activity over the vagal nerves and is thought to arise from an action of morphine on the brain stem.[186] It is not a constant finding in clinical circumstances, probably because other factors overshadow it. When hypotension is associated with bradycardia, however, it is often corrected by the administration of atropine or other anticholinergic drugs.

Histamine release and the associated hypotension are variable in both incidence and degree.[186-188] They are probably related to the dose and rate of morphine administration and to individual susceptibility to the histamine-releasing actions of the drugs. The degree of hypotension can be minimized by limiting the rate of morphine injection to 5 mg/min, by keeping the patient in a supine or legs-up position, and by maintaining a normal circulating blood volume. Hypotension resulting from histamine release can be corrected by vasopressor drugs. The administration of antihistamines is of no value in the treatment of hypotension and is not a practical approach to its prevention, since large doses administered prior to morphine only partially block the hypotensive response in animals and humans.[186,188,189] (It is conceivable that a combination of H_1 and H_2 histamine receptor blocking drugs could abolish this mechanism of morphine-induced hypotension.)

Only certain sympathetic nervous system functions are *selectively* impaired by morphine. One of the earliest clinical studies of morphine's cardiovascular effects demonstrated orthostatic hypotension in response to tilting.[190] More recently, Zelis et al. have shown that morphine reduces sympathetic tone to peripheral veins in humans, probably through an action within the central nervous system.[191] The CNS action is selective, since only certain sympathetic reflexes are impaired (e.g., venoconstriction to tilting or carbon dioxide inhalation), while others function normally (e.g., venoconstriction to a single deep breath or mental arithmetic).[192] Morphine does *not* block adrenergic receptors nor otherwise impair function in the peripheral components of the sympathetic nervous system.[193] Thus, hypotension resulting from decreased sympathetic tone and inhibition of certain sympathetic reflexes controlling venous capacitance and arteriolar resistance vessels can be both minimized and treated by maintaining the patient in a supine or legs-up position, by infusing intravenous fluids to restore an adequate circulating blood volume, and if necessary, by administering vasopressors. It is also important to assist ventilation in order to prevent the accumulation of carbon dioxide, because morphine blocks the sympathetically mediated venoconstrictor response to carbon dioxide, which is then unopposed in exerting its direct vasodilating effects.[192]

In addition to hypotension, the venodilating properties of morphine may be responsible for the increased requirements for intravenous fluid and blood transfusions as compared to patients anesthetized with halothane.[194] It also appears that the venodilating effect of morphine is dose-related, since Stanley et al. have shown that very large doses of morphine (8.6–11.0 mg/kg) result in even greater requirements of blood and fluid to maintain urine output.[195] Furthermore, patients receiving the huge doses become grossly edematous, develop metabolic acidosis, and are prone to hypotension, especially when their body position is changed.

Of equal or perhaps greater concern to the anesthesiologist is the development of hypertension and tachycardia in the patient with cardiac disease. These responses to noxious stimulation are likely to occur under light anesthesia of any type, including that produced primarily by morphine or one of its surrogates. Conahan et al.

have noted that while the incidence and severity of hypotension were almost the same in patients receiving either morphine or halothane during cardiac surgery, the occurrence of marked hypertension was associated primarily with morphine anesthesia (53 percent of 66 patients).[196] Arens et al. also noted a high incidence (35 percent) of hypertension and tachycardia in their series of patients anesthetized with morphine for coronary artery surgery.[197] It should be noted that the tachycardia and hypertension are *not* pharmacologic responses to morphine but rather responses to noxious stimulation that are not suppressed by morphine. Both the sympathetic nervous system and the renin–angiotensin mechanism contribute to the tachycardia and hypertension.[198,199] Very large doses of narcotic analgesics may reduce to some degree the incidence and severity of cardiovascular stimulation, but once the hypertension and tachycardia occur, additional doses of morphine are usually not able to restore the blood pressure and heart rate to normal. Stimulation of these mechanisms can be suppressed by deepening the level of general anesthesia, or the consequences of their stimulation can be overcome with adrenergic receptor blocking drugs and vasodilators (e.g., nitroglycerin, nitroprusside).

In summarizing the cardiovascular effects of morphine, it is also important to note what morphine does not do:

1. In concentrations likely to be achieved in vivo even following very large doses of morphine, direct myocardial and vascular smooth muscle depression is not likely. Direct depressant effects have been demonstrated in vitro only with extremely large concentrations (greater than 0.1 millimolar).[193,200–204]

2. Morphine does not sensitize the heart to catecholamines or otherwise predispose to dysrhythmias as long as its ventilatory depressant effects are compensated for by mechanical ventilation so that hypoxia and hypercarbia do not occur.

3. Morphine per se has relatively little effect on the circulating levels of catecholamines, renin, and angiotensin. The release of these substances increases in response to various stimuli, and morphine impairs neither the mechanisms of release nor the actions of these hormones. Pain is one such stimulus.

To the extent that morphine reduces pain, it may also modulate the release of these hormones.*

In regard to specific types of cardiac disease and the cardiovascular effects of morphine, the following are noteworthy:

1. Minimal alterations of cardiovascular function have been observed with careful administration of morphine to patients afflicted with valvular heart disease. In cases of aortic valvular insufficiency, morphine reduced systemic vascular resistance and increased cardiac output.[185]

2. It appears that morphine is also safe for patients with mitral valvular disease, even though they require a high venous filling pressure for maximal cardiac output; the circulating blood volume is high in such patients, and the venodilating effects of morphine are probably of relatively small magnitude.[13]

3. The basis of improvement in patients with pulmonary edema after they receive morphine is still not certain. Although the venodilating action of morphine has long been thought to be of major significance, a quantitative demonstration of its effect has not yet been made. Zelis et al. calculated that peripheral venodilation in the extremities could account for a withdrawal of less than 100 ml of blood from the central blood volume.[191] Their measurements and calculations did not include the splanchnic vascular bed. Recent studies of Green et al. demonstrated that in the dog, morphine in a dose of 4 mg/kg increased splanchnic venous resistance by constricting hepatic outflow vessels. As a result, blood was trapped in the liver and plasma was filtered at the liver sinusoids to produce ascites.[205A,206] The volume of ascites formed within a 15-minute period following morphine administration represented approximately 25 percent of the circulating blood volume of a normal dog.[207] A volume loss of this magnitude from the

---

* The sudden unmasking of pain by administration of a narcotic analgesic antagonist can lead to marked increases in sympathetic activity. This is the likely cause of ventricular fibrillation and death in patients given naloxone in the period following cardiac surgery.[205]

central circulation could contribute to a lessening of pulmonary edema.

4. In patients with coronary atherosclerotic heart disease, episodes of hypertension and tachycardia are detrimental because they increase myocardial work and oxygen demand in the face of fixed upper limit of oxygen supply. When such circumstances arise during morphine anesthesia, demand is likely to exceed supply even though morphine has been shown to produce a slight degree of coronary vasodilation, even in the absence of increased myocardial work.[208,209]

INTERACTIONS WITH OTHER DRUGS

As previously noted, nitrous oxide alone has a direct myocardial depressant effect and a sympathetic-stimulating action that tends to increase peripheral resistance. These same two features of nitrous oxide pharmacology are evident when it is added to morphine.[8,13,15] Since morphine is often used in patients with poor left ventricular function, the addition of nitrous oxide may reduce cardiac output and produce hypotension. These effects appear to result from nitrous oxide alone and not from its interaction with morphine.

Stoelting has suggested that the prior administration of thiamylal (4 mg/kg) for induction of anesthesia altered the hemodynamic responses to morphine.[210] Under the circumstances of his study the infusion of morphine (10 mg/min) up to a total dose of 1 mg/kg resulted in hypotension (16 percent) owing to a reduced stroke volume (36 percent) and cardiac index (42 percent). Systemic vascular resistance increased (35 percent). Similar effects did not occur when morphine was administered alone and have not been reported in the presence of other drugs or under clinical circumstances.

OTHER NARCOTIC ANALGESICS

Morphine is the most frequently used narcotic analgesic for cardiac surgical patients, and it has also been the most intensely studied. In general, other narcotic analgesics resemble morphine qualitatively in their pharmacologic actions, but studies of their effects in cardiac patients are limited in number and scope.

Meperidine (Demerol) was actually the first narcotic analgesic to be used as a primary anesthetic agent for cardiac surgery.[211] It differs from morphine in that it is approximately one-tenth as potent as an analgesic and has a shorter duration of action. A widespread clinical impression is that meperidine induces sleep more readily than does morphine, but there is no objective data to support this claim. Otherwise, its effects on the central nervous system are qualitatively identical to those of morphine.[180]

Like morphine, intravenously administered meperidine can produce hypotension. The hemodynamic changes contributing to hypotension include a negative inotropic effect, decreased arterial systemic vascular resistance, reduced venous return due to increased venous capacitance, and bradycardia.

In isolated cardiac tissue and in animals, meperidine has been shown to have a direct depressant effect on myocardial contractility.[203,212,213] Allowing for its weaker analgesic potency, Strauer has estimated that meperidine has a negative inotropic action 200 times more potent than morphine and that the concentrations of meperidine achieved in the intact subject are sufficient to cause myocardial depression.[203] Decreases in stroke volume and cardiac output and increases in right atrial pressure have been measured in patients by Rees et al.[214]

Orthostatic hypotension has been observed in volunteers given intravenous meperidine, which suggests that meperidine, like morphine, interferes with compensatory sympathetic reflexes.[186] Decreased arteriolar and venous tone have also been reported in human subjects.[215] The role of histamine in the hypotensive response is uncertain. Bradycardia has been associated with a decline in systolic blood pressure when 1 mg/kg doses of meperidine were injected intravenously in patients anesthetized with thiopental and nitrous oxide, but it was not evident in conscious volunteers given the same dose.[216] Much smaller doses (30 mg) given to patients anesthetized with halothane and nitrous oxide did not alter the heart rate but did produce a transient fall in cardiac output and a sustained rise in central venous pressure.[217] The latter patients were breathing spontaneously and became hypercarbic. In another study of conscious patients with chronic renal failure, meperidine (100 mg intravenously) produced a fall in systemic vascular resistance with little or no change in cardiac rate or output. The fall in resistance was associated with a slight degree of hypotension.[218] It appears that the hemodynamic alterations induced by meperidine are highly variable and strongly dependent on experimental conditions. Controlled studies are needed.

Meperidine has been used clinically for anesthetic purposes in initial doses of 1–3 mg/kg, supplemented as necessary with 0.3 mg/kg increments.

Fentanyl (Sublimaze) is 75 to 125 times more potent than morphine as an analgesic and has a shorter duration of action, at least after single doses. Pharmacokinetic data in humans and animals suggest that fentanyl can accumulate and exhibit a longer duration of action after large doses are administered.[219] Very large doses (50 μg/kg) have been used for anesthesia at European medical centers and are currently under investigation in the United States.

The cardiovascular effects of moderate doses of fentanyl (up to 10 μg/kg) administered intravenously to humans have been studied by several groups of investigators.[169,174,216,218,220] In subjects breathing spontaneously, there were no clinically significant changes in hemodynamic variables. Slight increases in stroke volume and cardiac output and a trend toward decreased systemic vascular resistance could be attributed to the accumulation of carbon dioxide as a result of ventilatory depression by fentanyl. A preliminary report by Stanley et al. and our own clinical experience indicate that very large intravenous doses of fentanyl (50 μg/kg) administered at a relatively rapid rate (100–250 μg/min) also have minimal effects on the cardiovascular system.[221] In comparison to the effects of morphine, histamine release is not evident, dilatation of venous capacitance vessels and the requirement for intravenous fluids appear to be less, bradycardia is more prominent but just as readily treated with anticholinergic drugs, and very large doses may provide greater stability of cardiovascular functions, especially in terms of lesser sympathetic responses to noxious stimulation.

Like morphine, fentanyl is a potent depressant of ventilation and can produce truncal rigidity and decreased thoracic compliance, especially when administered rapidly and in the presence of nitrous oxide.[182,183] Obviously, these ventilatory changes can influence cardiovascular function. Especially noteworthy is the impairment of the venous return of blood when positive pressure ventilation is applied in the face of a marked decrease in pulmonary compliance. Neuromuscular blocking drugs will relieve the rigidity, and anesthetic drugs (e.g., thiopental, enflurane, halothane) will probably prevent or reduce it.

Studies in dogs indicate that even very large doses of fentanyl do not impair myocardial contractility.[212,222–228] It is likely that the fentanyl concentrations achieved in intact animals and humans even after very large doses do not approach those shown to decrease contractility of isolated heart tissue in vitro.[202,203,213,229,230] In the intact animal, reduced cardiac output results from bradycardia and is associated with a proportionate fall in myocardial oxygen utilization and coronary blood flow. There is one report that fentanyl reduces splanchnic nerve activity, but the significance of this in terms of limiting sympathetic responses to noxious stimulation is uncertain.[228]

Additional experience with very large doses of fentanyl is required before it is possible to assign this narcotic analgesic a role in anesthesia for cardiac surgery. Several of the pharmacologic features described above may prove to be advantageous. They include lack of hypotension as a result of histamine release, suppression of sympathetic responses and the associated hypertension and tachycardia, and a relatively short duration of action, allowing for earlier discontinuation of ventilatory support in the postoperative period. Because it lacks any significant negative inotropic effect, fentanyl should be as useful as morphine in the patient with valvular heart disease. If indeed sympathetic responses to noxious stimulation can be suppressed by very large doses, fentanyl may be especially valuable for anesthesia in the patient with coronary artery disease and poor left ventricular function.

Ketamine

Ketamine (Ketalar, Ketaject) is unique among the anesthetic drugs currently in use because of the nature of its effects on the central nervous system and because it stimulates the cardiovascular system.[231,232] Ketamine has a very rapid onset of action (less than 1 minute) when injected intravenously, and its onset is only slightly less rapid after intramuscular injection (usually 2 to 4 minutes, occasionally up to

8 minutes). As a result, ketamine can be used for rapid induction of anesthesia, especially in patients for whom anesthetic drugs with cardiovascular-depressing properties are contraindicated. Ketamine can also be used for maintenance of anesthesia, but the indications for this use are limited because of emergence delirium, accumulation with prolonged recovery times after multiple doses, and undesirable degrees of cardiovascular stimulation.

The effects of ketamine result primarily from its action in the central nervous system and include profound analgesia, a cataleptic state, and increased muscle tone. The analgesia is thought to be greater for somatic than for visceral pain and can be achieved with low doses (0.3–0.5 mg/kg I.V.) that do not necessarily produce sleep or unconsciousness.[232,233] Analgesia outlasts the latter effects when they occur. The cataleptic state occurs after intravenous doses of 1–2 mg/kg. In this state the patient is noncommunicative, although he may appear to be awake and, in fact, may later have a vague recollection of the events transpiring while under the influence of ketamine. Larger doses may induce unconsciousness and result in amnesia for a period outlasting the return to consciousness. Muscle tone may be increased to the point of whole-body rigidity and can result in tightening of jaw muscles leading to airway obstruction; this can be reversed by the use of skeletal muscle relaxants or potent inhalational anesthetics. Ventilation is usually not depressed, although an occasional subject has become apneic for a brief period immediately following an intravenous injection of ketamine. Somatic reflexes (e.g., laryngeal, eyelid, corneal) are depressed only slightly, and a low incidence of aspiration has been reported.[234] Nevertheless, the usual precautions should be taken whenever possible to guard against vomiting and aspiration. Of still uncertain clinical value is the observation that ketamine reduces bronchospasm in patients with asthma; it may be chosen to reduce the incidence and severity of bronchospasm but probably should not be considered as a therapeutic agent for wheezing that develops during anesthesia.[235]

Recovery of consciousness after a single intravenous dose of moderate size is usually evident within 10 to 20 minutes, but the end point of ketamine's action is often difficult to determine. The patient may appear to be only vaguely aware of the surrounding environment, may exhibit any one of a variety of psychic reactions (e.g., delirium, restlessness, confusion), and may later complain of unpleasant or frightening dreams.

CARDIOVASCULAR EFFECTS

In both animals and humans, ketamine increases blood pressure, heart rate, and cardiac output.[236–239] Changes in stroke volume and systemic vascular resistance are variable, but under certain conditions, they too increase in response to ketamine.[238] The cardiovascular stimulating actions of ketamine follow a time course similar to that of its anesthetic effects, and there is substantial evidence that the cardiovascular stimulation results primarily from actions of ketamine within the central nervous system.[240,241]

The mechanisms of ketamine's cardiovascular stimulation are complex and include an action within the central nervous system to increase sympathetic outflow, desensitization or other impairment of baroreceptor reflexes,[242] and potentiation of norepinephrine by a cocaine-like action on adrenergic nerve terminals to prevent the reuptake and inactivation of catecholamines.[243] A central activation of the sympathetic nervous system seems to be the primary mechanism, because the cardiovascular stimulating actions of ketamine can be produced by injecting very small doses into the carotid artery.[240] Cardiovascular stimulation is reduced or eliminated by general anesthesia,[237,257] high levels of epidural anesthesia or spinal cord transection,[241,244] autonomic ganglionic blockade by hexamethonium,[245] or adrenergic receptor blockade by phentolamine.[246] Two studies have failed to demonstrate any alteration of the hemodynamic responses to ketamine by propranolol, but the experimental conditions, including the dose of propranolol, may have been inadequate to test its effect.[247,248] Further studies are needed. Increased circulating levels of epinephrine and norepinephrine are found after the injection of ketamine.[249–251]

Drugs with a cardiovascular stimulant action of their own (e.g., pancuronium) enhance the effects of ketamine.[252] With the exception of the potent volatile anesthetics, however, none of the other premedicant or anesthetic supplement drugs (e.g., droperidol) offers reliable protection against the cardiovascular stimulation by ketamine.[247,253,254]

Ketamine also has direct depressant effects on the heart. Ketamine reduces contractility in the isolated heart and in the patient under halothane anesthesia (which suppresses sympathetic stimulation by ketamine).[242,255-257] In addition, ketamine has an antiarrhythmic action, and cardiac dysrhythmias under ketamine anesthesia are rare.[242,256]

The best quantitative studies of the cardiovascular effects of ketamine in humans have been done by Tweed et al., who made measurements in patients undergoing diagnostic heart catheterization.[238] They gave a 2 mg/kg dose of ketamine intravenously 2 to 3 hours after a 5–20 mg intramuscular dose of diazepam. They found approximately a 30 percent increase in mean blood pressure, heart rate, and cardiac index within 5 minutes after injecting ketamine. These changes were associated with a marked increase in cardiac work and presumably with an equivalently marked increase in myocardial oxygen consumption.[252,257,258] For this reason, the use of ketamine in patients with coronary arterial occlusive disease is relatively contraindicated.

In another study by the same investigators, an analysis of the myocardial force–velocity relationships revealed that both contractility and preloading effects can be produced by ketamine.[239] Since it is not possible to predict which of these two effects will predominate in any particular patient, caution is advised in the choice of ketamine for patients with cardiac decompensation that may already reflect maximal utilization of the preloading (Frank-Starling) mechanism in an attempt to maintain cardiac output.

Muscle Relaxants

Indications for the use of muscle relaxants in cardiac surgery include: (1) facilitating tracheal intubation, (2) preventing body movements under light levels of general anesthesia, (3) arresting diaphragmatic motion that may hamper the surgeon, and (4) permitting controlled ventilation at a normal or elevated Pa_{CO_2}. The pharmacology of neuromuscular blockade is adequately reviewed in a number of textbooks concerned with anesthesiology and pharmacology. The focus of this discussion is on the cardiovascular effects of commonly used depolarizing (succinylcholine) and nondepolarizing skeletal muscle relaxants (d-tubocurarine, dimethyl tubocurarine, pancuronium, and gallamine).

d-Tubocurarine administered intravenously produces a dose-related degree of hypotension as a result of a decreased systemic vascular arterial resistance.[259-264] Two separate actions of d-tubocurarine contribute to its hypotensive effect: (1) blockade of sympathetic autonomic ganglia[265,266] and (2) histamine release.[266-269] d-Tubocurarine has little effect on myocardial function except perhaps for a slight increase in heart rate in response to hypotension.[263,264] These actions in humans are attributable primarily to d-tubocurarine per se,[270] although preservatives in the commercially prepared drug (benzyl alcohol, 4-chloro-3-methyl phenol, and chlorobutanol) have been implicated as cardiac depressants.[271]

The hypotensive effects of curare are enhanced by halothane and hypovolemia.[272-274] Pretreatment with promethazine, an antihistamine, is reported to prevent hypotension in approximately 50 percent of cases but is not recommended as a therapeutic measure.[275] Administration of any vasoconstrictor will readily overcome the hypotension induced by curare-like drugs.

Dimethyl tubocurarine (Metubine) is approximately 1.6 times more potent than d-tubocurarine as a neuromuscular blocking drug[276] but is considerably less potent as an inhibitor of vagal and sympathetic ganglionic transmission.[277,278] It also does not release histamine.[278] In accord with these pharmacologic properties, dimethyl tubocurarine produces minimal hemodynamic alterations in patients,[276,279] although some investigators have reported relatively small decreases in systemic vascular resistance compensated for by a rise in cardiac output, unless the patient was anesthetized with halothane.[279] Changes in heart rate are nil.[276,279,280]

Gallamine (Flaxedil) is noted for its ability to produce tachycardia.[261,281-283] Two mechanisms are contributory to this effect: (1) blockade of cholinergic receptors in heart innervated by the vagal nerves,[284] and (2) release of norepinephrine from cardiac adrenergic postganglionic nerve endings.[285] The norepinephrine releasing action is unique and limited to cardiac sympathetic nerves; no similar sympathomimetic action has been demonstrated in other tissues. Associated with the tachycardia is a rise in cardiac output, elevation of systolic blood pressure, and a decrease in peripheral vascular resistance.[261,283] Several investigators, however, have failed to demonstrate a positive inotropic effect of gallamine in patients anesthetized with halothane or in those with cardiac disease, and no effect on ventricular contractility was found in dogs.[286-288] There are scattered anecdotal reports that the cardiovascular responses to gallamine are unpredictable and that marked degrees of tachycardia and hypertension may occur in some patients.

Pancuronium (Pavulon) is a much more potent neuromuscular blocking drug than either *d*-tubocurarine or gallamine.[289] Its cardiovascular actions resemble those of gallamine; that is, pancuroniom has a tendency to increase heart rate and, as a result, to increase cardiac output and systemic blood pressure.[263,264,290-294] The intensity of these effects is less after pancuronium than after an equally paralyzing dose of gallamine.[295] A positive inotropic response to pancuronium has been both claimed and denied but is probably of no clinical significance in any event.[296] There is no significant alteration of peripheral vascular resistance by pancuronium.[263,264,290] In the usual clinical doses, it does not release histamine or interfere with transmission in autonomic ganglia.[297,298] We find the mild tachycardia induced by pancuronium to be useful in the anesthetic management of patients taking propranolol chronically. Heart rates increase transiently from the initial range of 40 to 60 up to 70 to 80 beats per minute without a marked increase in blood pressure.

Succinylcholine (Anectine) usually produces small and inconsistent effects on hemodynamics.[299] Much greater changes often result from stimuli associated with procedures such as endotracheal intubation.[300] Bradycardia occurs in certain circumstances after injection of succinylcholine. It can be dramatic in degree, is usually short-lived, and is readily reversed by atropine.[301,302] The mechanism is uncertain, although some predisposing factors are recognized: (1) the incidence is greater under cyclopropane or halothane anesthesia than with diethyl ether or thiopental;[303] (2) multiple injections have been implicated as a cause of an increased incidence and intensity of bradycardia;[304] and (3) a higher

incidence has been reported following experimental pretreatment with acetylcholine.[305] The latter two observations have led to the suggestion that metabolites of succinylcholine (choline or succinylmonocholine) may play a role in the bradycardic response. Pretreatment with hexafluorenium, a cholinesterase inhibitor, is reported to prevent the response but is not recommended in clinical practice. It has been shown that prior administration of a small dose of a nondepolarizing relaxant can prevent bradycardia from a second dose of succinylcholine.[306]

As a consequence of the depolarizing actions of succinylcholine, there is a release of potassium from cells and a rise of serum potassium levels of approximately 0.5 mEq/liter.[307] The shift of potassium from intracellular to extracellular fluid theoretically could be of concern in the digitalized patient, but in fact it appears to be clinically insignificant in the otherwise normal patient. Marked increases in serum potassium levels, leading to cardiac arrhythmias and ventricular fibrillation, have occurred in patients given succinylcholine after severe burns and trauma to large amounts of tissue or in those who have certain neurological diseases. Its use is contraindicated in such cases.[308]

The choice of muscle relaxants for cardiac surgery can be based, at least in part, on the patient's immediate cardiovascular status and on the direction of change that would be desirable. For example, an acutely hypotensive patient may benefit from the reflex stimulation associated with intubation, which can be accomplished rapidly with the aid of succinylcholine. A hypertensive patient may be the ideal subject for paralysis with *d*-tubocurarine. A patient with bradycardia from chronic propranolol therapy usually demonstrates a moderate and temporary increase in heart rate after pancuronium. Patients able to tolerate only minimal alterations of their hemodynamic status may be paralyzed with dimethyl tubocurarine, which appears to produce the least change in cardiovascular variables. All of these considerations have a theoretical basis but in practice are probably of minor significance in the overall management of most patients. Certainly, muscle relaxants should substitute neither for adequate levels of anesthesia nor for definitive and reliable therapy for cardiovascular problems.

REFERENCES

1. Chapman WP, Arrowood JG, Beecher HK: The anesthetic effects of low concentrations of nitrous oxide compared in man with morphine sulfate. J Clin Invest 22:871–875, 1943
2. Winter PM, Hornbein TF, Smith G: Hyperbaric nitrous oxide anesthesia in man: Determination of anesthetic potency (MAC) and cardiorespiratory effects. Abstracts, American Society of Anesthesiologists Meeting, October 1972, pp 103–104
3. Eisele JH, Smith NT: Cardiovascular effects of 40% nitrous oxide in man. Anesth Analg (Cleve) 51:956–961, 1972
4. Fukunaga AF, Epstein RM: Sympathetic excitation during nitrous oxide-halothane anesthesia in the cat. Anesthesiology 39:23–26, 1973
5. Millar RA, Warden JC, Cooperman LH, et al: Central sympathetic discharge and mean arterial blood pressure during halothane anesthesia. Br J Anaesth 41:918–928, 1969
6. Price HL, Helrich M: The effect of cyclopropane, diethyl ether, nitrous oxide, thiopental and hydrogen ion concentration on the myocardial function of the dog heart-lung preparation. J Pharmacol Exp Ther 115:206–216, 1955
7. Eisele JH, Reitan JA, Massumi RA, et al: Myocardial performance and N_2O analgesia in coronary-artery disease. Anesthesiology 44:16–20, 1976
8. Wong KC, Martin WE, Hornbein TF, et al: The cardiovascular effects of morphine sulfate with oxygen and with nitrous oxide in man. Anesthesiology 38:542–549, 1973
9. Hornbein TF, Martin WE, Bonica JJ, et al: Nitrous oxide effects on the circulatory and ventilatory responses to halothane. Anesthesiology 31:250–260, 1969
10. Smith NT, Eger-II EI, Stoelting RK, et al: The cardiovascular and sympathomimetic responses to the addition of nitrous oxide to halothane in man. Anesthesiology 32:410–421, 1970
11. Bahlman SH, Eger-II EI, Smith NT, et al: The cardiovascular effects of nitrous oxide-halothane anesthesia in man. Anesthesiology 35:274–285, 1971
12. Smith NT, Calverley RK, Prys-Roberts C, et al: Impact of nitrous oxide on the circulation during enflurane anesthesia in man. Anesthesiology 48:345–349, 1978
13. Stoelting RK, Gibbs PS: Hemodynamic effects of morphine and morphine-nitrous oxide in valvular heart disease and coronary-artery disease. Anesthesiology 38:45–52, 1973
14. McDermott RW, and Stanley TH: The cardiovascular effects of low concentrations of nitrous oxide during morphine anesthesia. Anesthesiology 41:89–91, 1974
15. Lappas DA, Buckley MJ, Laver MB, et al: Left ventricular performance and pulmonary circulation following addition of nitrous oxide to morphine during coronary-artery surgery. Anesthesiology 43:61–69, 1975
16. Bennett GM, Loeser EA, Kawamura R, et al: Cardiovascular responses to nitrous oxide during enflurane and oxygen anesthesia. Anesthesiology 46:227–229, 1977
17. Torri G, Damia G, Fabiani ML: Effect of nitrous oxide on the anaesthetic requirements of enflurane. Br J Anaesth 46:468–472, 1974
18. Wollman H and Smith TC: The therapeutic gases: Oxygen, carbon dioxide, and helium. *In* Goodman LS, Gilman A (eds): The Pharmacological Basis of Therapeutics (ed 5). New York, Macmillan, 1975, pp 881–899
19. Price HL, Cooperman LH, Warden JC, et al: Pulmonary hemodynamics during general anesthesia in man. Anesthesiology 30:629–636, 1969
20. Sheffer L, Steffenson JL, Birch AA: Nitrous oxide-induced diffusion hypoxia in patients breathing spontaneously. Anesthesiology 37:436–439, 1972
21. Freund FG, Martin WE, Wong KC, et al: Abdominal-muscle rigidity induced by morphine and nitrous oxide. Anesthesiology 38:358–362, 1973
22. Munson ES: Transfer of nitrous oxide into body air cavities. Br J Anaesth 46:202–209, 1974
23. Eger-II EI: Anesthetic Uptake and Action. Baltimore, Williams & Wilkins, 1974
24. Johnstone M: Halothane-oxygen: A universal anesthetic. Br J Anaesth 33:29–39, 1961
25. Johnstone M: The human cardiovascular response to fluothane anaesthesia. Br J Anaesth 28:392–410, 1956
26. Dykes MHM: Anesthesia and the liver. Int Anesth Clin, vol. 8, no. 2, 1970
27. Saidman LJ, Eger-II EI: Effect of nitrous oxide and of narcotic premedication on the alveolar concentration of halothane required for anesthesia. Anesthesiology 25:302–306, 1964
28. Miller RD, Way WL, Dolan WM, et al: The dependence of pancuronium- and *d*-tubocurarine-induced neuromuscular blockades on alveolar concentrations of halothane and forane. Anesthesiology 37:573–581, 1972
29. Stanley TH, Isern-Amaral J, Lathrop GD: The effects of morphine and halothane anesthesia on urine norepinephrine during and after coronary artery surgery. Can Anaesth Soc J 22:478–485, 1975
30. Prys-Roberts C, Greene LT, Medoche R: Studies of anaesthesia in relation to hypertension II:

Haemodynamic consequences of induction and endotracheal intubation. Br J Anaesth 43:531–546, 1971

31. Johnstone M: Some mechanisms of cardiac arrest during general anesthesia. Br J Anaesth 27:566–579, 1955

32. Price HL, Linde HW, Morse HT: Central nervous actions of halothane affecting the systemic circulation. Anesthesiology 24:770–778, 1963

33. Price HL, Price ML, Morse HT: Effects of cyclopropane, halothane and procaine on the vasomotor "center" of the dog. Anesthesiology 26:55–60, 1965

34. Skovsted P, Price ML, Price HL: The effects of halothane on arterial pressure, preganglionic sympathetic activity and barostatic reflexes. Anesthesiology 31:507–514, 1969

35. Millar RA, Warden JC, Cooperman LH, et al: Central sympathetic discharge and mean arterial pressure during halothane anesthesia. Br J Anaesth 41:918–928, 1969

36. Duke PC, Fownes D, Wade JG: Halothane depresses baroreflex control of heart rate in man. Anesthesiology 46:184–187, 1977

37. Garfield JM, Alper MH, Gillis RA, et al: A pharmacological analysis of ganglionic actions of some general anesthetics. Anesthesiology 29:79–92, 1968

38. Alper MH, Fleisch JH, Flacke W: The effects of halothane on the responses of cardiac sympathetic ganglia to various stimulants. Anesthesiology 31:429–436, 1969

39. Roizen MF, Moss J, Henry DP, et al: Effects of halothane on plasma catecholamines. Anesthesiology 41:432–439, 1974

40. Brown BR, Tatum EN, Crout JR: The effects of inhalational anesthetics on the uptake and metabolism of l-^{3}H-norepinephrine in guinea-pig atria. Anesthesiology 36:263–267, 1972

41. Goldberg AH, Ullrick WC: Effects of halothane on isometric contractions of isolated heart muscle. Anesthesiology 28:838–845, 1967

42. Price ML, Price HL: Effect of general anesthetics on contractile reponses of rabbit aorta strips. Anesthesiology 23:16–20, 1962

43. Burn JH, Epstein HG, Feigan GA, et al: Some pharmacological actions of Fluothane. In "Fluothane": A report to the medical research council by the committee on non-explosive anesthetic agents. Br Med J 2:479–490, 1957

44. Morrow DH, Morrow AG: The effect of halothane on myocardial force and vascular resistance. Anesthesiology 22:537–541, 1961

45. Eger-II EI, Smith NT, Stoelting RK, et al: Cardiovascular effects of halothane in man. Anesthesiology 32:396–409, 1970

46. Deutsch S, Linde HW, Dripps RD, et al: Circulatory and respiratory actions of halothane in normal man. Anesthesiology 23:631–638, 1962

47. Wyant GM, Merriman JE, Kilduff CJ, et al: The cardiovascular effect of halothane. Can Anaesth Soc J 5:384–402, 1958

48. Filner BE, Karliner JS: Alterations of normal left ventricular performance by general anesthesia. Anesthesiology 45:610–621, 1976

49. Shinozaki T, Mazuzan JE, Abajian J: Halothane and the heart. Br J Anaesth 40:79–88, 1968

50. Severinghaus JW, Cullen SC: Depression of myocardium and body oxygen consumption with fluothane. Anesthesiology 19:165–177, 1958

51. McGregor M, Davenport HT, Jegier W, et al: The cardiovascular effects of halothane in normal children. Br J Anaesth 30:398–408, 1958

52. Payne JP, Gardiner D, Verner IR: Cardiac output during halothane anesthesia. Br J Anaesthesiol 31:87–90, 1959

53. Lof B, Verner FR, Payne JP: Serial cardiac output estimations during anesthesia with Evans Blue dye dilution. Acta Anaesthesiol Scand 4:91–96, 1960

54. Grover FL, Webb GE, Bevis V, et al: Effects of morphine and halothane anesthesia on coronary blood flow. Ann Thorac Surg 22:429–435, 1976

55. Bland JHL, Lowenstein E: Halothane-induced decrease in experimental myocardial ischemia in the non-failing canine heart. Anesthesiology 45:287–293, 1976

56. Conahan JH, Ominsky AJ, Wollman H, et al: A prospective random comparison of halothane and morphine for open-heart anesthesia: One year's experience. Anesthesiology 38:528–535, 1973

57. Black GW, McArdle L: The effects of halothane on peripheral circulation in man. Br J Anaesth 34:2–10, 1962

58. Price HL: Calcium reverses myocardial depression caused by halothane: site of action. Anesthesiology 41:576–579, 1974

59. Prys-Roberts C, Gersh BJ, Baker AB, et al: The effects of halothane on the interactions between myocardial contractility, aortic impedance, and left ventricular performance. I: Theoretical considerations and results. Br J Anaesth 44:634–648, 1972

60. Delaney EJ: Cardiac irregularities during induction with halothane. Br J Anaesth 30:188–191, 1958

61. Dodd RB, Sims WA, Bone JH: Cardiac arrhythmias observed during anesthesia and surgery. Surgery 51:440–447, 1962

62. Michenfelder JD, Terry HR, Daw EF: Cardiac arrythmias during surgery and anesthesia. Surg Clin North Am 45:829–839, 1965

63. Raventos J: The action of Fluothane—a new volatile anaesthetic. Br J Pharmacol 11:394–410, 1956

64. Andersen N, Johansen SJ: Incidence of catecholamine induced arrhythmias during halothane anesthesia. Anesthesiology 24:51–56, 1963

65. Katz RJ, Matteo RS, Papper EM: The injection of epinephrine during general anesthesia with halogenated hydrocarbons and cyclopropane in man. Anesthesiology 23:597–600, 1962

66. Tucker WK, Ruckstein AD, Munson ES: Comparison of arrhythmic doses of adrenaline, metaraminol, ephedrine and phenylephrine during isoflurane and halothane anaesthesia in dogs. Br J Anaesth 46:392–396, 1974

67. Johnston RR, Eger-II EI, Wilson C: A comparative interaction of epinephrine with enflurane, isoflurane, and halothane in man. Anesth Analg (Cleve) 55:709–712, 1976

68. Cooperman LH, Engelman K, Mann PEG: Anesthetic management of pheochromocytoma employing halothane and beta-adrenergic blockade: A report of fourteen cases. Anesthesiology 28:575–582, 1967

69. Gold MI, Helrich M: Pulmonary mechanics during anaesthesia IV: Effect of intravenous isoprenaline in asthmatic patients. Br J Anaesth 41:834–839, 1969

70. Takaori M, Loehning RW: Ventricular arrhythmias during halothane anaesthesia: Effect of isoproterenol, aminophylline and ephedrine. Can Anaesth Soc J 12:275–280, 1965

71. Brodsky JB, Bravo JJ: Acute postoperative clonidine withdrawal syndrome. Anesthesiology 44:519–520, 1976

72. Goldberg LI: Anesthetic management of patients treated with antihypertensive agents or levodopa. Anesth Analg (Cleve) 51:625–632, 1972

73. Kaplan JA, Dunbar RW: Propranolol and surgical anesthesia. Anesth Analg (Cleve) 55:1–5, 1976

74. Prys-Roberts C, Meloche R, Foex P: Studies of anesthesia in relation to hypertension. I: Cardiovascular responses of treated and untreated patients. Br J Anaesth 43:122–136, 1971

75. Roberts JG, Foex P, Clarke TNS, et al: Haemodynamic interactions of high dose propranolol pretreatment and anesthesia in the dog. I. Halothane dose-response studies. Br J Anaesth 48: 315–325, 1976

76. Roberts JG, Foex P, Clarke TNS, et al: Haemodynamic interactions of high-dose propranolol pretreatment and anaesthesia in the dog. III: The effects of haemorrhage during halothane and trichloroethylene anaesthesia. Br J Anaesth 48:411–418, 1976

77. Prys-Roberts C, Roberts JG, Foex P, et al: Interaction of anesthesia, beta-receptor blockade and blood loss in dogs with induced myocardial infarction. Anesthesiology 45:326–339, 1976

78. Lucchesi BR: Cardiac actions of glucagon. Circ Res 22:777–787, 1968

79. Kaplan JA, Dunbar RW, Bland JW, et al: Propranolol and cardiac surgery: A problem for the anesthesiologist? Anesth Analg (Cleve) 54:571–578, 1975

80. Jones EL, Kaplan JA, Dorney ER: Propranolol therapy in patients undergoing myocardial revascularization. Am J Cardiol 38:696–700, 1976

81. Slogoff S, Keats AS, Hibbs CW, et al: Failure of general anesthesia to potentiate propranolol activity. Anesthesiology 47:504–508, 1977

82. Kopriva CJ, Brown ACD, Pappas G: Hemodynamics during general anesthesia in patients receiving propranolol. Anesthesiology 48:28–33, 1978

83. Shimosato S, Etsten B: Performance of the digitalized heart during halothane anesthesia. Anesthesiology 24:41–50, 1963

84. Morrow DH: Anesthesia and digitalis toxicity. VI: Effect of barbiturates and halothane on digoxin toxicity. Anesth Analg (Cleve) 49:305–309, 1970

85. Neigh JL, Garman JK, Harp JR: The electroencephalographic pattern during anesthesia with Ethrane: Effects of depth of anesthesia, $Paco_2$, and nitrous oxide. Anesthesiology 35:482–487, 1971

86. Gion H, Saidman LJ: The minimum alveolar concentration of enflurane in man. Anesthesiology 35:361–364, 1971

87. Fogdall RP, Miller RD: Neuromuscular effects of enflurane, alone and combined with d-tubocurarine, pancuronium, and succinylcholine, in man. Anesthesiology 42:173–178, 1975

88. Torri G, Damia G, Fabiani ML, et al: Uptake and elimination of enflurane in man: A comparative study between enflurane and halothane. Br J Anaesth 44:789–794, 1972

89. Chase RE, Holaday DA, Fiserova-Bergerova V, et al: The biotransformation of Ethrane in man. Anesthesiology 35:263–267, 1971

90. Maduska AL: Serum inorganic fluoride levels in patients receiving enflurane anesthesia. Anesth Analg (Cleve) 53: 351–353, 1974

91. Dobkin AB, Kim D, Choi JK, et al: Blood serum fluoride levels with enflurane (Ethrane) and isoflurane (Forane) anesthesia during and following major abdominal surgery. Can Anaesth Soc J 20:494–498, 1973

92. Calverley RK, Smith NT, Prys-Roberts C, et al: Cardiovascular effects of prolonged enflurane anesthesia in man. Abstracts, Annual Meet-

ing American Society of Anesthesiologists, Chicago, 1975, pp 57–58

93. Marshall BE, Cohen PH, Klingenmaier CH, et al; Some pulmonary and cardiovascular effects of enflurane (Ethrane) anaesthesia with varying $Paco_2$ in man. Br J Anaesth 43:996–1002, 1971

94. Graves CL, Downs NH: Cardiovascular and renal effects of enflurane in surgical patients. Anesth Analg (Cleve) 53:898–903, 1974

95. Millar RA, Warden JC, Cooperman LH, et al: Further studies of sympathetic actions of anesthetics in intact and spinal animals. Br J Anaesth 42:366–378, 1970

96. Skovsted P, Price HL: The effects of Ethrane on arterial pressure, preganglionic sympathetic activity, and barostatic reflexes. Anesthesiology 36:257–262, 1972

97. Merin RG, Kumazawa T, Luka NL: Enflurane depresses myocardial function, perfusion, and metabolism in the dog. Anesthesiology 45:501–507, 1976

98. Gothert M, Wendt J: Inhibition of adrenal medullary catecholamine secretion by enflurane. I: Investigations in vivo. Anesthesiology 46:400–403, 1977

99. Atlee JL, Rusy BF: Atrioventricular conduction times and atrioventricular nodal conductivity during enflurane anesthesia in dogs. Anesthesiology 47:498–503, 1977

100. Lippman M, Reisner LS: Epinephrine injection with enflurane anesthesia: Incidence of cardiac arrythmias. Anesth Analg (Cleve) 53:886–889, 1974

101. Knochigeri HN, Shaker MH, Winnie AP: Effect of epinephrine during enflurane anesthesia. Anesth Analg (Cleve) 53:894–897, 1974

102. Horan BF, Prys-Roberts C, Hamilton WK, et al: Haemodynamic responses to enflurane anaesthesia and hypovolemia in the dog, and their modification by propranolol. Br J Anaesth 49:1189–1197, 1977

103. Saidman LJ, Eger EI, Munson ES, et al: Minimum alveolar concentration of methoxyflurane, halothane, ether and cyclopropane in man: Correlation with theories of anesthesia. Anesthesiology 28:994–1002, 1967

104. Price HL: Volatile anesthetics: Ether, halothane, methoxyflurane, enflurane, and other halogenated volatile anesthetics. *In* Goodman LS, Gilman A (eds): The Pharmacological Basis of Therapeutics (ed 5). New York, Macmillan, 1975, pp 89–96

105. Halsey MJ, Sawyer DVM, Eger EI, et al: Hepatic metabolism of halothane, methoxyflurane, cyclopropane, Ethrane and Forane in miniature swine. Anesthesiology 35:43–47, 1971

106. Mazze RI, Shue GL, Jackson SH: Renal dys-

function associated with methoxyflurane anesthesia. JAMA 216:278–288, 1971

107. Walker JA, Eggers GWN, Allen CR: Cardiovascular effects of methoxyflurane anesthesia in man. Anesthesiology 23:639–642, 1962

108. Hudon F, Jacques A, Dery R, et al: Respiratory and hemodynamic effects of methoxyflurane anesthesia. Can Anaesth Soc J 10: 442–459, 1963

109. Black GW, McArdle L: The effects of methoxyflurane (Penthrane) on the peripheral circulation in man. Br J Anaesth 37:947–951, 1965

110. Libonati M, Cooperman LH, Price HL: Time-dependent circulatory effects of methoxyflurane in man. Anesthesiology 34:439–444, 1971

111. Merin RG, Borgstedt HH: Myocardial function and metabolism in the methoxyflurane-depressed canine heart. Anesthesiology 34:562–568, 1971

112. Skovsted P, Price HL: The effects of methoxyflurane on arterial pressure, preganglionic sympathetic activity and barostatic reflexes. Anesthesiology 31:515–521, 1969

113. Skovsted P, Price ML, Price HL: The effects of carbon dioxide on preganglionic sympathetic activity during halothane, methoxyflurane, and cyclopropane anesthesia. Anesthesiology 37:70–75, 1972

114. Saner CA, Foex P, Roberts JG, et al: Methoxyflurane and practolol: a dangerous combination? Br J Anaesth 47:1025, 1975

115. Kiersey DK, Bickford RG, Faulconer A: Electro-encephalographic patterns produced by thiopental sodium drug in surgical operations. Description and classification. Br J Anaesth 23:141–152, 1951

116. Etsten B, Li TH: Hemodynamic changes during thiopental anesthesia in humans: cardiac output, stroke volume, total peripheral resistance, and intrathoracic blood volume. J Clin Invest 34:500–510, 1955

117. Fieldman EJ, Ridley RW, Wood ER: Hemodynamic studies during thiopental sodium and nitrous oxide anesthesia in humans. Anesthesiology 16:473–489, 1955

118. Price HL, Helrich M: The effect of cyclopropane, diethyl ether, nitrous oxide, thiopental, and hydrogen ion concentration on the myocardial function of the dog heart-lung preparation. J Pharmacol Exp Ther 115:206–216, 1955

119. Greisherimer EM, Ellis DW, Baier HN, et al: Cardiac output by cuvette oximeter under thiopental. Am J Physiol 175: 171–172, 1953

120. Conway CM, Ellis DB: Hemodynamic effects of short-acting barbiturates. Br J Anaesth 41:534–542, 1969

121. List WF, Hiotakis K, Gravenstein JS: Die Wir-

kung von Tiopental auf die Myokard-Funktion. Anaesthetist 21:338–390, 1972

122. Dauchot PS, Rasmussen JP, Nicholson DH, et al: On-line systolic time intervals during anesthesia in patients with and without heart disease. Anesthesiology 44:472–480, 1976

123. Eckstein JW, Hamilton WK, McCammond JM: The effect of thiopental on peripheral venous tone. Anesthesiology 22:525–528, 1961

124. Watson WE, Seelye E, Smith AC: The action of thiopentone on the vascular distensibility of the hand. Br J Anaesth 34:19–23, 1962

125. Skovsted P, Price ML, Price HL: The effects of short-acting barbiturates on arterial pressure, preganglionic sympathetic activity and barostatic reflexes. Anesthesiology 33:10–18, 1970

126. Sonntag H, Hellberg K, Schenk H-D, et al: Effects of thiopental (Trapanal) on coronary blood flow and myocardial metabolism in man. Acta Anaesthesiol Scand 19:69–78, 1975

127. Sankawa H: Cardiovascular effects of propanidid and methohexital sodium in dogs. Acta Anaesthesiol Scand (Suppl) 17:55–57, 1965

128. Elder JD, Nagano SM, Eastwood DW, et al: Circulatory changes associated with thiopental anesthesia in man. Anesthesiology 16:394–400, 1955

129. Greenblatt DJ, Shader RI: Benzodiazepines. N Engl J Med 291:1011–1015, 1239–1243, 1974

130. Eisenberg L, Dwan AK: Neuroleptanaesthesia with diazepam-morphine in poor-risk surgical patients. Can Anaesth Soc J 18:465–471, 1971

131. Hatano S, Keane D, Wade MA, et al: Diazepam-pentazocine anaesthesia for cardiovascular surgery. Can Anaesth Soc J 21:586–599, 1974

132. Hatano S, Sadove MS, Deane DM, et al: Diazepam-ketamine anesthesia for open heart surgery; "micro-mini" drip administration technique. Anaesthetist 25:457–463, 1976

133. Stanley TH, Bennett GM, Loeser EA, et al: Cardiovascular effects of diazepam and droperidol during morphine anesthesia. Anesthesiology 44:255–258, 1976

134. Taub HA, Eisenberg L: A comparison of memory under three methods of anaesthesia with nitrous oxide and curare. Can Anaesth Soc J 22:298–306, 1975

135. Frumin MJ, Herekar VR, Jarvik ME: Amnesic actions of diazepam and scopolamine in man. Anesthesiology 45:406–412, 1976

136. Rao S, Sherbaniuk RW, Prasad K, et al: Cardiopulmonary effects of diazepam. Clin Pharmacol Ther 14:182–189, 1973

137. de Jong RH, Heavner JE: Diazepam prevents local anesthetic seizures. Anesthesiology 34:523–531, 1971

138. Dunbar RW, Boettner RB, Haley JV, et al: The effect of diazepam on the antiarrhythmic response to lidocaine. Anesth Analg (Cleve) 50:685–692, 1971

139. Baird ES, Hailey DM: Plasma levels of diazepam and its major metabolite following intramuscular administration. Br J Anaesth 45:546–548, 1972

140. Kaplan SA, Jack ML, Alexander K, et al: Pharmacokinetic profile of diazepam in man following single intravenous and oral and chronic oral administrations. J Pharm Sci 62:1789–1796, 1973

141. Langdon D: Thrombophlebitis following diazepam. JAMA 225:1389, 1973

142. Graham CW, Pagano RR, Katz RL: Thrombophlebitis after intravenous diazepam-can it be prevented? Anesth Analg (Cleve) 56:409–413, 1977

143. Dalen JE, Evans GL, Banas JS, et al: The hemodynamic and respiratory effects of diazepam (Valium). Anesthesiology 30:259–263, 1969

144. Kaplan SA, Jack ML, Alexander K, et al: Pharmacokinetic profile of diazepam in man following single intravenous and oral and chronic oral administrations. J Pharm Sci 62:1789–1796, 1973

145. Gyermek L: Clinical effects of diazepam prior to and during general anesthesia. Curr Ther Res 17:175–188, 1975

146. Knapp RB, Dubow H: Comparison of diazepam with thiopental as an induction agent in cardiopulmonary disease. Anesth Analg (Cleve) 49:722–726, 1970

147. Jenkison JL, MacRae WR, Scott DB, et al: Haemodynamic effects of diazepam used as a sedative for oral surgery. Br J Anaesth 46:294–297, 1974

148. Cote P, Gueret P, Bourassa MG: Systemic and coronary hemodynamic effects of diazepam in patients with normal and diseased coronary arteries. Circulation 50:1210–1216, 1974

149. Bianoc JA, Shanahan EA, Ostheimer GW, et al: Cardiovascular effects of diazepam. J Thorac Surg 62:125–130, 1971

150. Prindle KH, Gold HK, Cardon PV, et al: Effects of psychopharmacological agents on myocardial contractility. J Pharmacol Exp Ther 173:133–137, 1970

151. Abel RM, Staroscik RN, Reis RL: The effects of diazepam (Valium) on left ventricular function and systemic vascular resistance. J Pharmacol Exp Ther 173:364–370, 1970

152. Dhadphale PR, Behrendt DN, Jackson PF, et al: The effect of diazepam on contractility in the intact human heart. Abstract, American Society of Anesthesiologists Annual Meeting, New Orleans, 1977, pp 413–414

153. Ikran H, Rubin AP, Jewkes RF: Effect of diazepam on myocardial blood flow of patients

with and without coronary artery disease. Br Heart J 35:626–630, 1973

154. Abel RM, Reis RL, Staroscik RN: Coronary vasodilation following diazepam (Valium). Br J Pharmacol 38:620–631, 1970

155. Cote P, Campeau L, Bourassa MG: Therapeutic implications of diazepam in patients with elevated left ventricular filling pressure. Am Heart J 91:747–751, 1976

156. Katz J, Finestone SC, Pappas MT: Circulatory response to tilting after intravenous diazepam in volunteers. Anesth Analg (Cleve) 46:243–246, 1976

157. Abel RM, Reis RL, Staroscik RN: The pharmacological basis of coronary and systemic vasodilator actions of diazepam (Valium). Br J Pharmacol 39:261–274, 1970

158. Stoelting RK, King RD: Aortocoronary vein graft flow in response to peripheral venous administration of sodium nitroprusside or diazepam. Ann Thorac Surg 24:59–60, 1977

159. Gallon S, Dale GD, Lancee WJ: Comparison of lorazepam and diazepam as premedicants. Br J Anaesth 49:1265–1268, 1977

160. Dundee JW, Lilburn JK, Nair SG, et al: Studies of drugs given before anaesthesia XXVI: Lorazepam. Br J Anaesth 49:1047–1056, 1977

161. Fox JWC, Fox EJ, Crandell DL: Neuro-leptanalgesia for heart and major surgery. Arch Surg 94:102–106, 1967

162. Clark MM: Droperidol in preoperative anxiety. Anaesthesia 24:36–37, 1969

163. Morrison JD, Clarke RSJ, Dundee JW: Studies of drugs given before anaesthesia. XXI: Droperidol. Br J Anaesth 42:730–735, 1970

164. Lee CM, Yeakel AE: Patient refusal of surgery following Innovar premedication. Anesth Analg (Cleve) 54:224–226, 1975

165. AMA Drug Evaluations (ed 3). Littleton, Mass, Publishing Sciences Group, 1977, pp 302, 307

166. Yelnosky J, Katz R, Dietrich EV: A study of some of the pharmacological actions of droperidol. Toxicol Appl Pharmacol 6:37–47, 1964

167. Muldoon SM, Janssens WJ, Verbeuren TJ, et al: Alpha-adrenergic blocking properties of droperidol on isolated blood vessels of the dog. Br J Anaesth 49:211–216, 1977

168. Whitwam JG, Russell WJ: The acute cardiovascular changes and adrenergic blockade by droperidol in man. Br J Anaesth 43:581–590, 1971

169. Ferrari HA, Gorten RJ, Talton IH, et al: The action of droperidol and fentanyl on cardiac output and related hemodynamic parameters. South Med J 67:49–53, 1974

170. Graves CL, Downs NH, Browne AB: Cardiovascular effects of minimal analgesic quantities of innovar, fentanyl, and droperidol in man. Anesth Analg (Cleve) 54:15–22, 1975

171. McDonald HR, Baird DP, Stead BR, et al: Clinical and circulatory effects of neuroleptanalgesia with dehydrobenzperidol and phenoperidine. Br Heart J 28:654–672, 1966

172. Radnay PA, Rao DVS, Yun H, et al: Hemodynamic changes during induction of neurolept anesthesia for aortocoronary bypass surgery. Anesthesiol Rev 4:13–16, 1977

173. Dixon SH, Nolan SP, Stewart S, et al: Neuroleptanalgesia: effects of Innovar on myocardial contractility, total peripheral vascular resistance, and capacitance. Anesth Analg (Cleve) 49:331–335, 1970

174. Stoelting RK, Gibbs PS, Creasser CW, et al: Hemodynamic and ventilatory responses to fentanyl, fentanyl-droperidol, and nitrous oxide in patients with acquired valvular heart disease. Anesthesiology 42:319–324, 1975

175. Moran JE, Rusy BF, Vongvisces P, et al: Effects of halothane-oxygen and Innovar-nitrous oxide-oxygen on the maximum acceleration of left ventricular ejection and tension-time index in dogs. Anesth Analg (Cleve) 51:350–354, 1972

176. Stanley TH: Cardiovascular effects of droperidol during enflurane and enflurane-nitrous oxide anaesthesia in man. Can Anaesth Soc J 25:26–29, 1978

177. Becsey L, Malamed S, Radnay P, et al: Reduction of the psychotomimetic and circulatory side effects of ketamine by droperidol. Anesthesiology 37:536–542, 1972

178. Long G, Dripps RD, Price HL: Measurement of anti-arrhythmic potency of drugs in man: effects of dehydrobenzperidol. Anesthesiology 28:318–323, 1967

179. Bertolo L, Novakovic L, Penna M: Antiarrhythmic effects of droperidol. Anesthesiology 37:529–535, 1972

180. Jaffe JH, Martin WR: Narcotic analgesics and antagonists. In Goodman LS, Gilman A (eds): The Pharmacological Basis of Therapeutics (ed 5). New York, Macmillan, 1975, pp 245–283.

181. Lowenstein E: Morphine "anesthesia": A perspective. Anesthesiology 35:563–565, 1971

182. Gergis SD, Hoyt JL, Sokoll MD: Effects of Innovar and Innovar plus nitrous oxide on muscle tone and H-reflex. Anesth Analg (Cleve) 50:743–747, 1971

183. Sokoll MD, Hoyt JL, Gergis SD: Studies in muscle rigidity, nitrous oxide, and narcotic analgesic agents. Anesth Analg (Cleve) 51:16–20, 1972

184. Lappas DG, Geha D, Fischer JE, et al: Filling pressures of the heart and pulmonary circulation of the patient with coronary artery disease

after large intravenous doses of morphine. Anesthesiology 42:153–159, 1975

185. Lowenstein E, Hallowell P, Levine FH, et al: Cardiovascular response to large doses of intravenous morphine in man. N Engl J Med 25:1389–1392, 1969

186. Eckenhoff JE, Oech SR: The effects of narcotics and antagonists upon respiration and circulation in man. Clin Pharmacol Ther 1:483–524, 1960

187. Kayaalp SO, Kaymakcalan S: A comparative study of the effects of morphine in unanesthetized cats. Br J Pharmacol 26:196–204, 1966

188. Thompson WL, Walton RP: The elevation of plasma histamine levels in dogs following administration of muscle relaxants, opiates and macromolecular polymers. J Pharmacol Exp Ther 143:131–136, 1964

189. Hsu HO, Hickey RF, Forbes AR, et al: The effect of morphine on peripheral vascular resistance and capacitance in man. Abstracts, American Society of Anesthesiologists Annual Meeting, Chicago, 1975, pp 45–46.

190. Drew JH, Dripps RD, Comroe JH: Clinical studies on morphine. II The effect of morphine upon the circulation of man and upon the circulatory and respiratory responses to tilting. Anesthesiology 7:44–61, 1946

191. Zelis R, Mansour EJ, Capone RJ, et al: The cardiovascular effects of morphine: The peripheral capacitance and resistance vessels in human subjects. J Clin Invest 54:1247–1258, 1974

192. Zelis R, Flaim SF, Eisele JH: Effects of morphine on reflex arteriolar constriction induced in man by hypercapnia. Clin Pharmacol Ther 22:172–178, 1977

193. Flaim SF, Vismara LA, Zelis R: The effects of morphine on isolated cutaneous canine vascular smooth muscle. Res Commun Chem Pathol Pharmacol 16:191–194, 1977

194. Stanley TH, Gray NH, Isern-Amaral JH, et al: Comparison of blood requirements during morphine and halothane anesthesia for open-heart surgery. Anesthesiology 41:34–38, 1974

195. Stanley TH, Gray NH, Stanford W, et al: The effects of high-dose morphine on fluid and blood requirements in open-heart operations. Anesthesiology 38:536–541, 1973

196. Conahan TJ, Ominsky AJ, Wollman H, et al: A prospective random comparison of halothane and morphine for open-heart anesthesia: One year's experience. Anesthesiology 38:528–535, 1973

197. Arens JF, Benbow BP, Ochsner JL, et al: Morphine anesthesia for aortocoronary bypass procedures. Anesth Analg (Cleve) 51:901–909, 1972

198. Hasbrouck JD: Morphine anesthesia for open heart surgery. Ann Thorac Surg 10:364–369, 1970

199. Bailey DR, Miller ED, Kaplan JA, et al: The renin-angiotensin-aldosterone system during cardiac surgery with morphine-nitrous oxide anesthesia. Anesthesiology 42:538–544, 1975

200. Vasko JS: Effects of morphine on ventricular function and myocardial contractile force. Am J Physiol 210:329–334, 1966

201. Sullivan DL, Wong KC: The effects of morphine on the isolated heart during normothermia and hypothermia. Anesthesiology 38:550–556, 1973

202. Goldberg AH, Padget CH: Comparative effects of morphine and fentanyl on isolated heart muscle. Anesth Analg (Cleve) 48:978–982, 1969

203. Strauer BE: Contractile responses to morphine, piritramide, meperidine, and fentanyl: A comparative study of effects on isolated ventricular myocardium. Anesthesiology 37:304–310, 1972

204. Krishna G, Paradise RK: Effect of morphine on isolated human atrial muscle. Anesthesiology 40:147–151, 1974

205. Michaelis LL, Hickey PR, Clark TA, et al: Ventricular irritability associated with the use of naloxone hydrochloride. Ann Thorac Surg 18:608–614, 1974

205A. Green JF, Jackman AP, Krohn KA: The effects of morphine on the mechanical properties of the systemic circulation in the dog. Circ Res 42:474–478, 1978

206. Green JF, Jackman AP, Krohn KA: Mechanism of morphine-induced shifts in blood volume between extracorporeal reservoir and the systemic circulation of the dog under conditions of constant blood flow and vena caval pressures. Circ Res 42:479–486, 1978

207. Hoff HE, Deavers S, Huggins RA: Effects of hypertonic glucose and mannitol on plasma volume. Proc Soc Exp Biol 122:630–634, 1966

208. Leaman DM, Nellis SH, Zelis R, et al: Effects of morphine sulfate on human coronary blood flow. Am J Cardiol 41:324–326, 1978

209. Grover FL, Webb GE, Bevis V, et al: Effects of morphine and halothane anesthesia on coronary blood flow. Ann Thorac Surg 22:429–435, 1976

210. Stoelting RK: Influence of barbiturate anesthetic induction on circulatory responses to morphine. Anesth Analg (Cleve) 56:615–617, 1977

211. Bailey P, Gerbode F, Garlington L: An anesthetic technique for cardiac surgery which utilizes 100% oxygen as the only inhalent. AMA Arch Surg 76:437–440, 1958

212. Freye E: Cardiovascular effects of high doses of fentanyl, meperidine, and naloxone in dogs. Anesth Analg (Cleve) 53:40–47, 1974

213. Faulkner SL, Boerth RC, Graham TP: Direct myocardial effects of precatheterization medications. Am Heart J 88:609–614, 1974

214. Rees HA, Muir AL, MacDonald HR, et al: Circulatory effects of pethidine in patients with acute myocardial infarction. Lancet 2:863–866, 1967

215. Nadasdi M, Zsoter TT: The effect of meperidine on the peripheral circulation. Clin Pharmacol Ther 10:239–243, 1969

216. Tamminato T, Takki S, Toikka P: A comparison of the circulatory effects in man of the analgesics fentanyl, pentazocine and pethidine. Br J Anaesth 42:317–324, 1970

217. Stephen GW, Davie I, Scott DB: Circulatory effects of pentazocine and pethidine during general anesthesia with nitrous oxide, oxygen and halothane. Br J Anaesth 42:311–316, 1970

218. Mostert JW, Evers JL, Hobika GH, et al: Circulatory effects of analgesic and neuroleptic drugs in patients with chronic renal failure undergoing maintenance dialysis. Br J Anaesth 42:501–513, 1970

219. Murphy MR, Olson WA, Hug, Jr CC: Pharmacokinetics of ^{3}H-fentanyl in the dog anesthetized with enflurane. Anesthesiology 49:1978

220. Mostert JW, Evers JL, Hobika GH, et al: Cardiorespiratory effects of anaesthesia with morphine or fentanyl in chronic renal failure and cerebral toxicity after morphine. Br J Anaesth 43:1053–1060, 1971

221. Stanley TH, Webster LR: Anesthetic requirements and cardiovascular effects of fentanyl-oxygen and fentanyl-diazepam-oxygen anesthesia in man. Anesth Analg (Cleve) 57:411–416, 1978

222. Gardocki JF, Yelnosky J: A study of some of the pharmacologic actions of fentanyl citrate. Toxicol Appl Pharmacol 6:48–62, 1964

223. Laubie M, Schmitt H, Canellas J, et al: Centrally mediated bradycardia and hypotension induced by narcotic analgesics: Dextromoramide and fentanyl. Eur J Pharmacol 28:66–75, 1974

224. Ostheimer GW, Shanahan EA, Guyton RA, et al: Effects of fentanyl and droperidol on canine left ventricular performance. Anesthesiology 42:288–291, 1975

225. Eisele JH, Reitan JA, Torten M, et al: Myocardial sparing effect of fentanyl during halothane anaesthesia in dogs. Br J Anaesth 47:937–940, 1975

226. Liu W-S, Bidwai AV, Stanley TH, et al: Cardiovascular dynamics after large doses of fentanyl and fentanyl plus N_2O in the dog. Anesth Analg (Cleve) 55:168–172, 1976

227. Liu W-S, Bidwai AV, Stanley TH, et al: The cardiovascular effects of diazepam and pancuronium during fentanyl and oxygen anaesthesia. Can Anaesth Soc J 23:395–403, 1976

228. Patschke D, Gethmann JW, Hess W, et al: Hamodynamik, Koronardurchblutung und myokardialer Sauerstoffverbrauch unter hohen Fentanyl—und Firitramiddosen. Anaesthesist 25:309–317, 1976

229. Goldberg AH: Myocardial depression by fentanyl and morphine. Anesthesiology 38:600–602, 1973

230. Strauer BE: Myocardial depression by fentanyl and morphine. Anesthesiology 38:602–604, 1973

231. Wilson RD: Current status of ketamine, In Hershey SG (ed) Regional Refresher Courses in Anesthesiology, vol. 1. American Society of Anesthesiologists, 1973, pp 157–167

232. Dundee JW, Wyant GM: Intravenous Anesthesia. Edinburgh, Churchill Livingstone, 1974, pp 219–247

233. Sadove MS, Shulman M, Hatano S, et al: Analgesic effects of ketamine administered in sub-dissociative doses. Anesth Analg (Cleve) 50:452–457, 1971

234. Carson IW, Moore J, Balmer JP, et al: Laryngeal competence with ketamine and other drugs. Anesthesiology 38:128–133, 1973

235. Aviado DM: Regulation of bronchomotor tone during anesthesia. Anesthesiology 42:58–80, 1975

236. Virtue RW, Alanis JM, Mari M, et al: An anesthetic agent: 2-Orthochlorophenyl, 2-methylamino cyclohexanone HCL (CI-581). Anesthesiology 28:823–833, 1967

237. Kreuscher H, Gauch H: Die wirkung des Phencyclidinderivates Ketamine (CI-581) auf das kadiovasculare System des Menschen. Anesthetist 16:229–233, 1967

238. Tweed WA, Minuck M, Mymin D: Circulatory responses to ketamine anesthesia. Anesthesiology 37:613–619, 1972

239. Tweed WA, Mymin D: Myocardial force-velocity relations during ketamine anesthesia at constant heart rate. Anesthesiology 41:49–52, 1974

240. Ivankovick AD, Miletich DJ, Reimann C, et al: Cardiovascular effects of centrally administered ketamine in goats. Anesth Analg (Cleve) 53:924–931, 1974

241. Chodoff P: Evidence for central adrenergic action of ketamine: Report of a case. Anesth Analg (Cleve) 51:247–250, 1972

242. Dowdy EG, Kaya K: Studies of the mechanism of cardiovascular responses to CI-581. Anesthesiology 29:931–943, 1968

243. Miletich DJ, Ivankovic AD, Albrecht RF, et al: The effect of ketamine on catecholamine metabolism in the isolated perfused rat heart. Anesthesiology 39:271–277, 1973

244. Traber DL, Wilson RD: Involvement of the

sympathetic nervous system in the pressor response to ketamine. Anesth Analg (Cleve) 48:248–252, 1969

245. Traber DL, Wilson RD, Priano LL: Blockade of the hypertensive response to ketamine. Anesth Analg (Cleve) 49:420–426, 1970

246. Traber DL, Wilson RD, Priano LL: The effect of alpha-adrenergic blockade on the cardiopulmonary response to ketamine. Anesth Analg (Cleve) 50:737–741, 1971.

247. Bovill JG, Dundee JW: Attempts to control the cardiostimulatory effect of ketamine in man. Anesthesia 27:309–312, 1972

248. Traber DL, Wilson RD, Priano LL: The effect of beta-adrenergic blockade on the cardiopulmonary response to ketamine. Anesth Analg (Cleve) 49:604–613, 1970

249. Takki S, Bikki P, Jaattela A: Ketamine and plasma catecholamines. Br J Anaesth 44:1318–1322, 1972

250. Baraka A, Harrison T, Kachachi T: Catecholamine levels after ketamine anesthesia in man. Anesth Analg (Cleve) 52:198–200, 1973

251. Zsigmond EK: Guest discussion. Anesth Analg (Cleve) 53:931–933, 1974

252. Dundee JW: Ketamine. Proc R Soc Med 64:39–40, 1971

253. Bovill JG, Clarke RSJ, Dundee JW, et al: Clinical studies of induction agents. XXXVIII: Effects of premedicants and supplements on ketamine anesthesia. Br J Anaesth 43:600–608, 1971

254. Sadove MS, Hatano S, Redlin T, et al: Clinical study of droperidol in the prevention of side effects of ketamine anesthesia. A progress report. Anesth Analg (Cleve) 50:526–532, 1971

255. Traber DL, Wilson RD, Priano LL: Differentiation of the cardiovascular effects of CI-581. Anesth Analg (Cleve) 47:769–778, 1968

256. Goldberg AH, Keane PW, Phear WPC: Effects of ketamine on contractile performance and excitability of isolated heart muscle. J Pharmacol Exp Ther 175:388–394, 1970

257. Stanley TH: Blood-pressure and pulse-rate responses to ketamine during general anesthesia. Anesthesiology 39:648–649, 1973

258. Folts JD, Afonso S, Rowe GG: Systemic and coronary hemodynamic effects of ketamine in intact anesthetized and unanesthetized dogs. Br J Anaesth 47:686–694, 1975

259. Thomas ET: The effect of d-tubocurarine chloride on the blood-pressure of anesthetized patients. Lancet 2:772–773, 1957

260. Eger-II EI: Hypotension and the intravenous administration of d-tubocurarine. Anesthesiology 19:404–405, 1958

261. Smith NT, Whitcher CE: Hemodynamic effects of gallamine and tubocurarine administered during halothane anesthesia. JAMA 199:704–708, 1967

262. Longnecker DE, Stoelting RK, Morrow AG: Cardiac and peripheral vascular effects of d-tubocurarine in man. Anesth Analg (Cleve) 49:660–665, 1970

263. Stoelting RK: The hemodynamic effects of pancuronium and d-tubocurarine in anesthetized patients. Anesthesiology 36:612–615, 1972

264. Coleman AJ, Downing JW, Leary WP, et al: The immediate cardiovascular effects of pancuronium, alcuronium and tubocurarine in man. Anaesthesia 27:415–422, 1972

265. Hughes R, Chapple D: Effects of non-depolarizing neuromuscular blocking agents on peripheral autonomic mechanisms in cats. Br J Anaesth 48:59–68, 1976

266. McCullough LS, Reier CE, Delanunois AL, et al: The effects of d-tubocurarine on spontaneous postganglionic sympathetic activity and histamine release. Anesthesiology 33:328–334, 1970

267. Alam M, Anrep GV, Barsoum GS, et al: Liberation of histamine from the skeletal muscle by curare. J Physiol 95:148–158, 1939

268. Camroe JH, Dripps RD: The histamine-like action of curare and tubocurarine injected intracutaneously and intra-arterially in man. Anesthesiology 7:260–262, 1946

269. Lee DC, Johnson DL: Effects of d-tubocurarine and anesthesia upon cardiac output in histamine depleted dogs. Fed Proc 29:2804, 1970

270. Stoelting RK: Blood-pressure responses to d-tubocurarine and its preservatives in anesthetized patients. Anesthesiology 35:315–317, 1971

271. Dowdy EG, Holland WC, Yamanaka I, et al: Cardioactive properties of d-tubocurarine with and without preservatives. Anesthesiology 34:256–261, 1971

272. Johnstone M: The human cardiovascular response to Fluothane anesthesia. Br J Anaesth 28:392–410, 1956

273. Chatas GJ, Gottlieb JD, Sweet RB: Cardiovascular effects of d-tubocurarine during Fluothane anesthesia. Anesth Analg (Cleve) 42:65–69, 1963

274. Stoelting RK, Longnecker DE: Influence of end-tidal halothane concentration on d-tubocurarine hypotension. Anesth Analg (Cleve) 51:364–367, 1972

275. Stoelting RK, Longnecker DE: Effect of promethazine on hypotension following d-tubocurarine use in anesthetized patients. Anesth Analg (Cleve) 51:509–513, 1972

276. Hughes R, Ingram GS, Payne JP: Studies on dimethyl tubocurarine in anaesthetized man. Br J Anaesth 48:969–974, 1976

277. Hughes R, Chapple DJ: Cardiovascular and

neuromuscular effects of dimethyl tubocurarine in anaesthetized cats and rhesus monkeys. Br J Anaesth 48:847, 1976

278. McCullough LS, Stone WA, Delaunois AL, et al: The effect of dimethyl tubocurarine iodide on cardiovascular parameters, postganglionic sympathetic activity, and histamine release. Anesth Analg (Cleve) 51:554–559, 1972

279. Stoelting RK: Hemodynamic effects of dimethyl tubocurarine during nitrous oxide-halothane anesthesia. Anesth Analg (Cleve) 53:513–515, 1974

280. Zaidan J, Philbin DM, Antonio R, et al: Hemodynamic effects of metocurine in patients with coronary artery disease receiving propranolol. Anesth Analg (Cleve) 56:255–259, 1977

281. Kennedy BR, Farman JV: Cardiovascular effects of gallamine triethiodide in man. Br J Anaesth 40:773–780, 1968

282. Eisele JH, Marta JA, Davis HS: Quantitative aspects of the chronotropic and neuromuscular effects of gallamine in anesthetized man. Anesthesiology 35:630–633, 1971

283. Stoelting RK: Hemodynamic effects of gallamine during halothane-nitrous oxide anesthesia. Anesthesiology 39:645–647, 1973

284. Riker WF, Wescoe WC: The pharmacology of Flaxedil, with observations on certain analogues. Ann NY Acad Sci 54:373–394, 1951

285. Brown BR, Jr, Crout JR: The sympathomimetic effect of gallamine on the heart. J Pharmacol Exp Ther 172:266–273, 1970

286. Reitan JA, Fraser AI, Eisele JH: Lack of cardiac inotropic effects of gallamine in anesthetized man. Anesth Analg (Cleve) 52:974–979, 1973

287. Longnecker DE, Stoelting RK, Morrow AG: Cardiac and peripheral vascular effects of gallamine in man. Anesth Analg (Cleve) 52:931–935, 1973

288. Eriksen S, Hommelgard P, Videbaek J: Changes in myocardial performance induced by pancuronium and gallamine in hypercapnic and hypocapnic dogs. Br J Anaesth 49:1199–1206, 1977

289. Lund I, Stovner J: Dose–response curves for tubocurarine, alcuronium, and pancuronium. Acta Anaesthesiol Scand (Suppl) 37:238–242, 1970

290. Kelman GR, Kennedy BR: Cardiovascular effects of pancuronium in man. Br J Anaesth 43:335–338, 1971

291. Brown EM, Smiler BG, Plaza JA: Cardiovascular effects of pancuronium. Anesthesiology 38:597–599, 1973

292. Harrison GA: The cardiovascular effects and some relaxant properties of four relaxants in patients about to undergo cardiac surgery. Br J Anaesth 44:485–494, 1972

293. Loh L: The cardiovascular effects of pancuronium bromide. Anesthesia 25:356–363, 1970

294. Levin N, Dillon JB: Cardiovascular effects of pancuronium bromide. Anesth Analg (Cleve) 50:808–812, 1971

295. McIntyre JWR, Gain EA: Initial experience during the clinical use of pancuronium bromide. Anesth Analg (Cleve) 50:813–818, 1971

296. Seed RF, Chamberlain JH: Myocardial stimulation by pancuronium bromide. Br J Anaesth 49:401–406, 1977

297. Dobkin AB, Arandia HY, Levy AA: Effect of pancuronium bromide on plasma histamine levels in man. Anesth Analg (Cleve) 52:772–775, 1973

298. Buckett WR, Marjoribanks CEB, Marwick FA, et al: The pharmacology of pancuronium bromide (Org. NA 97), a new potent steroidal neuromuscular blocking agent. Br J Pharmacol Chemother 32:671–682, 1968

299. Graf K, Strom G, Wahlin A: Circulatory effects of succinylcholine in man. Acta Anaesthesiol Scand (Suppl) 14:1–48, 1963

300. Prys-Roberts C, Greene LT, Meloche R, et al: Studies of anesthesia in relation to hypertension. II: Haemodynamic consequences of induction and endotracheal intubation. Br J Anaesth 43:531–547, 1971

301. Phillips HS: Physiologic changes noted with the use of succinylcholine chloride as a muscle relaxant during endotracheal intubation. Anesth Analg (Cleve) 33:165–177, 1954

302. Leigh MD, McCoy DD, Belton MK, et al: Bradycardia following intravenous administration of succinylcholine chloride to infants and children. Anesthesiology 18:698–702, 1957

303. Williams CH, Deutsch S, Linde HW, et al: Effects of intravenously administered succinylcholine on cardiac rate, rhythm, and arterial blood pressure in man. Anesthesiology 22:947, 1961

304. Lupprian KG, Churchill-Davidson HC: Effect of suxamethonium on cardiac rhythm. Br Med J 2:1774–1777, 1960

305. Schoenstadt DA, Whitcher CE: Observations on the mechanism of succinylcholine-induced cardiac arrhythmias. Anesthesiology 24:358–362, 1963

306. Mathias JA, Evans-Prosser CDG, Churchill-Davidson HC: The role of the non-depolarizing drugs in the prevention of suxamethonium bradycardia. Br J Anaesth 42:609–613, 1970

307. Paton WDM: The effects of muscle relaxants other than muscular relaxation. Anesthesiology 20:453–463, 1959

308. Walts LF: Complications of muscle relaxants. In Katz, RL (ed): Muscle Relaxants, Monographs in Anesthesiology, Vol. I. New York, Excerpta Medica, 1975, pp 207–244.

Carl C. Hug, Jr., M.D., Ph.D.
Joel A. Kaplan, M.D.

2
Pharmacology—Cardiac Drugs

Many patients scheduled for cardiac surgery and anesthesia are dependent on the maintenance of a delicate balance of factors affecting cardiovascular function. They tolerate stress poorly and may exhibit sudden and severe alterations in cardiovascular function in response to anesthesia and surgery. Their survival depends on early recognition and prompt treatment by the anesthesiologist of detrimental cardiovascular responses. Modern anesthesiologists, like modern cardiologists, have at their disposal a vast array of drugs that can be used to restore the delicate balance in cardiovascular function. Used unwisely, however, these same drugs can further compromise cardiovascular function and survival of the patient.

Prudent use of cardiovascular drugs in the critically ill patient depends on a comprehensive knowledge of both pharmacology and the pathophysiology on which the drug effects are to be superimposed. This chapter emphasizes the pharmacologic facts essential to the use of cardiovascular drugs in the setting of anesthesia for cardiac surgery. Detailed considerations of pathophysiology are presented elsewhere in this text. The reader is referred to more general textbooks and reviews of pharmacology and anesthetic practices for the broader considerations of pharmacodynamics and therapeutic applica-

tions of the cardiovascular drugs in anesthesia (e.g., deliberate hypotension).

SYMPATHOMIMETICS

Sympathomimetic drugs include many naturally occurring (epinephrine, norepinephrine, and dopamine) and synthetic compounds. There are a number of important differences among the drugs, including their chemistry (catecholamine versus noncatecholamine), potency, and efficacy; their mechanism of action (direct interaction with adrenergic receptors versus indirect action by releasing endogenous catecholamines); their ability to stimulate the central nervous system; their tendency to elicit reflexes counteracting their direct effects; and their relative potency on different types of adrenergic receptors (alpha versus beta) and on the same type of receptor in different tissues (heart–B_1 versus lung–B_2). Knowledge of these sometimes subtle differences among sympathomimetic drugs is valuable in selecting the appropriate drug for optimal therapy, especially in critically ill patients with very limited tolerance of stress, including that imposed by drugs.

Understanding the effects of sympathomimetic drugs has been made simpler by employing the concept of receptors, that is, discrete sites on or within cells that have stereochemical characteristics that allow them to interact specifically with these drugs. Another useful advance has been the subdivision of adrenergic receptors into two primary groups: Alpha (α) and beta (β). As new information has accumulated, further subdivisions have evolved, β_1 and β_2, and a new type of receptor has been identified, dopaminergic. The locations of specific receptors are summarized in Table 2-1, along with the principal effects of receptor activation.[1,2]

Although all effects of sympathomimetic drugs may be clinically important at one time or another, those affecting the cardiovascular system are of primary interest to the anesthesiologist for the perioperative management of patients with cardiac disease. In cases involving patients with lung disease, the actions of sympathomimetic drugs on bronchial smooth muscle may also be important.

The principal cardiovascular effects of sym-

pathomimetic drugs include chronotropic, inotropic, and arrhythmogenic effects on the heart and alterations of smooth muscle activity in the vasculature. Again, a summary of these actions for any drug is facilitated by knowledge of its tendency to activate α, β, or both types of adrenergic receptors. Nevertheless, the net effect of any one drug on cardiac performance and blood pressure can be complex because of the reflex responses elicited even in normal subjects. The situation often becomes even more complex in the patient with cardiovascular disease who is taking one or more drugs chronically and is subjected to noxious stimulation and other alterations of biochemical and physiological mechanisms during anesthesia and surgery. To understand and to determine the beneficial and detrimental effects of these drugs in any single patient often requires full use of the sophisticated cardiovascular monitoring techniques now commonly available in operating rooms and intensive care facilities.

Table 2-1

Modulation of Effects or Organ Function by Activation of Autonomic Receptors

Effector Organ Responses	Adrenergic		Cholinergic (Muscarinic)
	Response	*Receptor*	
Heart			
Rate	↑	β_1	↓
Automaticity	↑	β_1	—
Contractility	↑	β_1	—
Arterioles—resistance			
Kidney	↑	α^*	—
Skeletal Muscle	↑ ↓	α β_2	—
Heart	↑ ↓	α $\beta_2{}^+$	
Lung			
Airway Resistance	↓	β_2	↑
Glandular Secretions	—	—	↑

    * Dopaminergic receptor activation produces vasodilation and decreases vascular resistance.

    + Coronary vascular resistance is primarily controlled by metabolism; coronary vasodilation occurs when cardiac work and metabolism increase.

Epinephrine

Epinephrine (Adrenalin) is the prototype drug among the sympathomimetics. It is synthesized, stored, and released from the adrenal medulla and some adrenergic nerve terminals in vivo. Its natural functions include the regulation of heart rate and contractility, vascular and other smooth muscle tone, glandular secretions, and various metabolic processes (e.g., glycogenolysis, lipolysis). It is the key hormonal element in the fight-or-flight responses to stress. Systemic administration of epinephrine is indicated in the therapy of cardiac failure, hypotension, and bronchospasm. Local infiltration and topical application have been used for hemostasis and to limit the systemic absorption of local anesthetics.[2]

The cardiovascular effects of epinephrine result from its direct stimulation of both α- and β-adrenergic receptors. Stimulation of cardiac β-adrenergic receptors results in an increased heart rate and force of contraction. Very small doses activate primarily β-adrenergic receptors in the vasculature. Moderate to large doses stimulate both α- and β-receptors, and the effects of α-receptor stimulation predominate in most vascular beds and in the cardiovascular system as a whole. The vasculature is constricted in the skin and in the kidneys and is dilated in skeletal muscle and splanchnic beds. The net hemodynamic effects of these actions of epinephrine in normal subjects are summarized in Table 2-2.

Table 2-2
Effects of Epinephrine on Resistance in Different Vascular Beds

	Alpha	Beta$_2$
Cerebral	±	—*
Coronary	↑	↓*
Pulmonary	↑ ↑	↓
Splanchnic	↑ ↑	±
Renal	↑ ↑	—
Skeletal muscle	↑	↓ ↓
Skin	↑	↓

Source: Modified from I. R. Innes and M. Nickerson. *In* L. S. Goodman and A. Gilman (eds.): *The Pharmacological Basis of Therapeutics.* New York, Macmillan, 1975, pp 404-444.

* Cerebral and coronary vascular tone is determined primarily by metabolic products.

The principal use of epinephrine in anesthesia for cardiac surgery is to increase cardiac output by increasing contractility of the failing heart. Intravenous bolus doses of 2–16 μg can provide a rapid, though transient stimulation of the heart. A sustained positive inotropic effect is achieved by continuous infusions of 2–20 μg/min in the average adult patient.[3]

Clinically, epinephrine appears to have a dose–response relationship as shown below:

Dose	Effect
1–2 μg/min	Primarily beta stimulation
2–10 μg/min	Mixed alpha and beta stimulation
10–16 μg/min	Primarily alpha stimulation

There are a number of side effects that can limit the usefulness of epinephrine as an inotropic agent, especially at the higher doses.[4] The development of tachycardia or dysrhythmias may interfere with cardiac output and limit the benefits from its inotropic effects. Ventricular dysrhythmias may be controlled if necessary by the simultaneous administration of lidocaine. The control of tachycardia is more difficult; digitalization of the patient may counteract the tachycardia to some degree and may also permit a lower dose of epinephrine to be used. Profound constriction of the renal arterioles will impair renal blood flow and function, and if continued for more than 12 to 24 hours, it will lead to renal failure, which is often irreversible. Similarly, vasoconstriction can limit blood flow to other tissues and lead to hypoxia, accumulation of an oxygen deficit, and metabolic acidosis (often not fully evident until perfusion of the tissue is restored). Although the overall increase in peripheral vascular resistance may contribute to elevation of blood pressure, nevertheless, it also limits the increase in cardiac output by epinephrine and substantially increases the work and oxygen demand of the heart. The simultaneous infusion of sodium nitroprusside (see below) to produce systemic vasodilation can be of benefit in improving cardiac output, limiting myocardial oxygen consumption, reducing peripheral vascular resistance, and restoring the perfusion of the kidneys and other tissues.[5]

The use of epinephrine in cardiogenic shock resulting from an acute myocardial infarction is relatively contraindicated because of the potential risk of extending the area of ischemia.[6,7] Although the increase in mean blood pressure may improve coronary perfusion, the increase in heart rate, myocardial contractile state, and ventricular wall tension (by virtue of increases in preload and afterload) all combine to increase myocardial oxygen utilization such that the increased demand is likely to greatly exceed the modest augmentation of supply.

Epinephrine is one of the principal drugs employed in the restoration of cardiac rate and contractility following cardiac arrest.[8] In this situation, intravenous bolus doses of 0.5–1 mg may be used to initiate spontaneous cardiac action or to convert fine ventricular fibrillation to a coarse pattern which is more easily defibrillated. In such circumstances, the primary objective is to restore the blood pressure needed for cerebral and coronary perfusion. Once that is accomplished, the long-term management of the patient should take the survival and function of other vital organs into account.

Norepinephrine

Norepinephrine (levarterenol) is the principal chemical transmitter released from peripheral adrenergic nerve endings. Its effects are qualitatively identical to epinephrine, but significant quantitative differences have been recognized.[2] Most notably, norepinephrine is a less potent stimulant of β-adrenergic receptors on vascular smooth muscle. It therefore tends to produce arteriolar constriction in all vascular beds and relatively greater increases in peripheral vascular resistance. In normal subjects, the hypertension resulting from the intense peripheral vasoconstriction by norepinephrine leads to baroreceptor activation and reflex slowing of the heart. As a consequence, cardiac output may be reduced, even though norepinephrine has direct actions on cardiac β-receptors to produce both positive chronotropic and inotropic responses in the isolated heart and in the subject given atropine.

Because of the profound vasoconstriction produced by norepinephrine, it would be expected to increase myocardial work and oxygen utilization in proportion to the elevated afterload. In cardiogenic shock norepinephrine has been infused to correct hypotension and thereby improve coronary perfusion and myocardial oxygen supply. It is reasoned further that myocardial work will be no greater than in normotensive patients.[7,9] It should be remembered, however, that norepinephrine is a potent cardiac stimulant when its direct actions are not overshadowed by baroreflex activation. In the hypotensive patient, baroreflex mechanisms would not be active.

Isoproterenol

Isoproterenol (Isuprel) is a synthetic and highly specific stimulant of β-adrenergic receptors but has no significant effect on α-receptors under clinical conditions. Among the catecholamines, it is the most potent cardiac stimulant, in part because it elicits no activation of baroreceptors. It increases heart rate, automaticity, and contractility. The net increase in cardiac output may be limited by impairment of cardiac filling by rate and rhythm changes as well as by decreased blood return to the heart. Isoproterenol dilates all vascular smooth muscle to produce marked reductions in systemic vascular resistance and an increased capacitance of veins.[2,4]

The principal clinical use of isoproterenol has been as a bronchodilator and cardiac stimulant. Drugs such as isoetharine and terbutaline, which stimulate β₂-receptors in bronchial smooth muscle more than β₁-receptors in the heart, have largely replaced isoproterenol as a bronchodilator. The availability of electrical pacemakers that can be inserted transvenously have supplanted isoproterenol in the management of complete heart block. Isoproterenol is still useful as an inotropic drug (1–5 μg/min in an average-sized adult).[10,11] Larger doses may have to be used in patients with partial β-receptor blockade. It is especially useful in certain cases of acute heart failure, such as that occurring in patients with valvular heart disease who may benefit from a relatively rapid heart rate and reduced peripheral resistance.[12] The major limitations are its tendency to produce tachycardia, dysrhythmias, and hypotension.[4] The combination of tachycardia (increased oxygen demand) and hypotension (decreased oxygen supply) may be detrimental in the patient with coronary atherosclerotic heart disease both before and after aortocoronary bypass surgery.[9,13]

We have occasionally combined isoproterenol and epinephrine in order to obtain greater degrees of cardiac stimulation and lesser increases in peripheral vascular resistance.

Dopamine

Dopamine (Intropin) itself is a chemical transmitter as well as an intermediate compound in the synthesis of norepinephrine and epinephrine.[1] Its role as a neurotransmitter has been defined at least in the basal ganglia of the brain.[14] Its transmitter functions in the peripheral parts of the nervous system are not fully understood, but specific dopaminergic receptors have been identified in the renal and mesenteric vascular beds and may also exist in the coronary circulation. These receptors are not affected by the usual α- and β- adrenergic receptor blocking drugs but are selectively blocked by butyrophenones (e.g., haloperidol) and by phenothiazines (e.g., chlorpromazine). Dopamine interaction with these receptors results in vasodilation of coronary, mesenteric, and renal arterioles.[15] In the kidney, dopamine is unique among sympathomimetic drugs in producing a naturetic effect, possibly as a result of an action on renal tubular cells, in addition to its effect of increasing renal blood flow.[16] Dopamine can also act directly on α- and β-adrenergic receptors and can release norepinephrine from nerve terminals.[17] The effects of large doses of dopamine (e.g., greater than 20 μg/kg/min) on α- adrenergic receptors in fact overshadow its actions on dopaminergic receptors and result in renal and mesenteric vasoconstriction similar to that produced by norepinephrine.[15,18]

The hemodynamic consequences of dopamine administration in moderate doses (up to 10 μg/kg/min) are an increase in cardiac output and a decrease in peripheral vascular resistance.[18] Its cardiac effects include increases in contractile force and rate as well as an increase in the incidence of dysrhythmias. Total peripheral resistance is not reduced by dopamine to the same extent as it is by isoproterenol, which dilates all vascular beds, but the distribution of blood flow is shifted favorably from skeletal muscle and skin to the mesentery and kidneys.[4,15-18] Compared to other catecholamines, moderate doses (i.e., up to 10 μg/kg/min) of dopamine seem to be ideal for the management of cardiac failure, since they can increase cardiac output and shift its distribution from nonvital to vital organs. There are limitations on its use in cardiogenic shock. Dopamine is a less potent cardiotonic than either isoproterenol or epinephrine, and if large doses (20–50 μg/kg/min) are required, they can produce the same side effects as the other catecholamines, namely intolerable degrees of tachycardia, dysrhythmias, and renal vasoconstriction.

Dobutamine

Dobutamine (Dobutrex) is a synthetic catecholamine recently released for clinical use. It is a potent inotropic stimulant with apparently fewer undesirable effects on heart rate and rhythm. It also is a potent stimulant of β_2-adrenergic receptors in certain vascular beds; unfortunately, it tends to redistribute blood flow to skeletal muscle at the expense of renal and visceral organs. Its overall effect on total peripheral resistance is moderate, so that only moderate increases in arterial blood pressure have been observed.[4,15,19,20]

Dobutamine has been used successfully in the therapy of low-output syndromes associated with chronic congestive heart failure,[21,22] myocardial infarction,[23] and open heart surgery.[3,24,24A] It may be less hazardous than other catecholamines as an arrhythmogenic agent in the presence of halogenated hydrocarbon anesthesia.[25,26] Table 2-3 shows the relative potencies of the five catecholamines.

Noncatecholamine Sympathomimetics

There are a large number of synthetic drugs with sympathomimetic effects based on direct interactions with adrenergic receptors, release of norepinephrine from nerve terminals (indirect action), or a combination of direct and indirect actions. Generally speaking, these drugs are much less potent than the catecholamines.[2] A few of these have been used in single bolus doses administered intravenously for their cardiotonic effects [e.g., 5–25 mg ephedrine, 7.5–15 mg mephentermine (Wyamine)]. Others have been used primarily as vasopressors for the temporary treatment of hypotension resulting from hypovolemia, anesthetic overdose, and other causes. The reader is referred to standard text-

Table 2-3
Relative Potencies of the Catecholamines

	Isoproterenol	Dobutamine	Dopamine	Epinephrine	Norepinephrine
Cardiac output	↑ ↑ ↑	↑ ↑ ↑	↑ ↑ ↑	↑ ↑	↑ ↔ ↓
Heart rate	↑ ↑ ↑	↑	↑ ↑	↑ ↑	↔ ↓
Mean arterial pressure	↓	↑	↑	↑ ↑	↑ ↑ ↑
Total peripheral resistance	↓ ↓	↑	↑	↑ ↑	↑ ↑ ↑
Renal blood flow	↓	↓	↑ ↑ ↑	↓ ↓	↓ ↓ ↓

Key:
↔   No change.
↑ ↑↑ ↑↑↑   Increase mild, moderate, marked.
↓ ↓↓ ↓↓↓   Decrease mild, moderate, marked.

books for a discussion of the pharmacology and clinical uses of these drugs.

METHOXAMINE AND PHENYLEPHRINE

Methoxamine (Vasoxyl) and phenylephrine (Neo-Synephrine) are of interest to the anesthesiologist because of their rather selective action on α-adrenergic receptors in vascular smooth muscle. They both produce a generalized peripheral vasoconstriction, resulting in an increased arterial blood pressure and decreased venous capacitance. Because of baroreceptor reflexes, cardiac rate and output decline. Both drugs are essentially devoid of positive inotropic and chronotropic effects, even in the isolated heart or in the presence of atropine in the intact subject.[2]

Phenylephrine (50–100 μg) and methoxamine (2–10 mg) can be administered intravenously as bolus doses to increase the venous return of blood to the heart and to temporarily raise peripheral vascular resistance in hypovolemic states and during the early phases of cardiopulmonary bypass perfusion. It is usually better to titrate the dosage in small increments according to the response of the patient since the effects are long lasting, especially those of methoxamine. Rarely is it necessary to administer a pure vasopressor over a prolonged period. Phenylephrine has been used as a continuous infusion (20–50 μg/min in an average adult) to sustain blood pressure during cardiopulmonary bypass and also during spinal anesthesia.

METARAMINOL

Metaraminol (Aramine) has both cardiotonic and vasopressor effects, although the latter predominate in normal subjects and reflexly lower heart rate and output. When the slowing of heart rate is prevented by atropine, metaraminol can increase cardiac output (similar to ephedrine). The inotropic effect is likely to occur in hypotensive patients. One disadvantage of this drug is related to its uptake by nerve endings whereby it then becomes a false transmitter, replacing the much more potent transmitter, norepinephrine. Sudden withdrawal of a metaraminol infusion can lead to profound hypotension until the nerve ending stores of norepinephrine are replenished, either by endogenous synthesis or by exogenously infused norepinephrine.[2]

ANGIOTENSIN

Angiotensin is a polypeptide capable of producing profound degrees of vasoconstriction by a mechanism not involving adrenergic receptors.[27] It has been infused (0.1–0.2 μg/kg/min) as an alternative to phenylephrine.

Table 2-4 shows the usual doses of the sym-

Table 2-4
Sympathomimetics

Drug	Dosage		Site of Action		Mechanism of Action
	Intravenous	*Infusion*	α	β	
Methoxamine (Vasoxyl)	2–10 mg	—	+ + + +		Direct
Phenylephrine (Neo-Synephrine)	50–500 μg	10 mg/500 ml 20 μg/ml 10–50 μg/min	+ + + +	±	Direct
Norepinephrine (levarterenol)	—	8 mg/500 ml 16 μg/ml 2–16 μg/min	+ + + +	+ + +	Direct
Metaraminol (Aramine)	100 μg	20–200 mg/500 ml 40–400 μg/ml 40–500 μg/min	+ + + +	+	Direct and indirect
Epinephrine (Adrenalin)	2–16 μg	4 mg/500 ml 8 μg/ml 2–20 μg/min	+ + +	+ + +	Direct
Ephredine	5–25 mg	—	+	+ +	Direct and indirect
Dopamine (Intropin)	—	400 mg/500 ml 800 μg/ml 2–30 μg/kg/min	+ +	+ + +	Direct
Dobutamine (Dobutrex)	—	250 mg/500 ml 2–20 μg/kg/min	+	+ + + +	Direct
Isoproterenol (Isuprel)	1–4 μg	2 mg/500 ml 4 μg/ml 1–5 μg/min		+ + + +	Direct

pathomimetics, as well as the relative sites and mechanisms of action.

SYMPATHETIC BLOCKING DRUGS

Excessive activity of the sympathetic nervous system can have a deleterious effect on cardiovascular function, especially in the patient with a limited cardiac reserve. Marked sympathetic stimulation is frequently evident as tachycardia and hypertension in patients subjected to noxious stimulation under light general anesthesia. Endotracheal intubation, skin incision, splitting of the sternum, and use of the electrocautery on subcutaneous tissue produce especially intense stimulation. Often, activation of the sympathetic system by these stimuli is brief in duration and followed by long periods of little or no stimulation. In patients sensitive to the cardiovascular depressant effects of potent general anesthetics, it may not be possible to deepen the level of anesthesia sufficiently to suppress the responses to intermittent, brief noxious stimulation. An alternative is to block transmission in the sympathetic nervous system (e.g., ganglionic blockade by trimethaphan) or to block effector organ responses to sympathetic impulses. Cardiac responses to sympathetic stimulation are mediated by β-adrenergic receptors, and peripheral vasoconstriction occurs by stimulation of α-adrenergic receptors. The only β-adrenergic blocker available in the United States is propranolol. Phentolamine is the only available short-acting α-adrenergic blocking drug. Chlorpromazine has α-adrenergic blocking effects, but its action can be long lasting and complicated by its many effects on other organ systems. Vasoconstrictor responses can also be inhibited by vasodilating drugs such as nitroglycerin and nitroprusside (see below).

Trimethaphan

Trimethaphan (Arfonad) is a drug capable of blocking transmission in all automatic ganglia, both sympathetic and parasympathetic. It can be used as an intravenous infusion (0.2–5 mg/min) titrated according to the response of the patient. Its duration of action is relatively short; recovery occurs approximately 5 to 15 minutes after the infusion is stopped.

Phentolamine

Phentolamine (Regitine) is an α-adrenergic receptor blocking drug with a rapid onset of action. Single bolus doses (1–3 mg) have a short duration of action that can be prolonged by repeated intravenous injections or a continuous infusion (0.1–0.5 mg/min) titrated to the hemodynamic responses of the patient. In addition to its blockade of α-adrenergic receptors, phentolamine has a vasodilating action on vascular smooth muscle not mediated by adrenergic receptors. It also causes cardiac stimulation exceeding that resulting from a reflex response to peripheral vasodilatation. The chronotropic response can be marked and may be the result of phentolamine-induced norepinephrine release from nerve endings; it has been associated with the appearance of dysrhythmias.[28]

Excessive hypotension resulting from either trimethaphan or phentolamine can be treated by: (1) positioning the patient to increase the venous return of blood to the heart, (2) rapidly infusing fluids or blood, (3) discontinuing the administration of other cardiovascular depressant drugs, and (4) administering a vasopressor such as phenylephrine. In the case of phentolamine, the dose of phenylephrine *may* be somewhat greater than usual because it has to compete with phentolamine for α-adrenergic receptors.

Propranolol

Propranolol (Inderal) blocks β-adrenergic receptors in all tissues and has other actions not mediated by adrenergic receptors (e.g., antiarrhythmic effects; see below). It is administered orally on a chronic basis in the therapy of angina pectoris, hypertension, hyperthyroidism, cardiac arrhythmias, and hypertrophic obstructive cardiomyopathies.[28,29] The anesthesiologist should be aware of the potential benefits and risks of continuing chronic propranolol therapy until the time of anesthesia and surgery;[30] these benefits and risks are discussed elsewhere in the text.

Intravenous injection of propranolol in the perioperative period is indicated for the control of supraventricular tachycardia and, in some cases, for the treatment of systolic hypertension not adequately controlled by other measures. Because of the risks of excessive cardiac depression and bronchoconstriction, the smallest effective dose of propranolol should be determined for each patient by administering incremental doses until the desired response is elicited. Generally, an initial intravenous dose of 0.25–1 mg is given and followed by additional doses up to an accumulative total of 3–5 mg over a 5- to 10-minute period. Seldom is 5 mg required for the acute control of tachycardia. Should the tachycardia recur, only small additional doses will be needed to regain control of the heart rate.

The effectiveness of propranolol as an antihypertensive agent is based on its reduction of cardiac output by decreasing heart rate (with large doses depressing contractility as well) and on its ability to block the release of renin by sympathetic nerve activity.[28,31] Dosage guidelines are the same as for the therapy of tachycardia. The use of propranolol as an antiarrhythmic drug is discussed below.

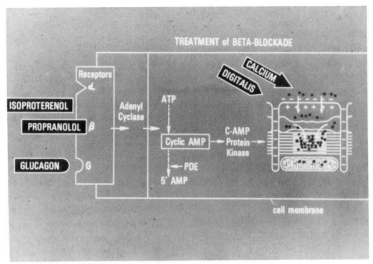

Fig. 2-1. Diagrammatic representation of β-adrenergic receptor blockade and its treatment. The block can be competitively antagonized with isoproterenol or bypassed with glucagon, calcium, or digitalis.

The principal undesired effects encountered in the intravenous administration of propranolol are bronchoconstriction and excessive cardiac depression. Since both of these effects result from the competitive blockage of β-adrenergic receptors, their treatment involves the use of larger than usual doses of isoproterenol* or the use of drugs that bypass the receptors. Aminophylline is a bronchodilator that acts beyond the β-receptors. Calcium, glucagon, and digoxin are effective inotropic drugs in the presence of β-receptor blockade. Glucagon also has positive chronotropic properties, and atropine can be used to block the vagal contribution to bradycardia (see Fig. 2-1).[32,33]

VASODILATORS

The concept of pharmacologically induced vasodilation has gained a place in the therapy of inadequate hemodynamic function. Vasodilators have recently been used in the treatment of re-

* Other catecholamines have the disadvantage of α-adrenergic receptor stimulation in vascular smooth muscle. Vasoconstrictive responses will be exaggerated by the larger doses of the catecholamines and by the blockade of β-receptors on vascular smooth muscle by propranolol.

fractory heart failure and myocardial ischemia (Table 2-5). There is substantial evidence that hemodynamic performance can be improved if systolic unloading is achieved. These drugs are now being used in the operating room and in the intensive care unit in many institutions. It must be emphasized that these drugs are *not* being used for deliberate hypotension; instead they are used to improve tissue perfusion.[34,35]

The rationale for vasodilator therapy is as

Table 2-5
Cardiac Indications for Vasodilator Therapy

I. Ischemic heart disease
   a. Elevated oxygen demand
   b. Hypertension
   c. Acute myocardial infarction
II. Heart failure
   a. Chronic intractable failure
   b. Complicated acute myocardial infarction
      1. Cardiogenic shock
      2. Acute mitral regurgitation
      3. Ruptured ventricular septum
   c. Mitral or aortic regurgitation
   d. Low-output syndrome after cardiopulmonary bypass

follows:[36]

1. Arterial vasodilation → reduction of mean arterial pressure (afterload) → decreased tension generated in the left ventricle during *systole* (decreased work) → decreased oxygen consumption by the left ventricle.
2. Venous vasodilation → peripheral pooling → decreased venous return to the heart (preload) → decreased diastolic left ventricular tension → decreased myocardial oxygen consumption.
3. Possible coronary vasodilation (redistribution of flow) → increased oxygen supply.

There are also three possible deleterious effects:

1. Reduction of mean arterial pressure leading to decreased coronary filling pressure.
2. Impairment of venous return to the point where cardiac output is inadequate.
3. Reflex increase in heart rate and increased myocardial oxygen demand.

Therefore, the safe use of these drugs in acutely ill patients requires extensive monitoring including the continuous measurement of arterial blood pressure, venous filling pressures, and the electrocardiogram. In addition, frequent determinations of cardiac output, arterial blood gases, and urine flow should be made.

Vasodilation can be produced by many drugs with varied sites of action and by different mechanisms. These are summarized in Table 2-6.[37–40] The vascular smooth muscle membrane is the ultimate target of adrenergic blocking agents, direct smooth muscle relaxants, and probably some of the other drugs. Figure 2-2 shows a modification of Needleman's postulated sites of action of these drugs.[41] In cardiac patients, the most commonly used intravenous va-

Table 2-6
Vasodilators: Sites and Mechanisms of Action

Site and Mechanism of Action	Drugs
Central nervous system—sympathetic inhibition	Halothane or enflurane
	Clonidine
	Chlorpromazine
Autonomic ganglia—sympathetic blockage	Trimethaphan
	Pentolinium
Adrenergic receptors on vascular smooth muscle	
Alpha blockade	Phentolamine
	Chlorpromazine
	Droperidol
Beta stimulation	Isoproterenol
	Dopamine
	Dobutamine
Vascular smooth muscle relaxation	Nitrates
	Nitroprusside
	Hydralazine
	Prazosin[37]
	Diazoxide
	Furosemide
Angiotensin inhibitor	Saralasin[38]
Not established	Hyperosmolar solutions[39] (glucose, mannitol, bicarbonate)
	Protamine[40]
	Methylprednisolone

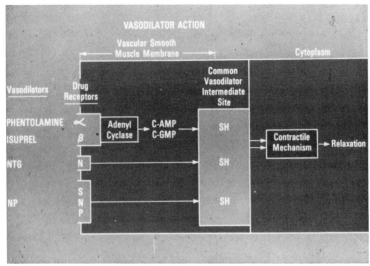

Fig. 2-2. Needlemen's schematic diagram of the interrelationship between vasodilators and tissue components. The xanthine drugs also act as vasodilators by blocking the breakdown of cyclic AMP to 5'-AMP.

sodilators are nitroprusside, nitroglycerin, and phentolamine (Table 2-7).

Nitroprusside

Sodium nitroprusside (Nipride) is used for the treatment of hypertensive crises and for the production of deliberate hypotension. Low-dose therapy for peripheral vasodilatation is a relatively new application. The drug effects both arterial and venous smooth muscle, but has no significant effect on other types of smooth muscle or on cardiac muscle. Its onset of action is immediate and very transient owing to its rapid metabolic breakdown.

The chemical formula of sodium nitroprusside is $Na_2Fe(CN)_5NO \cdot 2H_2O$. It can release cyanide ions spontaneously especially in the presence of sulfhydryl-containing compounds. Ordinarily cyanide released in the body is converted to thiocyanate by rhodonase enzymes found in the liver and other tissues, providing there is an adequate supply of thiosulfate. Thiosulfate availability is the rate-limiting factor in the conversion. Cyanide toxicity and death have been attributed to overdosage of nitroprusside and to inadequate levels of rhodonase activity and thiosulfate availability.[42] Thiocyanate toxicity can also occur, especially when nitroprus-

side is used for long-term therapy in patients with low cardiac output. In order to minimize the risk of toxicity with long-term therapy:

1. The rate of infusion should be limited to less than 8 $\mu g/kg/min$ and the total dose to less than 1 mg/kg/day;
2. Cyanide levels in the blood and urine should be measured; if any cyanide is detected, the nitroprusside infusion should be stopped and sodium thiosulfate (150 mg/kg) should be given intravenously;
3. Thiocyanate levels in the blood should also be determined; concentrations greater than 10 mg/100 ml have been associated with toxicity (fatigue, disorientation, psychosis, nausea, muscle spasm) and indicate the administration of nitroprusside should be discontinued.

The acute toxicity of nitroprusside is entirely secondary to excessive vasodilatation and hypotension.

Nitroprusside is a nonselective vasodilator and affects all vascular beds. Therefore, venous capacitance is increased and preload is decreased ($\downarrow$ LVEDP) while arteriolar and pulmonary resistances are also decreased, resulting in an increased cardiac output and decreased myocardial oxygen consumption (Table 2-8).[43,44]

Table 2-7
Intravenous Vasodilator Preparation and Dosage

Drug	Route	Preparation	Concentration	Dose		Comment
				Begin at	Progress to	
Sodium nitroprusside	I.V.	25–50 mg/500 ml	50 or 100 μg/ml	25 μg/min	100 μg/min	1. Intracoronary steal? 2. Potential cyanide toxicity
Phentolamine	I.V.	25 mg/250 ml	100 μg/ml	50 μg/min	500 μg/min	1. Decrease pulmonary vascular resistance and beta stimulation 2. Expensive
Nitroglycerin	I.V.	12 or 24 mg/220 ml	50 or 100 μg/ml	25 μg/min	300 μg/min	1. Not FDA approved 2. Minimal toxicity

Table 2-8
Vasodilator Actions

Drug	Venous	Arterial	MVO$_2$	LVEDP	CO
1. Nitrates					
a. Oral, sublingual, or topical	+++	±	↓	↓↓	↔
b. Intravenous	+++	+	↓	↓↓	↔ ↑
2. Nitroprusside	++	+++	↓	↓↓	↑↑
3. Phentolamine	+	+++	↓	↓	↑↑
4. Prazosin	++	+++	↓	↓↓	↑↑
5. Hydralazine	+	+++	↓	↓	↑↑

Nitroglycerin

Nitroglycerin is remarkably effective in the management of angina pectoris. A reduction in the myocardial oxygen consumption is the mechanism of its action. Its primary effect is on the venous capacitance vessels, resulting in peripheral pooling of blood and reduction of heart size and wall tension. At larger doses, and by the intravenous route, it also has an effect on arteriolar tone. Nitroglycerin has also been shown to cause a redistribution of coronary blood flow to subendocardial ischemic areas.[45-50]

Intravenous nitroglycerin has been used and studied since Christensson administered it to volunteers in 1969.[51] It has recently been the subject of a great deal of study in coronary care units. The advantages of the intravenous route are (1) greater control of the dose, (2) easy reversal, and (3) use in anesthetized patients. There have been no reports of toxicity except for hypotension with overdosage. Methemoglobin levels have been undetectable in the blood of our patients. The infusion is prepared by our hospital pharmacy in the following manner: 12 or 24 mg of nitroglycerin (20 or 40 tablets of 0.6 mg each) is dissolved in 20 ml of 0.9 percent sodium chloride. It is then sterilized by passage through a millipore filter. This solution is added to 220 ml of dextrose in water to provide a final nitroglycerin concentration of 50 or 100 μg/ml.[52]

In the past 2 years, studies in humans and animals have demonstrated that vasodilators decrease the extent of infarction as measured by creatine phosphokinase (CPK) levels, ST-segment changes, and improved systemic hemodynamics. Nitroglycerin has been used in most of these studies (both sublingual and intravenous), but some authors have used nitroprusside, phentolamine, and trimethapan.[53] Epstein has shown even better myocardial preservation with a combination of nitroglycerin and methoxamine.[54] The α-adrenergic agonist is added to maintain the coronary perfusion pressure. In a recent study by Chiariello and Maroko, nitro-

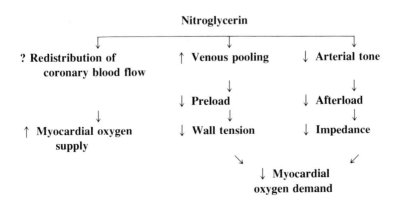

glycerin was found to decrease the area of damage of an infarction, but nitroprusside was found to *increase* it.[55] It was postulated that this resulted from nitroprusside causing an intracoronary steal of blood away from ischemic areas by arteriolar vasodilation. Nitroglycerin causes primary venous dilation and thus may not cause the same change in coronary hemodynamics.[56]

We feel that nitroglycerin may be the preferred vasodilator in patients with coronary artery disease for the following reasons:

1. It is easy to regulate the dose when given in a dilute intravenous solution.
2. Excessive hypotension is rare and recovery is rapid.
3. Minimal increases in heart rate occur.
4. It has no known toxicity.
5. It increases collateral circulation through the myocardium.
6. It redistributes blood flow to the subendocardium and does not produce an intracoronary steal.

Afterload Reduction in Heart Failure

A decrease in impedance to left ventricular ejection by afterload-reducing agents has recently been utilized in the management of acute congestive heart failure and low-output states. The mechanism of action of vasodilators in heart failure is fairly clear. Low-output states are characterized by increased total peripheral resistance secondary to sympathetic tone in order to support blood pressure in the face of a falling cardiac output. With the increased resistance and increased outflow impedance, left ventricular wall tension remains high during ejection, and stroke volume is therefore decreased. The vasodilators decrease the outflow impedance and thus allow for an increased stroke volume, decreased left ventricular chamber size, and decreased left ventricular work. Indeed, the increase in the stroke volume maintains the blood pressure in the face of a decreased total peripheral resistance.[57]

Guiha and others showed a dramatic improvement in hemodynamics in patients with congestive heart failure, using nitroprusside infusion at low doses (10–50 μg/min).[58] Cardiac output and renal function improved, while total peripheral resistance and pulmonary capillary

wedge pressure decreased and mean arterial blood pressure remained the same or increased. The benefits of vasodilators in patients with severe mitral or aortic regurgitation have been shown.[59,60] Sodium nitroprusside markedly increased the forward cardiac output and reduced the regurgitant flow. In the management of patients in *cardiogenic shock*, nitroprusside has become a useful adjunct to add to inotropic drugs such as dopamine. It is indicated if the patient is markedly vasoconstricted and has a high pulmonary capillary wedge pressure.

There is little information on the effect of vasodilators in those cases where difficulties are encountered *upon terminating cardiopulmonary bypass*. This is basically a form of cardiogenic shock. In 1974, Brown and Starek reported on a patient with severe mitral regurgitation whom they were unable to remove from cardiopulmonary bypass after a mitral valve replacement.[5] All the usual inotropes were tried, unsuccessfully. The blood pressure was 70 torr, left atrial pressure was 38 torr, and cardiac output was 1.8 liters/min. Then nitroprusside (100 μg/min) was administered in addition to epinephrine (20 μg/min) in an effort to unload the left ventricle. This was highly successful, and the patient was removed from bypass and survived the surgical procedure. We recently reported a case of triple coronary artery bypass along with mitral valve replacement where we were unable to discontinue bypass with the use of inotropic agents.[61] Nitroglycerin was added to decrease the left atrial pressure from 40 torr. It was immediately successful, with the left atrial pressure falling to 10 torr, and in combination with epinephrine, the patient was successfully weaned off bypass. Since then, we have used combinations of various inotropes and vasodilators to manage numerous patients in cardiogenic shock coming off cardiopulmonary bypass.[62,63]

CHOLINERGIC AND ANTICHOLINERGIC DRUGS

The uses of anticholinergic drugs for purposes of preanesthetic medication are well known and need not be reviewed in detail here. In addition to their inhibition of salivation, these drugs partially inhibit the secretion of gastric acid, decrease gastrointestinal motility, and tend to relax bronchial smooth muscle. Certain of the anticholinergic drugs also have effects on the central nervous system.[64] Most notable in the last regard is scopolamine, which produces sedation, amnesia, and in some cases, confusion and restlessness.[65] Because of the latter effects, it is seldom used alone but is often combined with narcotic analgesics and other sedatives. Its antiemetic actions are useful in combination with narcotic analgesics. Its amnesic effects interact additively or synergistically with diazepam.[66] It should be noted that the cardiovascular effects of premedicant doses of anticholinergic drugs are usually minimal because of the relatively small doses prescribed. Moreover, the duration of the cardiovascular actions of most of them is too short to extend beyond the preanesthetic period[67] (see Table 2-9).

Cholinergic innervation of the cardiovascular system is mediated primarily by the vagus nerve, which distributes cholinergic nerves to the sinoatrial and atrioventricular nodes and to the atria of the heart. There is no clinically significant innervation of the cardiac ventricles or of vascular smooth muscle by cholinergic nerves (although vascular smooth muscle has cholinergic receptors).[1] It is not surprising, therefore, that the therapeutic cardiovascular uses of these drugs are primarily related to disturbances of cardiac rate.

Edrophonium

Edrophonium (Tensilon) is a cholinergic drug that inhibits cholinesterase enzymes, including acetylcholinesterase, which hydrolyzes and thereby inactivates acetylcholine released by cholinergic nerve endings.[68] Although edrophonium has been used alone for the acute suppression of sinus and atrial tachycardias, it is probably more effective when combined with carotid sinus massage or other maneuvers that reflexly increase activity over the vagus nerves.[69] The use of this drug for the acute therapy of tachycardias has been largely supplanted by intravenous doses of propranolol. Edrophonium has been reported to cause severe bradycardia and even asystole in a few instances.[70] Because its inhibition of cholinesterase enzymes is nonselective, it interacts with muscle relaxants. Edrophonium prolongs the action of succinylcholine and antagonizes the action of nondepolarizing relaxants such as *d*-tubocurarine and pancuronium.

Atropine

Atropine is the prototype of anticholinergic drugs. It is used in the treatment of bradycardia mediated by the vagus nerves. Although small intravenous doses (0.2 mg) may elicit a brief increase in heart rate in some cases, complete blockade of cholinergic receptors requires doses as high as 2 to 3 mg. The duration of action of single intravenous doses is short, and additional injections may be required after 20 or 30 minutes.[64,67]

Atropine is also useful in the treatment of premature nodal or ventricular contractions and coupled beats when they are associated with a slow heart rate. In such cases, vagal activity slows the normal sinus pacemaker, and the slow heart rate permits secondary pacemakers to become dominant and escape rhythms to develop.[71]

The treatment of bradycardia associated with myocardial ischemia and acute infarction has been reviewed in detail by Dauchot and Gravenstein.[72] Under such circumstances, bradycardia may be benign or even beneficial. On the other hand, bradycardia may be associated with hypotension, escape rhythms, and conduc-

Table 2-9
Anticholinergic Drugs

Drug	Effects on			Duration of Action
	Salivation	*Heart Rate*	*CNS*	
Atropine	↓	↓ Low dose ↑ High dose	"Stimulation"	Short
Glycopyrolate	↓ ↓	↑	—	Long
Scopolamine	↓ ↓	—	"Depression"	Long

tion disturbances which may be corrected by the administration of atropine. Atropine is not a harmless drug, and the decision to use it should be based on considerations of both its potentially beneficial and its deleterious effects in the presence of an acute myocardial infarction.[73] The latter include the development of severe ventricular ectopic activity and lowering of the ventricular fibrillation threshold, exacerbation of myocardial ischemia and depression of left ventricular function, and extension of the area of infarction.

The responses to atropine can be variable and unpredictable. Occasionally, small intravenous doses elicit a transient bradycardia before the vagal blocking effect becomes evident.[72] The presence of toxic or near-toxic levels of digitalis may be manifested by an atropine-resistant bradycardia. A wide variety of factors, including other drugs, anesthesia, age, neurological or renal diseases, metabolic and endocrine disorders, and temperature, can affect the chronotropic responses to atropine. It is easy to overshoot the therapeutic objective with atropine if the vagal activity is masking a high sympathetic tone. The resulting tachycardia can have deleterious effects on cardiac function in all types of heart disease. For these reasons, it is wise to inject small incremental doses intravenously and titrate the total dose according to the response of the patient.[72] If a severe tachycardia results, it may be necessary to administer propranolol to control it. The intrinsic rate of a heart isolated from autonomic influences is usually between 80 and 100 beats per minute.

CARDIAC GLYCOSIDES

There are a number of digitalis derivatives that share the same pharmacologic actions and differ primarily in terms of potency and pharmacokinetics. The two most likely to be administered by an anesthesiologist are digoxin and ouabain. Ouabain is administered only by the intravenous route and has the most rapid onset and shortest duration of action among the cardiac glycosides. Digoxin is slightly slower in onset and somewhat longer lasting than ouabain, but digoxin has the advantage of being reliably effective after either intravenous or oral administration. Other digitalis preparations and derivatives are of interest to the anesthesiologist pri-

marily in the preoperative evaluation of a patient who has been taking them chronically (see Table 5-1 in Chapter 5).

From the point of view of the anesthesiologist, the most important actions of digoxin and the other glycosides on the cardiovascular system are those affecting cardiac contractility, conduction, and rhythm. The positive inotropic effect is usually at least potentially beneficial; the slowing of atrioventricular conduction can be beneficial in certain conditions but can be detrimental under some circumstances; and the production of cardiac dysrhythmias is always an undesirable effect of digitalis derivatives. The major problem with these drugs is the extremely narrow margin between doses that produce beneficial effects and those that cause toxicity. In the perioperative period, there is additional risk of digitalis toxicity because of the acute changes in electrolyte and acid-base balance, renal function, and drug interactions.

Digoxin will serve as the prototype for the discussion that follows. Qualitatively identical effects can be produced with any other cardiac glycoside, but there are important differences in the dosage requirements and in the onset and duration of action.[74-76] The following summary of digoxin pharmacology is based on several comprehensive reviews.[4,74-77]

Inotropic Effect

Digoxin produces a dose-related increase in myocardial contractility in both normal and failing hearts. Limits are imposed on the upper extension of the inotropic dose–response relationship by the development of ventricular dysrhythmias. The mechanism of the inotropic action has not been fully defined, but several facts are known. Digoxin acts directly on myocardial muscle and does not depend on the autonomic nervous system to increase contractility. It appears that digoxin increases the availability of ionized calcium to the contractile elements at the time of excitation–contraction coupling. The magnitude of the positive inotropic response depends on the contraction frequency and is lower on either side of an optimal rate. Both onset and magnitude of the response depend on the concentrations of cations—potassium, sodium, calcium, and magnesium. While there appears to be a number of close correlations between the inhibition of sodium-potassium-ATPase by digoxin and its inotropic actions, the fundamental basis of the relationship is not understood.[78]

The cardiac effects of digoxin can be described using the Frank-Starling relationship (see Figure 3-22 in Chapter 3). As the myocardial fiber lengthens (represented by an increased end-diastolic volume or pressure), the tension developed (and hence the work accomplished) increases. There is an optimal level in the relationship, beyond which further increases in end-diastolic pressure result in decreased work. By improving contractility, digoxin shifts the entire curve upward and to the left, so that for any given end-diastolic pressure, there is an increased amount of work performed. In other words, the pumping action of the heart is made more efficient. Another way of looking at myocardial contractility is in terms of the force–velocity relationship; digoxin increases the velocity of shortening of the muscle fiber for any given load (force) imposed on it. In most cases, we express this effect as an increased rate of pressure development (dP/dt).[76,77]

The hemodynamic consequences of the positive inotropic action of digoxin, including the total oxygen consumption by the heart, depend on the conditions existing when digoxin is administered and on the noncardiac actions and reflex effects induced by the drug. For example, there is no longer any doubt that digoxin increases myocardial contractility in *normal* animals and humans, but this may not be detected by the usual hemodynamic measurements for several reasons.[79] Digitalis acts in the central nervous system and directly on vascular smooth muscle to increase peripheral vascular resistance. These same actions lead to constriction of veins and, at least in animals, to pooling of blood in the portal venous system and decreased venous return to the heart. Probably the most important extracardiac hemodynamic changes are brought about reflexly as baroreceptors are activated in order to minimize increases in blood pressure by withdrawing sympathetic tone and increasing vagal activity to the heart. The reduced heart rate offsets increased contractility and prevents any increase in cardiac output. The net effect on myocardial work and oxygen consumption depends on the relative changes in heart rate and contractility as well as on the diastolic ventricular wall tension, which reflects both peripheral resistance (afterload) and central venous pressures (preload). A marked increase

in peripheral resistance and severe hypertension has been reported, and in such circumstances, oxygen demand by the heart is certain to increase dramatically.

In the patient with a *failing* heart, sympathetic nervous system activity is high. Digoxin improves myocardial contractility and cardiac output. As a result, reflex adjustments lead to a decrease in sympathetic activity and a fall in peripheral arterial resistance and venous tone. Pooling of blood in venous capacitance vessels reduces central venous pressure and blood volume. The improved contractility and reduction of both preload and afterload lead to a lower ventricular diastolic volume and wall tension. Moreover, the decrease in sympathetic tone leads to a reduced heart rate.* Hence, the work of the heart is more efficient, and oxygen consumption is reduced. At the same time, blood pressure is maintained and tissue perfusion improves as a result of the decreased sympathetic activity. With better perfusion, renal function increases, and a diuresis results, aided by the inhibition of renal tubular reabsorption of sodium by digoxin. The net effect of these changes induced by digoxin is a reduction of edema fluid and restoration of a more normal circulating blood volume.

Effects on Conduction and Heart Rate

The refractory period of specialized conduction tissue in the heart is increased and the conduction velocity reduced by digoxin. These effects are the result of two actions of digoxin—one occurs in the brain stem to increase vagal activity to the heart, and the other is a direct action on AV nodal tissue. The latter may in part reflect antagonism of adrenergic influence on the node. As a consequence of these actions, the P-R interval in the presence of a sinus rhythm is prolonged in proportion to the dose of digoxin, and toxic doses can produce complete heart block. In the presence of atrial fibrillation or flutter, the ventricular response can be slowed by digoxin. Slowing of the ventricular rate by this mechanism occurs in addition to

---

* In cases of atrial fibrillation associated with mitral valvular disease, the ventricular rate may also be slowed by the effects of digoxin on the atrioventricular conduction system.

that which results from reflex withdrawal of sympathetic activity as cardiac contractility increases and the circulatory state improves.

Dysrhythmias

Atrial and ventricular myocardial tissue exhibit considerably different responses to digoxin than does the specialized conduction tissue. Automaticity in ventricular tissue increases progressively with the dose and may be manifest initially as ventricular escape beats when conduction of supraventricular impulses through the AV node is slowed. When the ventricular refractory period and conduction both decrease at toxic doses of digoxin, the stage is set for reentry mechanisms, and ventricular fibrillation can result from one or more ectopic impulses. The enhancement of automaticity by digoxin may result from both its direct action on the myocardium as well as from the increase in sympathetic activity that occurs following toxic doses of digoxin. Automaticity can be further augmented by calcium and can be decreased by potassium. It should also be noted that the progressive increase in automaticity occurs as myocardial excitability is being reduced by progressively larger doses of digoxin. Hence, it is common to see multifocal premature ventricular contractions prior to the development of ventricular fibrillation.

Atrial responses to digoxin are a bit more complex, because in addition to the direct actions of digoxin, there are indirect actions mediated by the vagus nerve. In some cases, the direct action (increased refractory period) is opposed by the vagal mediated effects (decreased refractory period). In low doses, the vagal effects predominate, atrial excitability and conduction velocity increase, and the refractory period decreases. As a result of these actions, the average atrial rate will increase in the presence of atrial fibrillation because a greater number of impulses can be conducted through atrial tissue. Under most circumstances, the actions of digoxin on the AV node prevent any increment in ventricular rate in response to the increased atrial rate.

In higher doses, digoxin decreases atrial excitability and conduction to the point that impulses arising spontaneously in the sinus node no longer depolarize the surrounding atrial tissue and are not conducted to the AV node. The stage is thereby set for the appearance of junctional or ventricular rhythms.

These actions of digoxin on excitable membranes are related in a yet-undetermined manner to its inhibition of Na^+-K^+ ATPase.[78] This enzyme is an integral part of the transport mechanism maintaining the sodium and potassium ion gradients that determine the excitability and depolarization characteristics of myocardial cells. The potassium ion gradient is the primary determinant of resting membrane potential, and digoxin reduces the resting potential, thereby increasing excitability of the cell. Digoxin also increases the upward slope of phase 4 or spontaneous diastolic depolarization, so that automaticity is increased, and the cell may depolarize spontaneously as an independent ectopic focus out of phase with the orderly conduction of impulses from the normal pacemaker cells. Digoxin also affects the process of rapid depolarization which is dependent primarily on the inward diffusion of sodium ions. Digoxin's effect is evident as a decreased slope of the phase 0 or depolarization spike potential, and the depressed depolarization is reflected as a slowing of conduction. Phases 1, 2, and 3 of repolarization are altered by digoxin. The overall duration of the action potential is shortened, and the refractory period is decreased.

These electrophysiological effects of digoxin are also evident in the surface electrocardiogram (ECG) as a lengthened P-R interval (decreased AV conduction), shortened Q-T interval (more rapid repolarization), and ST-T-segment depression (altered slope of phase 1 and 2 repolarization). With toxic levels of digoxin, the ECG reveals the increased automaticity and impaired conduction as ectopic premature ventricular contractions, ventricular tachycardia, and fibrillation.

It is not surprising that alterations of electrolyte balance, particularly of potassium, have a marked influence on the development of dysrhythmias in the presence of digoxin.

Therapeutic Indications for Digoxin.[74–77, 80]

ACUTE HEART FAILURE

The use of digoxin in the perioperative period by the anesthesiologist is indicated by the diagnosis of acute heart failure in the absence of certain mechanical problems.* The development of congestive heart failure under anesthesia may indeed be acute as a result of exacerbation of preexisting disease, surgical stress, anesthetic overdose, fluid overload, intraoperative hypertension, and other causes of increased cardiac work, myocardial hypoxia, and infarction. The early diagnosis of acute failure in the anesthetized patient depends on careful monitoring of cardiovascular function, especially in terms of simultaneous and progressive changes in several cardiovascular measurements, including the responses to therapeutic interventions. For example, hypotension, low urine output, and an increasing alveolar-arterial oxygen gradient in the presence of a progressively rising pulmonary capillary wedge pressure are highly suggestive of the development of left ventricular failure. With such findings, digitalization of the patient with intravenous digoxin is indicated along with other therapeutic interventions (e.g., elimination of cardiac depressant anesthetics, administration of rapidly acting inotropic drugs and diuretics, reduced fluid infusion). As long as serum potassium levels are within normal limits and the digitalization is accomplished gradually, the risks are acceptable. It is particularly important to remember three facts:

1. The inotropic response to digoxin is dose-dependent, and significant improvement, albeit less than the maximal response, can be achieved with less than fully digitalizing doses.
2. The onset of action of digoxin administered intravenously is evident within 15 to 30 minutes, even though the peak effects may not be realized until 1½ to 5 hours later.
3. Lower concentrations of digoxin are required for the inotropic action than for the production of serious dysrhythmias.

* Mechanical problems include mitral stenosis, idiopathic hypertrophic subaortic stenosis (IHSS), constrictive pericarditis, and pericardial tamponade. In these cases, the primary problem is an obstruction to left ventricular filling or outflow rather than impairment of contractility. In IHSS, the increased contractility of the stenotic area may further impede ventricular outflow. In the *chronic* stages of these processes, pump failure may develop, and the use of digoxin may then be beneficial.

DISTURBANCES OF CARDIAC RHYTHM

Digoxin administered intravenously may be indicated for the control of supraventricular tachyarrhythmias because of its ability to block atrioventricular conduction and slow the ventricular rate. The specific types of atrial or nodal tachycardia include: (1) paroxysmal supraventricular tachycardia, (2) atrial flutter, (3) atrial fibrillation, and (4) Wolff-Parkinson-White syndrome. Several facts should be remembered in the use of digoxin for such dysrhythmias. Digitalis intoxication must be ruled out as the cause of the arrhythmia. Partial digitalization often improves the response to simpler means of vagal activation (e.g., carotid sinus pressure). Intravenous propranolol may be combined with digoxin to gain control of the tachycardia more rapidly and to reduce the effective doses (and hopefully the individual toxicity) of both drugs. Direct-current cardioversion in the presence of digoxin is hazardous because of the high risk of inducing ventricular fibrillation. Therefore, if cardioversion is to be considered, it should be attempted before administration of digoxin. Antiarrhythmic drugs such as quinidine and procainamide may be indicated for control of the supraventricular focus, but their administration can usually be delayed until the postoperative period.

MYOCARDIAL ISCHEMIA

Myocardial ischemia resulting from coronary insufficiency may be increased or decreased by digoxin depending on the functional state of the left ventricle. Changes in oxygen consumption are the net result of two opposing effects of digoxin: (1) increased contractility and (2) alterations of wall tension. In the failing heart, oxygen consumption may diminish or at least not increase in response to digoxin. Oxygen consumption always increases in the nonfailing heart following digoxin administration.

PROPHYLACTIC USE OF DIGOXIN

Prophylactic digitalization of the patient who is not in heart failure prior to surgery is controversial.[81-83] On the one hand, a patient with diminished cardiac reserve is predisposed to the development of failure as a result of the stress imposed by anesthesia and surgery, including the increased work of breathing in the postoperative period. Such patients may benefit from prophylactic digitalization, which not only increases their cardiac reserve but also reduces the likelihood of supraventricular tachycardia, which is tolerated poorly by diseased hearts. On the other hand, given the very narrow margin between effective and toxic doses of digoxin and the fact that anesthesia and surgery are often accompanied by acute changes in factors influencing the responsiveness of the patient to digoxin (e.g., fluid and electrolyte shifts, alterations of ventilation), prophylactic digitalization adds the risk of digitalis toxicity, which has been observed with increasing frequency among hospitalized patients. The risk is greater in the absence of a clear-cut end point of benefit (e.g., lessening failure, slowing of ventricular rate). In addition, the frequent occurrence of dysrhythmias during anesthesia and surgery in the absence of digitalis blurs the early recognition of digoxin toxicity from prophylactic administration in the preoperative period. An attempt to minimize the risk of toxicity by using lower doses of digoxin prophylactically also minimizes the benefits and creates an indefinite degree of digoxin activity.

One reasonable approach to the patient not in failure but with a lowered cardiac reserve is to take full advantage of the sophisticated monitoring techniques available for cardiac surgery in order to detect the need for digoxin as early as possible and then to measure its effects during rapid digitalization by the intravenous route in the intraoperative or postoperative periods.

Digoxin toxicity presents an especially difficult differential diagnosis in the perioperative period because the gastrointestinal and central nervous system signs and symptoms are either suppressed or their interpretation is complicated by the actions of drugs administered for anesthetic purposes.[84–86] Although alterations of cardiac rate and rhythm are among the earliest signs of digoxin intoxication, there are no unequivocal electrocardiographic features that distinguish the toxic effects of digoxin from those of anesthetic drugs, especially in the presence of intrinsic cardiac disease. Almost every form of rhythm disturbance has been attributed to digoxin toxicity at one time or other, including AV junctional escape beats and tachycardia, ventricular premature beats, bigeminy, trigeminy, tachycardia and fibrillation. The strongest (but not specific) evidence of digoxin toxicity is

found when atrioventricular block occurs along with increased automaticity of ectopic foci.

Perhaps it is fortunate that a specific etiologic diagnosis is not necessary for anesthesiologists to treat alterations of rate and rhythm that impair cardiac output in the anesthetized patient. Their initial treatment of bradycardia and ventricular dysrhythmias will probably involve the same therapeutic measures, including the choice of drugs, regardless of the primary cause. Their awareness of the potential contribution of digoxin to the problem should then lead them to investigate and to correct factors predisposing to the induction of dysrhythmias by digoxin (e.g., hypokalemia, acid-base imbalance, impaired renal function). Cardiopulmonary bypass does not cause any appreciable increase in digoxin excretion or loss. Renal function is altered during bypass and, as a consequence, serum K^+ and Mg^{++} levels are decreased, thereby predisposing the patient to the development of digitalis toxicity.[87]

The therapeutic measures for bradycardia include atropine (0.2–2.0 mg I.V.), correction of hypoxemia, reduction of partial pressures of inhalational anesthetics, potassium supplementation of hypokalemia, and insertion of transvenous or epicardial pacing wires if necessary to establish an adequate heart rate. In the case of serious ventricular rhythm disturbances, all of the above measures, except for pacing wires, are indicated. In addition, lidocaine (intravenous bolus doses of 1 mg/kg*) should be administered early for rapid control of ventricular dysrhythmias interfering with cardiac output. Also, factors increasing sympathetic nervous system activity should be corrected (e.g., hypercarbia, hypotension, noxious stimulation), and if necessary, propranolol (0.25–1 mg bolus doses, up to a total of 5 mg) can be given to reduce the responses to sympathetic stimulation. (The side effects of these drugs are discussed elsewhere in this chapter.) Magnesium sulfate has also

---

* While lidocaine suppresses ectopic foci and speeds conduction through the AV node (antidigoxin effects), it can lead to asystole if the ventricular ectopic focus is the only effective pacemaker. The threshold for CNS seizures induced by lidocaine is raised by many drugs used for anesthesia, including diazepam and nitrous oxide. Under the influence of these drugs, larger than customary doses of lidocaine may be used if needed to suppress the arrhythmia.

been recommended for treatment of these arrhythmias.[88] Should ventricular fibrillation occur, direct-current countershock is indicated, along with lidocaine to prevent the recurrence of dysrhythmias.

Once the rate and rhythm disturbances are controlled acutely, consideration can be given to longer-term therapeutic measures in consultation with the cardiologist who will assume responsibility for the patient in the postoperative period.

CALCIUM

Calcium is the fifth most abundant element in the body and plays a role in a number of physiological processes. More than 90 percent of total body calcium is incorporated as phosphate and carbonate salts in bone, which readily exchanges calcium with interstitial fluid and plasma. Concentrations of calcium in plasma are maintained around 5 mEq/liter, of which one-third is bound to protein, one-tenth is complexed with anions (e.g., phosphate, lactate, carbonate, citrate), and the remainder is ionized (normal range 2–2.3 mEq/liter, 1–1.5 millimols/liter, 4.0–4.6 mg/100 ml). Ionized calcium is the physiologically active form, and its concentration is greatly affected by pH, anions, and protein content of physiological fluids.[89] Only recently has the ionized calcium electrode been available to measure ionized calcium directly and specifically in biological specimens.[90]

Ionized calcium plays important roles in the electrophysiology of excitable membranes and in the contraction of all types of muscle. In fact, it appears that ionized calcium is a crucial element in coupling membrane excitation to the contractile processes in muscle cells. When the membrane depolarizes, ionized calcium is released from the sarcoplasmic reticulum into the cytoplasm where it complexes with tropin. Tropin complexed with calcium no longer inhibits the interaction between actin and myosin, and the muscle cell contracts. When the membrane repolarizes, calcium is removed from the cytoplasm and dissociates from tropin, which again is free to inhibit the interaction of actin and myosin, and the muscle fibril relaxes.[91]

Calcium influences the permeability of excitable membranes, especially in terms of stabilizing them against changes in their resting

potential. Calcium also plays a role in coupling secretion of neurotransmitters and hormones to excitation of the membranes of nerve endings and endocrine cells.[89] These functions are not as well understood as those for excitation–contraction coupling of muscle. One very important relationship is recognized, however, and that is the interaction between calcium and potassium ions. Equivalent effects on excitable membranes can be produced by either lowering calcium or raising potassium.[91,92]

In regard to the cardiovascular system, ionized calcium exerts a strong influence on cardiac contractility. On the one hand, acute reductions of ionized calcium, for example, by the rapid infusion of chelating agents (e.g., EDTA, citrate in banked blood) are associated with decreased cardiac stroke volume.[93–95] On the other hand, the intravenous injection of calcium produces a positive inotropic response manifested by increases in stroke volume and the velocity of ventricular pressure rise (dP/dt). Concomitantly, there are compensatory decreases in left ventricular end-diastolic pressure (LVEDP), heart rate, and total peripheral resistance.[96] These effects of calcium are usually transient as a result of the efficient exchange of calcium by bone.

Calcium also affects the electrophysiological properties of the heart and can produce sinus bradycardia (mediated by the vagus nerve), atrioventricular conduction block, and increased ventricular irritability. The most striking effect of calcium is on the plateau or phase 2 of the ventricular action potential; increased ionized calcium levels reduce the duration of phase 2, and hypocalcemic conditions lengthen it. There is a corresponding change in the Q-T interval of the ECG. All of these effects are accentuated in the presence of hypokalemia and digitalis.[97]

From a practical point of view, ionized calcium levels are important to anesthesiologists because the levels are influenced by conditions under their control or subject to therapy. Decreased levels of ionized calcium are found in respiratory and metabolic alkalosis, after correction of lactic acidosis, during rapid transfusion of citrated blood, and during hemodialysis.[90,98,99] If these conditions are associated with depressed cardiac function, the exogenous administration of calcium may prove of benefit, at least transiently. In many cases, however, the rapid release of calcium from bone can quickly replenish the total circulating level of calcium, and correction of the basic etiology is necessary for long-term restoration of normal concentrations of ionized calcium. The efficient uptake of calcium by bone and the rapid entry of calcium into equilibria with proteins and anions limit the duration of action of intravenous calcium supplements.

These same limitations apply to the use of intravenous calcium as an inotropic stimulant in normocalcemic states. Bolus doses of calcium chloride (3–7 mg/kg*) produce moderate increases in cardiac output for 15 to 30 minutes.[96] Additional doses are needed to maintain the effect for longer periods but are usually omitted in favor of other inotropic agents (e.g., digoxin, catecholamine infusion). The risk of dysrhythmias when calcium is administered to digitalized patients should be kept in mind and may contraindicate the use of calcium, especially in the presence of hypokalemia.[100]

It is common to administer 0.5–1 gm bolus doses of calcium chloride near the end of cardiopulmonary bypass to stimulate myocardial function which may be depressed by the use of hyperkalemic cardioplegia, by hypocalcemia secondary to the use of citrated blood, and by the use of bicarbonate for the correction of metabolic acidosis. It is worth noting that the level of ionized calcium may be stable in the presence of hemodilution, which reduces total serum calcium.

GLUCAGON

Glucagon is a polypeptide hormone synthesized in the pancreas and has widespread effects on several organ systems. Like the catecholamines, glucagon enhances the formation of adenosine 3', 5'-cyclic phosphate (cyclic AMP), which is thought to be the "second messenger" for stimulating a number of cellular processes. Unlike the catecholamines, glucagon does not act through adrenergic receptors. One of its

---

* Solutions of different salts of calcium contain different amounts of calcium.[101] Commercially available 10 percent calcium chloride contains 1.36 mEq of calcium per milliliter, 10 percent calcium gluconate contains 0.45 mEq/ml, and 23 percent calcium gluceptate contains 0.9 mEq/ml.[89] One milliequivalent of calcium is equivalent to 20 mg.

therapeutic indications as an inotropic agent is the presence of β-adrenergic receptor blockade by propranolol.[4,102–104]

Glucagon produces positive inotropic and chronotropic effects on the heart, independent of sympathetic nervous system function.[105] It has a decided advantage over the sympathomimetics in that it will enhance automaticity in the sinoatrial and atrioventricular nodes without increasing automaticity in the ventricle.[106] Moreover, glucagon can be used in the presence of digitalis without precipitating dysrhythmias.[105] Glucagon has been shown to have a coronary vasodilatory effect.[107–109] It is claimed that some portion of the coronary vasodilation results from a direct action on coronary vessels and is independent of its inotropic stimulation of the heart in animals.[4]

In humans, intravenous doses of 3–10 mg of glucagon have consistently produced positive chronotropic and inotropic effects.[4,104–106] The onset of action is evident within a few minutes and lasts approximately one-half hour. The effect can be extended by the intravenous infusion of approximately 66 μg/kg/min. There are some limitations to the effectiveness of glucagon as an inotropic drug. The tachycardia can be marked and may interfere with ventricular filling and cardiac output. Its potency and efficacy are more limited than those of the catecholamines and the cardiac glycosides. It is especially impotent in the chronically failed heart, perhaps as a result of a change in the receptor for glucagon.[4] In patients with atrial flutter or fibrillation the ventricular rate may increase rather suddenly as a result of the improvement of atrioventricular nodal transmission, especially if the rate was being controlled by propranolol prior to the injection of glucagon.[110] Glucagon should be avoided in patients with a pheochromocytoma because of its ability to release catecholamines from such tumors. Long-term infusions of glucagon can produce hypoglycemia because it stimulates the secretion of insulin. In such cases, the continuous intravenous infusion of glucose is indicated along with careful monitoring of serum glucose levels. The most common and dose-related side effects of nausea and vomiting are not a problem in the anesthetized patient but may present difficulties in patients confined to intensive care facilities.[4]

The principal cardiovascular indications for

glucagon therapy are in the management of acute heart failure and in cases where it is necessary to overcome cardiac depression by propranolol.[4,111-114]

ANTIARRHYTHMIC DRUGS

Much information is available concerning the electrophysiological properties of the normal heart and the effects of antiarrhythmic drugs on these properties. These drugs are used in patients with varying degrees of cardiac abnormalities, however, and in some cases, their effects are not predictable or even understandable. The latter is not surprising, since the mechanisms underlying cardiac arrhythmias have not been completely defined, and relatively little work has been done on the actions of antiarrhythmic drugs in abnormal myocardial tissue. For these reasons, the therapeutic choices of antiarrhythmic agents are still largely empirical and based on some general guidelines as to which drug is most often successful in controlling a particular type of dysrhythmia. In any particular patient, the final choice will be determined by which drug proves to be effective with minimal side effects.[32,115-118]

Antiarrhythmic drugs are of interest to anesthesiologists because some patients may have been taking these drugs chronically in the preoperative period. Fortunately, chronic oral administration of most of the currently available antiarrhythmic drugs (i.e., quinidine, procainamide, diphenylhydantoin) poses little threat to the safety of general (or regional) anesthesia. It is customary to continue the administration of these drugs up to the time of surgery and to resume their use in the immediate postoperative period. Propranolol and digoxin raise some concerns in the anesthesiologist's mind, and these are dealt with in other portions of this chapter.

Of course, the anesthesiologist is also interested in antiarrhythmic drugs because acutely developing abnormalities of cardiac rate and rhythm are frequently encountered in the anesthetized patient. The etiology of these disturbances often cannot be eliminated even when it is known, and the use of antiarrhythmic drugs becomes necessary. As in the case of chronic dysrhythmias, the choice of drug is largely empirical.

Electrophysiology of the Heart[119]

Myocardial cells have several important electrophysiological properties related to the development and treatment of dysrhythmias. *Automaticity* refers to the ability of the cell to undergo spontaneous depolarization. That is, the resting membrane potential gradually decreases in negativity until it reaches the threshold potential at which the all-or-none phenomenon of membrane depolarization takes place (see Fig. 4-2, Chapter 4). Under normal circumstances, automaticity is exhibited by cells in the sinoauricular node, atrioventricular node, and the specialized conducting tissues of the atria and ventricles (His bundle and Purkinje cells). In various abnormal states, any myocardial cell has the potential to become automatic and to initiate an ectopic impulse or beat.

Excitability refers to the ability of the myocardial cell to respond to a stimulus by depolarizing. One measure of excitability is the difference between the resting and threshold potentials of the cellular membrane. The smaller this difference, the more excitable (or irritable) is the cell. Cells undergoing spontaneous depolarization become progressively more excitable as the membrane potential approaches the threshold. Once a cell depolarizes, it is no longer excitable until the negative potential recovers to greater than threshold levels. That is, the cell is *refractory* to stimuli. The refractory period is divided into absolute and relative phases. In the latter phase, much greater than normal intensities of stimulation are required to excite the cell (i.e., to depolarize the membrane).

Conductivity of myocardial cells refers to the rate at which they are able to convey a stimulus from one cell to another. In the normal heart the conductivity of similar types of cells is the same, so that a wave of depolarization spreads evenly through the mass of myocardial muscle to produce a coordinated contraction of the myocardial cells. When the conductivity of similar type cells differs, impulses spread unevenly throughout the heart and may impair the contraction and pumping action of the heart. Another consequence of uneven spread of depolarization is the establishment of a circus movement of impulses in which an impulse spreads around a nonconductive area of myocardial tissue (e.g., scar, infarct, ischemic cells) and, upon returning to the initial site of excitation, finds it again excitable and able to conduct the impulse once more. The impulse thereby reenters successively each of the cells in the ring of conductive tissue. Maintenance of a circus movement is facilitated by slow conduction of the impulse by normal tissue around the nonconductive area and by a short refractory period in the normal cells. This circus movement, or reentry mechanism, is thought to be responsible for the persistence of dysrhythmic beating of the heart.

Another version of a circus movement involves the specialized conducting tissue of the atrioventricular node, specifically the Purkinje fibers. At points of branching of the fibers (see Fig. 4-16, Chapter 4) an impulse may be conducted by one branch but not by the other, which is refractory. The impulse from the conducting branch reaches the ventricular cells and is conducted to the terminus of the other branch, which is now excitable and able to conduct the impulse in a retrograde direction to the original branch point in the Purkinje fiber. If this point has recovered, another impulse will travel down the originally conductive branch and a circus or reentry mechanism is established.

Circus movements can be eliminated in several ways:

1. Restore normal conductivity in the abnormal, nonconductive tissue.
2. Speed conduction in the normal tissue so that the impulse reaches the initial site during its refractory period and therefore cannot reenter that cell.
3. Lengthen the refractory period of normally conducting cells so that the impulse cannot reenter them.

Mechanisms of Antiarrhythmic Drug Action[32,115,116,120,121]

All currently available drugs (except bretylium) depress automaticity in ectopic foci. That is, they decrease the rate of spontaneous depolarization by acting directly on the membranes of the abnormal cells. Their effects on normal pacemaker cells are more complex because in addition to their direct actions, they have potent effects on the autonomic nervous system. Spontaneous phase 4 depolarization is facilitated by increased sympathetic and decreased vagal activity and is depressed by increased vagal tone and the withdrawal of sympathetic influences. For example, quinidine and procainamide have atropinelike effects that oppose their direct actions on atrial and nodal pacemakers. Propranolol's blockade of β-adrenergic receptors reduces sympathetic tone and enhances its direct action in depressing spontaneous depolarization.

The effects of antiarrhythmic drugs on excitability and conduction in myocardial cells are even more complex. It has been noted that all the antiarrhythmic drugs have the effect of increasing the duration of the effective refractory period relative to the duration of the action potential. It is not yet clear, however, what, if any, bearing this ratio has on the propagation of dysrhythmias or the interruption of reentry mechanisms.

Another factor limiting the practical applications of basic knowledge about the electrophysiological effects of antiarrhythmic drugs is the lack of information concerning their actions in abnormal cells. For example, lidocaine speeds conduction and shortens the refractory period in normal tissue. In acutely ischemic myocardial tissue, however, lidocaine slows conduction and prolongs refractoriness. Since the action potential is shorter in the ischemic zone than in the normal zone, lidocaine reduces the disparity and improves the chances of a uniform spread of depolarization through myocardial muscle. At the same time, it suppresses automaticity in the ischemic cells and reduces the frequency of ventricular beats.[118]

Factors in the Choice of Antiarrhythmic Drugs[122]

Depending on the seriousness of the dysrhythmia, it may not be necessary to use an antiarrhythmic drug, especially if there are predisposing factors that can be eliminated rapidly. For example, it may be possible to correct dysrhythmias by improving ventilation to eliminate hypoxia and hypercarbia, by increasing anesthetic depth to eliminate responses to noxious stimulation, or by decreasing the anesthetic concentration to eliminate its excessive effects on the cardiovascular system. Often these simple measures are effective because they restore a normal balance of autonomic control over the heart. High levels of sympathetic stimulation increase automaticity of all myocardial cells, including those in ectopic sites. In the presence of strong vagal tone which suppresses normal atrial and nodal pacemakers, it is likely that sympathetic stimulation will produce ectopic beats. Moreover, dysrhythmias are likely to persist with combined vagal and sympathetic activity because of inhomogeneity among myocardial cells in terms of automaticity, excitability, and conductivity.

Heart rate has an important bearing on the development of ectopic beats. Heart rate is determined by the fastest pacemaker. Normally the rate of spontaneous depolarization is fastest in cells of the sinoatrial node and progressively slower in cells of the atrioventricular node, Purkinje system, specialized atrial conduction tissue, and atrial and ventricular myofibrils. When the dominant pacemaker is suppressed by vagal tone, hypoxia, or disease, the next fastest pacemaker assumes control. In some cases, it is possible to eliminate AV nodal or ectopic rhythms by stimulating the sinoatrial node with sympathomimetic drugs (e.g., isoproterenol) or, more often, by reducing vagal tone with atropine.

Hypotension and hypertension can predispose to the development of arrhythmias. The exact mechanisms are not proven, and in some cases, the blood pressure changes may be coincidental manifestations of the primary etiology (e.g., pheochromocytoma). It is easy to recognize that blood pressure has the potential to affect cardiac rate and rhythm through its effects on baroreceptor reflex mechanisms, coronary blood flow, ventricular work, and oxygen demand. Thus the incidence of dysrhythmias may be reduced by the use of vasodilator and pressor drugs to stabilize systemic blood pressure in a normal range.

Certain types of abnormal rates and rhythms are more dangerous than others and demand immediate intervention with antiarrhythmic drugs. Ventricular ectopic beats, especially those that occur during the repolarization phase ("R" on "T" in the ECG) and ventricular tachycardia have the potential for inducing ventricular fibrillation. Marked tachycardia of any type can interfere with the pumping action of the heart (inadequate filling time) and also create a marked imbalance in oxygen demand (increased with tachycardia) and supply (shortened diastolic coronary perfusion time).

Marked bradycardia contributes to reduced cardiac output and hypotension.

The drugs most likely to be used by the anesthesiologist are lidocaine for disturbances of ventricular rhythms, propranolol and digoxin for control of tachycardia, and atropine and sympathomimetics for bradycardia. With the exception of lidocaine, all of these drugs are discussed elsewhere in this chapter. A summary of the therapeutic applications of antiarrhythmic drugs is given in Table 4-3 in Chapter 4.

Lidocaine is a local anesthetic that has become the most widely used drug for the control of ventricular dysrhythmias encountered during cardiac surgery and in coronary care units.[32,122,123] It is administered intravenously in bolus doses of 1–1.5 mg/kg and has a very rapid onset of action. Because its duration of action is relatively short, it offers a number of advantages. Continuous intravenous infusions (1–5 mg/70 kg/min) are used to maintain its antiarrhythmic effect. The rate of infusion can be easily adjusted to the minimum required for suppression of dysrhythmias in each individual patient, thereby limiting the incidence and severity of toxic reactions. Should toxicity occur, it is relatively short-lived when lidocaine administration is reduced or discontinued.

The major toxicity and side effects of lidocaine are on the central nervous system and the heart. Stimulation of the CNS to the point of seizures occurs in a dose-related manner.* The threshold concentration of lidocaine for seizure activity is elevated by diazepam, nitrous oxide, and probably other general anesthetics. Thiopental has been used for rapid suppression of CNS stimulation by lidocaine.

Lidocaine causes little depression of the cardiovascular system when the sympathetic nervous system is functioning. When the heart is isolated from sympathetic innervation, its contractility is depressed by lidocaine. Because lidocaine suppresses automaticity in ventricular cells, it can produce asystole in the absence of a supraventricular pacemaker or with complete heart block. In the presence of atrial flutter,

---

* Plasma concentrations of 1.5–5 μg/ml are antiarrhythmic and can be achieved with infusion rates of 1.5–5 mg/70 kg/min. CNS stimulation becomes evident at plasma levels over 5 μg/ml, and seizures are frequent at plasma concentrations above 10 μg/ml unless CNS depressants are present.

lidocaine can cause alarming ventricular acceleration because of its ability to speed conduction
through the AV node.

Other Antiarrhythmic Drugs

Quinidine and procainamide have very similar actions on the electrophysiological properties of the heart.[32,121,122] Compared to lidocaine,
they have a broader spectrum of antiarrhythmic
effects and are useful in the treatment of atrial
flutter and fibrillation as well as ventricular dysrhythmias. They are rarely used in the anesthetized patient because of their side effects, which
include hypotension, paroxysmal tachycardia in
the presence of atrial flutter or fibrillation, and
a low incidence of ventricular fibrillation which
may occur after moderate doses.

Phenytoin (diphenylhydantoin) is an anticonvulsant drug that has proved useful in the
treatment of digitalis-induced dysrhythmias, especially ventricular tachycardia and paroxysmal
atrial tachycardia with AV block.[32,115]

The control of tachycardia can involve any
one of several drugs that are discussed elsewhere in this chapter. Sinus tachycardia induced
by increased sympathetic activity can be controlled with propranolol administered intravenously in increments of 0.25 to 0.5 mg up to a
total of 5 mg in adults. Edrophonium administered intravenously in 2 mg increments, up to a
total of 10 mg, has been used to interrupt episodes of paroxysmal atrial tachycardia. However, it has a short duration of action, it has not
been uniformly effective even when combined
with carotid sinus massage (with some risk of
compromising cerebral circulation), it has produced asystole even in moderate doses, and it
antagonizes the nondepolarizing type of skeletal
muscle relaxants. In the presence of atrial flutter
or fibrillation, digoxin is effective in slowing the
ventricular response by causing atrioventricular
block.

Bretylium is an antihypertensive agent that
has been effective in suppressing tachyarrhythmias arising after myocardial infarction. Its
mechanism of action and reliability as an antiarrhythmic agent are still under investigation. One
disconcerting finding is its enhancement of automaticity in specialized conducting tissue. Presumably this effect on automaticity is caused by
the release of catecholamines from adrenergic

nerve endings prior to the onset of antireleasing
effect of bretylium.[32]

DIURETICS

*Furosemide (Lasix) and ethacrynic acid
(Edecrin)* are potent diuretics that act primarily
in the ascending limb of Henle's loop to inhibit
sodium reabsorption. Furosemide is usually preferred because it has a broader dose–response
range and has fewer side effects than ethacrynic
acid.[124,125]

The anesthesiologist uses furosemide intravenously in noncardiac patients to increase the
flow of urine during oliguric states or in the
presence of a renal toxin (e.g., hemoglobinuria)
and to produce dehydration (e.g., in neurosur-
gery). Patients vary in their sensitivity to these
diuretics. For example, satisfactory diuresis has
been produced with furosemide in doses as small
as 0.15 mg/kg, while in other cases, 0.20–7 mg/
kg doses have been required. Graded responses
can be produced by varying the dosage; because
of the rapid onset of action, it is wise to begin
with the smallest dose and give progressively
larger doses at 15- to 20-minute intervals until
the desired response is obtained. In this way,
excessive diuresis can be avoided. It is noteworthy that the action of furosemide is not
markedly affected by acid-base, electrolyte, or
other metabolic disturbances. It is effective even
in the presence of reductions of glomerular filtration and partial renal failure.

Furosemide is used principally in patients
with congestive heart failure. Its ability to pro-
mote the rapid mobilization of edema fluid is
well known, as is its potential to produce alterations in electrolyte balance, especially hypokalemia. These diuretic actions are thoroughly
discussed in standard textbooks, along with the
common extrarenal side effects on hearing, the
gastrointestinal tract, and skin.

The cardiovascular effects of furosemide
are of special interest to the anesthesiologist
caring for patients with cardiac disease.[125–128]
Both furosemide and ethacrynic acid enhance
the digitalis-induced loss of potassium from myocardial cells and may facilitate the development
of dysrhythmias even in the presence of normal
levels of serum potassium. Both drugs produce
a marked systemic venodilation which precedes
the onset of diuresis. The rapid increase in pe-

ripheral venous capacitance and the associated reduction in blood return to the central circulation may explain the dramatic and immediate effects of these diuretics in acute pulmonary edema. Within 5 to 15 minutes following an intravenous dose of furosemide (0.5–1 mg/kg), the average left ventricular filling pressure fell from 20.4 to 14.8 mm Hg in one study of 20 patients.[126] It can be anticipated that the subsequent onset of diuresis will contribute to a reduction in circulating plasma volume and to the much more delayed resolution of radiological evidence of pulmonary congestion.[128] In the patient with coronary atherosclerotic heart disease and associated heart failure, both the acute and delayed mechanisms of reducing left ventricular filling pressures may also be beneficial in decreasing myocardial oxygen consumption.

Mannitol and other osmotic diuretics administered as hypertonic solutions can contribute to preservation of myocardial function through reductions in tissue ischemia. They can shrink edematous cells swollen with excessive fluid, they can improve blood flow compromised by tissue swelling, and they can limit the onset and extent of irreversible cell damage. These effects are particularly important during and following a period of interruption of coronary blood flow by arterial occlusive disease or surgical procedures.[129–131]

REFERENCES

1. Koelle GB: Neurohumoral transmission and the autonomic nervous system. *In* Goodman LS, Gilman A (eds): The Pharmacological Basis of Therapeutics. New York, Macmillan, 1975, pp 404–444
2. Innes IR, Nickerson M: Norepinephrine, epinephrine, and the sympathomimetic amines. *In* Goodman LS, Gilman A (eds): The Pharmacological Basis of Therapeutics. New York, Macmillan, 1975, pp 477–513
3. Steen PA, Tinker JH, Pluth JR, et al: Efficacy of dopamine, dobutamine, and epinephrine during emergence from cardiopulmonary bypass in man. Circulation 57:378–384, 1978
4. Lucchesi BR: Inotropic agents and drugs to support the failing heart. *In* Antonaccio M (ed): Cardiovascular Pharmacology. New York, Raven Press, 1977, pp 337–375
5. Brown DR, Starek P: Sodium nitroprusside-induced improvement in cardiac function in association with left ventricular dilation. Anesthesiology 41:521–523, 1974
6. Lesch M: Inotropic agents and infarct size: Theoretical and practical considerations. Am J Cardiol 37:508–513, 1976
7. Kones RJ: The catecholamines: Reappraisal of their use for acute myocardial infarction and low cardiac output syndromes. Crit Care Med 1:203–220, 1973
8. Standards for cardiopulmonary resuscitation (CPR) and emergency cardiac care (ECC). JAMA (Suppl) 227:833–868, 1974
9. Meuller H, Ayers SM, Gregory JJ, et al: Hemodynamics, coronary blood flow, and myocardial metabolism in coronary shock; response to *l*-norepinephrine and isoproterenol. J Clin Invest 49:1885–1902, 1970
10. Krasnow N, Rolett EL, Yurchak PM, et al: Isoproterenol and cardiac performance. Am J Med 37:514–525, 1964
11. Beregovich J, Reicher-Reiss H, Kunstadt D, et al: Hemodynamic effects of isoproterenol in cardiac surgery. J Thorac Cardiovasc Surg 62:957–964, 1971
12. Elliott WC, Gorlin R: Isoproterenol in treatment of heart disease: Hemodynamic effects in circulatory failure. JAMA 197:93–98, 1966
13. Holloway EL, Stinson EB, Derby GC, et al: Action of drugs in patients early after cardiac surgery. I. Comparison of isoproterenol and dopamine. Am J Cardiol 35:656–659, 1975
14. Iversen LL: Dopamine receptors in the brain. Science 188:1084–1089, 1975
15. Goldberg LI, Hsieh YY, Resnekov L: Newer catecholamines for treatment of heart failure and shock: An update on dopamine and a first look at dobutamine. Prog Cardiovasc Dis 19:327–340, 1977
16. McDonald RH Jr, Goldberg LI, McNay JL, et al: Effects of dopamine in man: Augmentation of sodium excretion, glomerular filtration rate, and renal plasma flow. J Clin Invest 43:1116–1124, 1964
17. Goldberg LI: Cardiovascular and renal actions of dopamine: Potential clinical applications. Pharmacol Rev 24:1–29, 1972
18. Goldberg LI: Dopamine—clinical uses of an endogenous catecholamine. N Engl J Med 291:707–710, 1974
19. Robie NW, Goldberg LI: Comparative systemic and regional hemodynamic effects of dopamine and dobutamine. Am Heart J 90:340–345, 1975
20. Meyer SL, Curry GC, Donsky MS, et al: Influence of dobutamine on hemodynamics and cor-

onary blood flow in patients with and without coronary artery disease. Am J Cardiol 38:103–108, 1976

21. Loeb HS, Bredakis J, Gunnar RM: Superiority of dobutamine over dopamine for augmentation of cardiac output in patients with chronic low output cardiac failure. Circulation 55:375–381, 1977

22. Leier CV, Webel J, Bush CA: The cardiovascular effects of the continuous infusion of dobutamine in patients with severe cardiac failure. Circulation 56:468–472, 1977

23. Gillespie TA, Ambos HD, Sobel BE, et al: Effects of dobutamine in patients with acute myocardial infarction. Am J Cardiol 39:588–594, 1977

24. Sakamoto T, Yamada T: Hemodynamic effects of dobutamine in patients following open heart surgery. Circulation 55:525–533, 1977

24A. Tinker JH, Tarhan S, White RD, et al: Dobutamine for inotropic support during emergence from cardiopulmonary bypass. Anesthesiology 44:281–286, 1976

25. Holloway GA, Frederickson EL: Dobutamine, a new beta agonist. Anesth Analg (Cleve) 53:616–622, 1974

26. Leighton KM, Bruce C: Dobutamine and general anesthesia: A study of the response of arterial pressure, heart rate, and renal blood flow. Canad Anaesth Soc J 23:176–184, 1976

27. Douglas WW: Polypeptides—angiotensin, plasma kinins, and other vasoactive agents; prostaglandins. In Goodman LS, Gilman A (eds): The Pharmacological Basis of Therapeutics. New York, Macmillan, 1975, pp 630–652

28. Nickerson M, Collier B: Drugs inhibiting adrenergic nerves and structures innervated by them. In Goodman LS, Gilman A (eds): The Pharmacological Basis of Therapeutics. New York, Macmillan, 1975, pp 533–564

29. Ahlquist RP: Present state of alpha and beta adrenergic drugs III. Beta blocking drugs. Am Heart J 93:117–120, 1977

30. Merin RG: Anesthetic management problems posed by therapeutic advances: III. Beta-adrenergic blocking drugs. Anesth Analg (Cleve) 51:617–624, 1972

31. Gross PF (ed): The Cardioprotective Action of Beta-Blockers, Facts and Theories. Baltimore, University Park Press, 1977

32. Lucchesi BR: Antiarrhythmic drugs. In Antonaccio M (eds): Cardiovascular Pharmacology. New York, Raven Press, 1977, pp 269–335

33. Kaplan JA, Dunbar RW: Propranolol and surgical anesthesia. Anesth Analg (Cleve) 55:1–5, 1976

34. Chatterjee K, Parmley WW: The role of vasodilator therapy in heart failure. Prog Cardiovasc Dis 19:301–325, 1977

35. Flaherty JT, Reid PR, Kelly OT, et al: Intravenous nitroglycerin in acute myocardial infarction. Circulation 51:132–139, 1975

36. Cohn JN, Franciosa JA: Vasodilator therapy of cardiac failure. N Engl J Med 297:27–31, 254–258, 1977

37. Awan NA, Miller RR, Mason DT: Comparison of effects of nitroprusside and prazosin on left ventricular function and the peripheral circulation in chronic refractory congestive heart failure. Circulation 57:152–159, 1978

38. Streeten DHP, Anderson GH, Freiberg JM, et al: Use of an angiotensin II antagonist (Saralasin) in the recognition of "angiotensinogenic" hypertension. N Engl J Med 292:657–662, 1975

39. Kaplan JA, Bush GL, Lecky JH, et al: Sodium bicarbonate and systemic hemodynamics in volunteers anesthetized with halothane. Anesthesiology 42:550–558, 1975

40. Jastrzebski J, Sykes MK, Woods DG: Cardiorespiratory effects of protamine after cardiopulmonary bypass in man. Thorax 29:534–538, 1974

41. Needleman P: Organic Nitrates. New York, Springer-Verlag, 1975, p 106

42. Davies DW, Greiss L, Kadar D, et al: Sodium nitroprusside in children: Observations on metabolism during normal and abnormal responses. Can Anaesth Soc J 22:553–560, 1975

43. Adams AP, Clarke TNS, Edmonds-Seal J, et al: The effects of sodium nitroprusside on myocardial contractility and haemodynamics. Br J Anaesth 46:807–817, 1974

44. Lappas DG, Lowenstein E, Waller J, et al: Hemodynamic effects of nitroprusside infusion during coronary artery operation in man. Circulation 54(Supp 3):4–10, 1976

45. Greenberg H, Dwyer EM, Jameson AG, et al: Effects of nitroglycerin on the major determinants of myocardial oxygen consumption. Am J Cardiol 36:426–432, 1975

46. Mason DT, Zelis R, Amsterdam EA: Actions of the nitrates on the peripheral circulation and myocardial oxygen consumption; significance in the relief of angina pectoris. Chest 59:296–305, 1971

47. Fam WM, McGregor M: Effect of nitroglycerin and dipyridamole on regional coronary resistance. Circ Res 22:649–659, 1968.

48. Goldstein RE, Stinson EB, Scherer JL, et al: Intraoperative coronary collateral function in patients with coronary occlusive disease. Circulation 49:298–308, 1974

49. Cowan C, Duran PVM, Corsini G, et al: The effects of nitroglycerin on myocardial blood flow in man. Am J Cardiol 24:154–160, 1969

50. Ludbrook PA, Byrine JD, Kurnik PB, et al: Influence of reduction of preload and afterload by nitroglycerin on left ventricular diastolic pressure-volume relations and relaxation in man. Circulation 56:937–943, 1977

51. Christensson B, Nordenfelt I, Westling H, et al: Intravenous infusion of nitroglycerin in normal subjects. Scand J Clin Lab Invest 23:49–53, 1969

52. Kaplan JA, Dunbar RW, Jones EL: Nitroglycerin infusion during coronary artery surgery. Anesthesiology 45:14–21, 1976

53. Chatterjee K, Parmley WW, Ganz W, et al.: Hemodynamic and metabolic responses to vasodilator therapy in acute myocardial infarction. Circulation 43:1183–1193, 1973

54. Epstein SE, Kent KM, Goldstein RE, et al: Reduction of ischemic injury by nitroglycerin during acute myocardial infarction. N Engl J Med 292:29–35, 1975

55. Chiariello M, Gold HK, Leinbach RC, et al: Comparison between the effects of nitroprusside and nitroglycerin on ischemic injury during acute myocardial infarction. Circulation 54:766–773, 1976

56. Mann T, Cohn PF, Holman BL, et al: Effect of nitroprusside on regional myocardial blood flow in coronary artery disease: Results in 25 patients and comparison with nitroglycerin. Circulation 57:732–737, 1978

57. Miller RR, Vismara LA, Williams DO, et al: Pharmacologic mechanisms for left ventricular unloading in clinical congestive heart failure: Differential effects of nitroprusside, phentolamine, and nitroglycerin. Circ Res 39:127–133, 1976

58. Guiha NH, Cohn JN, Franciosa JA, et al: Treatment of refractory heart failure with infusion of nitroprusside. N Engl J Med 291:587–592, 1974

59. Miller RR, Vismara LA, Demaria AN, et al: Afterload reduction therapy with nitroprusside in severe aortic regurgitation: Improved cardiac performance and reduced regurgitant volume. Am J Cardiol 38:564–567, 1976

60. Chatterjee K, Parmley WW, Swan HJC, et al: Beneficial effects of vasodilator agents in severe mitral regurgitation due to dysfunction of subvalvular apparatus. Circulation 48:684–690, 1973

61. Dunbar RW, Kaplan JA, King SB: Vasodilator treatment of heart failure after cardiopulmonary bypass. Anesth Analg (Cleve) 54:842–847, 1975.

62. Miller RR, Awan NA, Joye JA, et al: Combined dopamine and nitroprusside therapy in congestive heart failure. Circulation 55:881–884, 1977

63. Mikulic E, Cohn JN, Franciosa JA: Comparative hemodynamic effects of inotropic and vasodilator drugs in severe heart failure. Circulation 56:528–533, 1977

64. Innes IR, Nickerson M: Atropine, scopolamine, and related drugs. In Goodman LS, Gilman A (eds): The Pharmacological Basis of Therapeutics. New York, Macmillan, 1975, pp 514–532

65. Duvoisin RC, Katz R: Reversal of central anticholinergic syndrome in man by physostigmine. JAMA 206:1963–1965, 1968

66. Frumin MJ, Herekar VR, Jarvik ME: Amnesic actions of diazepam and scopolamine in man. Anesthesiology 45:406–412, 1976

67. Stoelting RK, Peterson C: Heart-rate slowing and junctional rhythm following intravenous succinylcholine with and without intramuscular atropine preanesthetic medication. Anesth Analg (Cleve) 54:705–709, 1975

68. Koelle GB: Anticholinesterase agents. In Goodman LS, Gilman A (eds): The Pharmacological Basis of Therapeutics. New York, Macmillan, 1975, pp 445–466

69. Moss AJ, Aledort LM: Use of edrophonium (Tensilon) in the evaluation of supraventricular tachycardias. Am J Cardiol 17:58–62, 1966

70. Rossen RM, Krikorian J, Hancock W: Ventricular asystole after edrophonium administration. JAMA 235:1041–1042, 1976

71. Hoffman BF, Cranefield PF: The physiological basis of cardiac arrhythmias. Am J Med 37:670–684, 1964

72. Dauchot P, Gravenstein JS: Bradycardia after myocardial ischemia and its treatment with atropine. Anesthesiology 44:501–518, 1976

73. Epstein SE, Goldstein RE, Smith ER, et al: The early phase of acute myocardial infarction: Pharmacological aspects of therapy. Ann Intern Med 78:918–936, 1973

74. Moe GK, Farah AE: Digitalis and allied cardiac glycosides. In Goodman LS, Gilman A (eds): The Pharmacological Basis of Therapeutics. New York, Macmillan, 1975, pp 653–682

75. Smith TW: Digitalis glycosides (parts 1 and 2). N Engl J Med 288:719–722, 942–946, 1973

76. Smith TW, Haber E: Digitalis (parts 1 to 4). N Engl J Med 289:945–952, 1010–1015, 1063–1072, 1125–1128, 1973

77. Mason DT, Amsterdam EA: Digitalis: Cardiovascular pharmacology and clinical application. In Bailey CP (ed): Advances in the Management of Clinical Heart Disease, vol 1. New York, Futura, 1976, pp 365–390

78. Schwartz A: Is the cell membrane Na^+, K^+—ATPase enzyme system the pharmacological receptor for digitalis? Circ Res 39:2–7, 1976

79. Mason DT: The cardiovascular effects of digitalis in normal man. Clin Pharmacol Ther 7:1–16, 1966

80. Cohn JN: Indications for digitalis therapy: A new look. JAMA 229:1911–1914, 1974

81. Deutsch S, Dalen JE: Indications for prophylactic digitalization. Anesthesiology 30:648–656, 1969

82. Selzer A, Cohn KE: Some thoughts concerning the prophylactic use of digitalis. Am J Cardiol 26:214–216, 1970

83. Johnson LW, Dickstein RA, Freuhan CT, et al: Prophylactic digitalization for coronary artery bypass surgery. Circulation 53:819–822, 1976

84. Beller GA, Smith TW, Abelmann WH, et al: Digitalis intoxication: A prospective clinical study with serum level correlations. N Engl J Med 284:989–997, 1971

85. Mason DT, Zelis R, Lee G, et al: Current concepts and treatment of digitalis toxicity. Am J Cardiol 27:546–559, 1971

86. Morrow DH: Anesthesia and digitalis toxicity, VI. Effect of barbiturates and halothane on digoxin toxicity. Anesth Analg (Cleve) 49:305–309, 1970

87. Coltart DJ, Chamberlain DA, Howard MR, et al: Effect of cardiopulmonary bypass on plasma digoxin concentrations. Br Heart J 33:334–338, 1971

88. Neff MS, Mendelssohn S, Kim KE, et al: Magnesium sulfate in digitalis toxicity. Am J Cardiol 29:377–382, 1972

89. Peach MJ: Cations: Calcium, magnesium, barium, lithium, and ammonium. In Goodman LS, Gilman A (eds): The Pharmacological Basis of Therapeutics. New York, Macmillan, 1975, pp 782–797

90. Robertson WG: Measurement of ionized calcium in body fluids—a review. Ann Clin Biochem 13:540–548, 1976

91. Nayler WG: Some factors in the maintenance and regulation of cardiac contractility. Circ Res 21 (Suppl 3):213, 1967

92. Logue RB, Robinson PH, Hatcher CR, et al: Medical management in cardiac surgery. In Hurst JW, Logue RB (eds): The Heart. New York, McGraw-Hill, 1978, pp 1777–1799

93. Denlinger JK, Nahrwold ML: Cardiac failure associated with hypocalcemia. Anesth Analg (Cleve) 55:34–36, 1976

94. Denlinger JK, Nahrwold ML, Gibbs PS, et al: Hypocalcemia during rapid blood transfusion in anaesthetized man. Br J Anaesth 48:995–1000, 1976

95. Olinger GN, Hottenrott DG, Muller DG, et al: Acute clinical hypocalcemic myocardial depression during rapid blood transfusion and postoperative hemodialysis. J Thorac Cardiovasc Surg 72:503–511, 1976

96. Denlinger JK, Kaplan JA, Lecky JH, et al: Cardiovascular responses to calcium administered intravenously to man during halothane anesthesia. Anesthesiology 42:390–397, 1975

97. Surawicz B: Effect of Ca^{++} on duration of Q-T interval and ventricular systole in dog. Am J Physiol 205:785–789, 1963

98. Pittinger C, Chang PM, Faulkner W: Serum ionized calcium: Some factors influencing its level. South Med J 64:1211–1215, 1971

99. Schaer H: Effects on ionized calcium of a correction of acidoses with alkalinizing agents. Br J Anaesth 48:327–332, 1976

100. Nola GT, Pope S, Harrison DC: Assessment of the synergistic relationship between serum calcium and digitalis. Am Heart J 79:499–507, 1970

101. White RD, Goldsmith RS, Rodriguez EA: Plasma ionic calcium levels following injection of chloride, gluconate, and gluceptate salts of calcium. J Thorac Cardiovasc Surg 71:609–613, 1976

102. Lucchesi BR: Cardiac actions of glucagon. Circ Res 22:777–787, 1968

103. Glick G, Parmley WW, Wechsler AS, et al: Glucagon: Its enhancement of cardiac performance and persistence of its inotropic action despite beta-receptor blockade with propranolol. Circ Res 22:789–799, 1968

104. Kones RJ, Phillips JH: Glucagon: Present status in cardiovascular disease. Clin Pharmacol Ther 12:427–444, 1971

105. Parmley WW, Glick G, Sonneblick EH: Cardiovascular effects of glucagon in man. N Engl J Med 279:12–17, 1968

106. Katz RL, Hinds L, Mills CJ: Ability of glucagon to produce cardiac stimulation without arrhythmias in halothane-anesthetized animals. Br J Anaesth 41:574–578, 1969

107. Goldschlager N, Robin E, Cowan CM, et al: The effect of glucagon on the coronary circulation in man. Circulation 40:829–837, 1969

108. Manchester JH, Parmley WW, Matloff JM, et al: Effects of glucagon on myocardial oxygen consumption and coronary blood flow in man and dog. Circulation 41:579–588, 1970

109. Rowe GG: Systemic and coronary hemodynamic effects of glucagon. Am J Cardiol 25:670–674, 1970

110. Whitsitt LS, Lucchesi BR: Effects of beta-receptor blockade and glucagon on the atrioventricular transmission system in the dog. Circ Res 23:585–595, 1968

111. Armstrong PW, Gold HK, Daggett WM, et al.: Hemodynamic evaluation of glucagon in symptomatic heart disease. Circulation 44:67–73, 1971

112. Parmley WW, Matloff JM, Sonnenblick EH: Hemodynamic effects of glucagon in patients following prosthetic valve replacement. Circulation 39, 40 (Suppl 1):I-163–167, 1969

113. Vaughn CC, Warner HR, Nelson RM: Cardiovascular effects of glucagon following cardiac surgery. Surgery 67:204–211, 1970

114. Ivankovic AD: Anesthetic management problems posed by therapeutic advances: Digitalis and glucagon. Anesth Analg (Cleve) 51:607–616, 1972

115. Moe GK, Abildskov JA: Antiarrhythmic drugs. *In* Goodman LS, Gilman A (eds): The Pharmacological Basis of Therapeutics. New York, Macmillan, 1975, pp 683–704

116. Gettes LS: The electrophysiologic effects of antiarrhythmic drugs. Am J Cardiol 28:526–535, 1971

117. Mason DT, Spann JF, Zelis R: The clinical pharmacology and therapeutic applications of antiarrhythmic drugs. Clin Pharmacol Ther 11:460–480, 1970

118. Kupersmith J: Antiarrhythmic drugs: Changing concepts. Am J Cardiol 38:119–121, 1976

119. Hoffman BF, Cranefield PF: Electrophysiology of the Heart. New York, McGraw-Hill, 1960

120. Trautwein W: Generation and conduction of impulses in the heart as affected by drugs. Pharmacol Rev 15:277–332, 1963

121. Mason DT, DeMaria AN, Amsterdam EA, et al: Antiarrhythmic agents: Mechanisms of action and clinical pharmacology. Drugs 5:261–291, 1973

122. Mason DT, DeMaria AN, Amsterdam EA, et al: Antiarrhythmic agents: Therapeutic considerations. Drugs 5:292–317, 1973

123. Collingsworth KA, Sumner MK, Harrison DC: The clinical pharmacology of lidocaine as an antiarrhythmic drug. Circulation 50:1217–1230, 1974

124. Mudge GH: Diuretics and other agents employed in the mobilization of edema fluid. *In* Goodman LS, Gilman A (eds): The Pharmacological Basis of Therapeutics. New York, Macmillan, 1975, pp 817–847

125. Gussin RZ: Renal physiology and pharmacology. *In* Antonaccio M (ed): Cardiovascular Pharmacology. New York, Raven Press, 1977, pp 45–81

126. Dikshit K, Vydan JK, Forrester JS, et al: Renal and extrarenal hemodynamic effects of furosemide in congestive heart failure after acute myocardial infarction. N Engl J Med 288:1087–1090, 1973

127. Seller RH, Banach S, Namey T, et al: Cardiac effect of diuretic drugs. Am Heart J 89:493–500, 1975

128. Austin SM, Schreiner BF, Kramer DH, et al: The acute hemodynamic effects of ethacrynic acid and furosemide in patients with chronic postcapillary pulmonary hypertension. Circulation 53:364–368, 1976

129. Leaf A: Cell swelling: A factor in ischemic tissue injury. Circulation 48:455–458, 1973

130. Willerson JT, Powell WJ Jr, Guiney TF, et al: Improvement in myocardial function and coronary blood flow in ischemic myocardium after mannitol. J Clin Invest 51:2989–2998, 1972

131. Weisfeldt ML, Scully HE, Selden AG, et al: Effect of mannitol on the performance of the isolated canine heart after fibrillatory arrest. J Thorac Cardiovasc Surg 66:290–299, 1973

Joel A. Kaplan, M.D.

3

Hemodynamic Monitoring

In patients with severe cardiovascular disease, adequate hemodynamic monitoring should be available at all times. Continuous measurements and recordings of all vital physiological parameters can now be obtained with modern catheters and electronic monitoring equipment. The development of dangerous hemodynamic events can be observed and corrected before they proceed to sudden catastrophic cardiac arrests. Thus the number of major cardiovascular complications should be reduced.

Many devices are currently available to monitor the cardiovascular system. These devices range from those that are totally noninvasive, such as the blood pressure cuff and electrocardiogram (ECG), to those that are extremely invasive, such as the Swan-Ganz catheter. In order to use the invasive monitors, the potential benefit to be gained from the information must heavily outweigh the risk of the procedure. In many patients with cardiac disease, the benefit obtained does in fact outweigh the risks, which explains the increasing utilization of invasive monitoring.

Standard monitors such as blood pressure, ECG, central venous pressure (CVP), urine output, temperature, and arterial blood gases are used in all patients undergoing cardiac surgery. Increasing use is being made of pulmonary artery catheters, left atrial pressure (LAP) catheters, cardiac output measurements, systolic time intervals, invasive measurements of myocardial contractility such as dP/dt, and indices of myocardial oxygenation. All of these measurements and their derivatives can be frequently obtained and recorded; however, interpretation of the complex data requires an astute clinician fully aware of the patient's overall condition and the problems inherent with the monitors. Wide application of computer technology in the future will undoubtedly help with some of the correlations of the data.

A modern anesthesia department utilizing sophisticated monitoring equipment requires the services of a complex electronic laboratory. Technicians and engineers are needed to modify and service the equipment at frequent intervals. An acute care laboratory in the operating room area is also needed to provide rapid information concerning arterial blood gases, electrolytes (Na^+, K^+, Ca^{++}), hematocrit, blood sugar, and oncotic pressure.

ARTERIAL BLOOD PRESSURE

The arterial blood pressure is a quantitative measurement used for assessment of the status of the cardiovascular system. The *mean arterial pressure* is the average pressure during a cardiac

71

cycle and is dependent on the cardiac output and peripheral resistance.[1] This relationship is expressed by the following formula:

$$MAP = CO \times TPR$$

which is the cardiovascular equivalent of Ohm's law of electricity:

$$E = I \times R$$

where MAP = mean arterial pressure, CO = cardiac output, TPR = total peripheral resistance, E = voltage, I = current, and R = resistance. The mean arterial pressure can be obtained by electrical damping or by calculation with the following formula:

$$MAP = DP + \tfrac{1}{3}(SP - DP)$$

where DP = diastolic pressure and SP = systolic pressure. The arterial pulse pressure is the difference between the systolic and diastolic pressure and is dependent on the stroke volume and arterial capacitance.

Indirect Measurement of Blood Pressure

Today the anesthesiologist depends primarily on techniques developed over 50 years ago, utilizing the Riva-Rocci occlusive cuff and ascultation of Korotkoff sounds. The cuff is inflated above systolic pressure and should be slowly deflated at 2–3 torr per beat for the most accurate measurement of the blood pressure. The systolic pressure may be obtained by observation of oscillations, by palpation of pulsations distal to the cuff, or by auscultation of the Korotkoff sounds. Van Bergen found that the oscillatory method correlated better with direct pressure measurements than did the standard Korotkoff sounds.[2] Blood pressure is most often obtained by the auscultatory method. The systolic blood pressure is the point at which Korotkoff sounds are first heard (phase 1). The diastolic blood pressure is more controversial and may be taken either at the end of phase 4 when the sounds disappear or between phases 3 and 4 when the sounds change quality.[3]

Other techniques to measure blood pressure indirectly are the oscillotonometer of von Recklinghausen, Doppler instruments, and plethys-mographs. The oscillotonometer is a double-cuff system that is accurate even at low pressures and has been useful during deliberate hypotension. The Doppler has been used successfully to monitor blood pressure in patients with low-output states and even during cardiopulmonary bypass.[4] A good correlation has been shown between aortic pressure and Doppler-measured peripheral arterial pressure.[5] Even noninvasive monitors can have serious complications associated with them, however. Gangrene of the thumb has been reported following the use of a photoelectric plethysmograph for pulse monitoring during anesthesia.[6]

It has been shown that there can be a considerable discrepancy between indirect and direct methods of blood pressure measurement. Some authors have found that direct measurements are usually higher than indirect, but others have found that the direct measurement may be higher or lower by a considerable amount. The discrepancy has been found to be the greatest in patients who are hypertensive, obese, hypothermic, or in shock.

Direct Measurement of Blood Pressure

Invasive arterial monitoring of blood pressure has become popular in recent years with the increased complexity of surgery and intensive care of critically ill patients. Catheters are placed in various arteries of the body for continuous beat-to-beat blood pressure monitoring and for multiple arterial blood gas measurements. Anesthetic procedures in which an arterial line may be indicated include the following:

1. Cardiac surgery with cardiopulmonary bypass
2. Major peripheral vascular surgery
3. Pulmonary resections
4. Intracranial operations
5. Major trauma procedures
6. Deliberate hypotension
7. Deliberate hypothermia

Surgical procedures in patients with any of the following abnormalities may also require an arterial cathether for careful monitoring:

1. Significant pulmonary disease
2. Cardiovascular disease

3. Severe metabolic derangements
4. Obesity

SITES AND METHODS OF DIRECT MONITORING

Radial artery. At the present time, the radial artery is the most commonly used artery for continuous blood pressure monitoring because it is easy to cannulate, it is readily accessible during surgery, and the collateral circulation is usually adequate and easy to check. The collateral circulation of the hand is formed by an arterial arcade on the palm of the hand where the radial and ulnar arteries come together. This collateral circulation is checked by performing an Allen's test prior to cannulation.[7] This test demonstrates that if the radial artery becomes thrombosed, adequate ulnar collateral flow is present to safely perfuse the hand. Palm showed that if there is adequate ulnar collateral flow, circulatory perfusion pressure to the fingers is also adequate following radial artery catheterization.[8] The Allen's test is performed by occluding both the radial and ulnar arteries and having the patient squeeze his fist until the hand blanches. Then the ulnar artery is released with the patient's hand open, and the color of the hand is observed. If the circulation is normal, color returns to the hand in less than 5 seconds. If the hand does not regain its color in 10 seconds, we consider it unsafe to cannulate the radial artery. It is important to prevent the patient from overextending the wrist; otherwise, a false abnormal result will be produced by occlusion of the transpalmar arch under the flexor retinaculum.[9] Some investigators have recently recommended the use of the Doppler finger pulse transducer, or the plethysmograph to check for adequate ulnar artery collateral circulation in anesthetized patients in whom an unanticipated radial artery catheter is needed.[10]

When selecting an artery for cannulation, it is preferable not to use a radial artery distal to a brachial artery cutdown site from a previous cardiac catheterization. We and others have found distorted pressures and early occlusion of these vessels.[11,12] Other factors that affect selection of a radial artery include:

1. Site of surgery: for example, for descending thoracic aortic aneurysms, we use the right radial artery, since the left subclavian artery may be occluded by the surgeons, and the left radial artery may be misleading.
2. Prior surgery on the hand.
3. Nondominant hand is the preferred side.
4. Preference of the surgeon and/or anesthesiologist.

Good technique is necessary to obtain a high degree of success in arterial catheterization.[13] The wrist should be sharply dorsiflexed over a pack of sponges and immobilized on a short arm board. It is helpful to draw the course of the artery for 1 inch and to be comfortably seated. A wheal of local anesthetic is raised over the artery, and a small skin nick is made with an 18-gauge needle. A short, 20-gauge, nontapered Teflon catheter is used, without a syringe attached, to make the puncture. The angle between the needle and the skin should be shallow (30° or less) and the needle advanced parallel to the course of the artery. When the artery is entered, reduce the angle between the needle and skin to 10° and try to thread the outer catheter off the needle while watching that blood continues to drip out of the needle hub (Fig. 3-1). Try not to puncture the back wall of the artery. If the blood should stop dripping, the needle has penetrated the back wall. The needle should be removed and the catheter pulled back until a brisk spurt of blood occurs and then advanced slowly up the artery. After insertion of the catheter, the wrist should be taken out of the dorsiflexed position, since continued dorsiflexion can lead to median nerve damage by stretching of the nerve over the wrist.

The catheter is attached via nondistensible tubing to the pressure transducer. A stopcock should not be placed directly on the catheter for at least two reasons: (1) it may become disconnected easily, and (2) constant manipulation of it will traumatize the artery. Instead, a short, 4-inch extension tubing with an attached stopcock is used (Fig. 3-2). The tubing is connected to a manifold which holds a series of pressure transducers and extension tubes (Fig. 3-3). The mechanical characteristics of this *connecting system* can markedly influence the fidelity of the arterial pressure trace and thus the systolic/diastolic digital displays. Most commonly, artifactual arterial traces are caused by "ringing" or "resonance" in the connecting system as it interacts with the mechanical characteristics of

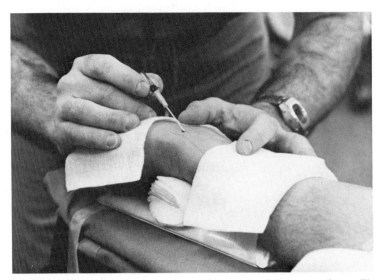

Figure 3-1. Placement of a percutaneous 20-gauge radial artery catheter. The artery has been entered and the catheter-needle unit is being gently threaded up the vessel. Note the position of the hand. The back wall of the artery has not been punctured.

the transducer and the dP/dt in the artery. Almost all the "ringing" artifacts are "false highs." Rarely, ringing or resonance can lead to a false low reading; the overwhelming number of false low readings are caused by a significant pressure gradient from the aortic arch to the radial artery.

The level of analysis necessary to understand the above-mentioned problems with the *connecting system* is quite complex. There are, however, some useful simple summary points:[14]

1. *No one component* (catheter, stopcock, tubing, etc.) is completely at fault. It is a total *system* problem.
2. Therefore, there is *no one solution*. In some instances, making the tubing softer may help, whereas in other instances, making it stiffer may help. In some cases, a bubble in the transducer dome may help by dampening the ringing, and in other cases, it may make it worse.
3. In general, most pressure systems can be made better by:
   a. Using the transducer with the highest frequency response (usually one of the modern small transducers);
   b. Keeping the tubing as short as possible (ideally 3–6 inches);
   c. Keeping the tubing, stopcocks, and domes *completely* free of bubbles.

Since we frequently must use a system that is already in existence and that cannot readily be changed, testing the fidelity of the arterial pressure tracing is necessary and can best be carried out by using the simple *return-to-flow method,* that is, using the appropriate blood pressure cuff pumped up until the pulsatile trace disappears and then slowly bleeding air from the cuff, reducing the pressure in the conventional manner and noting the pressure (on the mercury or dial manometer) at which the *first* pulsatile trace reappears on the oscilloscope screen. This is the best systolic pressure and should be very close to the same pressure at which the Korotkoff sounds are heard.

In addition to using the above method to check the *system*, the transducers themselves must of course be regularly calibrated with a mercury manometer at three or more pressures over their entire operating range (e.g., 0, 100, 200, 300).

The arterial line may be kept open by either intermittent flushing or a continuous infusion of heparinized solution. In the operating room, we prefer to flush the catheter intermittently with a small volume of heparinized solution (1 unit of

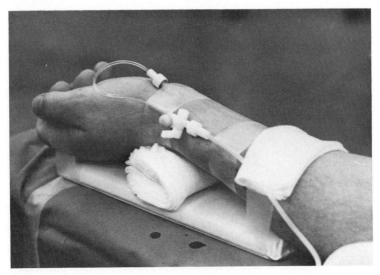

Fig. 3-2. The radial artery catheter is connected to a short, 4-inch extension tubing, not directly to a stopcock. The stopcock is removed from the catheter itself so that manipulations of the stopcock will not cause movement of the catheter in the vessel.

heparin per milliliter of saline). We flush with 2–3 ml of solution at a time to keep the catheter patent. Larger volumes may produce central arterial embolization and cerebral vascular accidents and thus must be avoided.[15] In the intensive care unit, the arterial line is kept open with a continuous flush device* at an infusion rate of 1–3 ml/hr. The infusion minimizes thrombus formation and helps prolong the usefulness of the catheter.[16] Gardner showed that pressure errors resulting from this flush system are clinically insignificant, averaging less than 2 percent.[17]

Thrombosis of the radial artery after cannulation is a common complication. The thrombi appear to be induced by the presence of the catheter itself, since the incidence of thrombosis increases with increasing duration of cannulation. In a study by Bedford, 18-gauge catheters in place for less than 20 hours induced a 25 percent incidence of thrombosis, while catheters in for longer durations (20 to 40 hours) resulted in 50 percent thrombosis.[18] The onset of thrombosis was frequently found to be delayed until some days after decannulation. There was a 10 percent incidence of minor vascular problems but no major complications, and 100 percent of the thrombosed vessels eventually recannulized.

* Sorenson Intra-Flo.

In other studies, nontapered 20-gauge Teflon catheters have had the lowest incidence of thrombosis (about 20 percent).[19] Bedford showed that the incidence of postcannulation radial artery occlusion could be decreased significantly by using 20-gauge cannulae instead of 18-gauge cannulae.[20] Tapered catheters tend to obstruct more of the vessel with their shoulders and therefore further reduce flow past the catheter. Teflon catheters appear to be less thrombogenic than polypropylene catheters.[21,22] Downs found 90 percent occlusion with polypropylene and only 29 percent with Teflon. Recently, it was found that the incidence of radial artery occlusion was also related to the radial artery diameter, with smaller vessels having a higher rate of occlusion. Wrist circumference can be used as a predictor of radial artery occlusion. Forty-seven percent of patients with a circumference of less than 18 cm sustained occlusion, while only 21 percent with a circumference greater than 18 cm had occlusion.[23]

It appears to be possible to remove some radial artery thrombi during decannulation. Bedford reported the technique of applying suction with a syringe to the hub of the radial artery catheter while it is being withdrawn.[24] In 9 of 19 patients with marked thrombus, the clot was successfully removed by aspiration. Feeley re-

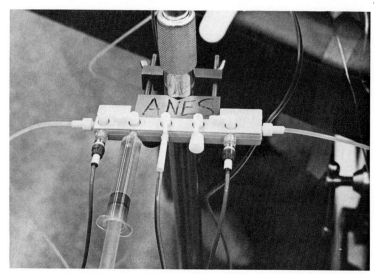

Fig. 3-3. Pressure transducers and extension tubing are connected to a manifold with five stopcocks. This allows for easy blood sampling and frequent flushing of the monitoring lines. The manifold must be maintained at the zero heart level. This is frequently done by attaching it to a pole directly on the operating table.

ported 4 cases of catheter thrombectomy to reestablish flow in thrombosed radial arteries.[25] A No. 3 French embolectomy catheter was inserted through an 18-gauge arteriotomy and the thrombus was removed. Then an 18-gauge catheter was reinserted through the same arteriotomy and monitoring continued. The new catheters worked satisfactorily for 32 to 72 hours in the 4 patients. This technique may be useful in long-term monitoring when the radial artery is felt to be the best site for blood pressure and gas measurements.

Numerous other complications of radial artery catheterization have been reported, including ecchymosis and hematoma formation at the puncture site, hand and wrist discomfort, arteriovenous fistulae or aneurysms, localized ischemia of digits, or embolic phenomena. Nine cases of proximal skin necrosis after radial artery catheterization have been reported.[26,27] These have occurred secondary to interference by the catheter and/or thrombus with the local cutaneous branches of the radial artery. Wyatt suggested cannulating as far distal as possible with a 20-gauge catheter to try to avoid this unfortunate complication. The radial artery catheter may also be the source of bacterial contamination. An outbreak of flavobacterium sepsis was traced to contaminated blood gas sy-

ringes, which in turn contaminated the stopcock and arterial catheter and ultimately led to positive blood cultures in 14 patients.[28]

Another technique of radial artery catheterization allows percutaneous insertion of a long catheter in order to obtain a central aortic tracing of arterial blood pressure. Gardner reported on 495 insertions of a 100-cm-long Teflon catheter through an 18-gauge thin-walled needle.[29] Ninety-two percent of the catheters were successfully placed in the radial artery, and only 2.9 percent could not be advanced into the subclavian artery. The advantages of a central arterial trace are that beat-to-beat determinations of stroke volume can be made by the pulse contour method and that the aortic pressure is more reliable than the radial artery pressure in certain patients with low-flow states. The main disadvantage is the increased incidence of complications. In Gardner's series, 3 patients required thrombectomies for complete arterial occlusion, and 1 patient required surgical removal of a catheter that was sheared off by the needle. The risk of retrograde arterial dissection by the catheter is also present during the insertion up the arm.

Ulnar artery. The ulnar artery may occasionally be cannulated instead of the radial artery. In a small percentage of patients, the regular Allen's test is inadequate; but when it is *reversed,* with the radial artery being released, the hand fills adequately. This shows radial artery dominance and, in this instance, it is preferable to cannulate the ulnar artery. This finding can be further confirmed with Doppler flow measurements over the radial and ulnar arteries. We use the same technique and equipment to cannulate the ulnar artery as we use for the radial artery.

Brachial or axillary arteries. The brachial or axillary arteries can also be cannulated for pressure measurements in the operating room or intensive care unit. The brachial artery has been shown to have a 17 percent incidence of obstruction after cardiac catheterization, with two-thirds being asymptomatic.[30] However, Barnes reported that hemodynamic complications resulting from brachial artery pressure monitoring are lower than those following cardiac catheterization.[31] Fifty-four patients had 18-gauge Teflon brachial artery catheters placed for monitoring during cardiac surgery without any of the patients developing evidence of obstruction of the brachial artery or distal ischemic symptoms during the 1 to 3 days of cannulation. About 10 percent of the patients in this group had a low output syndrome requiring inotropic therapy. Three patients developed localized obstruction of the radial or ulnar artery, however, probably secondary to embolic phenomena in spite of a continuous heparin infusion through the arterial catheter. None of these 3 patients developed ischemic symptoms in the hand.

Brachial artery cannulation may increase in popularity with the introduction of new in vivo blood gas analyzers that require insertion through 18-gauge catheters in high-flow vessels. Miniature polarographic oxygen electrodes are now clinically available and have been utilized during surgery. Recently, a new intravascular gas chromatographic system has been introduced that measures Pao_2 and $Paco_2$ every 4 minutes. This instrument allows simultaneous measurement of blood pressure and intermittent blood sampling and thus may find a role in the intensive care unit for chronically ill patients.*

The axillary artery has been recommended

* Sentorr system for blood gas analysis, Ohio Medical Products.

for long-term arterial pressure monitoring in the intensive care unit.[32] It allows freedom of the patient's hands and permits a large catheter to be placed in a central artery. Using the Seldinger technique, a 6- or 8-inch 18-gauge Teflon catheter can be inserted via the axillary artery into the aortic arch.[33] The left axillary artery is preferred to reduce the possibility of cerebral embolism off the catheter. The main complications reported have been related to axillary sheath hematomas with brachial plexus compression.

Femoral artery. Femoral artery catheterization may be used intraoperatively or in the postoperative period. This is a relatively simple technique in which the catheter may remain patent for a prolonged period of time. A 6- or 8-inch 18-gauge catheter is advanced up the artery without difficulty in most cases. If an obstruction is encountered in patients with arteriosclerosis, we have used a small J-wire to bypass the obstruction with a high degree of success. Ersoz reported prolonged femoral artery catheterization in 64 patients with no major complications during the 1 to 10 days of monitoring.[34] Twelve patients had minor complications, including decreased distal pulses and hematoma formation. None of the catheter sites became infected, but three of the catheter tips had positive cultures upon removal. The femoral artery is also a useful monitoring site during descending thoracic aorta aneurysm surgery. (See Chapter 10.) Using either partial left heart bypass or femoral-femoral bypass with the aorta cross-clamped, it is useful to monitor the blood pressure in the lower circulation to assess renal and spinal cord perfusion. Some surgeons are now using the Gott external shunt instead of cardiopulmonary bypass in these cases. It is necessary to measure pressure distal to the shunt, since kinking and partial occlusion of flow is a frequent problem with this technique.[35]

Dorsalis pedis artery. The two main arteries to the foot are the dorsalis pedis artery, which is a continuation of the anterior tibial artery extending from the ankle to the great toe, and the lateral plantar artery off the posterior tibial artery. These two vessels form an arterial arch on the foot that is similar to the one formed by the radial and ulnar arteries in the hand. The presence of collateral flow to the foot from the lateral plantar artery should be checked prior to cannulation of the dorsalis pedis artery. The test is performed by occluding both arteries and blanching the great toe by compressing it. The lateral plantar artery is released, and the toe should rapidly flush with color. It is not safe to cannulate the dorsalis pedis artery if color does not return to the toes within 10 seconds. The circulation may alternatively be checked using the Doppler flowmeter. It is recommended to catheterize this vessel with a 20-gauge Teflon catheter in a manner similar to that of the radial artery.

The dorsalis pedis artery appears to be a reasonable alternative to radial artery catheterization in patients undergoing surgical procedures in which the anesthesiologist is located along the patient's side. The vessel may not be palpable or present in 5 to 12 percent of patients, however.[36] This vessel probably should not be used in patients with diabetes or other peripheral vascular diseases. Youngberg demonstrated the safety of cannulating this artery.[37] In 26 patients who had catheters in the dorsalis pedis artery for 2 to 25 hours, the incidence of thrombosis was lower than that reported for radial artery catheters, and no major complications were observed.

It is important to realize that the pressure measured in the peripheral dorsalis pedis artery is different from a more central pressure. This is because the arterial pressure contour becomes progressively more distorted as the wave is transmitted down the arterial system. The high-frequency components such as the incisura disappear; the systolic peak increases, while the diastolic value decreases; and there is a transmission delay. These changes are due to decreased arterial compliance in the periphery and reflection and resonance of previous waves.[38] The systolic pressure is usually 10–20 torr higher in the dorsalis pedis artery than in the radial or brachial arteries, while the diastolic pressure is 15–20 torr lower.[37,39]

VENOUS PRESSURE MONITORING

Central Venous Pressure

The central venous pressure (CVP) is usually measured as an indication of right atrial and ventricular pressures. In order to do this, the catheter must lie within the thorax in a major vein or be in the right side of the heart. A reproducible landmark, such as the midaxillary line, must be used for repeated reference to the zero level, and the monitoring system (either water column or electronic) must be reliable. Electronic monitoring is preferable to a simple water manometer because it allows observation and diagnosis from the venous waves; respiratory fluctuations are easily observed; and it is quickly responsive to changes in pressure.

The normal venous tracing has three positive waves (a,c,v) and two negative ones (x,y).[40] These wave forms have a fixed relationship to the electrocardiogram and phonocardiogram (Fig. 3-4). The a wave is produced by right atrial contraction and begins before the first heart sound. When the atrium relaxes, the venous pulse descends and is interrupted by the second positive wave, the c wave. This is produced by the bulging of the tricuspid valve into the right atrium during the onset of ventricular contraction and occurs right after the first heart sound and QRS complex of the electrocardiogram. The x descent results from further atrial relaxation and downward displacement of the ventricle and tricuspid valve during ventricular systole. The v wave is formed by right atrial filling with a closed tricuspid valve, and the y descent, by opening of the tricuspid valve with blood flow into the right ventricle.

The a wave will be absent in patients with atrial fibrillation. Large a waves occur when there is increased resistance to right atrial emptying, as in tricuspid stenosis, right ventricular hypertrophy, pulmonary stenosis, or pulmonary hypertension. If the right atrium contracts when the tricuspid valve is still closed, a giant a wave or cannon wave will occur. This is frequently seen during anesthesia with enflurane when a nodal rhythm occurs (Fig. 3-5) and may produce a drop in blood pressure varying from 5 to 20 percent. Cannon waves may also be seen during ventricular arrhythmias and heart block. In patients with tricuspid regurgitation, the x descent disappears and is replaced by a large v wave.

The CVP is a useful monitor if the factors affecting it are realized and its limitations understood. The CVP reflects the patient's blood volume, venous tone, and right ventricular performance. It is also affected by central venous obstructions and alterations of intrathoracic pressure such as the increase caused by the use of positive end expiratory pressure. Serial meas-

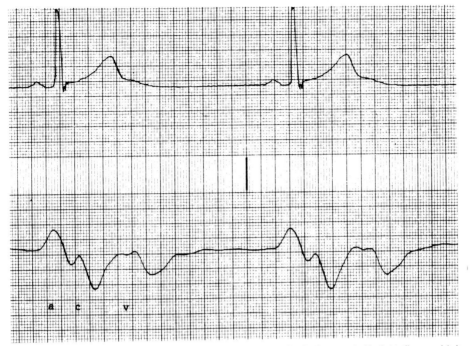

Fig. 3-4. A normal central venous pressure tracing is shown in the bottom half of the figure with its corresponding electrocardiogram in the top half. The a, c, and v waves on the venous pressure tracing are labeled. The x descent occurs between the c and v waves, while the y descent occurs after the v wave.

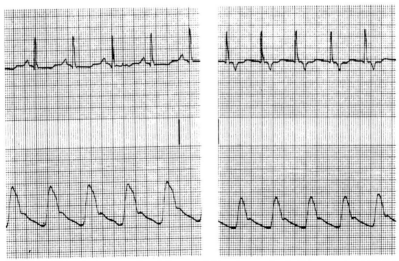

Fig. 3-5. The ECG on the top panel and the arterial tracing on the bottom panel are from a patient receiving enflurane anesthesia. The tracings on the left side show a blood pressure of 140/80 when the patient is in a sinus rhythm. The tracings on the right side show a blood pressure of 110/60 when the patient loses his atrial kick and is in a nodal rhythm. The CVP tracing at this time will show a cannon wave.

urements are more useful than an individual number, and the response of the CVP to a volume infusion is a very useful test of right ventricular function. A rapid infusion of 100–200 ml of fluid can be used to judge hemodynamic performance by observing how much of an increment it produces in the CVP and blood pressure. It must be remembered that the CVP reflects *right* heart performance and not left ventricular function. Therefore, it is possible to have a patient develop pulmonary edema with a normal CVP. Thus the combination of the CVP to monitor right atrial pressure and the esophageal stethoscope to monitor left atrial pressure (rales, S_3) is still a useful monitoring technique in patients with good left ventricular function.

Central venous pressure monitoring is indicated in:

1. Surgical procedures in which large volume shifts may occur (e.g., Whipple procedure)
2. Potentially hypovolemic patients (e.g., bowel obstruction)
3. Patients in shock
4. Massively traumatized patients
5. Some patients with preexisting cardiovascular disease undergoing surgery (others will require a Swan-Ganz catheter)

CVP catheters may even be preferred over-Swan-Ganz catheters in certain types of cardiac surgical patients—those with tricuspid valve disease, atrial septal defects or other congenital lesions—or in patients in whom autologous blood may need to be removed from the CVP catheter. Other indications for a CVP catheter include neurosurgical operations done in the sitting position with the possibility of air embolization, patients with poor peripheral veins, hyperalimentation, and rapid administration of fluid. Temporary transvenous cardiac pacemakers may also be placed using a central venous cannulation technique.

Many methods and routes of central venous catheterization have been described, together with their frequent and sometimes bizarre complications. Anesthesiologists should become experts on the introduction of these catheters via various techniques in order to give their patients the best possible care. They must understand and appreciate the risks of these techniques in order to avoid them and enjoy the benefits of this sophisticated method of monitoring.

INTERNAL JUGULAR VEIN

Cannulation of the internal jugular vein (IJV) was first described by English et al. in 1969 and since then has steadily increased in popularity to its present position, in our opinion, as the method of choice for CVP monitoring.[41] The technique is contraindicated in the hands of people not familiar with the anatomy, in anticoagulated patients, and in patients with prior surgery of the neck. Advantages of this technique are:

1. Ease of cannulation as a result of the constant relationships of the anatomic structures
2. A short, straight course to the right atrium that almost assures right atrial or superior vena cava localization of the catheter tip
3. Easy access from the head of the table
4. Fewer complications than subclavian catheterization

The IJV is located under the medial border of the lateral head of the sternocleidomastoid muscle (Fig. 3-6). The carotid artery is consistently deep and medial to the IJV. The right IJV is preferred, since this vein leads straight into the superior vena cava, the right cupula of the lung is lower than the left, and the thoracic duct is on the left side. The anatomy is demonstrated more easily in the awake patient who can make the sternocleidomastoid muscle stand out by momentarily lifting his head and tensing it. The cannulation is no more uncomfortable than starting a peripheral venous line and is well tolerated by awake, premedicated patients. The neck is extended and turned sharply to the left while the patient is placed in a 15° Trendelenberg position. The muscle borders should be identified and the location of the carotid artery noted (Fig. 3-7).

Three main routes of cannulation of the IJV have been described.[42] We strongly prefer the central route, which is described below.[43] After the skin is prepared, a wheal of local anesthetic is raised at the apex of the triangle formed by the two heads of the sternocleidomastoid muscle. This point is two to three fingerbreadths above the clavicle and well above the cupula of the right lung. The initial identifying venipuncture is made with a 1½-inch 22-gauge needle on a 5-ml syringe containing 1 ml of 1 percent lidocaine. With the skin tensed, the needle is ad-

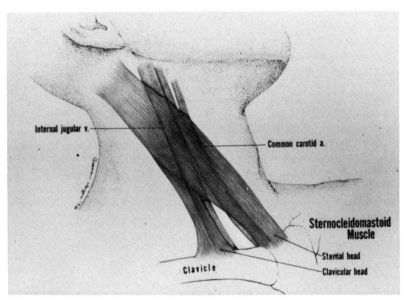

Fig. 3-6. A diagrammatic representation of the anatomy of the major structures in the region of the right internal jugular vein. Note that the internal jugular vein runs under the medial border of the clavicular head (lateral) of the sternocleidomastoid muscle. The carotid artery is deep under the sternal head (medial) of the sternocleidomastoid muscle.

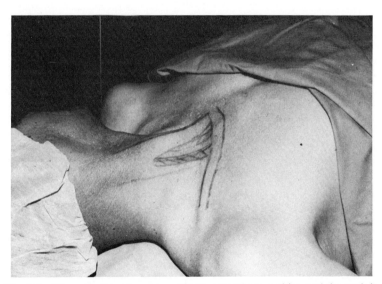

Fig. 3-7. The patient is placed in a 15° Trendelenberg position and the neck is extended and turned to the left. The sternocleidomastoid muscle and clavicle are outlined. Note the triangle formed by the junction of the medial and lateral heads of the sternocleidomastoid muscle. The carotid artery is shown to be medial and the internal jugular vein lateral. This anatomy is much more easily demonstrated in the awake, sedated patient.

vanced in a caudad direction at a 30° angle to the skin, away from the midline, and under the lateral head of the sternocleidomastoid muscle (Fig. 3-8). The needle tip should not enter the medial half of the sternocleidomastoid triangle where the carotid artery is located. Constant aspiration is maintained on the syringe as the needle is advanced into the vein at a depth of ½ to 1½ inches. If the vein is not found, a Valsalva maneuver by the patient will help distend it to a size of 2–3 cm and make location easier. After the vein is located, the skin is infiltrated with 1 ml of lidocaine and the needle removed. The skin should continue to be tensed by the left hand so that the underlying anatomy does not change position. A 14-gauge 8-inch intracath is then inserted at the same angle and depth into the vein (Fig. 3-9). Two "tissue pops" are noted at the prevertebral fascia and the vein, which is identified by a free return of dark venous blood up the catheter. It is not necessary to advance the needle down the vein. The catheter is advanced through the needle into the superior vena cava. The needle is then removed and the catheter protected with the plastic guard to avoid cutting it. The catheter is taped along the anterior border of the ear in a stable manner. The

tip of the 8-inch catheter is usually located at the junction of the superior vena cava and right atrium in the average adult (Fig. 3-10). A 12-inch catheter is used for placement in the right atrium. Using this technique, we have had over a 90 percent success rate of catheterization of the IJV and only a 1 to 2 percent incidence of carotid puncture in a teaching institution, with residents doing most of the catheterizations. In addition, we have seen no adverse sequelae to inadvertent carotid punctures.

The two other approaches described are the posterior and anterior routes. In the posterior route, the needle is introduced under the sternocleidomastoid muscle near the junction of the middle and lower thirds of its lateral border and is advanced toward the suprasternal notch.[44] In this technique, the needle is aimed in the direction of the carotid artery, and therefore the incidence of carotid artery puncture may be higher. In the anterior approach, the needle is inserted at the midpoint of the sternocleidomastoid muscle on its medial border and aimed toward the ipsilateral nipple.[45]

A new technique of IJV catheterization has recently been introduced in Canada by Boulanger.[46] The needle is introduced much higher on

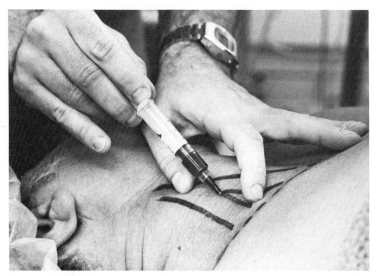

Fig. 3-8. The internal jugular vein is located with a 22-gauge needle on a 5-ml syringe. The skin puncture is made at the apex of the sternocleidomastoid triangle, which is usually two to three fingerbreadths above the clavicle (1½ to 2 inches) and lateral to the carotid pulse. The needle is advanced in a caudad direction at a 30° angle to the skin under the lateral head of the muscle while aspirating on the syringe.

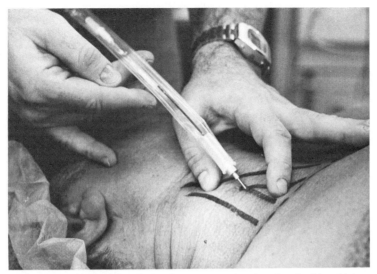

Fig. 3-9. The 22-gauge needle has been removed and replaced with a 14-gauge intracath needle at the exact same angle. The large needle is slowly advanced into the same depth as the 22-gauge needle, and the internal jugular vein is identified by the return of venous blood up the catheter.

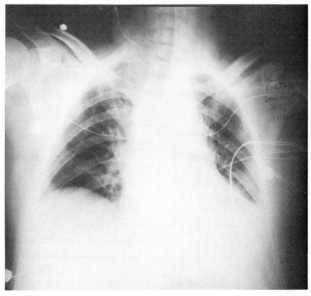

Fig. 3-10. The catheter is shown in the superior vena cava with the tip just above the right atria. X-ray localization of the catheter tip is not necessary for routine central venous pressure monitoring, since the right internal jugular vein, superior vena cava, and right atrium are in a straight line.

the medial border of the sternocleidomastoid muscle, at the level of the superior border of the thyroid cartilege. The needle is directed inferiorly and laterally under the posterior aspect of the muscle and meets the IJV at its widest diameter. The technique differs from those previously described by its high entry point, which further reduces the possibility of a pneumothorax, and its lateral, superficial path away from the carotid artery. Boulanger reported a 94 percent success rate, with a 2 percent incidence of carotid artery puncture. Our experience with this technique has been similar. We have found it to be technically more difficult than our usual technique described above, however.

Some authors have recommended additional techniques for cannulating the IJV in order to reduce the incidence of carotid artery puncture. Civetta recommended placing a 22-gauge spinal needle through the 14-gauge intracath needle, and Petty recommended leaving the small identifying needle in place while advancing the larger needle.[47,48] We have found that both of these techniques are awkward and do not guarantee avoidance of the carotid artery; therefore, we do not use either of them.

Many studies have verified the high degree of success in cannulating the IJV in the hands of experienced personnel. Vaughan reported a failure rate of only 2 in 227 adults (less than 1 percent), and 6.2 percent when including children 1 to 2 years of age.[49] Kuramoto found successful CVP catheterization via the right IJV in 96 percent of his adult patients and overall in 88 percent of IJV catheterizations versus only 70 percent using the basilic vein.[50] The success rate has been less in children, but with experience and proper equipment, it can be quite reasonable. Prince reported successful CVP catheterization in 68 percent of children 6 weeks to 2 years of age and in 82 percent in the 2- to 14-year-old group.[51] The rate of success was higher in infants weighing more than 10 kg and in patients with CVPs above 10 cm H_2O.

EXTERNAL JUGULAR VEIN

Cannulation of the external jugular vein (EJV) is our alternate method of choice when we cannot cannulate the right IJV. This vein contains valves that can make passing a catheter into the central circulation very difficult. Recently, however Blitt has introduced a J-wire EJV catheterization technique which makes this approach a reasonable alternative to the IJV.[52] This technique is based on the J-wire principle introduced by Baum in 1964 for retrograde catheterization of tortuous vessels during radiologic studies.[53] A 14- or 16-gauge $5\frac{1}{2}$ inch over-the-needle Teflon catheter is introduced into the external jugular vein. The needle is removed, and a 35-cm-long flexible J-wire is inserted through the catheter and rotated past venous valvular obstructions into the central circulation. This technique avoids insertion of a needle deep into the neck, and more than a 90 percent success rate of central venous catheter placement has been reported. Our success rate has not been this high, however, and it is therefore not our method of choice. In addition, we have not found this vein to be a good route for insertion of a Swan-Ganz catheter.

BASILIC AND CEPHALIC VEINS

When a neck vein is not available, we cannulate one of the arm veins and attempt to advance the catheter into the central venous circulation. The disadvantages of using the arm veins are the unreliability of obtaining a truly central catheter and being misled into thinking one has been obtained; the need for x-ray confirmation if right atrial location is required (e.g., sitting position); and the time delay in determining if the catheter is central.

A number of studies have examined the results of blind insertion of CVP catheters through the arm. Kellner found that 25 percent of the catheters were outside the central veins, with most of these passing up one of the jugular veins.[54] Fluctuation with respiration was found not to be a reliable sign of central location, since it was present in 21 percent of noncentral catheters. False high CVP readings of 2–6 torr were found in the noncentral catheters. Webre found that only 59 percent of arm catheters passed into the central circulation.[55] In the basilic vein, 65 percent of catheters passed central, while only 45 percent of those in the cephalic vein reached the central veins. Of the incorrectly placed catheters, 45 to 67 percent lay in the internal jugular veins.[56] Burgess has recently shown that turning the head of the patient toward the arm of insertion and placing the chin onto the ipsilateral shoulder during the threading of the catheter reduces the incidence of catheter passage up the internal jugular vein instead of into the central circulation.[57] Eighteen percent of catheters entered the IJV with the head in the midline, but only 4 percent entered when the head was turned. Central placement was successful in 80 percent of patients who had their heads turned during catheterization.

SUBCLAVIAN VEIN

The subclavian vein is readily available and has frequently been used for CVP catheterization in the past.[58] It has fallen into disfavor, however, because of the high incidence of major complications. It can be cannulated either from a supraclavicular or infraclavicular approach. Both methods have a high incidence of pneumothorax and the possibility of subclavian artery laceration.

COMPLICATIONS

All the methods of CVP monitoring mentioned above have the following potential complications:

1. Local and systemic infection
2. Thrombophlebitis
3. Mediastinal fluid infusion producing hydrothorax
4. Hematomas
5. Air embolism
6. Catheter shearing
7. Nerve injuries
8. Pericardial tamponade

Specific complications of internal jugular and subclavian venipuncture include:

1. Carotid or subclavian artery puncture: This can lead to significant hemorrhage from the subclavian artery into the chest, since it is difficult to compress this artery under the clavicle. Puncture of the carotid artery rarely causes problems if recognized immediately and compressed until the bleeding ceases in 10 to 15 minutes. Large hematomas can develop and endanger the airway, however. An arteriovenous fistula has been reported as a complication, as well as a chronic hematoma requiring surgical removal.[59,60]
2. Pneumothorax: This is much more common after subclavian puncture. It has been reported in 2 to 16 percent of attempted subclavian venipunctures but only rarely after jugular puncture. Cook, however, reported

a tension pneumothorax after IJV catheterization and general anesthesia.[61]
3. Nerve damage: If the needle is directed too far laterally in the neck, it is possible to injure the brachial plexus. A Horner's syndrome has been reported after puncture of the IJV.[62]
4. Thoracic duct injury: This can occur if the left IJV is used, and it is the main reason for preferring the right IJV. This can be a major complication requiring surgical intervention.[63]

Left Atrial Pressure

In patients with left-sided heart disease, the CVP cannot be reliably used as an estimate of left ventricular filling pressure. In these patients, it is necessary to monitor left atrial pressure (LAP) directly with a catheter in the left atrium or indirectly with a Swan-Ganz catheter in the pulmonary artery using the pulmonary capillary wedge pressure as an approximation of LAP. Measurement of left-sided filling pressures is indicated in patients with mitral and aortic valvular disease, coronary artery disease with poor left ventricular function, certain types of congenital heart disease, and in any patient in whom difficulty is encountered upon discontinuing cardiopulmonary bypass.

A 16-gauge 12-inch Teflon catheter is placed by the surgeon through a 14-gauge intracath needle or the previous vent site into the right superior pulmonary vein and advanced into the left atrium. A Teflon-pledgetted purse-string stitch is placed around the catheter to provide a surface for clotting upon removal of the catheter (Fig. 3-11). The catheter is brought out through the skin in the epigastric area and sutured in place. It is important to maintain positive airway pressure during insertion of the catheter in order to avoid the possibility of air entry into the pulmonary vein and thus to the left side of the heart, where it could embolize to the systemic circulation.

The left atrial catheter is an extremely informative monitor, but it is also quite risky and requires extreme caution in its use. The possibility of air embolism to the coronary or cerebral circulation is always present. This problem exists both upon insertion and during its continued use postoperatively in the intensive care unit. There is also the risk of clot formation on the

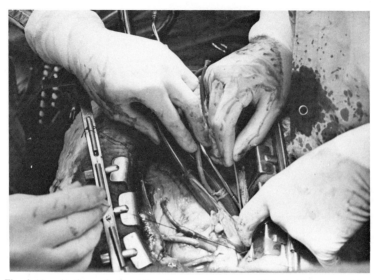

Fig. 3-11. At the end of cardiopulmonary bypass, a 12-inch 16-gauge catheter is placed by the surgeons into the right superior pulmonary vein and advanced into the left atrium for continuous measurement of left atrial pressure. The three aortocoronary bypass grafts can be seen as well as the cannulae for cardiopulmonary bypass.

catheter and subsequent embolization when the catheter is flushed or removed. Therefore, a continuous heparin infusion is necessary in an effort to avoid thrombus formation on the catheter tip in the postoperative period. There is also the risk of bleeding when the LAP catheter is removed postoperatively. It should therefore be removed while the chest tubes are still in place to diagnose and treat this problem.

In the past, CVP catheters were used to monitor patients with left-sided heart disease. The CVP has been shown to have a very poor correlation with the LAP in these patients, however. In 200 patients with mitral valve disease undergoing cardiac catheterization, the correlation coefficient of LAP and CVP was only 0.48.[64] Rapid changes in LAP induced by volume expansion, tachycardia, or vasoactive drugs frequently were not reflected in the CVP. When volume was infused in some of the patients, the LAP and CVP moved in *opposite* directions. This is supported by Sarnoff's previous work showing that there is no consistant relationship between right atrial pressure and left ventricular stroke work.[65] Other studies have shown the disparity between left and right ventricular function both in medical patients

with coronary artery disease and in surgical patients.[66-68]

Pulmonary Artery Pressure

One of the major advances in recent years in the care of the cardiac patient has been the introduction and extensive use of the Swan-Ganz flow-directed pulmonary artery catheter.[69] This catheter allows measurement of pulmonary artery systolic (PA_S), diastolic (PA_D), and mean pressures (PAP); pulmonary capillary wedge pressure (PCWP) which is also called pulmonary artery occluded pressure (PA_O); CVP; and cardiac output, using the thermal dilution technique. The PCWP has been shown to have a good correlation with direct LAP monitoring and thus can be used as a measure of the left ventricular filling pressure. The PCWP was within ±4 torr of LAP in 95 percent of 1620 simultaneous measurements in 43 patients after cardiac surgery.[70] Lappas showed an even better correlation, with the LAP-PCWP difference exceeding ±1 torr in only 10 percent of patients.[71] The relationship between LAP and PCWP may not be as close when the LAP exceeds 15 torr, however.[72] The PCWP also may not correlate as well with the LAP in patients on positive end expiratory pressure (PEEP) of more than 10 cm H_2O pressure. Lorzman showed a good correlation when PEEP was 5 cm H_2O or less (r = .83) but no significant correlation when PEEP was 10 cm H_2O or greater.[73] This may be a significant handicap in the postoperative care of these critically ill patients and needs to be examined further. When the catheter cannot be placed in a wedge position, the PA_D can also be used as an estimate of LAP with only a slightly lower degree of reliability.

The use of the Swan-Ganz catheter by the anesthesiologist has been a tremendous advance. It allows us to measure left-sided hemodynamics in the awake patient, during and after anesthetic induction, and in the prebypass period, as well as after bypass and postoperatively when the LAP is easily measured. This has contributed significantly to our understanding and care of these cardiac patients. It is indeed impressive to observe large changes in PAP and PCWP with almost no reflection in the CVP. The indications for catheterization of the pulmonary artery in the operating room are not clear at the present time however. Indications are still evolving and vary from hospital to hospital. Our present indications for the use of the Swan-Ganz catheter can be divided into cardiac surgical cases and noncardiac surgical cases (Tables 3-1 and 3-2).

There is a variety of equipment available to catheterize the pulmonary artery. For adult patients, the Swan-Ganz catheter comes in 5-Fr and 7-Fr sizes. The 5-Fr catheters only have one pressure lumen at the tip for pulmonary artery pressure, while the 7-Fr catheters have two pressure lumens (PAP at the tip and CVP port 30 cm back from the tip) and come with or without a thermistor located behind the balloon. A new 7-Fr multipurpose catheter will soon be available with two pressure lumens, with balloon and thermistor, and with electrodes at the atrial level for electrograms or atrial pacing.[75] There are also smaller catheters available for percutaneous use in children or for surgical use in which the catheters are brought out through the chest wall. The catheters may be introduced by a variety of techniques:

1. Venous cutdown in the anticubital fossae—original technique but rarely necessary any longer.

Table 3-1

Noncardiac Surgical Indications for Pulmonary Artery Catheterizations

1. Major surgery with large volume shifts in patients with known significant heart disease
2. Patients with severe coronary artery disease (e.g., recent infarction) for all surgical procedures
3. Sepsis with an unstable circulation
4. Patients requiring inotropes, vasodilators, or the intra-aortic balloon pump for heart failure
5. Massive trauma cases
6. Patients in shock
7. Surgery of the aorta requiring cross-clamping[74]
8. Patients in respiratory failure undergoing surgery
9. Patients with suspected or diagnosed pulmonary emboli
10. Cirrhotic patients undergoing portal systemic shunts

2. Percutaneously via a large intravenous catheter—the 5-Fr catheter fits through a 12-gauge cannula, and the 7-Fr will fit through a 10-gauge cannula.
3. Percutaneously in a central vein (IJV or subclavian) using a dilator set* and a modified Seldinger technique.[33]

Table 3-2

Cardiac Surgical Indications for Pulmonary Artery Catheterization

1. Patients undergoing coronary revascularization who have:
   a. Poor left ventricular function—EF < .4 or LVEDP > 18 torr
   b. A recent acute myocardial infarction
   c. A complication such as acute mitral insufficiency, ventricular septal rupture, or a ventricular aneurysm
2. Mitral or aortic valve replacement
3. Pulmonary hypertension
4. Combined lesions such as coronary stenosis and valvular heart disease
5. Complex lesions such as idiopathic hypertrophic subaortic stenosis (IHSS)

* UMI Intro-set, 8-Fr, 8-inch, Universal Medical Instrument Corp.

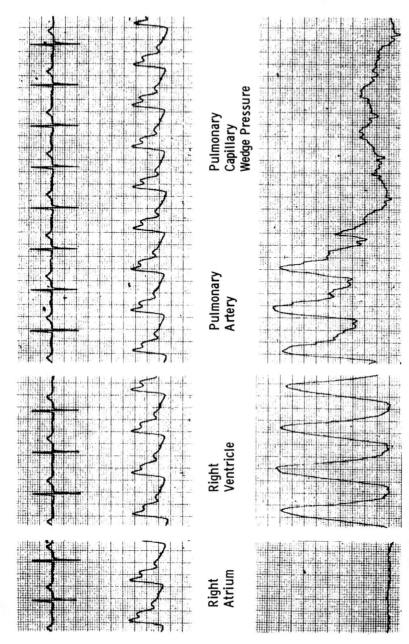

Right   **Right**   **Pulmonary**   **Pulmonary**
Atrium   **Ventricle**   **Artery**   **Capillary**
                                                Wedge Pressure

Fig. 3-12. The electrocardiogram and arterial pressure tracings are shown on the top and the venous pressure tracing as the Swan-Ganz catheter is advanced is shown on the bottom panel. Starting from the left, the catheter enters the right atrium and the pressure changes to a large pulsatile tracing when the catheter enters the right ventricle. Notice that the right ventricular end-diastolic pressure is very low, as was the right atrial pressure. When the catheter enters the pulmonary artery, the pulmonary artery diastolic pressure is elevated because of the interposition of the valve. This is frequently the key sign that the pulmonary artery has been entered. The catheter is then advanced into the pulmonary capillary wedge position.

It is also necessary to have high-frequency pressure transducers, a calibrated oscilloscopic display, and preferably, a recorder for observation of wave forms during the passage of the catheter through the right side of the heart. The normal intracardiac pressures are shown in Table 3-3.[76] The wave forms observed during passage of the Swan-Ganz catheter are shown in Figure 3-12. The right atrial trace is seen at 25–35 cm, right ventricle at 35–45 cm, pulmonary artery at 45–55 cm, and wedge at 50–60 cm using the IJV approach.

The preferred method of insertion of a Swan-Ganz catheter utilizes the right IJV and a modified Seldinger technique. This technique has the advantages of speed of insertion and a high success rate. Zaidan reported the mean time from catheterization of the IJV to passing the Swan-Ganz catheter into the pulmonary artery wedge position was 2.6 minutes, with 72 percent placed in under 2 minutes.[77] We have found that the time for the entire procedure averages about 15 minutes after a little practice. The success rate was 97 percent (74 of 76) in Zaidan's study. Premature ventricular contractions (PVCs) were the most common complication, occurring in 58 percent of his patients.

Table 3-3
Intracardiac Pressures

Cardiac Location	Normal Pressures (torr)	
	Mean	*Range*
RA	5	1–10
RV	25/5	15–30/0–8
PA S/D	23/9	15–30/5–15
PAP	15	10–20
PCWP	10	5–15
LAP	8	4–12
LVEDP	8	4–12

The patient is first attached to an electrocardiograph for continuous monitoring throughout the procedure. The anatomy of the neck is defined, and a surgical prep and draping is performed. The right IJV is identified with a 22-gauge needle as in the CVP cannulation technique (see above). Then an 18-gauge, thin-walled, 2½-inch Teflon catheter is placed into the vein and threaded down the vessel for a short distance (Fig. 3-13).[77A] This is a key step to be sure that the catheter threads easily and that

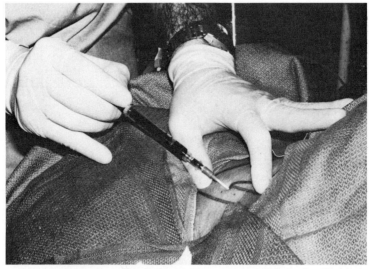

Fig. 3-13. The patient's right neck is sterilely prepped while he is sedated, and local anesthesia is used. The internal jugular vein has previously been identified with a 22-gauge needle. The 22-gauge needle has then been replaced with an 18-gauge, thin-walled, 2½-inch Teflon catheter, which is slowly advanced down the internal jugular vein.

blood can be freely aspirated from the vein. The reason this step is so important is that the rest of the procedure is *blind* and the introducer can inadvertently be passed into other structures if this step is incorrectly performed. The catheter introduction set is used at this point. The guide wire's flexible end is passed through the 18-gauge catheter into the superior vena cava, and the 18-gauge catheter is removed (Fig. 3-14). The wire must advance easily without too much resistance or one should not proceed to the next step. The skin hole around the guide wire is enlarged with a No. 11 scapel blade to allow introduction of the dilator set. The dilator set consists of an internal vessel dilator and an external 10-gauge catheter sheath. This combination is passed into the IJV over the guide wire by a twisting motion until the catheter sheath is in the superior vena cava (Fig. 3-15). Then the 7-Fr Swan-Ganz catheter, which has been filled with fluid and attached to a transducer, is passed through the sheath into the superior vena cava, with the tip pointed up toward the pulmonary outflow tract (Fig. 3-16). The Swan-Ganz catheter is advanced about 20 cm into the superior vena cava and then 1 cc of air is put into the balloon to allow it to float into the right ventricle. When it reaches the right ventricle, 1.5 cc of air is put into the balloon to totally cover the tip of the catheter in an effort to reduce ventri-

cular arrhythmias. The location of the catheter tip is determined by the venous pressure tracing as shown above. If multiple PVCs or runs of ventricular tachycardia occur with the catheter in the right ventricle, lidocaine (50–100 mg) can be used to suppress them. In some instances, the augmented stroke volume after the PVC will float the balloon into the pulmonary artery. A large inspiration by the patient can also be used to augment the stroke volume and help pass the catheter into the pulmonary artery. If the catheter does not enter the pulmonary artery by 60 cm, it should be brought back into the right atrium and another pass made. Excessive coiling of the catheter in the right ventricle should be avoided to prevent catheter knotting. When the pulmonary artery is entered, the tracing will change and the diastolic pressure will become elevated. The catheter is further advanced into the wedge position with 1.5 cc of air in the balloon; letting the air out of the balloon will show a pulmonary arterial tracing. The balloon should be left deflated and should be inflated only for short periods of time to measure the PCWP. The pulmonary artery oscilloscopic tracing should be constantly monitored to make sure the catheter does not float out into a constant wedge position and possibly infarct an area of the lung. After proper positioning, the catheter sheath should be removed from the IJV but

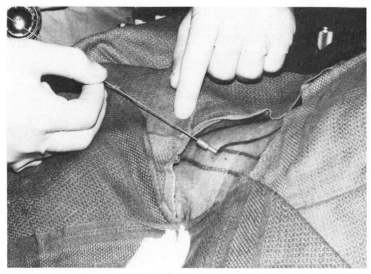

Fig. 3-14. The guide wire easily slides through the 18-gauge catheter and into the superior vena cava. Then the introductory Teflon catheter is removed and the skin hole is enlarged with a No. 11 scalpel blade.

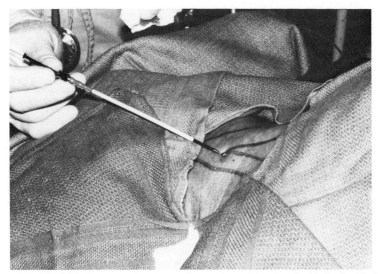

Fig. 3-15. The dilator set is advanced over the guide wire. Inside is the black vessel dilator and outside is the 10-gauge catheter sheath. The white sheath is advanced all the way into the vena cava, and then the wire and dilator are removed.

left under the skin to keep a few centimeters of the catheter sterile for additional manipulations if they are needed. Most often, the catheter has to be pulled back a short distance, as any extra catheter in the right ventricle floats out into the pulmonary artery.

A chest x-ray should be obtained postoperatively in all patients to check the position of the Swan-Ganz catheter. Benumof found that most of the catheters pass into the right middle or lower lobes.[78] We have also found most of the catheters to be in these lobes. The catheters

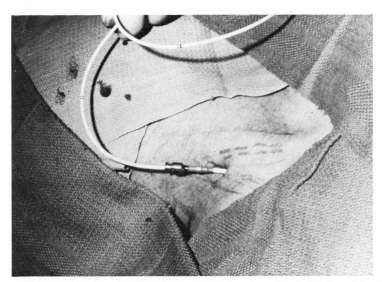

Fig. 3-16. The 7-French Swan-Ganz catheter has been filled with heparinized saline and attached to a venous pressure transducer. The balloon was checked with 1–2 cc of air. Then the catheter is advanced through the catheter sheath into the pulmonary artery.

seem to work best if located proximally in either of these lobes and worst if located in the left lung because of the inherent curvature of the 7-Fr Swan-Ganz catheter. We have found the most ideal position is to have the tip in the right middle or lower lobe, within 5 to 6 cm of where it is seen crossing the catheter passing through the right atrium on the chest x-ray (Fig. 3-17). This places the tip of the catheter in the proximal third of the right lung on the chest x-ray.

As would be expected, many problems can be anticipated with the use of right heart catheterization with the Swan-Ganz catheter. The following complications have been reported:[79]

A. Immediate
1. Supraventricular and ventricular arrhythmias on insertion: Katz reported a 17 percent incidence of PVCs on passing the catheters and 1 case of ventricular tachycardia and fibrillation.[80] Geha reported a persistent supraventricular arrhythmia;[81] and Abernathy reported a case of third-degree heart block and death.[82]

2. Other complications associated with cannulation of central veins: e.g., arterial puncture, air emboli, etc. (see CVP above).

B. Long term
1. Balloon rupture: This is not uncommon when the catheters have been left in place for more than a few days or when the balloon is inflated with more than 1.5 cc of air. Small volumes of air injected into the pulmonary artery will be of no consequence, and rupture can be diagnosed if the injected air cannot be withdrawn. In patients with right-to-left shunts, carbon dioxide should be used for inflation, and great care must be taken not to rupture the balloon, with the attendant possibility of systemic gas embolization.

2. Pulmonary infarction: Foote reported a 7.2 percent incidence of ischemic infarction of the lung in 125 patients with Swan-Ganz catheters.[83] This incidence can be markedly reduced by continuously monitoring the pulmonary artery

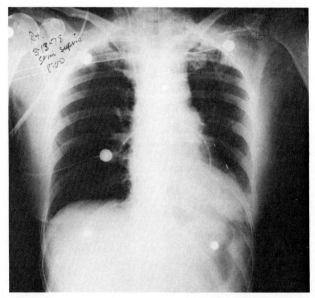

Fig. 3-17. The Swan-Ganz catheter is shown to have passed through the right internal jugular vein, down the superior vena cava, through the right atrium and right ventricle, and out into the right pulmonary artery. Note that the tip is just somewhat slightly beyond the point where the catheter crosses the superior vena cava. This is ideal positioning of the Swan-Ganz catheter.

trace for inadvertent wedging and by frequent checks of the catheter tip position by chest x-ray. The largest pulmonary infarctions can be induced by leaving the balloon inflated, and therefore this should be avoided (Fig. 3-18).

3. Pulmonary rupture: Rapid inflation of the balloon can damage the pulmonary artery wall and lead to production of hemoptysis or hemorrhage.[84] This can be avoided by slow inflation of the balloon to the minimum volume necessary to wedge it.

4. Knotting: This is more likely with the smaller 5-Fr catheters, which are very flexible.[85] Knotting has been reported and will be more common if the catheter is advanced excessively in the right ventricle when one is unable to pass it out into the pulmonary artery.[86] The catheter should not be advanced further than 60 cm from the right IJV or more than 15 cm once it enters the right ventricle if it does not pass into the pulmonary artery.

5. Formation of thrombotic endocardial vegetations: These were found in 4 of 24 patients in one series and in 5 of 413 in another recently reported series.[87,88]

6. Infections: Both local and generalized systemic infections have been reported in patients with Swan-Ganz catheters in place.[89] Such infections require removal of the catheter.

7. Erroneous diagnosis from malfunctioning catheters: Malfunctions of the catheter and balloon can lead to spurious numbers for the PCWP and incorrect treatment of the patient. Shin reported on the problem of eccentric inflation of the balloon, with the catheter tip impinging on the pulmonary artery wall.[90] This causes "pseudo-wedging" of the catheter and an incorrect estimate of LAP. This can be avoided, to some degree, by always being sure the PCWP is less than the $\overline{PAP}$ and similar to the PA_D pressure. Large errors have also been reported in measuring cardiac outputs by the Fick technique with incorrect blood sampling via the pulmonary artery catheter.[91]

CARDIAC OUTPUT MEASUREMENT

The cardiac output is the amount of blood pumped to the peripheral circulation by the heart per minute. It is a measurement that reflects the status of the *entire circulatory system,* not just the heart. It is governed by autoregulation from the tissues. Cardiac output is affected by a number of peripheral factors, but severe cardiac dysfunction may serve to limit it. The cardiac output equals the stroke volume per beat times the heart rate per minute:

$$CO = SV \times HR$$

Normal average values are a cardiac output of 5-6 liters/min in a 70-kg man, with a stroke volume of 60-90 ml per beat and a heart rate of 80 beats per minute. In order to compare patients of different body sizes, the cardiac output may be corrected in relation to body surface area, and this is the cardiac index which equals the cardiac output divided by the body surface area:

$$CI = \frac{CO}{BSA}$$

The normal value for a 70-kg man is 3–3.5 liters/min/m².[92] A normal person has a tremendous reserve capacity in his ability to increase the cardiac output, with some people attaining outputs of 25–30 liters/min. Factors controlling the cardiac output include venous return to the heart, peripheral vascular resistance, peripheral tissue oxygen need, blood volume, body position, pattern of respiration, heart rate, and myocardial contractility. The heart rate is affected by the central and autonomic nervous systems, and the stroke volume, by the preload, afterload, and myocardial contractility.

Cardiac output monitoring during and after cardiac surgery has recently been increasing in frequency. Serial measurements can be used to assess the general status of the circulation and to determine the appropriate hemodynamic therapy and the subsequent response to the intervention. This is especially important in patients requiring treatment with inotropes, vasodilators, and aortic counterpulsation.

The measured cardiac output value is important, but equally useful are the parameters that may be determined once the cardiac output

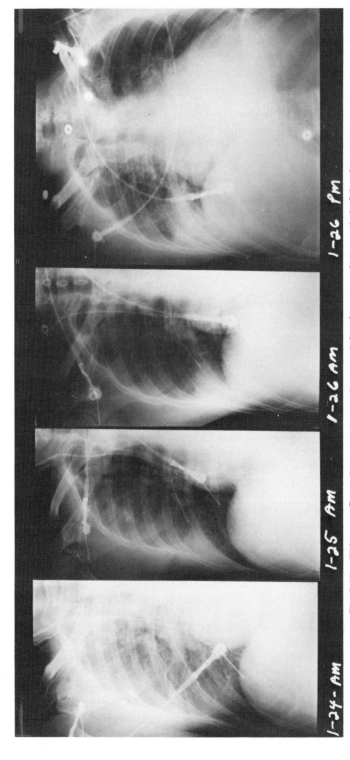

Fig. 3-18. This x-ray figure demonstrates a pulmonary infarction over a 2-day period of time because the Swan-Ganz catheter was too far out in the periphery of the right lung. The second panel, labeled 1-25, shows a triangular-shaped pulmonary infarction. The next two films show evolution of this infarction in a severely ill patient.

Table 3-4
Derived Parameters

Formula	Units	Normal Value
$SV = \dfrac{CO}{HR} \times 1000$	ml/beat	60–90
$SI = \dfrac{SV}{BSA}$	ml/beat/m^2	40–60
$LVSWI = \dfrac{1.36(\overline{MAP} - PCWP)}{100} \times SI$	gram-meters/m^2	45–60
$RVSWI = \dfrac{1.36(\overline{PAP} - PCWP)}{100} \times SI$	gram-meters/m^2	5–10
$TPR = \dfrac{\overline{MAP} - CVP}{CO} \times 80$	dynes-sec/cm^{-5}	900–1500
$PVR = \dfrac{\overline{PAP} - PCWP}{CO} \times 80$	dynes-sec/cm^{-5}	50–150

is known. These parameters include the peripheral and pulmonary resistances, stroke volume, and left ventricular stroke work. These values can then be used to determine ventricular function by deriving Starling curves (see below). Formulas for these parameters, units, and normal values are shown in Table 3-4.

These parameters can be rapidly calculated in the operating room or in the intensive care unit and used to help manage the patient. A cardiac slide rule* can be used to calculate CI, SV, SI, and TPR when CO, MAP, HR and BSA are known (Fig. 3-19). We have found a programmable calculator† to be even more useful in managing the patients. (Fig. 3-19). This can be programmed to give SV, SI, CI, RVSWI, LVSWI, LVMWI, Starling point, PVR and TPR when the HR, $\overline{MAP}$, $\overline{PAP}$, PCWP, CO, and BSA are entered.

There are many techniques currently available to measure cardiac output. The thermal dilution method, employing the Swan-Ganz catheter, is the method of choice for measuring cardiac outputs in the clinical setting. With this technique, multiple outputs can be obtained at frequent intervals; arterial blood withdrawal and reinfusion is not required; the indicator is inert 5 percent dextrose in water; and, in addition,

the catheter allows measurement of filling pressures of both the right and left sides of the heart. Calibration for measurements by this technique is simple to perform, highly reproducible and does not require blood withdrawal. Also, the technique is very suitable to computer analysis, since there is little recirculation of the indicator.

Swan, Ganz, and Forrester introduced their catheter for the thermal dilution method in 1971 and first documented the accuracy and reproducibility of the system.[93,94] They found that thermal-dilution-measured flow was accurate to within 2.2 percent of known pump flow in vitro, with a correlation coefficient of 0.993. In 20 patients, they found the standard deviation of triplicate measurements was 4.6 percent in the range of 2–8 liters/min. Weisel compared the thermal dilution method to the indocyanine green method in 83 subjects and found an excellent correlation ($r = .990$).[95] Kohanna also found a high correlation between dye and thermal dilution cardiac outputs in patients after cardiac surgery ($r = .90$).[96] He felt that the thermal dilution method was more accurate at low outputs (less than 2.0 liters/min), since there is no recirculation of indicator and the indicator curve is sharp and well defined.

In order to get the high rate of reproducibility reported above, the technique of measurement must be standardized. The injectate temperature and volume, as well as the speed of injection, should be carefully controlled and du-

---

* Cardiac Slide Rule, Lexington Instrument Corp., 241 Crescent Street, Waltham, Massachusetts.
† Hewlett-Packard 65 Programmable Calculator.

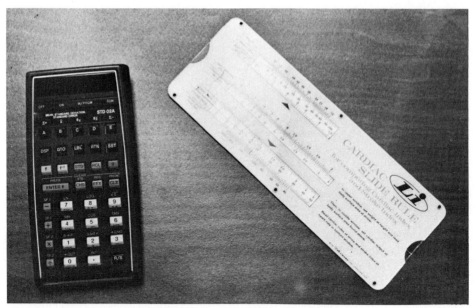

Fig. 3-19. The Lexington Instruments Cardiac Slide Rule is demonstrated as well as the Hewlett-Packard 65 Programmable Calculator that we use for our hemodynamic determinations.

plicated. The most reproducible results have been obtained using injections of 10 ml of cold (0°–2°C) 5 percent dextrose in water. All measurements should be made in duplicate or triplicate during the same phase of respiration. Needed equipment includes a sterile system for maintaining the cold syringes at 0°–2°C, a cardiac output computer, and precise temperature measurements of the injectate and the patient. Additional pieces of equipment that may be used are a mechanical injector for greater reproducibility and a recorder for observation and calculation of the curves.

The 7-Fr Swan-Ganz thermal dilution catheter contains two fine wires that extend the length of the catheter and terminate in a thermistor embedded in the catheter wall just proximal to the balloon. The principle of measurement is similar to the dye dilution method of cardiac output measurements (see below), except that the cold solution acts as the indicator. A known change in the temperature of the blood is induced at one point in the circulation, and the resulting change in temperature is detected at a point downstream. The baseline pulmonary artery body temperature is recorded in the computer, the cold solution is then injected via the CVP port into the right atrium, and the resulting temperature change is detected by the thermistor in the pulmonary artery. A typical thermal dilution temperature time curve, which is similar to a dye dilution curve except for the absence of recirculation and a more protracted downslope is shown in Figure 3-20. The thermistor has a linear relationship between temperature and electrical resistance. It acts as a variable resistor in a Wheatstone bridge, which is balanced before each measurement. The change in temperature alters the resistance and thus the output from the bridge, which is amplified and recorded, and the cardiac output calculated by the computer.[97]

Thermodilution cardiac outputs may also be used in pediatric cardiac surgery. A 4-Fr double lumen catheter may be passed by the surgeon into the pulmonary artery through the right atrium or ventricle. Another technique involves placing a small thermistor in the pulmonary artery and injecting through a separate right atrial catheter. A standard cardiac output computer can be used with a 2-ml aliquot of cold 5 percent dextrose in water. Colgan found a correlation coefficient of 0.976 between this technique and dye dilution in 8 infants and children.[98]

Other methods to measure cardiac output include the standard Fick and dye dilution tech-

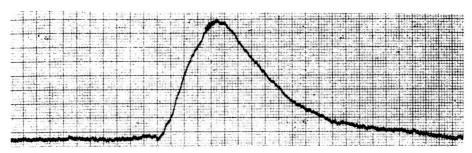

Fig. 3-20. A typical thermodilution cardiac output curve is demonstrated. Note that there is no recirculation peak.

niques and direct flowmeter techniques, including the Doppler and aortic pulse contour measurements. The Fick technique is the standard for steady-state measurements of cardiac output and is said to be accurate to within ±10 percent. The Fick principle states:

$$CO = \frac{V_{O_2}}{A - V_{O_2} \text{ difference}}$$

where CO = cardiac output in milliliters per minute,

V_{O_2} = uptake of oxygen per minute in milliliters per minute,

$A - V_{O_2}$ = arteriovenous oxygen difference in milliliters per milliliter of blood.

The technique is complex and cumbersome, however, involving both the collection of expired gases and right heart catheterization to obtain mixed venous blood.

The indicator dilution method using indocyanine green dye had been the most popular technique of cardiac output measurement prior to the thermal dilution method. This technique consists of rapid injection of a precise amount of dye into the central venous circulation, where the indicator passes rapidly through the heart and lungs and into the arterial circulation, where it is detected by sampling arterial blood and passing it through a densitometer. Recirculation of the indicator is one of the main problems of the technique, since it makes calculation of the area under the primary circulation curve more difficult. A typical dye dilution curve is shown in Figure 3-21 with the recirculation hump.

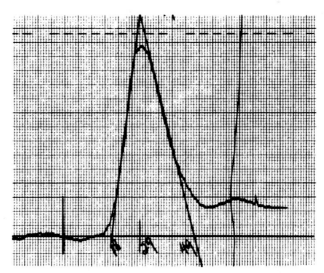

Fig. 3-21. A typical dye dilution curve is shown. There is a recirculation peak. Also, some of the lines have been drawn over it for calculation of the cardiac output by the fore-and-aft triangle method.

The area under the curve must be calculated to derive the cardiac output. This may be done by the following methods:

1. Exponential extrapolation using the *method of Hamilton*, where

$$CO = \frac{I \times 60}{A \times Cal\ f}$$

where I = amount of dye injected,
   Cal f = calibration factor converting the recorder deflection to the concentration of dye,
      A = area plotted on semilogarithmic paper.

2. The *fore-n-aft triangle method*, where

$$CO = \frac{I \times 51.4}{PC \times T_{50} \times Cal\ f}$$

where PC $\times$ T_{50} = area (Fig. 3-21)
      PC = peak concentration of the dye in millimeters,
      T_{50} = time span in seconds from PC_{50} on the ascent to PC_{50} on the descent of the curve.

Bradley found that this rapid method of calculation gave very good correlation with the laborious Hamilton method.[99]

3. *Cardiac output computer methods* to give on-line computation of the dye dilution curves. Carey studied two commercially available computers in 1971 and compared them with arithmetic calculation.[100] He found that one machine had a net error of +11 percent and the other, of −22 percent, and he thus stated that there was a need for improving the technology. Another method of cardiac output measurement using computers is the *aortic pulse contour analysis*. This allows on-line measurement of stroke volume; however, this technique makes assumptions concerning the distensibility of the systemic arterial bed that may not be valid with certain therapeutic interventions, e.g., sodium nitroprusside. Therefore, this technique has been questioned by some and has not gained great popularity.

MEASUREMENTS OF VENTRICULAR FUNCTION

Two categories of measurement techniques are included in this section: (1) ventricular function curves, and (2) contractility measurements. First it is necessary to define some terms that are common in cardiac physiology.[101,102]

Preload is determined by the intraventricular *volume*. This is the initial stretch on the ventricular muscle. Clinically, it is measured by using ventricular *pressure*, which assumes that the ventricular compliance is relatively normal. Occasionally, this can be an incorrect assumption, and misleading information can be obtained. Left ventricular end-diastolic pressure (LVEDP) can be measured with a catheter in the left ventricle, but this is usually done only at cardiac catheterization. Clinically, we use the LAP, PCWP, or PA_D to reflect left ventricular

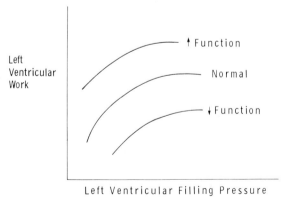

Left Ventricular Work

↑Function

Normal

↓Function

Left Ventricular Filling Pressure

Fig. 3-22. A typical Starling curve is shown. The normal curve is shown in the middle with a hyperfunctioning curve above and a hypofunctioning curve below.

preload and the CVP to measure right ventricular preload.

Afterload is the systolic ventricular wall tension. This is affected by the aortic blood pressure, ventricular radius at end-diastole (preload), and the wall thickness. This demonstrates the complex interaction of the cardiovascular system where the preload is part of the definition of the afterload. Clinically, we measure the MAP, TPR, and PCWP to assess the afterload of the heart.

Contractility (inotropy) describes the force–velocity relationship of muscle contractions at a fixed preload and afterload. This is a difficult parameter to measure clinically, since most of the techniques are unable to hold preload and afterload constant.

Ventricular Function Curves

Multiple measurements of cardiac output and its derivatives, along with ventricular filling pressures, allow the construction of Starling ventricular function curves to aid in patient care. The Frank-Starling mechanism of the heart relates the filling volume of the heart (preload) to the stroke work of the corresponding ventricle. Stroke volume is a function of the diastolic fiber length, with increases in fiber length causing increases in stroke volume up to a certain point. It is possible to overdistend the ventricular muscle and then decrease the stroke volume (descending limb of the curve). A typical Starling curve is shown in Figure 3-22. Preload can be expressed on the horizontal axis as PCWP, and ventricular work, on the vertical axis as LVSWI. These are both measurements of left ventricular function. They could be replaced by CVP and RVSWI to measure right ventricular function. It is not accurate, however, to mix one measurement from each side of the heart, e.g., CVP and LVSWI. Interventions that increase contractility shift the curve up and to the left. Disease states or drugs that depress the heart shift the curve down and to the right.[103]

Ventricular performance curves have been used to define the status of the cardiovascular system and to define the level of the contractile state in a number of studies. Crexells found optimal ventricular performance at a PCWP of 14–18 torr after acute myocardial infarction.[104] Forrester and Swan have used performance curves to divide patients into subsets, after infarction, with different therapies and results according to the subset.[105] Weisel and Gudwin recommend using left ventricular function curves for the management of critically ill medical and surgical patients.[95,106] We have found the use of serial hemodynamic measurements, including Starling curves, to be very useful in a number of situations in the operating room and the intensive care unit.

TREATMENT OF PATIENTS IN HEART FAILURE

Heart failure in patients can occur postoperatively in the intensive care unit or intraoperatively either before or after cardiopulmonary bypass. (Fig. 3-23). A patient may be at point 1 with the following hemodynamics: blood pressure (BP), 80/40 torr; heart rate (HR), 90; cardiac index (CI), 2.0 liters/min/m²; and total peripheral resistance (TPR), 3500 dynes-sec/cm⁻⁵. These values can all be rapidly obtained with the Swan-Ganz catheter and a programmable calculator. If the patient is given an inotropic agent such as dopamine (5–10 µg/kg/min), he will probably move up and to the left (point 2) with an increase in blood pressure and cardiac index. The measurements are needed to document the therapeutic response, however. A vasodilator such as nitroprusside will decrease the TPR, reducing the afterload, and the patient will move up and to the left (point 3) with an increase in blood pressure and cardiac index. If too much nitroprusside is given, however, the patient will lose too much preload and move to point 6 without an increase in blood pressure or cardiac index. A volume infusion will increase the preload and move him from point 6 back to point 3, but this obviously requires close monitoring. Some patients will get the best response from a combination of an inotrope and a vasodilator and move the furthest up and to the left to point 5. It is necessary to add one agent at a time, measure the response, and then add the second drug in this complex pharmacologic scheme of treatment. This technique of treatment maximizes the contractility while minimizing the afterload.[107]

GUIDING THERAPY WITH THE INTRA-AORTIC BALLOON

Serial hemodynamic measurements during aortic counterpulsation have been very helpful.[108] These patients are frequently receiving ino-

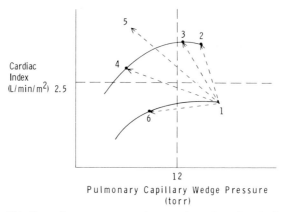

Fig. 3-23. This figure demonstrates a patient at #1 on a hypofunctioning Starling curve. Five therapeutic interventions are made, and the results are demonstrated on the Starling curve. These therapeutic interventions are labeled 2, 3, 4, 5, and 6. See the text for full explanation.

tropes, vasodilators, and positive pressure ventilation along with the balloon support. Specific serial measurements are necessary to be able to judge the effects of each therapy. We have also found the measurements useful in helping to decide if the patient needs the balloon preoperatively or if he is a reasonable risk for anesthesia without counterpulsation, e.g., a patient with four-vessel coronary artery disease, EF = .3, and LVEDP = 20 torr at cardiac catheterization. We bring the patient to the operating room and measure his hemodynamics before deciding if the balloon is indicated. If his BP = 90/60, CI = 3.0 liter/min/m², TPR = 2000 dynes-sec/cm⁻⁵, and he is at point 4 on the above curve, we would give him volume to improve his hemodynamics and not use the balloon. If his BP = 90/60, but his CI = 2.0 liters/min/m², his TPR = 3500 dynes-sec/cm⁻⁵, and he is at point 1, we would consider the balloon or a vasodilator before the surgical procedure.

GUIDING THERAPEUTIC DECISIONS COMING OFF CARDIOPULMONARY BYPASS

Patients are frequently hypotensive at the end of bypass. Additional hemodynamic measurements can take the guesswork out of this difficult situation. For example, if the BP = 80/50, HR = 85, and PCWP = 15 torr, what is the problem? Is the patient dilated with a low peripheral resistance or is his heart not working well? The cardiac output and derived values can give the answer. If his CO = 6.5 liters/min, his TPR will be under 1000 dynes-sec/cm⁻⁵, and he needs a small dose of an alpha constrictor such as phenylephrine. If his CO = 2.5 liters/min, his TPR will be over 3000 dynes-sec/⁻⁵, and he needs an inotrope or a vasodilator or both.

GUIDING THERAPY DURING ANESTHESIA

It is useful to know the patient's left ventricular function at many critical times during surgery because the anesthesia will vary depending on this factor. Two examples will help to explain this:

1. A patient becomes hypertensive during coronary artery surgery with morphine and nitrous oxide anesthesia. If his cardiac output and ventricular function are good, then a myocardial depressant such as halothane is a proper choice to control the blood pressure. If cardiac output is low, however, and TPR is high, a vasodilator such as nitroprusside is a better choice.

2. During aortic aneurysm surgery, there is frequently hypotension after releasing the aortic cross-clamp. Measurements of hemodynamics can rapidly assess whether this is secondary to vasodilation or myocardial depression and guide appropriate therapy for each individual patient.

Measurements of Contractility

The contractile state of the heart is only one of several determinants of its ability to eject blood. The cardiac output and the heart's contractile state cannot be related to one another in a simple manner. Measurements of cardiac output alone are of limited value in deducing the myocardial contractility. It is important to realize the difference between cardiac output and myocardial contractility and not to equate the two.[109]

Considerable controversy exists over the definition and measurement techniques of myocardial contractility. Many techniques have been proposed to measure this elusive factor, and all have had their problems, since most of the techniques are also affected by changes in preload, afterload, and heart rate. Some of these techniques are highly invasive, while others are totally noninvasive.

INVASIVE TECHNIQUES

Force–velocity curve. The force–velocity curve is the basic measurement based on Hill's model of contraction of an isolated muscle. There is an inverse relationship between force and velocity in cardiac muscle. Velocity decreases as the total load (preload and afterload) increases. The maximum velocity of shortening is called V_{max} and is a good measurement of contractility. It is derived by extrapolating the curve to zero load. Positive inotropic interventions shift the curve up and to the right and raise V_{max}.[110] Even V_{max}, however, has been questioned as to its validity as a pure measure of contractility.[111]

Walton-Brodie strain gauge arch. The strain gauge arch can be sutured to the surface of the ventricle to measure contractile force. This technique was used by Morrow to measure the effects of halothane on the intact human heart while on cardiopulmonary bypass.[112]

Rate of pressure development (dP/dt). The rate at which ventricular pressure rises (the first derivative of the ventricular pressure) is called dP/dt and is expressed in millimeters of mercury per second. The normal range is 800–1700 mm Hg/sec.[113] This number can now be obtained during cardiac surgery or catheterization using catheters with microtransducers at their tip which are inserted into the left ventricle and attached to an external differentiating circuit. Many studies have shown that when contractility is augmented, the dP/dt increases. Examples of left ventricular pressure and dP/dt tracings are shown in Figure 3-24. However, dP/dt is also affected by changes in preload, afterload, and heart rate. Increases in any of these three factors also increase dP/dt.[114] This problem has been partially solved by using a series of correction factors. The best measurement is dP/dt/CPIP, where CPIP is the common peak isovolemic pressure. This is the peak pressure common to both the control measurement and the measurement after the intervention. This factor corrects any differences in afterload but not in preload or heart rate, which still must be held relatively constant.[115]

Electromagnetic flowmeters and ultrasound velocity probes. Tomlin has found a good correlation between indices derived from velocity and flow of blood compared to dP/dt.[116] Noble has shown that the maximum acceleration of aortic blood flow is a good measurement of contractility which is relatively independent of preload and afterload.[117] These relatively new techniques may have a lot to offer in the future.

Angiography. Left ventriculography is an important part of a cardiac catheterization and can provide useful information about ventricular function.[118] The ejection fraction is a measurement of overall systolic function and is the difference between the end-diastolic volume and the end-systolic volume. Normal ventricles eject more than 55 percent of their volume (ejection fraction = .55). Abnormalities of left ventricular wall motion can also be observed at catheterization. Inward motion of a wall segment may be totally impaired (akinetic) or partially impaired (hypokinetic). Segments that bulge outward during systole are called dyskinetic. Potential reversibility of these abnormal wall segments is often tested for with nitroglycerin or postextrasystolic potentiation. These measurements are more sensitive measures of myocardial function than is the resting cardiac output, and they are therefore frequently seen to be abnormal in patients with normal cardiac outputs.

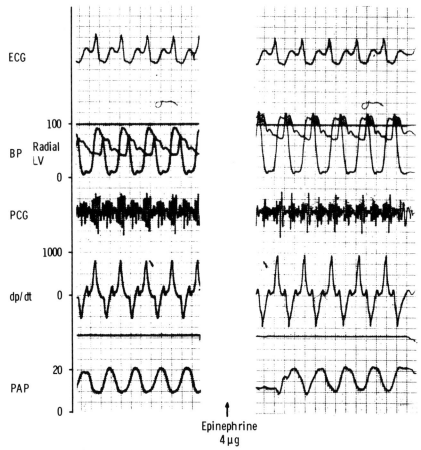

ECG

BP Radial
    LV

PCG

dp/dt

PAP

Epinephrine
4 µg

Fig. 3-24. Hemodynamic responses of a patient during cardiac surgery are demonstrated. The panel on the left was before the administration of 4 µg of epinephrine and the panel on the right after it. Note that the dP/dt changed from 800 to about 950. This was associated with an increase in the radial artery and left ventricular blood pressures to about 110–120 torr. Also shown are the electrocardiogram, phonocardiogram, and pulmonary artery pressure tracings.

NONINVASIVE TECHNIQUES

Systolic time intervals (STI). These measure the phases of left ventricular systole in man and are determined from simultaneous high-speed recordings of the electrocardiogram, phonocardiogram, and an arterial pressure tracing (Fig. 3-25). Total electromechanical systole (QS_2) is the interval from the onset of the QRS complex on the ECG to the first major deflection of the second heart sound. The left ventricular ejection time (LVET) is the phase of systole when the ventricle ejects blood into the aorta and is measured from the beginning of the arterial upstroke to the dicrotic notch. The pre-ejection period (PEP) is the interval from onset of ventricular depolarization to the beginning of ejection and is derived by subtracting the LVET from the QS_2.[119] These intervals vary with heart rate, and therefore Weissler developed correction factors to adjust for this fact.[120] An ECG lead showing a clear onset of the QRS complex is selected. A chest phonocardiogram is used over the upper precordium when possible. During thoracic surgery an esophageal phonocardiogram is used, similar to the one described by Tonnesen.[121] We use a miniature hearing-aid microphone with a frequency response of 50–15,000 Hz and filter this to the 25–200 Hz range to detect the second heart sound, which has a frequency range of 100–150 Hz. Tonneson showed a good correlation between the time in-

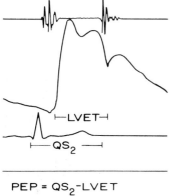

PEP = QS$_2$-LVET

Derived Intervals

PEP/LVET

1/PEP^2

EF = 1.125 - 1.250 PEP/LVET

Fig. 3-25. High-speed recordings of the phonocardiogram, arterial pressure tracing and electrocardiogram are demonstrated. Measurement of the QS$_2$ and LVET is shown. The PEP is derived by subtracting the LVET from the QS$_2$. Further derived intervals are shown at the bottom of the figure.

tervals recorded using the esophageal phonocardiogram versus a chest microphone. Central aortic, carotid, or subclavian arterial tracings are preferred, but more peripheral arterial tracings have been used in some studies. The PEP has been found to be the best of the measured STIs as an estimate of contractility. It changes inversely to the dP/dt measurement, and there is a direct correlation between the externally derived STIs and internal measures of left ventricular function.[122,123] The PEP/LVET ratio shows an even better relation to internal measurements. Increases in contractility decrease the PEP, increase the LVET, and decrease the PEP/LVET ratio from its normal value of 0.35. With decreased left ventricular performance, the PEP increases, LVET shortens, and PEP/LVET increases. These correlate closely with a decreased stroke volume, cardiac output, and ejection fraction. The closest correlation (r = .90) was found between PEP/LVET and the ejection fraction. Garrard even proposed a regression formula for noninvasively deriving the ejection fraction from the STIs:[124]

$$EF = 1.125 - 1.25 \ PEP/LVET$$

A new indirect index of contractility using the PEP along with PCWP has been described by Diamond. The mean electromechanical $\Delta P/\Delta T$ is derived as follows:

$$\frac{\Delta P}{\Delta T} = \frac{DP - PCWP}{PEP}$$

where DP = diastolic blood pressure,
PCWP = wedge pressure,
PEP = preejection period.

This index had a correlation with dP/dt of 0.96 in a study of 18 patients.[125]

Several studies have shown that the STIs, especially PEP, are influenced by changes in the preload and afterload. The PEP is lengthened by increased afterload and shortened by increased preload. PEP/LVET is somewhat less affected by these changes but is still altered. Reitan proposed the use of 1/PEP^2, which correlated well with peak ascending aortic blood flow.[126] Peak blood flow acceleration is minimally affected by changes in loading conditions, and therefore 1/PEP^2 may be the STI least affected by these factors.

The STIs have been used to study patients with coronary artery disease, acute infarctions, and valvular heart disease. They have also been used in clinical studies of drug effects and comparisons of anesthetic agents.[127] Table 3-5 summarizes the factors affecting STIs. Recently, attempts have been made to use STIs as on-line monitors of ventricular function during anesthesia and surgery.[128] In the future, these may provide the anesthesiologist with additional clinically useful information about the cardiovascular system.

Ballistocardiogram (BCG). The BCG is a complex apparatus designed to record body motion produced by cardiovascular phenomena. The BCG was studied extensively by Starr, and Harrison showed a good correlation between the I-J wave of the BCG and dP/dt.[129] In recent years, however, there has arisen a fair amount of skepticism and criticism concerning the merits and uses of this technique.[130] In anesthesia, the BCG has been used to measure contractility during hemodynamic studies of anesthetic agents in volunteers by one group of investigators.[131]

Table 3-5
Systolic Time Intervals: Influencing Factors

	QS$_2$	PEP	LVET	PEP/LVET
1. Tachycardia				
a. Spontaneous	↓	↓	↓	
b. Atrial pacing	↓	→	↓	
c. Vagal blockade	↓	→	↓	
d. Adrenergic stimulation	↓	↓	↓	
2. Increased afterload	↑	↑	↑	
3. Increased preload	→	↓	↑	↓
4. Inotropes	↓	↓	↕	
5. Beta blockade	→	↑	↕	↑
6. Decreased left ventricular performance	→	↑	↓	↑
7. A.S. and/or A.I. without CHF	↑	↓	↑	↓
A.S. and/or A.I. with CHF	→	↑	↓	↑
A.S. and/or M.I. with CHF	→	↑	↓	↑
8. Chronic hypertension without CHF	→	→	→	
Chronic hypertension with CHF	→	↑	↓	↑
9. Acute myocardial infarction with CHF	↓	↑	↓	↑
10. LBBB	→	↑	→	↑
RBBB	→	→	→	
11. Advanced age	↑	↑	↑	
12. Upon assuming an erect posture	↓	↑	↓	↑
13. 4–8 PM diurnal cycle	↓	→	↓	↑

Code:
  ↑ *Increased time interval*
  ↓ *Decreased time interval*
  → *Unchanged time interval*

Echocardiography. Echocardiography is a relatively new technique that has become extremely popular in modern cardiology but is only beginning to be applied to the field of anesthesiology. It could prove very useful in studies of anesthetic agents and ventricular function. The echocardiogram is useful for measuring right or left ventricular function (ejection fraction or wall motion), analyzing valve function, and detecting pericardial effusions.[132]

Radioisotopic techniques. Measurements of ventricular function, including the ejection fraction, can be obtained using radiopharmaceuticals, such as labeled albumin, and a scintillation counter.[133] The use of mobile scintillation counters and computers makes these measurements available at the bedside of the sickest patient. It is not unreasonable to expect an expansion of the uses of this technique in the future.

Electrocardiogram. The ECG in patients with coronary artery disease may prove useful as a simple, noninvasive guide to assessment of left ventricular function.[134] Askenazi correlated the sum of R waves in leads AVL, AVF, and $V_1 - V_6$ (ΣR) with the ejection fraction. Among patients with ΣR less than 4.0 Mv, the PVC augmented ejection fraction was less than 0.45 in 73 percent; while in patients with ΣR of 4.0 Mv or more, the augmented ejection fraction was greater than 0.45 in 93 percent.

HEMODYNAMIC MEASUREMENTS OF MYOCARDIAL ISCHEMIA

There is a delicate balance between the myocardial oxygen supply and the oxygen demand in patients with coronary artery disease. (Figure 3-26) The myocardial oxygen supply depends on the following factors:

  1. Coronary blood flow
      a. Patency of coronary arteries

   b. Aortic diastolic blood pressure
   c. Intracavitary end-diastolic pressure
   d. Diastolic filling time
2. Oxygen content of coronary artery blood
   a. Hemoglobin content
   b. Arterial oxygen tension (Pao_2)
   c. Position of the hemoglobin-dissociation curve

Determinants of the myocardial oxygen demand (myocardial oxygen consumption {MVO_2}) include:[135,136]

1. Systolic wall tension
   a. Aortic systolic blood pressure
   b. Left ventricular end-diastolic pressure
   c. Ventricular volume
2. Contractile state of the myocardium
3. Heart rate
4. Other less important factors
   a. Basal cost—oxygen use of the non-
       beating heart
   b. Oxygen cost of depolarization
   c. Direct metabolic cost of catecholamines
   d. Activation cost of calcium
   e. Energy of maintenance of the active state
   f. Fenn effect—cost of shortening against a load

These factors affecting the oxygen supply and demand of the myocardium are becoming increasingly important, since we can now measure many of the variables and influence the myocardial oxygen balance. For example, Braunwald has shown that positive inotropic drugs such as norepinephrine, calcium, or digitalis increase both dP/dt (contractility) and MVO_2 to a similar degree. In addition, negative inotropic drugs such as propranolol or procaine similarly decrease both dP/dt and MVO_2.

Measurements of Myocardial Oxygen Supply

CORONARY BLOOD FLOW (CBF)

Coronary blood flow is regulated by the following equation:

$$\dot{Q} = \frac{\Delta P}{R}$$

where $\dot{Q}$ = coronary blood flow,
ΔP = driving pressure across the coronary vascular bed,
R = total coronary resistance.

Total coronary resistance is made up of:[137]

1. Basal resistance tone in diastole.
2. Autoregulatory resistance—major factor affecting the tone of the vessels; under the control of the autonomic nervous system and local metabolites.
3. Compressive resistance—caused by compression of the coronary vessels by intracavitary pressure. This is especially im-

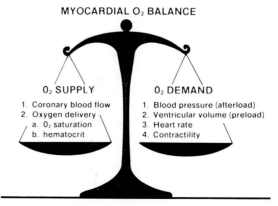

MYOCARDIAL O_2 BALANCE

O_2 SUPPLY
1. Coronary blood flow
2. Oxygen delivery
   a. O_2 saturation
   b. hematocrit

O_2 DEMAND
1. Blood pressure (afterload)
2. Ventricular volume (preload)
3. Heart rate
4. Contractility

Fig. 3-26. The myocardial oxygen balance between the oxygen supply and oxygen demand is demonstrated. Those factors affecting the oxygen supply and oxygen demand are listed on each side.

portant in the subendocardium during systole when the vessels are obstructed secondary to this pressure.

Coronary artery disease with its *stenotic resistance* obviously must also be considered. Flow through stenotic areas is reduced only with severe stenosis (above 60 to 70 percent) and is compensated to some degree by a decreased autoregulatory resistance. Stenosis of the vessel is critical when about 90 percent of the lumen is occluded, and CBF markedly falls. Coronary collateral blood flow may also compensate for decreased CBF to an area of the heart. Collateral flow may be either (1) intercoronary, i.e., connect capillary beds of two different coronary arteries; or (2) intracoronary, i.e., connect vessels within the same capillary bed. The rapidity of coronary occlusion appears to play a role in the development of these collateral channels.

There are regional differences in myocardial blood flow that make studies of CBF more difficult. Subendocardial ischemia and infarctions are seen earlier and more commonly than transmural damage, probably because of the coronary flow pattern relative to the needs of the myocardium. In patchy diseases such as coronary artery disease, the disorders of blood flow are typically regional. Thus, measurement of CBF should measure total as well as regional CBF.

Methods of measuring *total* CBF include:[138]

1. Venous sampling techniques: These techniques are based on the Fick principle using inert gases, where

$$CBF = \frac{\text{myocardial inert gas uptake}}{\text{arteriovenous difference of the inert gas}}$$

   Commonly used gases include nitrous oxide, krypton, xenon, hydrogen, and helium. Kety and Schmidt first used this technique with nitrous oxide for measurement of cerebral blood flow. The gases are inhaled, and blood levels of the gases are measured in arterial and coronary sinus blood. CBF for normal patients is 70–90 ml/min/100 gm, while patients with coronary artery disease have values averaging 58 ml/min/100 gm.[139,140]

2. Precordial counting techniques: This is analogous to the above technique and is based on the residue detection of a radioisotope indicator rather than on outflow detection in the coronary sinus. The indicator, xenon, is injected directly into the coronary artery.

3. Coronary sinus thermodilution: Ganz designed a 7-Fr catheter for percutaneous insertion into the coronary sinus to measure total CBF.[141] The principle and operation are similar to the thermal dilution cardiac output measurements. In 14 patients studied by Ganz, the coronary sinus outflow averaged 122 ml/min. This predominantly represents flow from the left coronary system.

4. Absolute flow of the entire heart with isotope counting: Radioactive isotopes of potassium or rubidium are injected into the left atrium and detected by a scinticamera. The advantage of this is that it measures total CBF in milliliters per minute without regard for the unknown myocardial mass.

Methods of measuring *regional* CBF are rapidly being developed and offer an exciting new look at coronary artery disease.[142]

1. Steady imaging: This approach is used when the myocardial distribution of the indicator is assumed to be constant. The distribution of the indicator is proportional to the distribution of the CBF. Particulate indicators are most often used, consisting of microspheres of human albumin labeled with isotopes of iodine (^{131}I) or technicium (^{99m}Tc) and ranging in size from 10–30 μ. The indicators are detected by scanners or scinticameras and tell the location of poorly perfused areas or changes in the distribution of the coronary blood flow.

2. Dynamic imaging: Xenon^{133} or thallium is used and is detected by computer analysis of scinticamera pictures. This dynamic study allows regional flow measurement during exercise or drug intervention and permits the evaluation of the site and degree of ischemia as well as response to therapy.

3. Measurement of flow through coronary bypass grafts: This has been measured primarily with electromagnetic flowmeters in the operating room. A number of groups have correlated intraoperative flow measurements with graft patency. Flows of less than 40 ml/min have been associated with increased graft closure. Other groups, including ours, have found these measurements to be very unreliable, however, and

have abandoned the routine intraoperative use of them.

The coronary blood flow depends on the patency of the coronary arteries as well as upon the aortic diastolic blood pressure, diastolic filling time, and the ventricular end-diastolic pressure. The coronary perfusion pressure includes two of these factors and is defined as

$$CPP = DP - LVEDP$$

where CPP = coronary perfusion pressure,
DP = diastolic pressure,
LVEDP = left ventricular end-diastolic pressure.

The *diastolic pressure time index* (DPTI) includes all three of the factors affecting coronary blood flow. This index was introduced by Hoffman and Buckberg in 1974[143,144] (Fig. 3-27). Philips has described a simple clinical formula for deriving the DPTI:[145]

$$DPTI = (\overline{DP} - \overline{LAP}) \times T_D$$

where $\overline{DP}$ = diastolic pressure,
$\overline{LAP}$ = left atrial pressure,
T_D = diastolic time.

Detrimental effects on coronary blood flow can easily be seen in Figure 3-27. A drop in the $\overline{DP}$ will decrease the DPTI and CPP. The other key factor, however, which is not always recognized, is that an increase in the left ventricular filling pressure (LVEDP, LAP, or PCWP) will also decrease the DPTI and CPP, as well as increasing the myocardial oxygen demand. Thus, an increase in the LVEDP is detrimental in two ways: (1) decreased coronary blood flow and (2) increased MVO_2, thus explaining the severe ischemia seen with overdistention of the left ventricle. Tachycardia is also extremely detrimental because it (1) decreases coronary filling time, and thus DPTI, and (2) increases oxygen demand. Subendocardial ischemia is easily produced by a combination of tachycardia and elevated LVEDP.

Oxygen delivery by the coronary circulation is extremely important because of the extensive oxygen extraction by the heart. Certainly, hypoxia must be avoided in patients with coronary artery disease, and frequent measurements of arterial blood gases are indicated to check the Pa_{O_2}.

The effect of the Pa_{CO_2} on the coronary circulation has only recently been recognized. Lowering the Pa_{CO_2} has been shown to reduce the CBF (Fig. 3-28).

EFFECTS OF IABP ON MYOCARDIAL OXYGEN SUPPLY (DPTI) AND DEMAND (TTI)

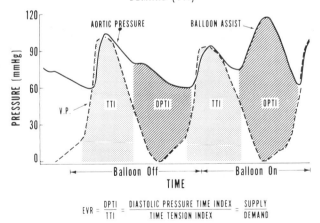

$$EVR = \frac{DPTI}{TTI} = \frac{DIASTOLIC\ PRESSURE\ TIME\ INDEX}{TIME\ TENSION\ INDEX} = \frac{SUPPLY}{DEMAND}$$

Fig. 3-27. The diastolic pressure time index and tension time index areas are shown on the figure. From these the endocardial viability ratio (EVR) is calculated. Effect of the IABP on the endocardial viability ratio is demonstrated. (Reproduced from Bolooki H: Clinical Application of the Intraaortic Balloon Pump, Futura Publishing Co., 1977, with permission of the author and publisher.)

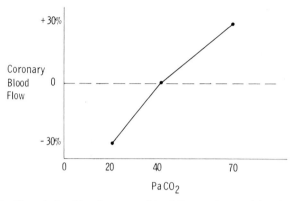

Fig. 3-28. The relationship of coronary blood flow to the arterial carbon dioxide tension is demonstrated. By reducing the $Paco_2$ from 40 down to 20, the coronary blood flow is decreased by about 30 percent. (Adapted from a personal communication by P. Foex.)

Other factors that shift the hemoglobin-dissociation curve to the left should also be avoided in order to maximize the oxygen transport to the myocardium. Therefore, alkalosis, hypoxia, and hypocarbia should all be checked for and avoided in the blood gases. With each blood gas sample, a hematocrit reading should be obtained to avoid intraoperative anemia and preserve the oxygen carrying capacity.

Measurements of Myocardial Oxygen Demand

The four major factors involved are (1) systolic blood pressure and (2) LVEDP (these two together make up the left ventricular wall tension), (3) contractility, and (4) heart rate. In our experience, increases in MVO_2 are more often the cause of ischemia in the operating room than are decreases in oxygen supply. In most cases, ischemia occurs when the MVO_2 exceeds the critical CBF level of the patient with coronary stenosis. There are a series of indices designed to look at these factors, but no one index accounts for all of them.

RATE PRESSURE PRODUCT (RPP)

The RPP, reflecting MVO_2, is obtained by multiplying the systolic blood pressure by the heart rate:

$$RPP = SBP \times HR$$

For example, 15,000 = 150 × 100 (some authors

divide the product by 100):

$$RPP = \frac{SBP \times HR}{100}$$

for example,

$$150 = \frac{150 \times 100}{100}$$

The RPP has been a valuable tool to cardiologists conducting exercise tolerance tests. It holds a relatively constant relationship to the onset of anginal pain. Robinson showed that 20,000 was the RPP at which patients most often have the onset of pain.[146] He correlated RPP with onset of pain but did not report onset of ischemic changes on the ECG. Gobel has shown that the RPP correlates well with myocardial oxygen consumption during exercise in patients with ischemic heart disease ($r = .83$).[147]

Cokkinos showed that there is a constant MVO_2 for each patient at which angina will occur.[148] Each of his patients developed angina at a constant RPP regardless of whether the RPP was produced by augmentation of heart rate (pacing) or blood pressure (angiotensin). The onset of angina was at a RPP of 23,000, and 10 of 12 patients had ischemic ST-segment changes at this level. However, Loeb demonstrated that at similar increases in MVO_2, stress of increased heart rate led to more myocardial ischemia than stress of increased blood pressure.[149]

We have used the RPP intraoperatively as

a guide to MVO_2 during coronary artery surgery. We attempt to keep this below the patient's preoperative maximum RPP while in the hospital. A multiplier circuit has been added to our monitoring equipment so that a continuous RPP is displayed on a digital readout (Fig. 3-29). In a recent study, the RPP was correlated with ischemic changes on the electrocardiogram.[150] (Also see Chapters 4 and 7). All patients whose RPPs were over 12,000 showed ischemic ECG changes in the V_5 lead during the prebypass period of coronary artery surgery. In the group of patients who showed no ischemic changes, the RPP was below 12,000 at all times. In the group of patients with ischemic changes, most had a RPP above 12,000, but some had lower RPPs. This last group can probably be accounted for by the fact that the RPP does not reflect left ventricular end-diastolic volume or pressure at all, both of which are also important in determining the MVO_2. On the basis of this information, we monitor the RPP in all patients with coronary artery disease and maintain it less than 12,000 during surgery; especially during periods of stress such as endotracheal intubation. In the past, large increases in the RPP were associated with ischemia during intubation under too light an anesthetic.

TRIPLE INDEX (TI)

The TI is used in an effort to include the left ventricular end-diastolic volume or pressure in our assessment of the MVO_2. The formula we use is

$$TI = SBP \times HR \times PCWP$$

and we try to keep this index under 150,000. We have found that in some cases the TI will be elevated by an increase in the PCWP when the RPP would not show the increased MVO_2. An elevated LVEDP (PCWP) can also cause regional ischemia of the subendocardium by compression of the small coronary arterioles. These cases are relatively rare, however, and the RPP demonstrates most cases of increased MVO_2.

TENSION TIME INDEX (TTI)

The TTI has been studied extensively by Sarnoff and Braunwald.[151] It is defined as the product of the heart rate and the area under the systolic portion of the aortic pressure curve, or more simply as

$$TTI = MSP \times \text{duration of systole}$$

where MSP = mean systolic pressure.

Sarnoff showed a close relationship between the TTI and MVO_2 in a dog model. Others however, have shown the TTI to correlate less well with the MVO_2 than the RPP.[152]

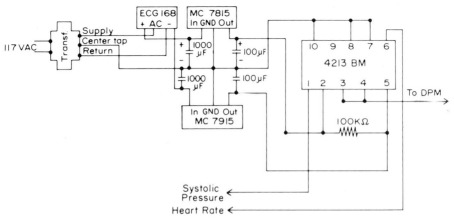

Fig. 3-29. Multiplier and power supply wiring diagram for our rate pressure product digital meter is demonstrated. (This unit was designed and built by Mr. Earl Lerette at Emory University Hospital.)

ENDOCARDIAL VIABILITY RATIO (EVR)

The EVR was proposed by Hoffman and Buckberg to measure *subendocardial* ischemia.[143,144] It compares the ratio of the myocardial oxygen supply to the oxygen demand. To assess the oxygen supply, the DPTI is used, and for oxygen demand, the TTI is utilized.

$$\frac{DPTI}{TTI} = \frac{oxygen\ supply}{oxygen\ demand}$$

(See Fig. 3-27). In most studies, these areas under the systolic and diastolic curves have been measured by planimetry. Recently, Philips described a formula for deriving the EVR from the arterial and PCWP (LAP) traces.[145]

$$EVR = \frac{DPTI}{TTI} = \frac{(\overline{DP} - \overline{LAP}) \times T_D}{\overline{SP} \times T_s}$$

where $\overline{DP}$ = mean diastolic pressure,

$\overline{LAP}$ = mean left atrial pressure (or PCWP),

$\overline{SP}$ = mean systemic arterial pressure,

T_D = diastolic time,

T_s = systolic time.

Note the change in the TTI formula. Sarnoff described the mean *systolic* pressure, but this formula used the mean *systemic* pressure, which is obviously a lower pressure. A commercially available computer can now be used to calculate the EVR off the arterial and pulmonary artery traces using the above formula.

A normal EVR is 1.0 or above where the DPTI equals or exceeds the TTI. When the EVR

Table 3-6
Effects of IABP on the Endocardial Viability Ratio

1. ↑ DPTI
2. ↓ TTI
3. ↓ LAP
4. ↓ HR
5. ↑↑ EVR

is less than 0.7, Hoffman and Buckberg found that the left ventricular endocardial blood flow fell in proportion to the epicardial flow (decreased endo/epi ratio) indicating subendocardial ischemia. The endo/epi ratio fell whether the decreased EVR was secondary to decreased diastolic pressure, increased left atrial pressure, or increased heart rate.

The EVR was described as being useful to detect subendocardial ischemia *after* cardiopulmonary bypass, and we would agree with this use. In patients with coronary artery disease (before bypass grafts), however, the concept of the EVR reflecting subendocardial ischemia is open to debate. We have not found the EVR to correlate closely with ischemic ECG changes in the prebypass period.

It has been shown that Isuprel can lead to myocardial ischemia. The DPTI is decreased as a result of a decreased DP and an increased HR; and the TTI is increased owing to the increased HR. Table 3-6 shows how the IABP can help the subendocardial blood flow and why Philips recommended monitoring of the EVR to determine when to use the IABP.[153]

REFERENCES

1. Berne RM, Levy MN: Cardiovascular Physiology. St Louis, CV Mosby, 1977, pp 99–114

2. Van Bergen FH, Weatherhead DS, Treloar AE, et al: Comparison of indirect and direct methods of measuring arterial blood pressure. Circulation 10:481–490, 1954

3. Whitcher C: Blood pressure measurement. *In* Belville JW, Weaver CS (eds): Clinical Physiology. London, McMillan, 1969, pp 85–124

4. Waltemath CL, Preuss ED: Determination of blood pressure in low flow states by the doppler technique. Anesthesiology 34:77–79, 1971

5. Harken AH, Smith RM: Aortic pressure versus doppler measured peripheral arterial pressure. Anesthesiology 38:184–186, 1973

6. Lebowitz MH: Gangrene of the thumb following the use of the photoelectric plethysmograph during anesthesia. Anesthesiology 32:164–167, 1970

7. Allen EV: Thromboangiitis obliterans: Methods of diagnosis of chronic occlusive arterial lesions distal to the wrist with illustrated cases. Am J Med Sci 178:237–244, 1929

8. Palm T: Evaluation of peripheral arterial pressure in the thumb following radial artery cannulation. Br J Anaesth 49:819–824, 1977

9. Greenhow DE: Incorrect performance of Allen's test—ulnar artery flow erroneously presumed inadequate. Anesthesiology 37:356–357, 1972

10. Brodskay J: A simple method to determine patency of the ulnar artery intraoperatively prior to radial-artery cannulation. Anesthesiology 42:626–627, 1975

11. Mundth ED, Austen WG: Postoperative intensive care in the cardiac surgical patient. Prog Cardiovasc Dis 11:229–261, 1968

12. Ryan JF, Raines J, Dalton BC, et al: Arterial dynamics of radial artery cannulation. Anesth Analg (Cleve) 52:1017–1025, 1973

13. Kaplan JA, Miller ED: Radial artery catheterization. Anesthesiol Rev, January 1976, pp 21–23

14. Frazier WT: Personal communication

15. Lowenstein E, Little JW, Lo HH: Prevention of cerebral embolization from flushing radial artery cannulae. N Engl J Med 285:1414–1415, 1971

16. Downs JB, Chapman RL, Hawkins IF, et al: Prolonged radial artery catheterization. Arch Surg 108:671–673, 1974

17. Gardner RM, Bond EL, Clark JS: Safety and efficacy of continuous flush systems for arterial and pulmonary catheters. Ann Thorac Surg 23:534–538, 1977

18. Bedford RF, Wollman H: Complications of radial artery cannulation. Anesthesiology 38:228–236, 1973

19. Kin JM, Arakawa K, Bliss J: Arterial cannulation: Factors in the development of occlusion. Anesth Analg (Cleve) 54:836–840, 1975

20. Bedford RF: Radial artery function following percutaneous cannulation with 18-gauge and 20-gauge catheters. Anesthesiology 47:37–39, 1977

21. Downs JB, Rackstein AD, Klein EF, et al: Hazards of radial artery catheterization. Anesthesiology 38:283–286, 1973

22. Bedford RF: Percutaneous radial artery cannulation, increased safety using Teflon catheters. Anesthesiology 42:219–222, 1975

23. Bedford RF: Wrist circumference predicts the risk of radial-arterial occlusion after cannulation. Anesthesiology 48:377–378, 1978

24. Bedford RF: Removal of radial artery thrombi following percutaneous cannulation for monitoring. Anesthesiology 46:430–432, 1977

25. Feeley TN: Reestablishment of radial artery patency for arterial monitoring. Anesthesiology 46:73–75, 1975

26. Wyatt R, Glover I, Cooper EJ: Proximal skin necrosis after radial artery cannulation. Lancet 1:1135–1138, 1974

27. Johnson RW: A complication of radial artery cannulation. Anesthesiology 40:598–600, 1974

28. Stamm WE, Colella JJ, Anderson RL, et al: Indwelling arterial catheters as a source of nosocomial bacteremia. N Engl J Med 292:1099–1102, 1975

29. Gardner RM, Schwartz R, Wong HC, et al: Percutaneous in-dwelling radial artery catheters for monitoring cardiovascular function. N Engl J Med 290:1227–1231, 1974

30. Barnes RW, Petersen JL, Krugmire BB, et al: Complications of brachial artery catheterization: Prospective evaluation with the doppler ultrasonic detector. Chest 66:363–367, 1974

31. Barnes RW, Foster EJ, Jansen GA, et al: Safety of brachial artery catheters as monitors in the intensive care unit—prospective evaluation with the Doppler ultrasonic velocity detector. Anesthesiology 44:260–264, 1976

32. Adler DC, Bryan-Brown CW: Use of the axillary artery for intravascular monitoring. Crit Care Med 1:148–150, 1973

33. Seldinger SI: Catheter replacement of the needle in percutaneous arteriography: New technique. Acta Radiol 39:368–376, 1953

34. Ersoz CJ, Hedden M, Lain L: Prolonged femoral artery catheterization for intensive care. Anesth Analg (Cleve) 49:160–164, 1973

35. Kopman EA, Ferguson TB: Intraoperative monitoring of femoral artery pressure during replacement of aneurysms of the descending thoracic aorta. Anesth Analg (Cleve) 56:603–605, 1977

36. Barnhorst BA, Boener HB: Prevalance of generally absent pedal pulses. N Engl J Med 278:264–265, 1968

37. Youngberg JA, Miller ED: Evaluation of percutaneous cannulation of the dorsalis pedis artery. Anesthesiology 44:80–83, 1976

38. Remington JW: Contour changes of the aortic pulse during propagation. Am J Physiol 199:331–334, 1960

39. Johnstone RE, Greenhow DE: Catheterization of the dorsalis pedis artery. Anesthesiology 39:654–655, 1973

40. Hurst JW, Schlant RC: Examination of veins. In Hurst JW, Logue RB (eds): The Heart (ed 4). New York, McGraw-Hill, 1978, pp 193–201

41. English IC, Frew RM, Pigott JF, et al: Percutaneous catheterization of the internal jugular vein. Anaesthesia 24:521–531, 1969

42. Defalque RJ: Percutaneous catheterization of the internal jugular vein. Anesth Analg (Cleve) 53:116–121, 1974

43. Kaplan JA, Miller ED: Internal jugular vein catheterization. Anesthesiol Rev, May 1976, pp 21–23

44. Jernigan WR, Gardner WC, Mahr MM, et al: Use of the internal jugular vein for placement

of central venous catheters. Surg Gynecol Obstet 130:520–524, 1973

45. Mostert JW, Kenny GM, Murphy GP: Safe placement of cardiovascular catheters into the internal jugular vein. Arch Surg 101:431–432, 1970

46. Boulanger M, Delva E, Patiement JM: Une nouvelle voie D'Abord de la veine jugularie interne. Can Anaesth Soc J 23:609–615, 1976

47. Civetta JM, Gabel JC, Gemer M: Internal jugular vein puncture with a margin of safety. Anesthesiology 36:622–623, 1972

48. Petty C: Alternate methods of internal jugular venapuncture for monitoring central venous pressure. Anesth Analg (Cleve) 54:157, 1975

49. Vaughan RW, Weyjandt GR: Reliable percutaneous central venous pressure measurement. Anesth Analg (Cleve) 52:709–716, 1973

50. Kuramoto T, Sakav T: Comparison of success in jugular versus basilic vein techniques for central venous pressure catheter positioning. Anesth Analg (Cleve) 54:696–697, 1975

51. Prince SR, Sullivan RL, Hackel A: Percutaneous catheterization of the internal jugular vein of infants and children. Anesthesiology 44:170–174, 1976

52. Blitt CD, Wright WA, Petty WC, et al: Cardiovascular catheterization via the external jugular vein: A technique employing the J-wire. JAMA 229:817–818, 1974

53. Baum S, Abrams HL: A J-shaped catheter for retrograde catheterization of tortuous vessels. Radiology 83:436–437, 1964

54. Kellner GA, Smart JF: Percutaneous placement of catheters to monitor "central venous pressure." Anesthesiology 36:515–516, 1972

55. Webre DR, Aren JF: Use of cephalic and basilic veins for introduction of cardiovascular catheters. Anesthesiology 38:389–392, 1973

56. Johnston AOB, Clark RG: Malpositioning of cardiovascular catheters. Lancet 2:1395–1397, 1972

57. Burgess GE, Marino RJ, Peuler MJ: Effect of head position on the location of venous catheters inserted via the basilic vein. Anesthesiology 46:212–213, 1977

58. Defalque RJ: Subclavian venapuncture: A review. Anesth Analg (Cleve) 47:677–682, 1968

59. Ortiz J, Dean WF, Zumbro GL, et al: Arteriovenous fistula as a complication of percutaneous internal jugular vein catheterization. Milit Med 141:171, 1976

60. Brown CS, Wallace CT: Chronic hematoma—a complication of percutaneous catheterization of the internal jugular vein. Anesthesiology 45:368–369, 1976

61. Cook TL, Dueker CW: Tension pneumothorax following internal jugular cannulation and general anesthesia. Anesthesiology 45:554–555, 1976

62. Parikh RK: Horner's syndrome: A complication of percutaneous catheterization of the internal jugular vein. Anaesthesia 27:327–329, 1972

63. Khalil KG, Parker FB, Mukherjee M, et al: Thoracic duct injury: A complication of jugular vein catheterization. JAMA 221:908–909, 1972

64. Bell H, Stubbs D, Pugh D: Reliability of central venous pressure as an indicator of left atrial pressure. Chest 59:169–173, 1971

65. Sarnoff SJ, Berglund E: Ventricular function. I. Starling's law of the heart studied by means of simultaneous right and left ventricular function curves in the dog. Circulation 9: 706–718, 1954

66. Forrester JS, Diamond G, McHugh TJ, et al: Filling pressures in the right and left sides of the heart in acute myocardial infarction. N Engl J Med 285:190–193, 1971

67. Civetta JM, Gabel JC, Laver MB: Disparate ventricular function in surgical patients. Surg Forum 22:136–139, 1971

68. Toussaint GPM, Burges JS, Hampson LG: Central venous pressure and pulmonary capillary wedge pressure in critical surgical illness. Arch Surg 109:265–269, 1974

69. Swan HJC, Ganz W, Forrester JS, et al: Catheterization of the heart in man with the use of a flow directed balloon tipped catheter. N Engl J Med 283:447–451, 1970

70. Humphrey CB, Oury JH, Vrigilo RW, et al: An analysis of direct and indirect measurement of left atrial filling pressures. J Thorac Cardiovasc Surg 41:643–647, 1976

71. Lappas D, Lell WA, Gabel JC, et al: Indirect measurement of left atrial pressure in surgical patients—pulmonary capillary wedge pressure and pulmonary artery diastolic pressure compared with left atrial pressure. Anesthesiology 38:394–397, 1973

72. Walston A, Kendall ME: Comparison of pulmonary wedge and left atrial pressure in man. Am Heart J 86:159–164, 1973

73. Lorzman J, Powers SR, Older T, et al: Correlation of pulmonary wedge and left atrial pressure: A study in the patient receiving positive end-expiratory pressure ventilation. Arch Surg 109:270–277, 1974

74. Carroll RM, Laravso RB, Schauble JF: Left ventricular function during aortic surgery. Arch Surg 111:740–743, 1976

75. Mantle JA, Massing GK, James TN, et al: A multipurpose catheter for electrophysiologic and hemodynamic monitoring plus atrial pacing. Chest 72:285–290, 1977

76. Kelman GR: Applied Cardiovascular Physiol-

ogy. London, Appleton-Century-Crofts, 1971, p 53

77. Zaidan J, Lowenstein E, Hallowell P, et al: Routine use of the Swan-Ganz flow-directed pulmonary artery catheter in adult cardiac surgical patients: Time for insertion, success rate, and the incidence of complications in 76 consecutive attempts. Presented at the American Society of Anesthesiologists annual meeting, 1975

77A. Kaplan JA, Miller ED: Insertion of the Swan-Ganz catheter. Anesthesiol Rev, November 1974, pp 22-25

78. Benumof JL, Saidman LJ, Arkin DB, et al: Where pulmonary artery catheters go: Intrathoracic distribution. Anesthesiology 46:336-338, 1977

79. Pace NL: A critique of flow-directed pulmonary artery catheterization. Anesthesiology 47:455-465, 1977

80. Katz JD, Cronau LH, Barash PG, et al: Pulmonary artery flow-guided catheters in the perioperative period: Indications and complications. JAMA 237:2832-2834, 1977

81. Geha DG, Davis NJ, Lappas DG: Persistant atrial arrhythmias associated with placement of a Swan-Ganz catheter. Anesthesiology 39:651-653, 1973

82. Abernathy WS: Complete heart block caused by the Swan-Ganz catheter. Chest 65:349, 1974

83. Foote GA, Schabel SI, Hodges M: Pulmonary complications of the flow-directed balloon tipped catheter. N Engl J Med 290:927-931, 1974

84. Lapin ES, Muriaz JA: Hemoptysis with flow-directed cardiac catheterization. JAMA 220:1246, 1972

85. Buckbinder N, Ganz W: Hemodynamic monitoring: Invasive techniques. Anesthesiology 45:146-155, 1976

86. Lipp H, O'Donoghue K, Resenekov L: Intracardiac knotting of a flow-directed balloon catheter. N Engl J Med 284:220, 1971

87. Greene JF, Cummings KC: Aseptic thrombotic endocardial vegetations. JAMA 225:1525-1526, 1973

88. Pace NL, Horton W: In-dwelling pulmonary artery catheters: Relationship to aseptic thrombotic endocardial vegetations. JAMA 233:893-894, 1975

89. Greene JF, Fitzwater JE, Colemmer TP: Septic endocarditis in in-dwelling pulmonary artery catheters. JAMA 233:891-892, 1975

90. Shin B, McAslan TC, Ayella RJ: Problems with measurements using the Swan-Ganz catheter. Anesthesiology 43:474-476, 1975

91. Suter PM, Lindauer JM, Fairley HB, et al: Errors in data derived from pulmonary artery blood gas values. Crit Care Med 3:175-181, 1975

92. Guyton AC, Jones EC, Holman TG: Circulatory Physiology: Cardiac Output and Its Regulation (ed 2). Philadelphia, WB Saunders, 1973, pp 9-11

93. Ganz W, Donoso R, Marcus HS, et al: A new technique for measurement of cardiac output by thermodilution in man. Am J Cardiol 27:392-396, 1971

94. Forrester JS, Ganz W, Diamond G, et al: Thermodilution cardiac output determinations with a single flow-directed catheter. Am Heart J 83:306-311, 1972

95. Weisel RD, Berger RL, Hectman HB: Measurement of cardiac output by thermodilution. N Engl J Med 292:682-684, 1975

96. Kohanna FH, Cunningham JN: Monitoring of cardiac output by thermodilution after open heart surgery. J Thorac Cardiovasc Surg 73:451-457, 1977

97. Ganz W, Swan HJC: Measurement of blood flow by thermodilution. Am J Cardiol 29:241-246, 1972

98. Colgan FJ, Stewart S: An assessment of cardiac output by thermodilution in infants and children following cardiac surgery. Crit Care Med 5:220-225, 1977

99. Bradley EC, Barr JW: Fore-n-aft triangle formula for rapid estimation of curves. Am Heart J 78:643-648, 1969

100. Carey JS, Williamson H, Scott CR: Accuracy of cardiac output computers. Ann Surg 174:762-768, 1971

101. Braunwald E, Ross J, Sonnenblick EH: Mechanisms of Contraction of the Normal and Failing Heart (ed 2). Boston, Little, Brown, 1976

102. Sonnenblick EH, Strobeck JE: Derived indices of ventricular and myocardial function. N Engl J Med 296:978-982, 1977

103. Sarnoff SJ: Myocardial contractility as described by ventricular function curves: Observations on Starling's law of the heart. Physiol Rev 35:107-122, 1955

104. Crexells C, Chatterjee K, Forrester JS, et al: Optimal level of filling pressure on the left side of the heart in acute myocardial infarction. N Engl J Med 289:1263-1266, 1973

105. Forrester JS, Diamond G, Chatterjee K, et al: Medical therapy of acute myocardial infarction by application of hemodynamic subsets. N Engl J Med 295:1356-1362, 1404-1413, 1976

106. Gudwin AL, Goldstein CR, Cohn JD, et al: Estimation of ventricular mixing volume for prediction of operative mortality in the elderly. Ann Surg 168:183-192, 1968

107. Cohn JN, Franciosa JA: Vasodilator therapy of

heart failure. N Engl J Med 297:27–31, 254–258, 1977

108. Dilley RB, Ross J, Bernstein EF: Serial hemodynamics during intraaortic balloon counterpulsation for cardiogenic shock. Circulation 47, 48 (Suppl 3):99–104, 1973

109. Braunwald E: On the difference between the heart's output and its contractile state. Circulation 43:171–174, 1971

110. Sonnenblick EH, Parmley WE, Urshel CW: The contractile state of the heart as expressed by force velocity relationships. Am J Cardiol 23:488–503, 1969

111. Pollack GH: Maximum velocity as an index of contractility in cardiac muscle: A critical evaluation. Circ Res 26:111–127, 1970

112. Morrow DH, Morrow AG: The effects of halothane on myocardial contractile force and vascular resistance: Direct observations made in patients during cardiopulmonary bypass. Anesthesiology 22:537–541, 1961

113. Gleason WL, Braunwald E: Studies on the first derivative of the ventricular pressure pulse in man. J Clin Invest 41:80–90, 1962

114. Wallace AG, Skinner NS, Mitchell JH: Hemodynamic determinents of the maximal rate of rise of left ventricular pressure. Am J Physiol 205:30–36, 1963

115. Braunwald E, Ross J, Gault JH, et al: Assessment of cardiac function. Ann Intern Med 70:369–399, 1969

116. Tomlin PJ, Duck F, McNulty M, et al: A comparison of methods of evaluating myocardial contractility. Can Anaesth Soc J 22:436–448, 1975

117. Nobel M, Trenchard D, Guz A: Left ventricular ejection in conscious dogs: I. Measurement and significance of the maximum acceleration of blood from the left ventricle. Circ Res 19:139–147, 1966

118. Alderman EL: Angiographic indicators of left ventricular function. JAMA 236:1055–1058, 1976

119. Weissler AM: Systolic time intervals. N Engl J Med 296:321–324, 1977

120. Weissler AM, Harris WS, Schoenfled CD: Systolic time intervals in heart failure in man. Circulation 37:149–159, 1968

121. Tonnesen AS, Gabel JC, Cooper JR, et al: Intraesophageal microphone for phonocardiographic recording. Anesthesiology 46:70–71, 1977

122. Martin CE, Shaver JS, Thompson ME: Direct correlation of external systolic time intervals with internal indices of left ventricular function in man. Circulation 44:419–431, 1971

123. Talley RL, Meyer JF, McNay JL: Evaluation of the pre-ejection period as an estimate of myocardial contractility in dogs. Am J Cardiol 27:384–391, 1971

124. Garrard CL, Wessler AM, Dodge HT: The relationship of alterations in systolic time intervals to ejection fraction in patients with cardiac disease. Circulation 42:455–462, 1970

125. Diamond G, Forrester JS, Chatterjee K, et al: Mean electromechanical $\Delta P/\Delta T$. Am J Cardiol 30:338–341, 1972

126. Reitan JA, Smith NT, Barrison VS, et al: The cardiac preejection period. Anesthesiology 36:76–80, 1972

127. Lewis RP, Rittgess SE, Forrester WF, et al: A critical review of the systolic time intervals. Circulation 56:146–158, 1977

128. Dauchot PJ, Rasmussen JP, Nicholson DH, et al: On-line systolic time intervals during anesthesia in patients with and without heart disease. Anesthesiology 44:472–480, 1976

129. Harrison WK, Friessenger GC, Johnson SL, et al: Relation of the ballistocardiogram to left ventricular pressure measurements in man. Am J Cardiol 23:673–678, 1969

130. Eddleman EE, Harrison WK, Jackson WDH, et al: A critical appraisal of ballistocardiography. Am J Cardiol 29:120–122, 1972

131. Stevens WC, Cromwell TH, Halsey MJ, et al: The cardiovascular effects of a new inhalation anesthetic, Forane, in human volunteers at constant arterial carbon dioxide tension. Anesthesiology 35:8–16, 1971

132. Wexler LF, Pohost GM: Hemodynamic monitoring: Non-invasive techniques. Anesthesiology 45:156–183, 1976

133. Pitt B, Strauss HW: Evaluation of ventricular function by radioisotopic techniques. N Engl J Med 296:1097–1099, 1977

134. Askenazi J, Parisi AF, Cohn PF, et al: Value of the QRS complex in assessing left ventricular ejection fraction. Am J Cardiol 41:494–499, 1978

135. Braunwald E: Control of myocardial oxygen consumption: Physiologic and clinical considerations. Am J Cardiol 27:416–432, 1971

136. Hoffman JIE, Buckberg GD: The myocardial supply:demand ratio. A critical review. Am J Cardiol 41:327–332, 1978

137. Klocke FJ, Mates RE, Copely DP, et al: Physiology of the coronary circulation in health and coronary artery disease. *In* Yu PN, Goodwin JF (eds): Progress in Cardiology. Philadelphia, Lea and Febinger, 1976, pp 1–17

138. Klocke FJ: Clinical measurements of coronary blood flow. *In* Yu PN, Goodwin JF (eds): Progress in Cardiology. Philadelphia, Lea and Febinger, 1976, pp 91–130

139. Rowe GG, Thomsen JH, Stenlund RR: A study

of hemodynamics and coronary blood flow in man with coronary artery disease. Circulation 39:139–148, 1969

140. Rowe GG, Castillo CA, Afonso S: Coronary flow measured by nitrous oxide method. Am Heart J 67:457–468, 1964

141. Ganz W, Tamura K, Marcus HS: Measurements of coronary sinus blood flow by continuous thermodilution in man. Circulation 44:181–195, 1971

142. Maseri A: Radioactive tracer techniques for evaluating coronary blood flow. *In* Yu PN, Goodwin JF (eds): Progress in Cardiology. Philadelphia, Lea and Febinger, 1976, pp 141–168

143. Hoffman JIE, Buckberg GD: Regional myocardial ischemia—causes, prediction, and prevention. Vasc Surg 8:115–130, 1974

144. Hoffman JIE, Buckberg GD: Pathophysiology of subendocardial ischemia. Br Med J 1:76–79, 1975

145. Philips PA, Marty AT, Miyamoto AM: A clinical method of detecting subendocardial ischemia after cardiopulmonary bypass. J Thorac Cardiovasc Surg 69:30–39, 1975

146. Robinson BF: Relation of heart rate and systolic blood pressure to the onset of pain and angina pectoris. Circulation 25:1073–1083, 1967

147. Gobel FL, Nordstrom LA, Nelson RR, et al: The rate pressure product as an index of myocardial oxygen consumption during exercise in patients with angina pectoris. Circulation 57:549–556, 1978

148. Cokkinos DV, Voridis EM: Constancy of rate-pressure-product in pacing induced angina pectoris. Br Heart J 38:39–42, 1975

149. Loeb HS, Saudye A, Croke RP, et al: Effects of pharmacologically induced hypertension on myocardial ischemia and coronary hemodynamics in patients with fixed coronary obstruction. Circulation 57:41–46, 1978

150. Kaplan JA, Jones EL: Monitoring of myocardial ischemia during coronary artery surgery. Abstract presented at the American Society of Anesthesiologists annual meeting, 1977

151. Sarnoff SJ, Braunwald E, Welch GH, et al: Hemodynamic determinants of oxygen consumption of the heart with special reference to the tension time index. Am J Physiol 192:148–156, 1958

152. Monroe RG: Myocardial oxygen consumption during ventricular contraction and relaxation. Circ Res 14:294–300, 1964

153. Philips PA, Bregman D: Intraoperative application of intraaortic balloon counterpulsation determined by clinical monitoring of the endocardial viability ratio. Ann Thorac Surg 23:45–51, 1977

Joel A. Kaplan, M.D.

4
Electrocardiographic Monitoring

The electrocardiogram (ECG) is a graphic representation of the electrical potential produced by the heart and its conduction system. The ECG is being used more and more by the anesthesiologist, and therefore a better and more detailed understanding of it is required. All preoperative patients over the age of 40 years and all those below 40 years with cardiac disease need an ECG. The ECG is being used with increasing frequency during anesthesia and postoperatively in the recovery room and intensive care unit. In addition, during postoperative rounds the anesthesiologist is faced with the interpretation of ECGs. Table 4-1 points out some of the areas of usefulness of the ECG.

BASIC ELECTROPHYSIOLOGY

The electrical conduction system of the heart and its anatomic relationships are shown in Figure 4-1.

The primary function of the sinoatrial (SA) node is the initiation of the cardiac impulse. It consists of a bundle of specialized neural tissue that lies on the endocardial surface of the right atrium at the junction of the superior vena cava and right atrial appendage.[1] The SA node is the pacemaker of the heart because it has the most rapid spontaneous phase 4 depolarization of any normal cardiac tissue (Fig. 4-2).

If the SA node fails to function, a secondary slower pacemaker will take over. The SA node normally fires 60 to 100 impulses per minute, while the atrioventricular node (AV) will fire 45 to 50 times per minute, and the ventricular Purkinje system will fire 30 to 40 times per minute. Thus the rate will become slower as the pacemaker moves further down, away from the SA node.[2] The SA nodal impulse spreads through the internodal pathways and atrial muscle, providing the P wave of the ECG, and arrives in the AV node. This specialized neuromuscular tissue is located on the endocardial surface on the right atrial side of the interatrial septum near the tricuspid valve and just inferior to the opening of the coronary sinus. The rapidly moving impulse is abruptly delayed in the AV node because of its complex conducting system. The delay in the AV node is normally 70-100 msec. The impulse next arrives at the bundle of His, located on the right side of the atrial septum immediately above the interventricular septum. The right and left bundle branches arise from the bifurcation of the lower part of the bundle of His in the membranous portion of the interventricular septum and are located on either side of the interventricular septum. These are the most rapidly conducting tissues of the heart, and the passage of the impulse through them does not even appear on the usual surface ECG. The left bundle divides into the anterior or superior

117

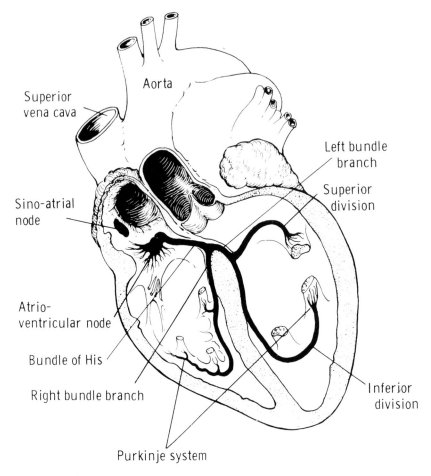

Illustration of Conduction System

ELECTRICAL CONDUCTION THROUGH THE HEART

Fig. 4-1. The electrical conduction system of the heart is demonstrated (Reproduced from Goldman MJ: Principles of Clinical Electrocardiography, Los Altos, Lange, 1976, with permission of author and publisher.)

division and the posterior or inferior division. After passing through the bundles, the impulses arrive in the Purkinje system, which covers the subendocardial surfaces of both ventricles. Then the impulse passes from the endocardial to the epicardial surface of the ventricular muscle, producing the QRS complex of the ECG.[3]

The ECG is the recording of the electrical forces produced by the heart. This may be on a written record as from an ECG machine or on an oscilloscopic tracing in the operating room or intensive care unit. The normal ECG tracing and definition of wave forms and intervals are shown in Figure 4-3. The P wave represents atrial depolarization. Atrial repolarization is usually not seen, but there is a T_a wave buried in the QRS complex. The QRS complex is ventricular depolarization and the T wave is ventricular repolarization. The U wave sometimes follows the T wave and should have the same polarity as the T wave. Its precise significance is uncertain, but it most likely represents phase 3 repolari-

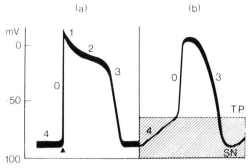

Fig. 4-2. Action potential of a ventricular muscle is shown in panel A and that of the sinoatrial node in panel B. The threshold potential (TP) is shown as −70 mV. Phases 1–4 of the action potential are demonstrated. (Reproduced from Krikler DN: The Paroxysmal Supraventricular Tachyarrhythmias. *In* Yew and Goodwin (eds): Progress in Cardiology, Philadelphia, Lea and Febiger, 1976, with permission of author and publisher.)

Table 4-1
Uses of the Electrocardiogram

I. *Preoperatively*
1. Rate and rhythm disturbances
2. Ischemic heart disease
3. Chamber enlargement
4. Heart block
5. Electrolyte and/or drug effects
6. Pericardial disease
II. *Intraoperatively*
1. Arrhythmia detection
2. Ischemia detection
3. Electrolyte changes
4. Pacemaker function
III. *Postoperatively*
1. Arrhythmia detection
2. Myocardial infarction

zation of the Purkinje system. The P-R interval should be less than 0.20 seconds, the QRS interval less than 0.10 seconds, and the Q-T interval less than one-half the R-R interval.

ELECTROCARDIOGRAPHIC LEAD SYSTEMS

The usual ECG lead system is composed of five electrodes, one on each extremity and one on the chest. The right leg lead serves only as an inactive ground electrode. Each lead measures the electrical potential between two of the electrodes or between one electrode and a combination of the others. Figure 4-4 shows Ein-

thoven's triangle and the standard limb leads.

The three standard limb leads are the most useful leads overall. Most arrhythmias and heart blocks can be diagnosed from them. Lead I connects the right and left arms; lead II, the right arm and left leg; and lead III, the left arm and left leg. The electrodes can be attached anywhere on the extremities or on the trunk at the root of the extremity, e.g., shoulder. The polarity of the leads is also shown in Figure 4-4.

The standard limb leads have disadvantages: (1) each is derived from two points (bipolar) distant from the heart, and (2) all three leads are in the same frontal body plane.[4] Additional information can be obtained by placing electrodes closer to the heart or around the thorax. The precordial V leads are unipolar, using the four extremity electrodes to form a

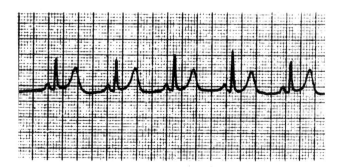

Fig. 4-3. A normal electrocardiogram is demonstrated with the P, QRS, and T waves. P-R interval and Q-T intervals are also shown.

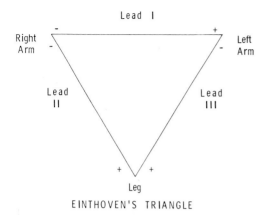

EINTHOVEN'S TRIANGLE

Fig. 4-4. Einthoven's triangle is demonstrated. The three standard leads are shown, as well as their electrical polarity.

central indifferent terminal, and then an active exploring electrode is placed at one of the six usual chest lead positions. The V_1 lead has the active electrode to the right of the sternum in the fourth interspace; V_2 is to the left of the sternum in the fourth interspace; V_4 is in the midclavicular line in the fifth interspace; V_3 is halfway between V_2 and V_4; V_5 and V_6 are in the fifth interspace in the anterior axillary and midaxillary lines, respectively. These leads are most helpful in diagnosing rotational changes of the heart, ventricular hypertrophy, bundle branch patterns, and ischemia of the anterior, anteroseptal, and lateral areas of the ventricles. Precordial mapping techniques have recently been used to localize and quantitate myocardial ischemia and infarction. Systems of 30 leads and more have been used by various investigators. Maroko described a "35-lead blanket" consisting of five vertical rows (A—E) with seven leads on each row (V_1-V_7).[5,6]

During exercise stress testing, other lead systems have been used to identify ischemia.[7] Many of these have used a bipolar lead system, with the positive electrode in the V_5 position. The CM_5 lead has the positive electrode at V_5 and the negative electrode on the upper sternum (manubrium); while the CS_5 lead has the negative electrode just below the right clavicle. The CM_5 is the most popular lead for stress testing because of its simplicity (two electrodes) and high incidence of positive findings.

Unipolar augmented limb leads are also used and are labeled AVR, AVL, and AVF. In these, the electrodes from two extremities (e.g., right arm and left arm) are made the central inactive terminal, and the other extremity (left leg) is the active electrode—this example being the AVF lead. These leads make up the algebraic parts of the standard bipolar limb leads as follows:

$$\text{Lead I} = \text{AVL} - \text{AVR}$$
$$\text{Lead II} = \text{AVF} - \text{AVR}$$
$$\text{Lead III} = \text{AVF} - \text{AVL}$$

Unipolar esophageal leads have been used to record atrial complexes and diagnose arrhythmias. The active electrode is placed in the esophagus and thus the posterior surface of the left ventricle and the atrioventricular junction can be explored.[8]

The MCL_1 lead is popular for cardiac monitoring, arrhythmia detection, and conduction disturbance monitoring in coronary care units.[9] The MCL_1 lead is a modified lead V_1, which is the best single lead to detect arrhythmias. This is a bipolar lead, with the positive electrode to the right of the sternum in the fourth interspace (V_1 position), while the negative electrode is placed near the left shoulder under the left clavicle. A typical tracing of an MCL_1 lead is shown in Figure 4-5.

Another lead that can be examined when trying to record clear atrial complexes (P waves) takes advantage of the atrial vector forces which are oriented anteriorly, inferiorly, and leftward. The right arm electrode is placed just to the right of the manubrium of the sternum, and the left arm electrode, on the zyphoid sternum.

Intracardiac electrocardiography has also been used for diagnostic purposes, since it is relatively easy to obtain. In the past, a long central venous pressure catheter was filled with hypertonic saline and advanced into the cardiac chambers. The catheter was attached to the V lead of the ECG by an alligator clip. When the catheter reached the superior vena cava, the ECG tracing looked like a normal lead AVR with inverted P, QRS, and T waves. In the high right atrium, the P wave was large and deeply inverted; in mid-atrium, the P was biphasic; and in the low atrium it was upright. When the ventricle was entered, the QRS complex became very large.[10] Recently, a multipurpose pulmonary artery catheter with atrial ECG or pacing

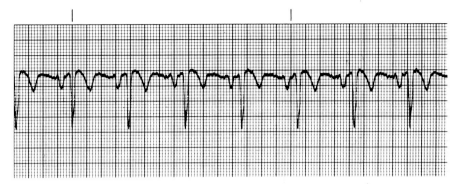

Fig. 4-5. A typical tracing of an MCL_1 lead is taken from a patient in the intensive care unit. Note the inversion of all the waves.

electrodes has become available.[11] The catheter permits monitoring of a bipolar atrial electrograph and diagnosis of complex arrhythmias with two electrodes located at 25 and 27 cm from the tip.

A further diagnostic ECG step is to record the bundle of His electrograph using an intracardiac catheter.[12,13,14] This part of conduction in the heart is so rapid that it does not appear on the standard ECG. In patients with intact atrioventricular conduction, the P-R interval can be subdivided into two subintervals:

1. P-H interval—from the atrial complex to the His bundle electrogram, which reflects AV nodal conduction time.
2. H-R interval—from the His bundle to the ventricular complex, which reflects conduction time in the His bundle, and the bundle branches.

This may be used to localize heart blocks to certain areas of the conduction system or diagnose the mechanism of complex arrhythmias.

A SYSTEMATIC APPROACH TO THE ELECTROCARDIOGRAM

In examining an ECG, the following features should always be checked:

1. Heart rate
2. Rhythm
3. Axis of the heart
4. P wave
5. P-R interval
6. QRS complex and interval
7. ST segment
8. T wave
9. U wave
10. Q-T interval

Heart Rate

ECG paper usually has interval markers in the margin at 3-second intervals. One method of rapidly obtaining the heart rate is to count the number of cycles in 6 seconds and multiply by 10. The thick lines on the ECG paper are 0.2 seconds (one-fifth of a second) apart, and the thin lines are 0.04 seconds apart, with a usual paper speed of 25 mm/sec. Marriott has described a rapid system to estimate the heart rate based on the thick one-fifth of a second lines.[4] Since there are 300 fifths in a minute (5×60), if the number of fifths of a second between two beats is counted and divided into 300, the heart rate is determined. Actually, this is a lot simpler than it sounds! For example, if there are two large boxes between consecutive QRS complexes, the heart rate is $300 \div 2 = 150$. In fact, a simple system of recall of this is as follows on the ECG strip (Fig. 4-6).[4] This system is useful only if the rhythm is regular. It is best to find two beats on the heavy lines to be exact. It can be estimated, however, if the second beat is between two lines, e.g., if the second beat occurred at point A, the heart rate is about 87 beats per minute.

Rhythm

The key question is whether or not the rhythm is regular. If it is irregular, is there any pattern to the irregularity? Also, it must be as-

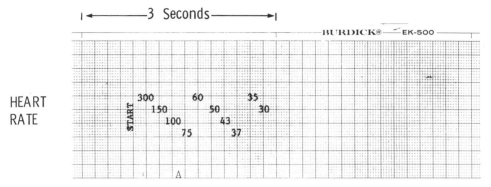

Fig. 4-6. A strip of electrocardiographic paper is shown. A 3-second interval is used to determine the heart rate. If the first QRS complex occurs on the start line, a second complex occurring on the designated lines will have the heart rates shown. This is an adaptation of Marriott's system for determining heart rates.

certained if there is one P wave for each QRS complex. This will be discussed in more detail in the section below on arrhythmias.

Axis of the Heart

The axis of the heart describes the orientation of the heart's electrical activity in the frontal plane. The axis can be determined off the three standard limb leads and the augmented limb leads. The Einthoven triangle is rearranged so that the leads bisect each other (Fig. 4-7).

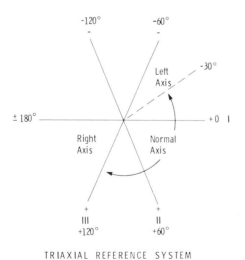

TRIAXIAL REFERENCE SYSTEM

Fig. 4-7. Einthoven's triangle rearranged so that the three leads bisect each other to form the triaxial reference system. The normal axis is clearly demonstrated as well as left axis and right axis deviations.

The normal axis is from $-30°$ to $+110°$. An abnormal left axis shift is from $-30°$ to $-90°$, and an abnormal right axis shift is from $+110°$ to $+180°$.[2] The system may be made more sophisticated and complex by adding in the augmented limb leads. The electrical axis is easily derived by measuring the net height of the QRS complexes in the limb leads (Fig. 4-8). These are plotted on the axial system and perpendicular lines are erected. A line from the center of the system to the intersection describes the axis of the heart.

P and T wave axes can be derived in the same manner. Abnormal right axis deviation may be caused by right bundle branch block, right ventricular hypertrophy, respiratory changes, or inferior wall myocardial infarction. Abnormal left axis deviation may result from left bundle branch block, ischemic heart disease, or ectopic beats.

P Wave

The P wave is normally upright, except in AVR and sometimes in lead III. The P wave is inverted when an abnormal conduction pathway exists or an atrial site other than the SA node is the pacemaker. Its amplitude should not exceed 2.5 mm, and its duration should not exceed 0.11 seconds. Increased amplitude or width indicate atrial hypertrophy. There are a few specific configurations seen in the P wave that are diagnostic (Figs. 4-9 and 4-10):

1. P-mitrale—wide and notched P waves, with

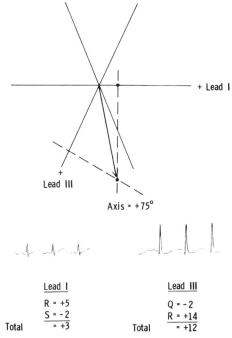

Axis = +75°

Lead I		Lead III	
R = +5		Q = -2	
S = -2		R = +14	
Total	= +3	Total	= +12

Fig. 4-8. The electrical axis is calculated off the triaxial reference system. The net height of the QRS complexes in leads I and III are calculated and marked on the triaxial reference system and then perpendicular lines are erected to the point where they cross. The axis is determined from the center of the system to the point of crossing. In this case, an axis of +75 ° is demonstrated.

the P being taller in lead I than in lead III (left atrial hypertrophy).

2. P-pulmonale—tall pointed P waves are seen, with the P in lead III being taller than in lead I (right atrial hypertrophy).

P-R Interval

The P-R interval occurs from the beginning of the P wave to the beginning of the QRS complex and is normally 0.12 to 0.20 seconds at normal heart rates. It is prolonged in first-degree heart block and in patients taking digitalis. It is shortened in junctional rhythms, Wolff-Parkinson-White syndrome, and Lown-Ganong-Levine syndrome.

QRS Complex and Interval

The normal duration is 0.05 to 0.10 seconds, and above 0.12 seconds is indicative of abnormal intraventricular conduction. Low voltage in all three standard leads (less than 5 mm) may be seen in myxedema, heart failure, pericardial effusions, diffuse coronary artery disease, or emphysema. Voltage criteria can be used to diagnose left and right ventricular hypertrophy (LVH and RVH). LVH is diagnosed by any one of the following criteria (Fig. 4-11):

1. S_{V_1} and $R_{V_5} \geq 35$ mm
2. $R_{AVL} \geq 12$ mm
3. Any precordial lead deflections ≥ 30 mm

LVH may occur with "strain," which is probably caused by associated ischemia or conduction abnormalities. In leads V_5 and V_6, the ST segments are depressed and the T waves are deeply depressed. This is most often produced by hypertension or aortic stenosis.

RVH is diagnosed by a reversal of the normal precordial pattern. The R waves are large in the right precordial leads, and the S waves are large in the left precordial leads. If the R:S ratio exceeds 1 in V_1, RVH is present (Fig. 4-

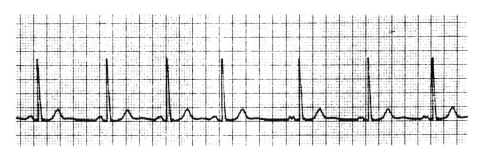

Fig. 4-9. This ECG demonstrates P-mitrale. There is a wide-notched P wave demonstrated in this lead I.

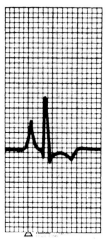

Fig. 4-10. P-pulmonale is demonstrated. A tall, pointed P wave is seen in lead III.

12). This is frequently associated with a right axis deviation and a right bundle branch block, especially in patients with mitral stenosis. Other causes of RVH are congenital heart disease and emphysema.

The Q wave is the first wave of the QRS complex, if it is negative in direction. Pathologic Q waves should be over 0.04 seconds in width and should be bunched in a "pattern." For example, inferior infarctions show Q waves in II, III, and AVF; and anterolateral infarcts in I, AVL, and V_4-V_6.

ST Segment

The point at which the ST segment takes off from the QRS complex is called the J (junction)-point. Normally it is isoelectric with the TP segment. It may normally be elevated less than 1 mm in standard and precordial leads, however. It is never normally depressed. The level of the ST segment relative to the TP segment should be observed, as well as its shape and slope. Upsloping, downsloping, horizontal ST segment depression, and J-junction depression may have different meanings (see the section on ischemia). Occasionally, the T_a wave may be seen to alter the ST segment.

T Wave

The T wave is normally upright in leads I, II, and V_{3-6}, inverted in AVR, and variable in the other leads. It normally does not exceed 5 mm in height in standard leads or 10 mm in precordial leads. Larger T waves may be indicative of myocardial ischemia or hyperkalemia.

U Wave

The U wave is best seen in lead V_3 and has the same polarity as the T wave. It is enlarged in hypokalemia and inverted in ischemia.

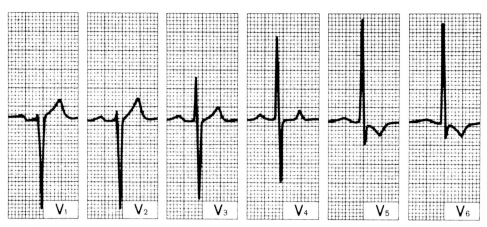

Fig. 4-11. An ECG of left ventricular hypertrophy is demonstrated. The S wave in V_1 plus the R wave in V_5 equal more than 35 mm. (Reproduced from the Electrocardio-Guide, produced by Merck, Sharp and Dohme, with permission.)

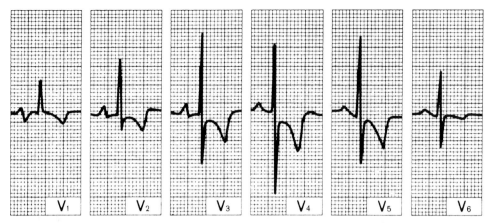

Fig. 4-12. The precordial leads in a patient with right ventricular hypertrophy are demonstrated. The R:S ratio exceeds 1 in lead V_1. (Reproduced from the Electrocardio-Guide, produced by Merck, Sharp and Dohme, with permission.)

Q-T Interval

The Q-T interval is measured from the beginning of the Q wave to the end of the T wave. It should be less than one-half of the preceding R-R interval and is affected by heart rate. It is called the Q-T$_c$ when corrected for heart rate. It is prolonged by hypocalcemia, quinidine, procainamide, and myocarditis. It is shortened by digitalis, hypercalcemia, and hyperkalemia.

ELECTROCARDIOGRAPHIC MONITORING IN THE OPERATING ROOM

The ECG monitor is almost routine in today's operating room and is certainly routine in all patients with cardiac disease. It is useful for monitoring arrhythmias, ischemia, heart block, and drug and electrolyte effects. It does not give any useful information about myocardial function or cardiac output, however. Arrhythmia detection has been the main function of the ECG in the operating room, with lead II being the most commonly used lead.[15] Lead II has frequently been selected, since a good P wave is seen, and junctional or ventricular rhythms are easy to identify. The reported incidence of arrhythmias during surgery ranges from 10 to more than 60 percent of the cases.[16] At the present time, many patients with coronary artery disease are coming to surgery, and the ECG is equally useful to diagnose ischemic changes. A precordial lead (V_5) has been very useful in diagnosing ischemia during surgery.[17] Figure 4-13 shows the location of the V_5 lead and the lead selector box from which one of seven leads can be selected (I, II, III, AVR, AVL, AVF, V_5). We presently display two simultaneous leads (II, V_5) in all patients with coronary artery disease. This allows us to look at both the left and right sides of the coronary circulation.

During surgery, the ECG is read off an oscilloscope and may be recorded if indicated. All operating rooms where cardiac surgery is performed should have ECG recording capabilities, and portable recorders should be available to all other operating rooms for interesting diagnostic problems. The recorder is needed to make accurate measurements of the ST-segment changes and accurate diagnosis of complex arrhythmias. In addition, the recorder is frequently needed to be sure artifacts are not being read off the oscilloscope. The recorder should make the tracing directly from the patient without first going through the oscilloscope's filter circuits.

Artifacts on the oscilloscope can be a major problem and lead to incorrect diagnoses.[18] Unfortunately, most physicians do not know enough about the electronics of the monitors to be able to distinguish these artifacts from real changes. The low-frequency filters of the ECG circuitry are the main source of the problem, since these can be selected by the physician or nurse using the equipment. The *diagnostic* mode

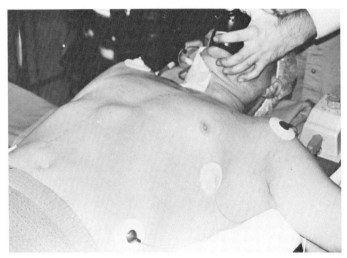

Fig. 4-13. The location of the four standard electrodes are shown on the shoulders and hips. The V₅ electrode is in the fifth intercostal space in the anterior axillary line. It is covered with a small piece of steri-drape so that the surgeons may prep right over it. The lead selector switchbox is shown by the patient's left shoulder.

on monitors filters frequencies below 0.14 Hz. A second mode frequently available is called the *monitor* mode, and this filters all frequencies below 4 Hz. The diagnostic mode should be used (especially for recording ST-segment changes), but unfortunately it is susceptible to baseline wandering caused by respiration, movement, or poor electrode contact. As more filtration is added (monitor mode), the baseline becomes more stable, but the ECG complex becomes more distorted. The P and T waves may be decreased in amplitude, but the main problem is change in the ST segment. As isoelectric ST segment may be elevated or depressed, resembling ischemic changes. Elevated or depressed ST segments may also be shifted toward the isoelectric line (Fig. 4-14). High-frequency filters are less of a problem. They are usually set at about 50 Hz so as to eliminate 60-cycle interference. Arrhythmias have also been inappropriately diagnosed as a result of ECG artifacts. Broken electrode wires have been reported to produce an ECG pattern mistaken for atrial flutter.[19] Also, hypothermia with shivering has been

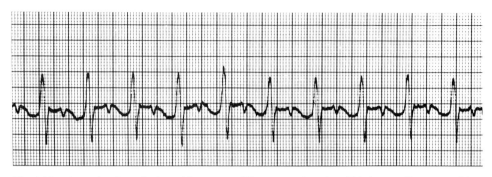

Fig. 4-14. A regular sinus rhythm with apparent ST-segment elevation. This is an artifact created by switching from the diagnostic to the monitoring mode on the operating room oscilloscope. This could be corrected back to normal by switching back to the lower frequency filter.

reported to be misdiagnosed as atrial flutter.[20] Artifacts produced by the roller pumps on cardiopulmonary bypass can also create an ECG pattern that looks like atrial flutter (Fig. 4-15).

Another electrical problem with ECG monitoring in the operating room is the electrocautery. When the cautery is used, the standard ECG is totally lost as a result of the electrical interference. The interference is a combination of radiofrequency current (800-2000 kHz), ac line frequency (60 Hz), and low frequency (0.1-10 Hz). Doss has shown that it is possible to modify the ECG preamplifiers so they will function well in the presence of the electrocautery.[21] It is surprising that this has not been done to more monitoring units designed for use in the operating room.

In addition to the usual causes of ECG changes that may occur during surgery, there are mechanical factors that can also affect the ECG.[21A] Respiratory variation can affect the height of the QRS complex which is most marked in leads III and AVF. This is caused either by a shift of the mediastinum with respirations or by a change in volume of the heart with the respiratory effects of venous return. Studies have shown that increases in the ventricular end-diastolic volume lead to increased height of the QRS complex, and hemorrhage leads to a decreased height of the QRS.[22,23] Catheters or wires in the heart frequently lead to arrhythmias. This is seen with placement of the Swan-Ganz catheter, where premature ventricular contractions are very common (58 percent as reported by Zaidan). There are also ECG changes related to age alone.[24] There is a decreasing amplitude of the QRS and T waves with

increasing age, and increasing PVCs occur over the age of 40 years.

CARDIAC ARRHYTHMIAS

Arrhythmia detection has been and still is the most important use of the ECG during and after surgery. Intraoperative arrhythmias were reported in the early 1900s, but the first large series of ECG studies during anesthesia was reported in 1936 by Kurtz.[25] In 109 patients, he found that sinus arrhythmia, extrasystoles, and downward displacement of the pacemaker site predominated and that 79 percent of the patients developed some rhythm disturbance during surgery. More recent studies, as summarized by Katz, have found the incidence of intraoperative arrhythmias to vary from 16.3 to 61.7 percent.[26] Bertrand studied 100 patients, using continuous electromagnetic tape recording during surgery, and reported an 84 percent incidence of supraventricular and ventricular arrhythmias.[27] Arrhythmias were most common at the times of intubation and extubation of the trachea. Patients with preexisting cardiac disease had a higher incidence of ventricular arrhythmias (60 percent versus 37 percent) then patients without known heart disease. Twenty-four of 25 patients with heart disease had a rhythm disturbance during surgery. In a study of patients undergoing cardiac surgery, Angelini reported that 29 of 50 patients (58 percent) having valve surgery and 35 of 78 patients (45 percent) having coronary revascularization developed significant postoperative arrhythmias.[28] These arrhythmias tended to correlate with the severity of the heart dis-

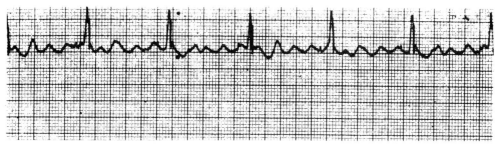

Fig. 4-15. This is an electrocardiogram of a patient shortly after he was placed on cardiopulmonary bypass. He is in a sinus rhythm, but it appears to be atrial flutter because of the artifact of the roller pumps appearing on the electrocardiogram.

ease, prolonged the hospital stay, and were responsible for up to 80 percent of the surgical mortality. Factors that may contribute to the etiology of perioperative arrhythmias are shown in Table 4-2.

Hypercarbia, hypocarbia, and hypoxia have all been shown to precipitate the development of arrhythmias, especially with the use of halothane or cyclopropane anesthesia.[29] Edwards showed that hyperventilation to a $Paco_2$ of 30 or 20 torr (pH 7.51 and 7.61) lowered a normal serum potassium level (4.03 mEq/liter) to 3.64 and 3.12 mEq/liter, respectively.[30] If serum and total body potassium start at lower levels, it is possible to decrease the serum potassium level into the 2 mEq/liter range by hyperventilation and precipitate severe cardiac dysrhythmias. Koehstrop recently showed that drugs such as cocaine and ketamine, which block the uptake of norepinephrine, can facilitate the development of epinephrine-induced arrhythmias.[31] Endotracheal intubation is probably the most common cause for arrhythmias during surgery, and Fox recently reported on the severe hypertension and arrhythmias that can occur during this procedure.[32] Many ECG abnormalities have been reported with intracranial pathology, especially subarachnoid hemorrhages, including changes in Q-T intervals, development of Q waves, ST-segment changes, U waves, and all types of arrhythmias.[33] The mechanism of the arrhythmias appears to be caused by changes in the autonomic nervous system. Dental surgery has been one of the types of surgery most often associated with arrhythmia formation.[34] Junctional rhythms are very common and may be caused by stimulation of the autonomic nervous system via the fifth cranial nerve.

Table 4-2

Factors Leading to Perioperative Arrythmias

1. Anesthetic agents[14]
2. Abnormal arterial blood gases[29,30]— $\downarrow Po_2$, $\uparrow Pco_2$, $\downarrow Pco_2$
3. Endogenous or exogenous catecholamines[31]
4. Endotracheal intubation[32]
5. Electrolyte imbalance[30]
6. Reflexes—vagal, occulocardiac[26]
7. Central nervous system stimulation[33]
8. Location of surgery—dental[34]
9. Preexisting cardiac disease[27]

Arrhythmias may also be *corrected* by general anesthesia, however. Borg and others have reported the disappearance of chronic arrhythmias following the induction of general anesthesia.[35] This could result from the relief of anxiety and loss of sympathetic stimulation; from an antiarrhythmic property of the anesthetic agent itself; or from the correction of abnormalities of respiration, blood gases, and electrolytes.

Physiological Basis of Cardiac Arrhythmias

Arrhythmias may result from abnormalities of impulse formation (automaticity), or impulse conduction (block, reentry), or both.[36] The cells of the SA node undergo a rapid spontaneous phase 4 depolarization and are thus the pacemakers of the normal heart, while ventricular cells normally do not (Fig. 4-2). If, however, the higher pacemaker cells do not fire, the lower cells will undergo slow spontaneous phase 4 depolarization and take over as pacemakers. Factors that selectively decrease the rate of phase 4 depolarization of the higher pacemaker sites while the lower cells are unaffected favor the movement of the pacemaker to a lower area in the heart. In addition, factors that increase the spontaneous phase 4 depolarization of a lower pacing site favor the takeover of these as the cardiac pacemaker.[37] Factors tending to slow pacemaker sites above the AV node are primary vagal influences such as digitalis, parasympathomimetic drugs, and halothane. Factors that tend to enhance automatic pacemaker activity below the AV node are catecholamines, hypercarbia, hypoxia, and digitalis overdose. Therefore, the combination of halothane to depress the atrial pacemaker and hypercarbia to increase ventricular automaticity may lead to ventricular arrhythmias. Increased automaticity is usually caused by an increase in the slope of phase 4 depolarization, but it may also be caused by an increase in the resting membrane potential or a decrease in the threshold potential (Fig. 4-16A).

Abnormal impulse conduction is the second major mechanism of arrhythmia formation. There may be a localized depression of excitability, leading to a form of blocked conduction (e.g., Wenchebach phenomenon), or abnormal conduction circuits may be formed. The most common form of abnormal conduction is called

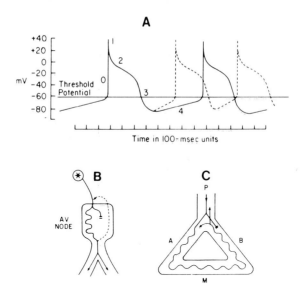

Fig. 4-16. Figure 4-16A shows an action potential and demonstrates an increase in slope of phase 4 depolarization. Figure 4-16B demonstrates the reentry mechanism for supraventricular tachyarrhythmias. Figure 4-16C demonstrates the reentry mechanism for ventricular tachyarrhythmias. See the text for details. (Reproduced from Lurie AJ: Rapid overdrive pacing for refractory tachyarrhythmias in patients after open heart surgery. J Thorac Cardiovasc Surg 72:458, 1976, with permission of author and publisher.)

reentry excitation.[36,38,39] For an impulse to complete a reentrant circuit, it must be unidirectionally blocked, travel slowly over another pathway, and reexcite in a retrograde manner the tissue proximal to the block after its refractory period. This results in a coupled premature contraction. The two key features are slow conduction and unidirectional block of the AV node or Purkinje network. This may be the mechanism of most arrhythmias. The reentry mechanism for supraventricular tachyarrhythmias is shown in Figure 4-16B. The impulse comes from the SA node and is partially blocked in the AV node. The block is shown as ≠. The retrograde reentry is shown as the dashed line.

The mechanism of ventricular tachyarrhythmias is shown in Figure 4-16C. The impulse comes down the Purkinje fibers and is blocked at ≠ in limb B. It continues in the other limb and reenters past the unidirectional block. This mechanism is used to best explain ventricular bigeminy and can also be used to explain self-sustaining tachyarrhythmias such as paroxysmal atrial tachycardias.

The mechanism of action of the antiarrhythmic drugs can be integrated with the above discussion. All the commonly used antiarrhythmic drugs suppress automaticity in pacemaker fibers by decreasing the slope of phase 4 spontaneous depolarization. Group I drugs (quinidine, procainamide, and propranolol) decrease reentry by converting the unidirectional block to a total bidirectional block by decreasing conduction. Group II drugs (lidocaine and diphenylhydantoin) decrease reentry by increasing membrane response and thus eliminating the unidirectional block.[40]

Approach to Arrhythmias

The best leads in order of preference to diagnose arrhythmias are as follows:[41]

1. V_1—Use four-limb electrodes and the V electrode placed in the fourth intercostal space to the right of the sternum. This requires a five-electrode system, however. It shows a good atrial deflection and QRS complex.
2. MCL_1 (Modified chest lead one)—A three-electrode system is most easily set up by placing the left arm electrode under the left

clavicle (negative electrode); the left leg electrode in the V_1 position in the fourth intercostal space to the right of the sternum (positive electrode); and the right arm electrode in the usual position (ground). The lead selector switch is placed on lead III.

3. II—Standard lead II is the third choice. It reflects a good atrial deflection but not necessarily a good QRS complex.

There are six key diagnostic questions to ask:[42]

1. What is the heart rate?
2. Is the rhythm regular?
3. Is there one P wave for each QRS? Is there block?
4. Is the QRS complex normal?
5. Is the rhythm dangerous?
6. Does the rhythm require treatment?

Diagnosis and Treatment

SUPRAVENTRICULAR
ARRHYTHMIAS

Sinus arrhythmia. The sinus node irregularly forms impulses. There are two types of sinus arrhythmias: (1) the first type varies with respiration (heart rate accelerates with inspiration), and (2) the second has no relationship to respiration (rare type).

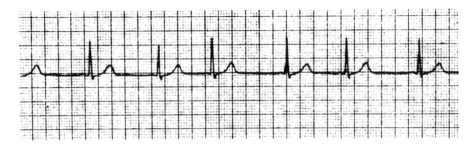

1. Heart rate—60- 100 beats per minute
2. Rhythm—irregular
3. P:QRS—1:1; all P waves the same
4. QRS complex—normal
5. Significance—normal finding; do not confuse with more serious problems
6. Treatment—none

Premature atrial contractions (PAC). Premature atrial contractions arise from an atrial focus other than the SA node and therefore are ectopic. They discharge the atria before the next SA nodal impulse and are therefore premature. They are recognized by a premature, abnormally shaped P wave and usually a normal QRS complex. They tend to reset the SA node and cause a slight pause but not a full compensatory pause.

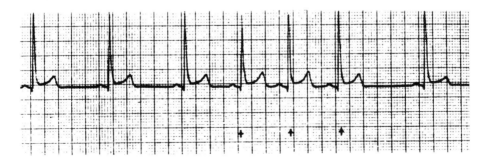

1. Heart rate—variable, depending on frequency of PACs.
2. Rhythm—irregular.
3. P:QRS—usually 1:1. The P waves have various shapes and may even be lost in the

QRS or T waves. Occasionally, the P wave will be so early as to find the ventricle refractory. Then it will not be conducted and will have no QRS complex.

4. QRS complex—usually normal. Occasion-

ally, the PAC may find part of the ventricular conduction system refractory. Then it will travel down an aberrant pathway and create an abnormal QRS complex. This is called a premature atrial contraction with *ventricular aberration* and can be very easily confused with a premature ventricular contraction.

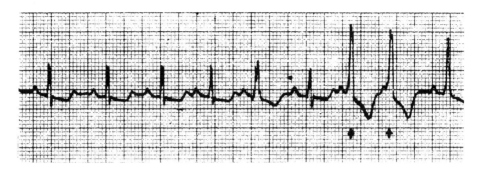

The following points are helpful in distinguishing a PAC with aberration from a PVC: (1) there is a preceding P wave that is usually abnormally shaped; (2) the complex is frequently of a right bundle branch configuration; (3) there is an rSR' in V_1; and (4) the initial vector force is *identical* with the preceding beat but is usually the opposite with a PVC.

5. Significance—usually not dangerous, but very frequent PACs can lead to other supraventricular tachyarrhythmias.

6. Treatment—usually none; rarely, digitalis or propranolol if the arrhythmia is causing poor hemodynamic function.

Sinus bradycardia. The discharge site is the SA node but at a slower than normal rate. Occasionally other pacemaker sites will try to take over and cause "premature" beats, e.g., PVCs.

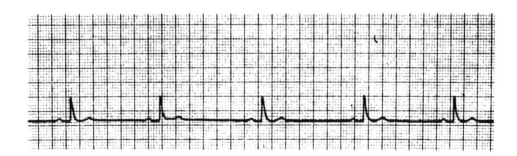

1. Heart rate—40-60 beats per minute. In patients taking chronic propranolol therapy, we have redefined this arrhythmia as a heart rate less than 50 beats per minute.

2. Rhythm—regular, except for premature "escape" beats that occasionally occur.

3. P:QRS—1:1.

4. QRS complex—normal.

5. Significance—This is the goal for patients treated with propranolol for ischemic heart disease. It may be seen with acute inferior myocardial infarction and with many drugs, e.g., morphine and neostigmine. It is of little significance unless it is affecting peripheral perfusion or is associated with hypotension or PVCs. Heart rates below 40 beats per minute are rarely tolerated very long and require treatment. This may be part of the "sick sinus syndrome" in which sinus node dysfunction can precipitate bradycardia, heart block, various tachyarrhythmias, or alternating bradytachyarrhythmias.[43]

6. Treatment—usually none; atropine (0.3-2.0 mg I.V.) if associated with hypotension or PVCs. Rarely, isoproterenol infusion (4 μg/ml) or a pacemaker will be required.

Atrial pacemaker is demonstrated below.

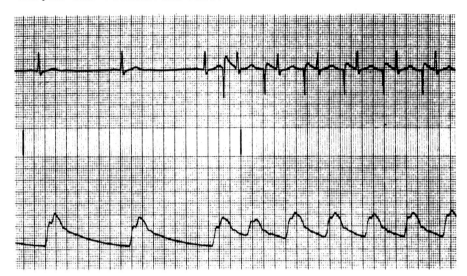

Sinus tachycardia. The discharge site is the SA node but at a faster than normal rate. This is a very common arrhythmia during and after surgery. Determining its cause is frequently the main problem. Included among the possible etiologies are pain, hypovolemia, fever, emotion, heart failure, and hyperthyroidism.

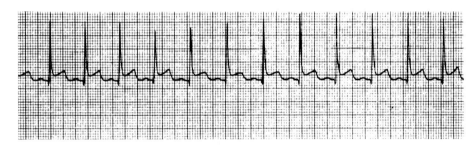

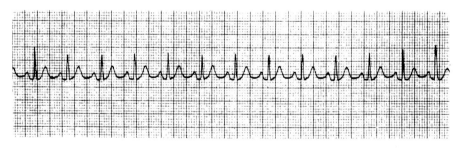

1. Heart rate—above 100 beats per minute. The top rate is 150-170 beats per minute, which is usually seen with a high fever.
2. Rhythm—regular.
3. P:QRS—1:1.
4. QRS complex—normal.

5. Significance—Prolonged rapid heart rates in patients with underlying heart disease can precipitate congestive heart failure. The fast heart rate decreases coronary perfusion time which can cause secondary ST-T-wave changes and can precipitate angina pectoris

in patients with coronary artery disease (see top figure above). The usual problem is finding the underlying cause of the problem; light anesthesia and hypovolemia are the most common intraoperative causes.

If the heart rate is *150 beats per minute,* it can be a major diagnostic problem. This is a common heart rate for three arrhythmias: (1) sinus tachycardia; (2) paroxysmal atrial tachycardia (PAT); and (3) atrial flutter with 2:1 block.

There are three diagnostic maneuvers to try to separate these three arrhythmias:

a. Carotid sinus massage—A sinus tachycardia will gradually slow and then speed up again, or it will be unaffected; a PAT will usually break and revert to sinus rhythm or it will be unaffected; and atrial flutter with 2:1 block will usually increase the heart block and make the atrial flutter waves more obvious.
b. Edrophonium (Tensilon)—5- 10 mg I.V. will accentuate the carotid massage effects.

c. Atrial or esophageal ECG leads to see the P waves better.
6. Treatment—treat the underlying cause. While determining the cause, propranolol may be used in patients with ischemic heart disease or in those who develop ST-T-wave changes, in an effort to prevent further myocardial ischemia.

Paroxysmal atrial tachycardia (PAT). PAT is a run of rapidly repeated supraventricular premature beats from a site other than the SA node. This rhythm is frequently very rapid and can lead to severe ST-T-wave changes that may persist even after the rate slows (the posttachycardia syndrome). This arrhythmia is frequently seen in patients with the Wolff-Parkinson-White (WPW) syndrome in which an abnormal conduction pathway is present (bundle of Kent). This pathway can be identified by epicardial mapping and bundle of His studies.[44] This arrhythmia may be called a chaotic atrial mechanism (CAM) if the P waves are constantly changing configuration and the atrial rate is irregular.[45]

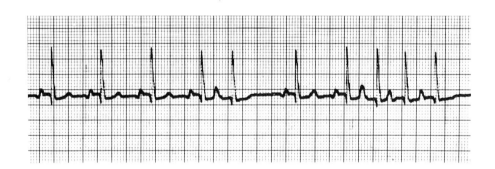

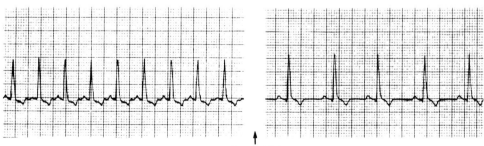

↑
Carotid
Massage

1. Heart rate—150-250 beats per minute.
2. Rhythm—usually regular except for CAM.
3. P:QRS—1:1; P waves frequently abnormal.
4. QRS complex—normal; ST-T depression common.
5. Significance—may occur under anesthesia and produce severe hemodynamic deterioration.[46] This can be precipitated by changes in the autonomic nervous system, drug effects, or volume shifts. It may be seen in 5 percent of normal young adults and many patients with WPW. It may be associated with atrioventricular block owing to the fast atrial rate and slow AV conduction. PAT with 2:1 block represents digitalis intoxication in 50 percent of the cases. CAM is usually seen in elderly patients with advanced heart disease.
6. Treatment—This arrhythmia frequently has to be treated because of its rapid rate and associated poor hemodynamic function.
   a. Carotid sinus massage is frequently effective but should only be applied to one side and should be used carefully in elderly patients with cerebrovascular disease.[47,48] Eyeball pressure to achieve vagal stimulation should not be used (see above figure).
   b. Edrophonium (Tensilon) (5-10 mg I.V.) slowly given frequently increases vagal tone enough to make carotid massage effective.[49]
   c. If the patient is hypotensive, an α-adrenergic stimulator such as phenylephrine can be used in 100 μg doses to increase

the blood pressure and achieve a reflex vagal showing.
   d. Propranolol (0.5 mg) will frequently slow the PAT and may be used in combination with digitalis (propranolol, 0.5 mg, and digoxin, 0.25 mg).[50]
   e. Lidocaine (50-100 mg) may be tried and may work if the mechanism of the arrhythmia and conduction are over an anomalous pathway.[51]
   f. Rapid overdrive pacing may be used to "capture" the ectopic focus and then the rate progressively slowed.[52]
   g. Cardioversion with appropriate synchronization may occasionally be required. This is used less now than in the past, since propranolol is so effective.[53]
   h. Quinidine and procainamide have also frequently been used in the past, especially for prevention of these episodes in patients with WPW.
   i. Surgery is now occasionally used to excise the aberrant conduction pathway of the bundle of Kent in patients with WPW who have frequent attacks of PAT, even when receiving maximal medical therapy.[54]

Atrial flutter. Atrial flutter represents a *faster discharge* from an irritable focus in the atria than does a rapid atrial tachycardia. It is usually associated with AV block, since the atrial rate is so fast. Classical saw-toothed flutter waves (F waves) are usually present.

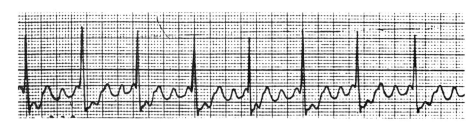

1. Heart rate—atrial rate, 250-350 beats per minute; a ventricular rate, around 150 beats per minute.
2. Rhythm—Atrial rhythm is regular, but ventricular may be regular if a fixed block or irregular if a variable block exists.
3. P:QRS—usually 2:1 block, with atrial rate of 300 and a ventricular rate of 150, but it

may vary between 2:1 and 8:1. F waves best seen in leads V_1 and II.
5. Significance—usually associated with severe heart disease.
6. Treatment—Two main forms of treatment are used. If the rhythm is being tolerated, it can be treated pharmacologically with digitalis and propranolol, which will slow it and

possibly convert it to atrial fibrillation. If there is acute hemodynamic deterioration, cardioversion using very low voltage (10–40 w/sec) is effective in more than 90 percent of cases.

Atrial fibrillation. Atrial fibrillation is an excessively rapid and irregular atrial focus. There are no P waves on the ECG but rather, a fine fibrillatory activity called "f" waves. This is the most irregular rhythm and is thus called irregularly irregular. It is frequently associated with a pulse deficit.

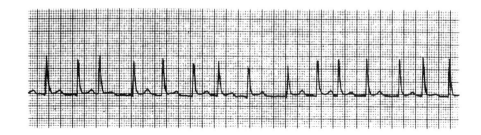

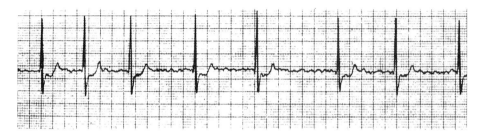

1. Heart rate—atrial rate, 350–500 beats per minute; ventricular rate, depending on treatment, 60–170 beats per minute.
2. Rhythm—irregularly irregular.
3. P:QRS—P waves absent and replaced with f waves or no obvious atrial activity at all.
4. QRS complex—normal, may have some aberrancy.
5. Significance—Usually associated with severe heart disease. Loss of atrial contraction tends to decrease cardiac output.[55] This rhythm must be differentiated from (1) atrial flutter with varying block (atrial fib-flutter), (2) frequent premature beats, (3) sinus rhythm with varying block, (4) gross sinus arrhythmia, and (5) wandering atrial pacemaker.[4] Atrial fibrillation or flutter commonly occurs during cannulation of the right atrium for cardiopulmonary bypass.
6. Treatment—Digitalis is usually used to slow the ventricular response. Propranolol may also be added. In atrial fibrillation of recent onset, especially after cardiac surgery, cardioversion may be used to reestablish sinus

rhythm. Lidocaine should be avoided or used cautiously in patients with atrial fibrillation, since it can markedly increase atrioventricular conduction and lead to an accelerated ventricular response.[56] Internal cardioversion should be used if this rhythm occurs during cannulation for bypass.

Junctional rhythm (nodal). The impulse arises in the AV junctional tissue. It travels down into the ventricles in the normal fashion and travels retrograde into the atrium (the P wave may be distorted). There are three varieties of this rhythm:[57]

A. High-nodal rhythm: the impulse reaches the atrium before the ventricle, and therefore the P wave precedes the QRS but has a shortened P-R interval (less than 0.1 second).
B. Midnodal rhythm: the impulse arrives in the atrium and the ventricle at the same time, and the P wave is lost in the QRS.
C. Low-nodal rhythm: the impulse reaches the

ventricle first and then the atrium, so that the P wave follows the QRS complex.

NODAL BIGEMINY

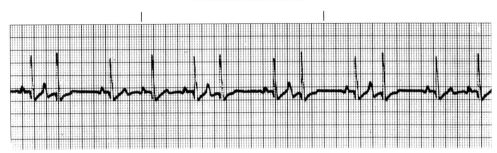

1. Heart rate—variable, 40–180 beats per minute; nodal bradycardia to nodal tachycardia.
2. Rhythm—regular.
3. P:QRS—1:1, but appears variable depending on the location of the P wave.
4. QRS complex—normal, unless altered by the P wave.
5. Significance—Junctional rhythms are common under anesthesia (about 20 percent of the cases), especially with halogenated anesthetic agents or the ether drugs. The nodal rhythm frequently decreases blood pressure and cardiac output by about 15 percent, but it can decrease it by up to 30 percent in patients with heart disease.[58]

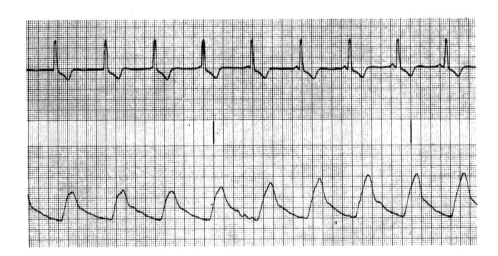

6. Treatment—Usually no treatment is required, and the rhythm reverts spontaneously. If hypotension and poor perfusion are associated with the rhythm, treatment is indicated. Atropine, ephedrine, or isoproterenol can be used in an effort to increase the activity of the SA node so it will take over as the pacemaker. A small dose of succinylcholine (10 mg I.V.) may revert a nodal rhythm to a sinus rhythm during anesthesia with halothane or enflurane.[59] This probably works as a result of succinylcholine's effect as a sympathetic ganglionic stimulator.

Wandering atrial pacemaker. Multiple irritable sites of the atria or AV node act as the pacemaker. The wandering atrial pacemaker is a variety of a junctional rhythm.

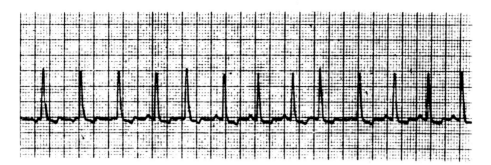

1. Heart rate—usually under 100 beats per minute.
2. Rhythm—somewhat irregular.
3. P:QRS—variable; may be 1:1, but P waves may be lost in the QRS (junctional rhythm) or even occur afterward (retrograde conduction).
4. QRS complex—usually normal unless the P wave distorts it.
5. Significance—usually not dangerous, but may lead to a decreased blood pressure and cardiac output when "atrial kick" is lost before the QRS complex.
6. Treatment—usually none. Correct blood gases if abnormal. Administer atropine if the rate is too slow.

Premature nodal contractions (PNC). The premature discharge originates in the AV junctional tissue. The P wave may be inverted or lost in the QRS complex. The irritable focus may cause a single premature beat (PNC) or a run of premature beats (AV nodal tachycardia).[60]

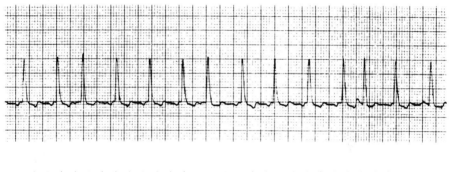

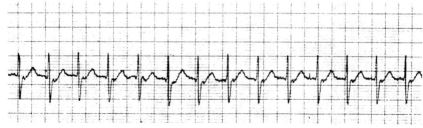

1. Heart rate—depends on frequency of PNCs.
2. Rhythm—irregular.
3. P:QRS—usually 1:1, but the P wave may be lost in or occur after the QRS.
4. QRS complex—usually normal, but possibly altered by P wave.
5. Significance—usually of no significance, but nodal tachycardia is frequently poorly tolerated and requires treatment.
6. Treatment—usually none. PNCs may be treated with digitalis or propranolol. Nodal tachycardia can also be controlled by propranolol.

VENTRICULAR ARRHYTHMIAS

Premature ventricular contractions (PVC). PVCs are premature ectopic beats arising from a focus below the AV junction and are one of the most common arrhythmias seen in anesthesia and in patients with cardiac disease. They are usually identified by being premature, having a wide QRS complex, an ST segment that slopes in the opposite direction from the QRS, and a compensatory pause associated with these premature beats. There is no P wave visible with these beats in most situations. Interpolated PVCs occur between two normal beats, and there is no compensatory pause. Usually, PVCs are coupled to regular beats (fixed coupling); occasionally, however, they are not coupled and thus fire off at their own rate. This latter pattern is called *parasystole* (variable coupling) and is identified by an irregular interval between the normal beat and the PVCs.

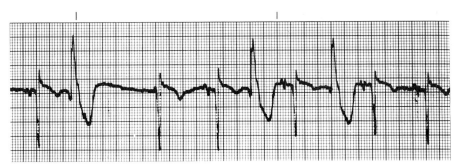

1. Heart rate—depends on the frequency of the PVCs.
2. Rhythm—irregular.
3. P:QRS—no P waves are seen.
4. QRS complex—wide and bizarre, with a width of over 0.12 seconds. The T wave is directed in the opposite manner.
5. Significance—potentially a very dangerous arrhythmia that can proceed to ventricular tachycardia or fibrillation. The most dangerous forms are multiple PVCs, multifocal PVCs (many irritable sites), coupled PVCs (bigeminy), short runs of PVCs (more than three in a row is frequently considered ventricular tachycardia), or the R-on-T phenomenon (PVCs near the vulnerable period which can precipitate ventricular fibrillation). The PVCs may also decrease coronary blood flow and saphenous vein bypass graft blood flow.[61]

6. Treatment—The first step is to correct any underlying abnormalities such as a low potassium or a low arterial oxygen tension. Lidocaine is the treatment of choice with an initial dose of 1.5 mg/kg intravenously as a bolus. Recurrent PVCs can be treated with a lidocaine infusion (1-4 mg/min) or with procainamide, quinidine, propranolol, or bretylium.

Ventricular tachycardia. Ventricular tachycardia is a run of rapidly repeated ectopic beats that can be life-threatening. Diagnostic criteria include the presence of (1) fusion beats—the ventricle is activated partially by the atrial impulse and partially by the ventricular impulse; (2) capture beats—these are conducted SA nodal beats; and (3) AV dissociation, in which unrelated P waves can be identified.

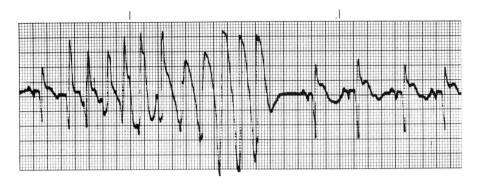

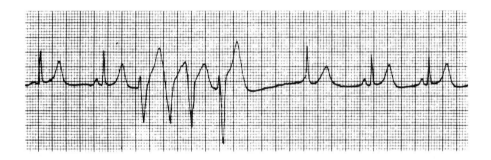

1. Heart rate—100-250 beats per minute.
2. Rhythm—usually regular but may be irregular if the ventricular tachycardia is paroxysmal
3. P:QRS—no fixed relationship (ventricular tachycardia is a form of atrioventricular dissociation). The P waves can be seen marching through the QRS complex.
4. QRS complex—wide; over 0.12 seconds in width, with P waves marching through.
5. Significance—Acute onset is life-threatening and requires immediate treatment. Many patients have chronic ventricular tachycardia and tolerate it quite well, however.[62]
6. Treatment—A lidocaine bolus will frequently convert this to sinus rhythm. Cardioversion is needed in some patients.

Ventricular fibrillation. In ventricular fibrillation, the ventricles discharge in a completely chaotic asynchronous fashion without effective output. There is no clear-cut ventricular complex seen on the ECG. The most important conditions precipitating this arrhythmia are myocardial ischemia, electrolyte imbalance, hypoxia, hypothermia, slow conduction, and drugs that increase automaticity.[63] In order to produce better operating conditions for the surgeon, ventricular fibrillation may be induced in certain situations by passing a small, low-voltage, direct current through the heart (electrical fibrillator).

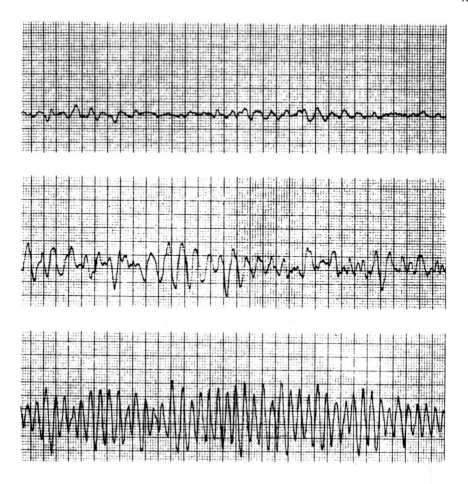

1. Heart rate—rapid and grossly disorganized.
2. Rhythm—totally irregular.
3. P:QRS—none are seen.
4. QRS complex—not present.
5. Significance—there is no effective cardiac output, and life must be sustained by artificial means (external message or extracorporeal circulation). This has been a great fear in anesthesia since Guedel reported it in 1936.[64]
6. Treatment—Cardiopulmonary resuscitation must be initiated immediately, but defibrillation is the standard definitive treatment. The external dosage is 200-400 w/sec, and the internal electrical dosage is 10-60 w/sec. This is frequently unsuccessful if electrolytes or acid-base status is out of balance.

Pharmacologic therapy has occasionally been successful with propranolol, bretylium, or lidocaine even when defibrillation has not been successful.[65,66]

Ventricular asystole. No ventricular activity is present in ventricular asystole. This is a bad sign in association with a cardiac arrest. Occasionally, patients have had transient atrioventricular standstill lasting up to 20 seconds as a result of vagal stimuli or drugs, which produced cerebral ischemia and required resuscitation.[67] During cardiac surgery, asystole is frequently produced by injecting hypothermic, hyperkalemic cardioplegic solutions into the coronary circulation to reduce oxygen requirements.

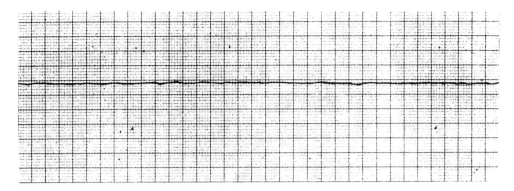

1. Heart rate—none present.
2. Rhythm—straight line on the ECG; must be sure ECG is not disconnected from the patient.
3. P:QRS—none present.
4. QRS complex—absent.
5. Significance—second most common rhythm associated with a cardiac arrest (ventricular fibrillation is first). Difficult to treat, and an attempt should be made to convert it to ventricular fibrillation.
6. Treatment—Maintain cardiopulmonary resuscitation while administering calcium chloride, isoproterenol, epinephrine, $NaHCO_3$, and inserting a transvenous pacemaker.

TREATMENT OF ARRHYTHMIAS

Antiarrhythmic drugs (see Chapter 2 for further details). Table 4-3 shows the commonly used drugs along with their dosage, classification, and toxicities.

Cardiac pacing (see Chapter 9 for details). Temporary pacemakers have been used instead of or along with drug therapy to treat tachyarrhythmias in many cases. The pacer "captures" the rhythm by pacing the heart at rates which are at least 10 beats per minute faster than the intrinsic rate.[52] Once the single focus of pacemaker stimulation is established, it is sometimes possible to slow the rate of pacing to a near normal heart rate.

This use of cardiac pacing has been a very helpful technique in cardiac surgical patients in whom temporary atrial and ventricular pacing wires have been left on their hearts after surgery. Lurie reported the use of ventricular over-

drive pacing to treat both ventricular and supraventricular tachyarrhythmias in patients with arrhythmias refractory to conventional therapy.[39] Waldo used rapid atrial pacing to interrupt atrial flutter in 30 postoperative patients.[72] It is necessary to have one of the new atrial pacemakers that can generate stimuli at 800 beats per minute, since the atrial flutter rate is generally 250-350 beats per minute. He found that if the heart was paced 10 beats per minute faster for up to 30 seconds, the rhythm could be captured.

Transesophageal atrial pacing has also been reported as a method to override both supraventricular and ventricular arrhythmias.[73] Montoyo reported 22 patients treated with an esophageal electrode without complications. In 17 patients, atrial pacing was achieved; and in 6 patients the rhythm reverted to a normal sinus mechanism.

Cardioversion. Since its introduction by Lown in 1962, direct current cardioversion has been widely utilized in the treatment of cardiac arrhythmias.[74] It is used to treat ventricular tachycardia and acute or chronic atrial fibrillation or flutter. Cardioversion (countershock) is performed by using a *synchronized dc shock* applied either directly to the heart or through the chest wall. Pulse discharge is synchronized to occur within 20 msec of the peak of the R wave on the ECG, thereby avoiding the ventricular vulnerable period at the peak of the T wave.[75] The shock depolarizes all the fibers that are excitable at that instant and allows for restoration of a normal sinus rhythm. Synchronization is important to avoid inadvertent ventricular fibrillation, which will occur about 2 percent of the time in nonsynchronized cardio-

Table 4-3
Antiarrhythmic Drugs[68,69]

Drug	Class	Indication	Intravenous Dose	Blood Level Desired	Toxicity
Propranolol (Inderal)	I	All tachycardias: digitalis toxicity	0.5 mg q 5 min → 5 mg	50 ng/ml	Bronchospasm; hypotension; AV block; heart failure
Procainamide (Pronestyl)	I	Ventricular arrhythmias	100 mg q 5 min → 1000 mg; or infusion, 1–4 mg/min	4–6 mg/liter	Hypotension; lupus; widened QRS complex
Quinidine (Quinaglute)	I	Atrial and ventricular arrhythmias	200 mg *P.O.* (not I.V.)	4–8 mg/liter	Fever; chill; nausea; diarrhea
Disopyramide (Norpace)	I	Atrial and ventricular arrhythmias	150 mg q 6 hr *P.O.* (not I.V.)	2–4 μg/ml	Heart block: anticholinergic symptoms
Lidocaine (Xylocaine)	II	Ventricular arrhythmias	50–100 mg; or infusion, 1–4 mg/min	2–5 μg/ml	Drowsiness; seizures; hypotension
Diphenylhydantoin (Dilantin)	II	Ventricular arrhythmias; digitalis toxicity	100 mg q 5 min → 500 mg	8–16 μg/ml	Hypotension; hematologic effects; nystagmus; ataxia
Bretylium (Bretylol)	III	Ventricular arrhythmias	5 mg/kg	—	Hypotension
Digoxin	Glycoside	Supraventricular tachycardias	0.25–0.5 mg → 1.5 mg	2 ng/ml	Heart block; PVCs
Ouabain	Glycoside	Supraventricular tachycardias	0.1–0.2 mg → 1.0 mg	—	Heart block; PVCs
Atropine	Parasympatholytic	Bradycardia	0.3 → 2 mg	—	Dryness; fever; coma
KCl[70]	Electrolyte	Ventricular arrhythmias; digitalis toxicity	40 mEq/hr; or 2 mEq bolus	K^+ = 3.5–4.5 mEq/liter	Heart block; asystole
MgSO$_4$[71]	Electrolyte	Ventricular arrhythmias; digitalis toxicity	6 gm (49 mEq)	Mg^{++} = 1.6–2.0 mEq/liter	Neuromuscular blockade
CaCl$_2$	Electrolyte	Asystole	500–1000 mg	Ca^{++} = 2.0–2.2 mEq/liter	Ventricular fibrillation

version.[76] All recent cardiovertor/defibrillator machines have a synchronizer switch that must be turned on to achieve synchronization.

Internal direct cardioversion requires much lower energy levels than does external cardioversion. For *external* cardioversion, the paddles are placed in the same position as for defibrillation—one paddle over the apex of the heart and the other to the right of the sternum. Atrial flutter is the easiest rhythm to convert and usually requires about 50 w/sec externally. For atrial fibrillation or ventricular tachycardia, 200 w/sec externally frequently works, but 300 or 400 w/sec may be required. For *internal* cardioversion, the paddles are placed across the atria for treatment of supraventricular arrhythmias (Fig. 4-17) and on the ventricles for treatment of ventricular tachycardia or fibrillation. All supraventricular tachycardias are treated with 10 w/sec; ventricular arrhythmias are also initially treated with 10 w/sec, but it may be necessary to increase to 50-60 w/sec.

We have found internal cardioversion to be very useful during cardiac surgery. Atrial arrhythmias are frequently produced by the cannulation of the right atrium for cardiopulmonary bypass. The arrhythmias are often very rapid and poorly tolerated by these cardiac patients. The occurrence of these arrhythmias appears to be more frequent in patients with right coronary artery disease, hypovolemia, hypokalemia, or with "rough" surgeons. If cannulation is almost complete, we prefer to go right onto bypass to support the circulation. If cannulation is not completed, however, we prefer to cardiovert the patient immediately back into sinus rhythm rather than begin pharmacologic therapy.

Elective external cardioversion is indicated for patients with recent onset (less than 1 year) atrial fibrillation or flutter. We prefer to wait at least 3 weeks to cardiovert postoperative open heart patients. Contraindications include long-term atrial fibrillation, underlying heart block, recent systemic embolization, a giant left atrium, or digitalis toxicity. Digitalis intoxication is especially important, since cardioversion of these patients can produce serious arrhythmias or even a resistant ventricular fibrillation.[77] Therefore, digitalis is discontinued 24 to 48 hours prior to elective cardioversion. Quinidine is frequently begun at this time in an effort to maintain sinus rhythm after the cardioversion. Anticoagulants are used only for patients with a prior history of embolization.

Numerous methods of anesthesia have been described for cardioversion, including rapid acting barbiturates, diazepam, and methoxyflurane analgesia. Thiopental (50–100 mg) or methohexital (20–50 mg) are frequently used to achieve a rapid level of light anesthesia.[78,79] The goal is light anesthesia with loss of the cyelid reflex and a rapid return of consciousness after the car-

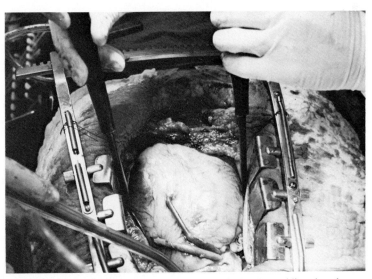

Fig. 4-17. Internal cardioversion is demonstrated with the paddles placed across the atria. The three aortocoronary bypass grafts can be seen in place.

dioversion. This should be done only in the operating room area (recovery room or holding area), where further equipment and personnel are available. An anesthetic machine, oxygen, suction, and cardiac drugs must be prepared and readily available. In the past few years, diazepam has become a popular drug to achieve amnesia and sedation for cardioversion.[74,80] It is administered in 5-mg intravenous increments every 1 to 2 minutes up to a maximum of 25 mg or an end point of somnolence, slurred speech, and loss of coordinated eye movement. Orko found the mean dose of diazepam required was 0.32 mg/kg in 50 patients he studied.[80] Using this dose, 2 of 50 patients became apneic and required positive pressure ventilation. Amnesia is not guaranteed with diazepam, since Orko reported that 37 percent of the patients recalled the electric shock. Ventricular arrhythmias including ventricular fibrillation have also been reported upon administration of diazepam prior to the countershock.[81] In many centers, diazepam is administered by a cardiologist without an anesthesiologist being present. We believe it is safer for an anesthesiologist to administer the diazepam and to monitor the patient for apnea, airway obstruction, arrhythmias, and level of consciousness. Reier has also reported the use of methoxyflurane analgesia for cardioversion in 20 patients.[82] A disposable inhaler was used to provide conscious analgesia and amnesia without surgical anesthesia or hemodynamic effects.

Many complications of cardioversion have been reported, and the anesthesiologist should be prepared for them (Table 4-4).

Defibrillation. In 1899, Prevost and Batelli, in France, observed that an electric shock

Table 4-4
Complications of Cardioversion

1. Ventricular tachycardia and fibrillation—1-2%
2. Various arrhythmias
3. Bradycardia or asystole
4. Transient ST-segment elevation
5. Pulmonary edema—1-2%[83]
6. Systemic emboli—less than 1%
7. Skeletal muscle damage leading to elevated SGOT, LDH, CPK—20%
8. Hypoventilation

could cause ventricular fibrillation and a second shock could stop it. In 1933, Kouwenhoven confirmed that a dog with a fibrillating heart could be converted to regular sinus rhythm by an electric countershock. In 1940, Wiggers studied ventricular fibrillation and showed that an alternating current (ac) shock could stop it, and he termed this a countershock. The first successful human defibrillation was performed by Beck in 1947 with an ac defibrillator.[76] Alternating current defibrillators are not presently used for the following reasons:

1. Their bulk and weight
2. Production of myocardial damage
3. Less power than direct current (dc) defibrillators
4. Long discharge time
5. Inability to synchronize
6. Greater operator hazard
7. More violent skeletal muscle contraction

In 1966, Nachlas demonstrated the superiority of dc over ac defibrillators. Direct current defibrillators have the following advantages:

1. Small size and portability
2. Ability to synchronize
3. More powerful and shorter discharge time (3-5 msec)
4. More effective than ac defibrillators

To terminate ventricular fibrillation, a dc shock is the recommended treatment. For external defibrillation in an adult over 50 kg, the full output of 400 w/sec should be used. For a child or small adult weighing less than 50 kg, 3.5-6.0 w/sec/kg should be used.[84] The standard electrode positions should always be used: one electrode just to the right of the upper sternum below the clavicle, and the other electrode just to the left of the cardiac apex or left nipple. Standard electrode paste may be used, but saline-soaked gauze sponges are also excellent conductors. For internal defibrillation, the smallest possible "dose" of electricity should be used to reduce myocardial damage. Most hearts can be defibrillated with 5-20 w/sec, but some hypertrophied ventricles may require up to 60 w/sec.[85]

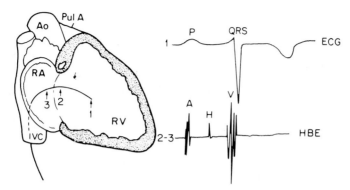

Fig. 4-18. An intracardiac electrocardiographic lead is shown coming up through the inferior vena cava, the right atrium, and across the tricuspid valve, with the tip in the right ventricle. A normal ECG is shown as well as the intracavitary His bundle electrograph. Normal a, h, and v waves are demonstrated. (Reproduced from Akhtar M: Clinical use of His Bundle electrocardiography. Am Heart J 91:520, 1976, with permission of author and publisher.)

Chest thump. The chest thump was recommended to treat ventricular tachycardia by Pennington in 1970.[86] He reported its use in terminating 12 episodes of ventricular tachycardia in 5 patients with coronary heart disease. The chest thump is performed by hitting the midsternum with a fist raised 12 inches off the chest. It is not a smash, but a moderate thump and should be delivered only one time. This will deliver 4-5 w/sec of energy, which may convert ventricular tachycardia to sinus rhythm. This small energy discharge works by interrupting a reentrant mechanism in a manner similar to how a pacemaker spike converts an arrhythmia. The present American Heart Association recommendations are to use a chest thump only in two situations: (1) a witnessed cardiac arrest and (2) a monitored cardiac arrest. In both of these situations, the heart is oxygenated, and the thump can be applied within 15 seconds of the arrest. If it fails to convert the arrhythmia to regular sinus rhythm, cardiopulmonary resuscitation should be immediately instituted.

HEART BLOCKS—DIAGNOSIS AND TREATMENT

Two types of blocks will be discussed in this section: (1) intraventricular conduction disturbances and (2) atrioventricular heart block.

Bundle of His electrographs have greatly improved our understanding of AV conduction. A normal ECG and a His bundle electrograph (HBE) are shown in Figure 4-18 along with their recording locations. The normal intervals are as follows:[87]

1. The P-H interval—from the onset of P wave to the His complex (normal = 119 ± 38 msec). This complex is made up of:
   a. A-H interval—from the atrial electrograph to the His complex (normal = 92 ± 38 msec).
   b. P-A interval—from the onset of the P wave to the atrial electrograph (normal = 27 ± 18 msec).
2. H-R or H-V interval—from the His complex to the R wave or ventricular electrograph (normal = 43 ± 12 msec).

Intraventricular Conduction Disturbances

LEFT BUNDLE BRANCH BLOCK (LBBB)

The impulse reaches the ventricles exclusively through the right bundle branch, and there is a wide QRS complex of more than 0.12 seconds and a wide notched R wave seen in leads I, AVL, and V_6. Also, there is no Q wave in V_6.

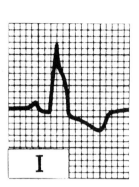

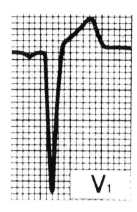

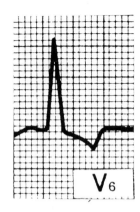

The most important leads to study in bundle branch blocks are I, V_1 and V_6. The pattern of LBBB in V_6 is similar to LVH but exaggerated. The QRS complex interval is longer, and the ST-T changes are more pronounced owing to the slow conduction in LBBB. A similar pattern with a QRS duration of less than 0.12 seconds (0.10 to 0.11) occurs when there is an incomplete

LBBB. The H-V interval is almost always prolonged in the LBBB.

RIGHT BUNDLE BRANCH BLOCK (RBBB)

The QRS complex exceeds 0.11 seconds, leads V_1-V_3 have broad RSR´complexes, and leads I and V_6 have wide S waves.

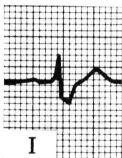

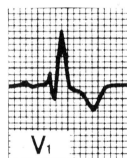

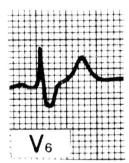

An incomplete RBBB is diagnosed if the QRS duration is 0.09 to 0.10 seconds with the RBBB configuration. Unlike LBBB, which is always associated with heart disease, RBBB may be of no clinical consequence. Its overall incidence is about 1 percent in hospitalized patients. Incomplete RBBB is frequently present in patients with elevated right ventricular pressures, e.g., chronic lung disease or atrial septal defects.

HEMIBLOCKS

Hemiblock is the term used for blockage of one of the two main divisions of the *left* bundle branch. If both divisions are blocked, then LBBB exists. Even though hemiblocks are a form of intraventricular block, the QRS complex is not prolonged. The order and direction of ventricular activation is altered, but the time

required for depolarization is not markedly prolonged. Marriott's criteria for a left anterior hemiblock (LAH) are as follows:[4]

1. Left axis deviation greater than −60°
2. Small Q in lead I, small R in III
3. Normal QRS duration

The criteria for left posterior hemiblock (LPH) are as follows:[4]

1. Right axis deviation greater than +120°
2. Small R in lead I, small Q in III
3. Normal QRS duration
4. No RVH

The hemiblocks can occur by themselves, but LAH and LPH are frequently associated with RBBB to form a bilateral bundle branch block. Hearts with RBBB and LAH progress to complete heart block (trifascicular block) in only

10 percent of patients, while hearts with RBBB and LPH usually proceed to complete heart block.[88,89]

The anesthesiologist must be concerned with these conduction defects because of the possibility of complete heart block developing during or after anesthesia and the need to decide if a pacemaker is indicated in the perioperative period. Rooney studied 27 patients undergoing surgery who had RBBB and LAH.[90] None of these patients developed further conduction problems, and routine use of a pacemaker was found not to be needed. Patients with RBBB and LPH are more controversial.[91] If they are symptomatic, it is our feeling that they possibly should have a temporary pacemaker placed before major surgical procedures.

INTERMITTENT BLOCK

Rate-related bundle branch blocks are not uncommon and have been reported during general anesthesia.[92] When a critical heart rate is exceeded, conduction through a diseased bundle branch can become blocked. Heart rates above 120 beats per minute can produce either RBBB or LBBB and can be mistaken for a ventricular tachycardia since both have wide QRS complexes and abnormal ST-T changes.

Atrioventricular Heart Block (AV Block)

AV block may be incomplete or complete. First- and second-degree AV blocks are incomplete, while third-degree AV block is complete heart block.

FIRST-DEGREE HEART BLOCK

First-degree heart block is a delay in passage of the impulse through the AV node with the P-R interval greater than 0.21 seconds. The A-H interval is prolonged on the His bundle electrograph.

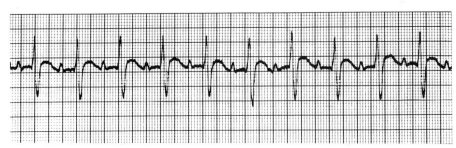

1. Heart rate—normal.
2. Rhythm—regular.
3. P:QRS—1:1 with no dropped beats.
4. QRS complex—normal.
5. Significance—may be normal; seen in patients taking digitalis or those with rheumatic fever.
6. Treatment—usually none. The P-R interval may be shortened with atropine or catecholamines.

SECOND DEGREE HEART BLOCK

There are two types of second-degree block:

1. Mobitz type I block—reflects disease of the AV node.
2. Mobitz type II block—reflects disease of the His bundle-Purkinje tissues.

In both of these blocks, some P waves are not followed by QRS complexes.

Mobitz I block (Wenckebach). There is a progressive lengthening of the P-R interval until a QRS complex is dropped. The Mobitz I block is relatively benign, frequently reversible (e.g., digitalis intoxication), and does not require a pacemaker.

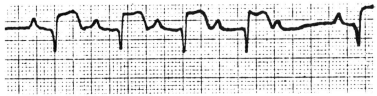

1. Heart rate—Atrial rate is normal, and the ventricular rate depends on the degree of AV block.
2. Rhythm—irregular ventricular response as a result of the varying P-R interval.
3. P:QRS—more P waves than QRS complexes.
4. QRS complex—normal.
5. Significance—generally caused by digitalis toxicity or myocardial infarction. It is transient and does not require pacing.

6. Treatment—Discontinue digitalis, and if the rate is very slow, atropine, isoproterenol, or pacing can be used.

Mobitz II block. The Mobitz II block is the less common and more serious form of second-degree heart block. P waves occur without subsequent QRS complexes. These are just "dropped beats" without any lengthening of the P-R interval.

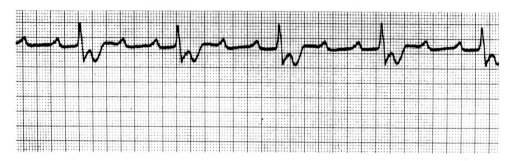

1. Heart rate—Atrial rate is normal, and the ventricular rate depends on the number of dropped beats.
2. Rhythm—irregular ventricular response as a result of the irregularly dropped beats.
3. P:QRS—more P waves than QRS complex. The P-R intervals are normal when present.
4. QRS complex—normal, but a bundle branch block is frequently present.
5. Significance—This is seen only when the block occurs in the His-Purkinje system and has a serious prognosis, since it frequently progresses to complete heart block.

6. Treatment—Atropine or isoproterenol can usually restore 1:1 conduction. Pacemaker insertion should be considered for major surgery.

THIRD-DEGREE HEART BLOCK (COMPLETE HEART BLOCK)

In third-degree heart block, no impulses from the atrium can reach the ventricle, and the ventricles act as the pacemaker of the heart. There is no relationship between the P waves and QRS complexes.

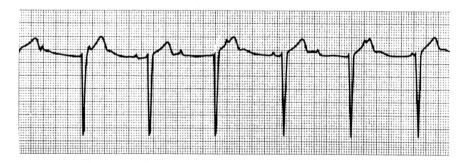

1. Heart rate—30-40 beats per minute.
2. Rhythm—regular.
3. P:QRS—no relationship; more P waves than QRS complexes.
4. QRS complex—may be normal if the pacer

site is in the AV node but usually is widened to longer than 0.12 seconds with the pacer site in the ventricle.
5. Significance—The heart rate is too slow to maintain adequate cardiac output, and syn-

cope (Stokes-Adams syndrome) and heart failure will occur.

6. Treatment—pacemaker. Atropine or isoproterenol may temporarily increase the heart rate.

ISCHEMIA AND INFARCTION

Electrocardiographic monitoring of myocardial ischemia is a relatively new technique in the operating room. Studies of intraoperative ECG monitoring by Cannard in 1960 and Russell in 1969 did not even mention the use of the ECG to diagnose ischemia; they only discussed the use of the ECG to diagnose arrhythmias.[15,16] In recent years, coronary artery disease has become the number one health problem in the United States. Patients admitted for all types of surgical procedures have significant coronary artery disease, and many have histories of acute myocardial infarctions or angina pectoris. In these patients, the ECG should be used to identify myocardial ischemia during the stresses of anesthesia and surgery, as well as for arrhythmia recognition. It is important to realize that a substantial number of patients with severe coronary artery disease may have a normal resting ECG. Benchimol found that 17 of 106 patients with documented triple-vessel coronary artery disease had normal resting ECGs.[93] Therefore, it is important to monitor the ECG for ischemic changes in all patients with potential coronary artery disease (e.g., obese or hypertensive patients); probable coronary artery disease (e.g., patients with atherosclerosis undergoing vascular surgery, such as a carotid endarterctomy); or known coronary artery disease.

The cardiologist frequently states in his consultations for all patients with coronary artery disease that the ECG should be monitored. However, he has never told the anesthesiologist or surgeon the specific techniques that he has learned during exercise stress testing, e.g., lead placement, criteria for the diagnosis of ischemia. Until recently, therefore, the older ECG lead systems designed primarily for arrhythmia detection have been used during surgery when monitoring of ischemic changes was desired.

Lead Systems

As early as 1931, it was noted that the precordial leads gave a greater sensitivity in detecting ST-segment depression of ischemic origin than did the standard leads.[7] Since then, a number of lead systems have been developed to monitor myocardial ischemia, and they have been studied extensively during stress testing. Blackburn has done many studies of the lead systems and found that the most sensitive exploring electrode was at the V_5 chest position.[94] He showed that 89 percent of the ST-segment information contained in a conventional 12-lead ECG is found in lead V_5. Mason studied 174 patients using a multiple lead ECG during exercise, and he found that leads V_4, V_5, and V_6 were the most valuable and lead I the least informative.[95] Of the 56 patients with a positive test, 30 had "anterior" ischemia (V_3-V_6), 8 had "inferior" ischemia (II, III, AVF), and 18 had a combined pattern. As can be seen from this study, isolated anterior wall (V_1-V_2) or inferior wall ischemia can still be missed by single V_5 lead monitoring. Because of this factor, most authors have recommended the observation of multiple leads when monitoring for myocardial ischemia.

It was not until 1976 that any information on the use of precordial leads for monitoring of ischemia during anesthesia first appeared. Dalton recommended placing a sterile spinal needle in the V_4 or V_5 position after the skin was "prepped" for cardiac surgery.[96] Kaplan recommended that a multiple lead ECG system be used in all patients with coronary artery disease.[17] Four disposable electrocardiographic pads are placed on the extremities, and a fifth is placed in the V_5 position covered with a small piece of steri-drape (Fig. 4-13). The V_5 lead and steri-drape are placed *prior to the induction of anesthesia* and can be "prepped over" by the surgical team. We have found that this lead does not interfere with the majority of cardiac surgery, which is performed through a median sternotomy. We have observed many instances of severe ischemic changes in V_5 both before and after the skin prep, when little was seen in the other leads (Fig. 4-19).

Using the five electrodes, we can select seven different ECG leads to observe (I, II, III, AVR, AVL, AVF, or V_5). All seven leads are observed prior to the start of anesthesia and *recorded* for later reference. In patients undergoing coronary revascularization, we record all seven leads and then simultaneously display two leads (V_5 and II) using two different

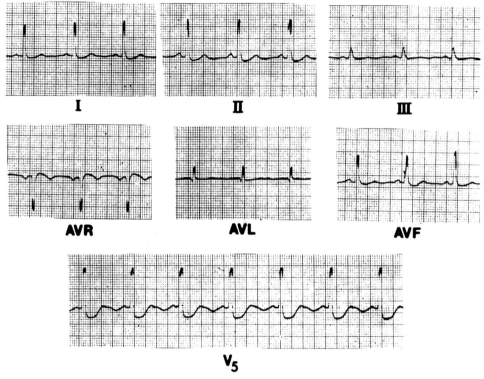

Fig. 4-19. Electrocardiogram associated with mild hypotension (90/50) upon opening the pericardium. V_5 shows severe ST-segment depression, while only minimal ST-segment changes are present in leads I, II, III and AVF. (Reproduced from Kaplan JA: The precordial electrocardiographic lead (V_5) in patients with coronary artery disease. Anesthesiology 45:570, 1976, with permission of author and publisher.)

ECG channels (Fig. 4-20). This allows us to look at the anterior and inferior walls of the heart at the same time. Robertson has shown that there is some degree of correlation between the site of coronary artery obstruction and the lead in which ischemia is detected.[97] ST-segment changes in leads II, III and AVF correspond to disease of the right coronary artery; and ischemic changes in V_4-V_6 indicate disease of the left anterior descending or circumflex coronary artery. We recently had a patient who suddenly developed isolated ST-segment elevation in V_5 after a four-vessel bypass procedure (Fig. 4-21). Reexploration demonstrated an occluded anterolateral obtuse marginal graft, which demonstrated the anatomic specificity of the anterior lead. The correlation between ECG zonal ischemia and coronary anatomy is not always this precise, however.

We prefer the five-electrode system discussed above, including the true V_5 lead. Some operating room ECG systems have only three or four electrode wires, however. A modification of the V_5 lead can be readily used in those cases, as is frequently done during exercise stress testing. The most popular modified leads during stress testing have been the CM_5 and CS_5 bipolar leads, in which the negative electrode is at the upper sternum (manubrium) in CM_5 or under the right clavicle in the CS_5, with the positive electrode at the V_5 position. These leads are more convenient than V_5 because they require fewer wires. They are good leads for detection of ischemia, but Froelicher has recently shown that they are not as good as V_5.[98] In the operating room, the right arm electrode can be placed just under the clavicle or on the right shoulder, and the left arm electrode placed in the V_5 position. Then lead I can be selected to observe the anterior heart wall (a modified CS_5), and lead II for the inferior wall. Another alternative in a four-electrode system is to place the left arm lead in the V_5 position and observe lead AVL, which will be a modified V_5 lead.

ST-Segment Changes

The criteria for ischemic changes on the ECG are still not entirely agreed upon. There is more agreement than there has been in the past, however, as a result of extensive studies during exercise stress testing. Surgery and anesthesia are certainly a good stress test for the patient with coronary artery disease, and we therefore believe that exercise testing information is transferable to the operating room. When patients with coronary artery disease are exercised, the first abnormality seen is depression of the J-point (the J-point is where the QRS joins the ST segment).[7] This J-point depression evolves into a progressively more depressed horizontal ST segment, and then anginal pain may frequently

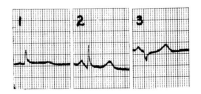

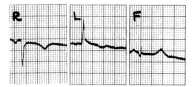

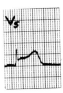

Fig. 4-21. An intraoperative ECG tracing of our seven standard leads. From 3 to 4 mm of horizontal ST-segment elevation are shown only in V_5. Minor 1-mm changes are seen in the other leads (Reproduced from Kaplan JA: Diagnostic value of the V_5 precordial lead. Anesth Analg, 57:364, 1978, with permission of author and publisher.)

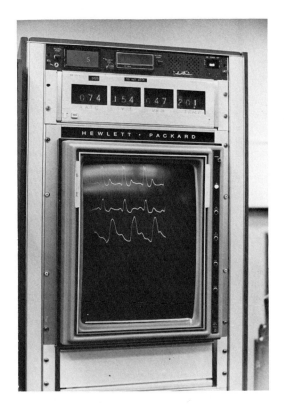

Fig. 4-20. A simultaneous display of leads V_5 (top) and lead II (bottom) are shown. Also demonstrated are the arterial trace, digital readouts, and the rate pressure produce meter on the upper center panel.

occur. The pain always *follows* the ST-segment depression, however. At the end of the test, the ST segment may either return to the upsloping J-point depression or convert to a downsloping ST segment with a deeply inverted T wave. Significant myocardial ischemia is defined as greater than 1 mm of horizontal or downsloping ST-segment depression measured from a point 0.06 seconds from the J-point. Downsloping ST-segment depression, beginning from 1.0 mm depression at the J-point, is the most specific sign of myocardial ischemia. There is general agreement that an increased magnitude of ST-segment depression denotes an increased degree of ischemia. J-point depression with upsloping ST segments may reflect ischemia but is not a specific sign. Also, T wave changes may reflect ischemia but again are not specific.[99–101] All ST-segment elevations of greater than 1.0 mm are considered significant. This is a manifestation of a more severe myocardial ischemia reflecting transmural, rather than subendocardial ischemia.[102] In patients with Prinzmetal angina

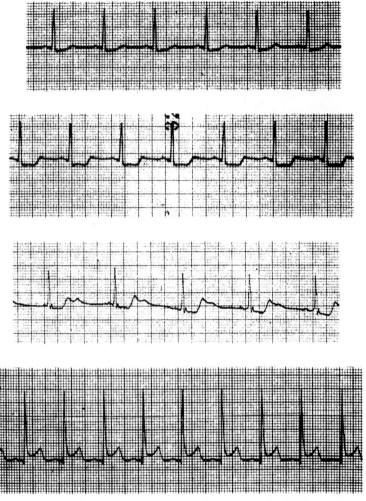

Fig. 4-22. ST-segment changes of myocardial ischemia are demonstrated. The top panel shows J-point depression and upsloping ST-segment depression. The second panel shows horizontal ST-segment depression of ischemia. The third panel shows downsloping ST-segment depression of ischemia. And the fourth panel shows ST-segment elevation of the ischemia.

(coronary spasm), the ST segments are also elevated with pain (Fig. 4-22).

The ST segments and T waves can be affected by many factors other than myocardial ischemia.[103] These other factors produce the "nonspecific ST-T-wave changes." Drugs that can affect the ST segments include digitalis, diuretics which deplete potassium, and reserpine. Hypokalemia or glucose infusion can affect the ST segment by altering the membrane-potassium relationships. The ST segments may appear to be depressed by the T_a wave of atrial repolarization and altered by conduction disturbances such as LBBB or WPW. ST-segment depression and T wave inversion have been reported with changes in respirations alone.[104]

Myocardial Infarction

The classic ECG pattern of ischemia progresses to infarction as follows:

1. ST-segment depression and T wave inversion—possible ischemia.

2. ST-segment elevation—pattern of injury.
3. Q wave appearance—pattern of necrosis; only the Q waves are diagnostic of definite infarction.

The Q waves are diagnostic if they are more than 0.03 seconds in width; the ST-segment elevation shows an upward convexity; and the T waves are symmetrical and pointed (Fig. 4-23). These *indicative* changes of an infarction are seen in the leads of the ECG facing the necrotic area. The opposite surface of the heart shows *reciprocal* changes consisting of an increased height of the R wave, depressed ST segments, and tall upright T waves.

The location of myocardial infarctions are described by the "wall" of the heart they affect.[4] These are only approximations, however, since there are no clear-cut boundaries between areas of the heart. The four walls usually referred to are anterior, lateral, inferior, and posterior (Table 4-5).

Acute myocardial infarctions tend to evolve electrocardiographically through various stages. Soon after the onset of pain, the ST segments are elevated, and the T waves are taller and upright (hyperacute changes); then the T waves become symmetrically inverted (coving) as the ST segments return to baseline; finally, the T waves return to their baseline position. The Q waves usually appear within 12 to 24 hours of the infarction but may be delayed to a much later time. Persistent ST elevation is usually caused either by pericarditis or by a ventricular aneurysm (Fig. 4-24).

Not all infarctions are as easy to diagnose as it would appear from the above discussion, and in some cases, the diagnosis is made from the history and enzyme studies, not from the ECG. Some of these difficult situations are pa-

Table 4-5
Location of ECG Changes with Different Myocardial Infarctions

Location of Infarction	Indicative Changes	Reciprocal Changes
Anterior	V_1-V_4, I, AVL	II, III, AVF
Lateral	V_5-V_6, I, AVL	V_1, AVR
Inferior	II, III, AVF	V_1-V_4, I, AVL
Posterior	None	V_1-V_2

tients with LBBB, previous infarctions, lack of development of Q waves (loss of R waves only), or subendocardial infarctions. The diagnosis of an acute subendocardial infarction depends on the following factors (Fig. 4-25):

1. The clinical history of chest pain
2. ST-segment depression and symmetrical T wave inversion in the precordial leads
3. No Q wave development
4. Elevation of the CPK enzyme and the CPK-MB isoenzyme

Myocardial infarctions after coronary artery revascularization have been extremely difficult to define and diagnose. This partially accounts for the great variability of infarction rates reported among different institutions, ranging from 5 to 40 percent. The two primary techniques for detecting perioperative infarctions have been (1) development of new Q waves on the ECG and (2) elevation of serum enzymes. In the past, less specific enzymes, such as LDH or SGOT, were studied. In one study, elevation of at least two enzymes was noted in patients with acute myocardial infarctions to levels of SGOT

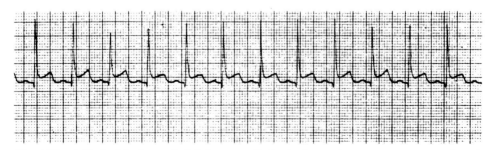

Fig. 4-23. A V_5 lead is demonstrated from a patient who has undergone an acute anterolateral infarction. There are Q waves present and ST-segment elevation.

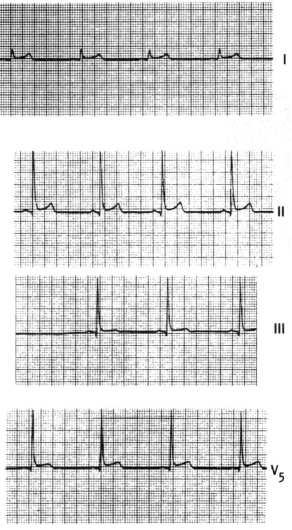

Fig. 4-24. Persistent ST-segment elevation is seen in leads I, II, III, and V$_5$ in a patient with chronic pericarditis.

greater than 200, LDH greater than 400, or CPK greater than 800.[105]

Recently, the myocardial isoenzymes of creatine phosphokinase (CPK-MB) and of lactic dehydrogenase (LDH$_1$) have been used for much greater specificity. The LDH$_1$ isoenzyme is predominately myocardial but is also present in red blood cells, kidney, brain, stomach, and pancreas. Therefore, it has not correlated with acute infarctions as well as the CPK-MB isoenzyme, which is only found in the heart. The normal total CPK is less than 40 mIU/ml and

CPK-MB is 2 ± 1 mIU/ml. During an acute infarction, the total CPK frequently exceeds 800 and the peak CPK-MB has been found to range from 25 to 400 mIU/ml.[106] The initial CPK-MB is detectable within 3 hours after the onset of chest pain, and peak values usually occur within 12 hours. Dixon studied a series of 100 patients undergoing coronary revascularization and divided them into three groups according to the presence or absence of postoperative CPK-MB.[107] Group I (49 patients) had no CPK-MB postoperatively and had a peak total CPK of

PATIENT 1

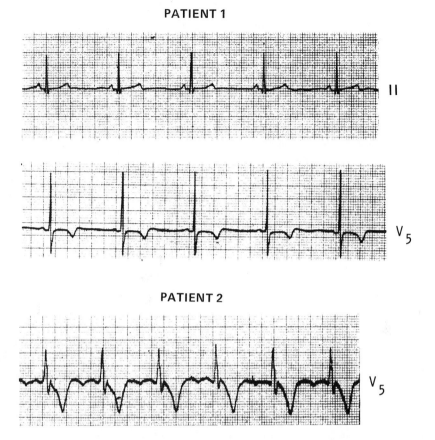

Fig. 4-25. Two patients with subendocardial myocardial infarctions are demonstrated. In patient 1, top, there is symmetrical T wave inversion demonstrated only in lead V_5. In patient 2, bottom, there is severe symmetrical T wave inversion demonstrated in V_5. Neither patient showed the development of Q waves or ST-segment elevation.

about 900 and peak LDH of 500; group II (4 patients) had CPK-MB in a low concentration (less than 40 mIU/ml) for only 1 day and peak total CPK of about 650 and LDH of 400; group III (17 patients) had CPK-MB activity ranging from 40 to 400 mIU/ml and lasting 31 hours and peak total CPK of 1100 and LDH of 500. These groups correlated with the ECG findings as well. Groups I and II had no ECG changes, while group III had changes characteristic of acute infarctions.

The other standard method of diagnosing an infarction after coronary artery surgery is by the appearance of new Q waves on the ECG. Sternberg found that new Q waves correlated well with the appearance of localized abnormalities of left ventricular wall motion on repeat

cardiac catheterization.[108] Basson, however, reported that all new Q waves may not be a new infarction but just an "unmasking" of a preexisting inferior infarction by anterior wall ischemia.[109] To complicate things even further, Kennedy reported the disappearance of Q waves after coronary revascularization as a result of either reperfusion of an ischemic area or a "cancelling effect" of new perioperative myocardial damage upon the old ECG evidence of a myocardial infarction.[110] Rigihetti compared the ECG changes with CPK-MB measurements and concluded that (1) new Q waves on the ECG *underestimate* the incidence of myocardial damage after coronary artery surgery; (2) CPK-MB alone *overestimates* the incidence of infarction; and (3) the two techniques should possibly be combined along with a ^{99m}Tc pyrophosphate myocardial scan to best detect perioperative infarction.[111]

QRS and ST-Segment Mapping Techniques

The amount of myocardium that ultimately becomes ischemic or necrotic appears not to be fixed at the onset of ischemia. This is an important concept, because it means that appropriate interventions can reduce the final size of the necrotic area. In order to measure the area of ischemia and evaluate therapeutic interventions, the following four mapping techniques have been developed primarily by Muller, Maroko, and Braunwald:[112]

1. Epicardial ST-segment mapping
2. Epicardial QRS mapping
3. Precordial ST-segment mapping
4. Precordial QRS mapping

The epicardial techniques were used first in animals, and then the precordial techniques were compared to them in animals and applied to patients. A good correlation was shown in all cases between the epicardial and precordial techniques ($r = .92$).[113]

ST-segment mapping, also sometimes called TQ-ST-segment mapping, is the most commonly used and debated form of mapping. Models of partial thickness myocardial ischemia have been developed to explain ST-segment changes. Subendocardial ischemia with normal subepicardial blood flow produced subendocardial ST elevation but epicardial and precordial ST-segment depression. Epicardial and precordial ST-segment depression represents reciprocal subendocardial ST elevation as long as a layer of nonischemic muscle is present. When the ischemia becomes transmural, however, epicardial and precordial ST-segment elevation occurs.[114,115] Altered ion transport across the ischemic myocardial cell membrane appears to be the cause of the change in current responsible for the ST-segment elevation. A reduction of intracellular potassium or an excess of extracellular potassium is critical to the generation of the elevated ST segment.[116] The ST-segment elevation seen on the ECG is made up of two components:[117]

1. True ST-segment elevation from the original TQ-segment baseline, which is the less important factor.
2. Apparent ST-segment elevation resulting from depression of the TQ segment, which is the predominant factor.

Conventional capacitor-coupled ECG amplifiers do not permit differentiation of ST-segment elevation from TQ-segment depression.

Epicardial ST-segment mapping has been used to evaluate most potential therapeutic interventions in dogs with acute coronary occlusion (Maroko dog model) (Fig. 4-26).[118] An occlusion is placed on the left anterior descending coronary artery of the dog, and the ST-segment elevation in multiple epicardial sites is determined 15 minutes after the occlusion. The occlusion is then released, and the heart is allowed to recover for 1 hour. The procedure is then repeated, but in the presence of the intervention under study. The mean ST-segment elevation (ST) and the sum of ST elevation in all epicardial leads (ΣST) are then compared between the control and intervention studies (Fig. 4-27). Hillis and Braunwald have recently summarized all the data on interventions that have been obtained by this technique.[116] They divided treatments into those that *increased* myocardial injury after coronary artery occlusion either by increasing MVO$_2$ (e.g., isoproterenol) or by decreasing myocardial oxygen supply (e.g., nitroprusside); and those that *decreased* myocardial injury either by decreasing MVO$_2$ (e.g., propranolol, nitroglycerin) or by increasing myocardial oxygen supply (e.g., intra-aortic balloon counterpulsation). Bland showed that halothane decreased the extent of ST-elevation (ΣST) after an acute occlusion of a coronary artery.[119]

Epicardial QRS mapping is a relatively newer technique than ST-segment mapping. Hillis has recently shown that QRS mapping can also be used to assess interventions to modify myocardial necrosis.[120] He demonstrated by this technique that both propranolol and hyaluronidase are beneficial to the ischemic myocardium. Q wave development ($\triangle$Q), R wave fall ($\triangle$R), and their combinations ($\triangle$R + $\triangle$Q) at 24 hours were correlated with the extent of necrosis measured by CPK-MB.

Precordial ST-segment mapping has had the greatest clinical application of these techniques. A 35-lead electrode blanket was developed by

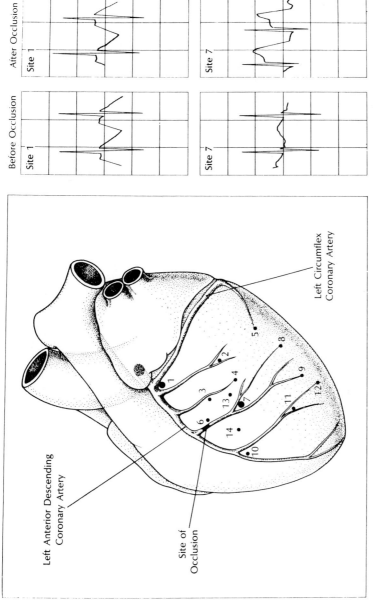

Fig. 4-26. The Maroko dog model is demonstrated. A branch of the left anterior descending coronary artery is occluded and epicardial ST-segment mapping is performed. An affected site, site 7, which became ischemic, is demonstrated as well as an unaffected site, site 1. (Reproduced from Braunwald E: Protection of the ischemic myocardium. *In* The Myocardium: Failure and Infarction, New York, H. P. Publishing Co., 1974, with permission of the author and publishers.)

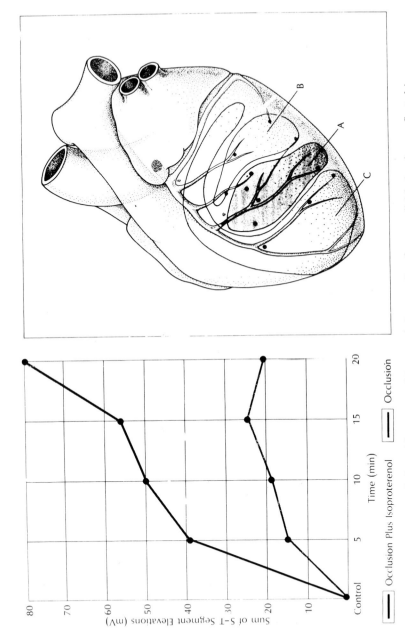

Fig. 4-27. Infusion of isoproterenol increased the severity of myocardial ischemia as reflected in the sum of the ST-segment elevation recorded after coronary occlusion. After occlusion, the sum ranged from 15–25 mV; while, after occlusion plus isoproterenol, it ranged from 40–80mV. (Reproduced from Braunwald E: Protection of the ischemic myocardium. *In* The Myocardium: Failure and Infarction, New York, H. P. Publishing Co., 1974, with permission of the author and publishers.)

Maroko to record precordial maps in patients. Interventions such as propranolol, counterpulsation, nitroglycerin, and oxygen have been shown to reduce ST-segment elevation.[121] Maroko has recently used precordial QRS mapping to demonstrate the beneficial effects of hyaluronidase in 91 patients with acute anterior wall myocardial infarction.[122]

There are many limitations and controversies associated with the TQ-ST mapping techniques. The greatest limitation is that they can only be used in patients with anterior or lateral ischemia. They provide information only about the therapeutic response of the epicardial half of the anterior left ventricular wall. In addition, they cannot be used in patients with intraventricular conduction defects since these markedly affect the ST segment. The areas of controversy involve validation of this method in relation to other techniques measuring infarct size[123] and questions about the technical limitations and electrophysiology involved in the technique.[124]

Further modifications of precordial mapping will almost certainly occur. It may be possible to reduce the number of leads without a loss of information. In the operating room, it may be found necessary to monitor more than V_5 alone. Possibly V_3-V_6 and leads above and below them (nine precordial leads) will be needed to detect all anterior ischemia. Evaluation of the inferior side of the heart using leads II, III, and AVF needs further study, since early claims of beneficial therapeutic effects were made on the basis of ST-segment changes in a full 12-lead ECG. Foerster has shown that the ST-segment vector in the vectorcardiogram (VCG) correlated with the ΣST segments derived from epicardial mapping.[125] This may develop into a useful tool, since it only requires three Frank XYZ leads, and the VCG has been shown to be superior to the scalar ECG in detecting areas of ischemia.

OTHER CONDITIONS AFFECTING THE ELECTROCARDIOGRAM

Effects of Drugs on the Electrocardiogram[4,126]

DIGITALIS

Digitalis preparations have many effects on the ECG. The usual effects include the prolongation of the P-R interval to a first-degree heart block but no change in the QRS complex. Marked ventricular repolarization effects include: (1) depression of the ST segment, (2) decreased amplitude of the T wave and sometimes inversion of the T wave, (3) shortening of the Q-T_c interval, and (4) increase of the U wave amplitude.

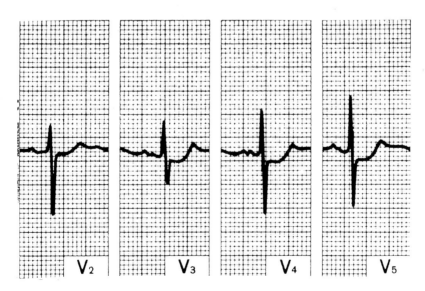

V_2 V_3 V_4 V_5

As a result of increased automaticity of ectopic pacemaker fibers, digitalis intoxication can produce almost any arrhythmia. The most common arrhythmias seen with toxicity are PVCs of multifocal origin which proceed to ventricular bigeminy. The most characteristic supraventricular arrhythmia is PAT. This is frequently associated with atrioventricular block, since digitalis prolongs AV conduction. All forms of heart block have been produced by digitalis toxicity, the most common being a Mobitz type I block.

QUINIDINE

Therapeutic doses of quinidine decrease the upslope of the action potential and decrease automaticity. It may prolong the P wave and P-R interval, but increasing doses always prolong the QRS complex. At high plasma levels, the QRS complex can be widened by 50 percent. The ST segments may be depressed, the T wave depressed or inverted, and the U waves increased, as with digitalis. With quinidine, however, the $Q-T_c$ interval lengthens, while it shortens with digitalis. Two types of toxic reactions may occur: (1) dose-dependent widening of the QRS, heart block, and severe bradycardia; and (2) dose-independent ventricular ectopy resulting from reentry promoted by slow conduction.

PROCAINAMIDE AND OTHER CARDIAC DRUGS

The effects of procainamide are very similar to those of quinidine, but since procainamide is frequently given intravenously and is a shorter-acting drug, its effects on the ECG appear sooner and last for a shorter period of time. Therapeutic doses of lidocaine, diphenylhydantoin, and propranolol have no definite effects on the ECG. Diuretics have no direct effect on the ECG but can affect it profoundly by altering electrolytes. Moreover, the antihypertensive drugs do not affect the ECG directly, but only through changes in electrolytes and the autonomic nervous system.

PSYCHOTROPIC DRUGS

Several phenothiazines produce dose-dependent abnormalities of ventricular repolarization. These are most commonly seen with thioridazine (Mellaril) but are also seen with chlorpromazine and other major tranquilizers. Widening of the $Q-T_c$ interval and T wave and increased U wave amplitude are seen, but no changes occur in the P, QRS, or ST segment. Ectopic rhythms have also been reported, probably secondary to reentry. Imipramine hydrochloride, the non-MAO inhibitor antidepressant drug, has been associated with marked ECG changes. It prolongs the $Q-T_c$ interval, depresses the ST segment and T waves, widens the QRS complex, and produces supraventricular and ventricular arrhythmias.

Effects of Electrolytes on the Electrocardiogram[126,127]

Since depolarization and repolarization of myocardial cells depend on potassium, calcium, and magnesium ion, it would be expected that abnormalities of these electrolytes would markedly affect the ECG.

POTASSIUM

The ECG is the best measurement of the relationship between intracellular and extracellular potassium. Hypokalemia produces characteristic changes on the ECG. When the serum potassium is reduced to 3-3.5 mEq/liter, the T wave is lowered and a tall U wave is seen. This appears to prolong the Q-T interval but, in fact, does not; it is the fused Q-TU interval that is observed. When the serum potassium is under 3 mEq/liter, the ST segment is also depressed.

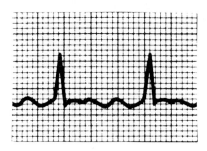

Hyperkalemia can produce profound changes on the ECG. Narrowing and peaking of the T wave, along with shortening of the Q-T interval, are seen when the serum potassium level reaches 6.0 mEq/liter. This is due to an increased velocity of repolarization. When the serum potassium level exceeds 6.5 mEq/liter, the QRS complex begins to widen and simulates a left bundle branch block. The P-R interval increases when the potassium level exceeds 7 mEq/liter, and by a potassium level of 8.8 mEq/liter, the P wave is lost. Potassium levels greater than 10-12 mEq/liter produce ventricular asystole or fibrillation.

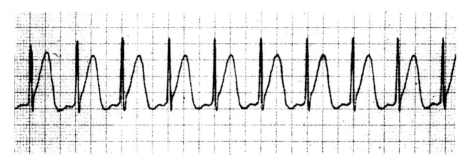

High levels of potassium also block AV conduction, and this is now being seen with increasing frequency since hyperkalemic solutions are being used to arrest the heart on cardiopulmonary bypass. In this situation, the potassium frequently has to be driven into the cells to reestablish the membrane potential and allow repolarization and conduction. This is done by administering either calcium chloride, sodium bicarbonate, or glucose and insulin.

CALCIUM AND MAGNESIUM

Hypocalcemia prolongs the Q-T interval by elongating the ST segment. This must be differentiated from the prolonged Q-U interval of hypokalemia. In patients with a low ionized calcium, the U wave is usually absent. In hypercalcemia, the Q-T interval is shortened, and the proximal limb of the T wave abruptly rises to its peak. In animal experiments, the pattern of hypocalcemia is exaggerated by hypomagnesemia and corrected by hypermagnesemia. Early magnesium deficiency is characterized by tall, peaked T waves (not narrow as in hyperkalemia) and a

normal Q-T interval. Later changes include a prolonged P-R interval, widened QRS, ST segment depression, and low T waves.[128]

Effects of Hypothermia on the Electrocardiogram[129,130]

The ECG findings of hypothermia can be quite marked. As the temperature decreases, there is a progressive slowing of the sinus rate, inversion of the T waves, and prolongation of the P-R, QRS, and Q-T intervals. Atrial fibrillation or flutter is frequently encountered, and ventricular arrhythmias appear below 30°C. Further decreases below 28°C produce ventricular fibrillation. In addition, a secondary deflection at the end of the QRS complex called the J wave, Osborn wave, or "camel hump" is frequently seen. The figure below demonstrates progressive hypothermic changes on the ECG. The top panel is at 37°C; the second panel at 29°C demonstrates the "camel hump"; the third and fourth panels show coarse and fine ventricular fibrillation which occurred at 27°C.

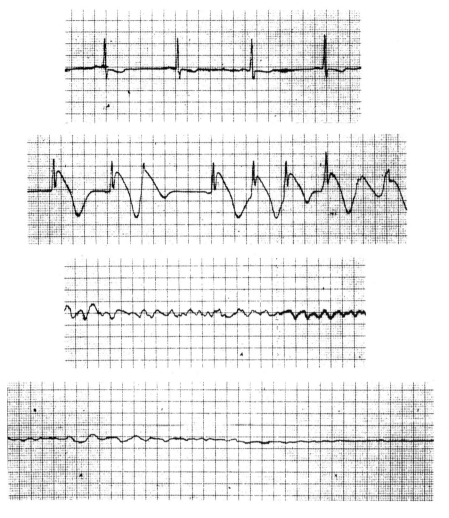

The abnormal Osborn wave is seen in hypothermia below 28°C, but is not diagnostic, since it has also been reported with central nervous system disease.[131]

REFERENCES

1. Titus JL: Normal anatomy of the human conduction system. Anesth Analg (Cleve) 52:508-514, 1973
2. Goldman MJ: Principles of Clinical Electrocardiography. Los Altos, Calif, Lange, 1976
3. Castellanos A, Myerburg RJ: The resting heart. *In* (Hurst JN, Logue RB) The Heart (ed 4). New York, McGraw-Hill, 1977, pp 298-312
4. Marriott JHL: Practical Electrocardiology (ed 5). Baltimore, Williams & Wilkins, 1972
5. Maroko PR, Libby P, Covell JW, et al: Precordial S-T segment elevation mapping: An atraumatic method for assessing alterations on the extent of myocardial ischemic injury. The effects of pharmacologic and hemodynamic interventions. Am J Cardiol 29:223-230, 1972
6. Muller JE, Maroko PR, Braunwald E: Evaluation of precordial ECG mapping as a means of assessing changes in myocardial ischemic injury. Circulation 52:16-27, 1975
7. Ellestad MH: Stress-testing: Principles and Practice. Philadelphia, FA Davis, 1975, pp 25-46
8. Kistin AD, Bruce JC: Simultaneous esophageal

and standard ECG leads for the study of cardiac arrhythmias. Am Heart J 53:65-73, 1957

9. Marriott HJL, Fogg E: Constant monitoring for cardiac dysrhythmias and blocks. Mod Concepts Cardiovasc Dis 39:103-108, 1970

10. Richards CC, Freeman A: Intra-atrial catheter placement under ECG guidance. Anesthesiology 25:388-391, 1964

11. Mantel JA, Massing GK, James TN, et al: A multipurpose catheter for electrocardiographic and hemodynamic monitoring plus atrial pacing. Chest 72:285-290, 1977

12. Akhtar M, Damato AN: Clinical uses of His bundle electrocardiography. Part I. Am Heart J 91:520-526, 1976

13. Goldreyer BN: Intracardiac ECG in the analysis and understanding of cardiac arrhythmias. Ann Intern Med 77:117-136, 1972

14. Atlee JL, Rusy BF: Ventricular conduction times and AV nodal conductivity during enflurane anesthesia in dogs. Anesthesiology 47:498-503, 1977

15. Cannard TH, Dripps RD, Helwig J, et al: The ECG during anesthesia and surgery. Anesthesiology 21:194-202, 1960

16. Russell PH, Coakley CS: Electrocardiographic observation in the operating room. Anesth Analg (Cleve) 48:784-788, 1969

17. Kaplan JA, King SB: The precordial electrocardiographic lead (V_5) in patients who have coronary artery disease. Anesthesiology 45:570-574, 1976

18. Arbeit SR, Rubin IL, Gross H: Dangers in interpreting the ECG from the oscilloscope monitor. JAMA 211:453-456, 1970

19. Rubenfine M, Rosenzweig S: ECG artifacts simulating atrial flutter. JAMA 220:1130, 1972

20. Borrello G: ECG artifacts simulating atrial flutter. JAMA 223:439, 1973

21. Doss JD, McCabe CW, Weiss GK: Noise free ECG data during electrosurgical procedures. Anesth Analg (Cleve) 52:156-160, 1973

21A. Goldberg E: Mechanical factors and the ECG. Am Heart J 93:629-644, 1977

22. Manoach M, Gitter S, Grossman E, et al: Influence of hemorrhage on the QRS complex of the ECG. Am Heart J 82:55-61, 1971

23. Voukydis PC: Effect of intracardiac blood on the ECG. N Engl J Med 291:612-616, 1974

24. Simonson E: The effect of age on the ECG. Am J Cardiol 29:64-73, 1972

25. Kurtz CM, Bennett JH, Shapiro HH: ECG studies during surgical anesthesia. JAMA 106:434-440, 1936

26. Katz RL, Bigger JT: Cardiac arrhythmias during anesthesia and operation. Anesthesiology 33:193-213, 1970

27. Bertrand CA, Steiner NV, Jameson AG, et al: Disturbances of cardiac rhythm during anesthesia and surgery. JAMA 216:1615-1617, 1971

28. Angelini L, Feldman MI, Lufschonowski R, et al: Cardiac arrhythmias during and after heart surgery: Diagnosis and management. Prog Cardiovasc Dis 16:469-495, 1974

29. Ayres SM, Grace WJ: Inappropriate ventilation and hypoxemia as causes of cardiac arrhythmias: The control of arrhythmias without antiarrhythmic drugs. Am J Med 46:495-505, 1969

30. Edwards R, Winnie AL, Ramamurthy S: Acute hypocapnic hypokalemia: An iatrogenic anesthetic complication. Anesth Analg (Cleve) 56:786-792, 1977

31. Koehntop DE, Liao JC, Van Bergen FH: Effects of pharmacologic alterations of adrenergic mechanisms by cocaine, tropolone, aminophylline, and ketamine on epinephrine-induced arrhythmias during halothane-nitrous oxide anesthesia. Anesthesiology 46:83-93, 1977

32. Fox EJ, Sklar GS, Hill CH, et al: Complications related to the pressor response to endotracheal intubation. Anesthesiology 47:524-525, 1977

33. Smith M, Ray CT: Cardiac arrhythmias, increased intracranial pressure, and the autonomic nervous system. Chest 61:125-133, 1972

34. Alexander JP: Dysrhythmia and oral surgery. Br J Anaesth 43:773-778, 1971

35. Borg DE: Paradox of cardiac arrhythmias in anaesthesia. Br J Anaesth 41:709-710, 1969

36. Cranefield PF, Wit AL, Hoffman BF: Genesis of cardiac arrhythmias. Circulation 47:190-204, 1973

37. Morrow DH, Logic JR: Management of cardiac arrhythmias during anesthesia. Anesth Analg (Cleve) 48:748-754, 1969

38. Moe GK, Mendez C: Physiologic basis of premature beats and sustained tachycardia. N Engl J Med 288:250-253, 1973

39. Lurie AJ, Salel AF, Vera Z, et al: Rapid overdrive pacing for refractory tachyarrhythmias in patients after open heart surgery. J Thorac Cardiovasc Surg 72:458-463, 1976

40. Rosen M, Hoffman BF: Mechanism of action of antiarrhythmic drugs. Circ Res 32:1-14, 1973

41. Schamroth L: How to approach an arrhythmia. Circulation 47:420-425, 1973

42. Hampton AG: Monitoring and dysrhythmia recognition in advanced life support. American Heart Association, Advanced Life Support Course

43. Slapa WJ: The sick sinus syndrome. Am Heart J 92:648-660, 1976

44. Moore EN, Spear JF, Boineau JP: Recent electrocardiographic studies of the Wolff-Parkinson-White syndrome. N Engl J Med 289:956-963, 1973

45. Kones RJ, Phillips JH: Chaotic atrial mecha-

nisms: Characteristics and treatment. Crit Care Med 2:243-249, 1974

46. Sprague DH, Mandel SD: Paroxysmal supraventricular tachycardia during anesthesia. Anesthesiology 46:75-77, 1977

47. Braunwald E, Sobel BE, Braunwald NS: Treatment of paroxysmal supraventricular tachycardia by electrical stimulation of the carotid sinus nerves. N Engl J Med 281:885-887, 1969

48. Askey JM: Hemiplegia following carotid sinus stimulation. Am Heart J 31:131, 1946

49. Cantwell JD, Dawson JE, Fletcher GF: Supraventricular tachyarrhythmias: Treatment with edrophonium. Arch Intern Med 130:221-224, 1973

50. Chung EK: Tachyarrhythmias in Wolff-Parkinson-White syndrome: Antiarrhythmia drug therapy. JAMA 237:376-379, 1977

51. Rosen KM, Denes P, Wu D, et al: Conversion of paroxysmal supraventricular tachycardia due to a concealed extranodal pathway with an intravenous bolus of lidocaine. Chest 71:78-80, 1977

52. Escher DJW, Furman S: Emergency treatment of cardiac arrhythmias: emphasis on use of electrical pacing. JAMA 214:2028-2034, 1970

53. Kleiger RE: Cardioversion of paroxysmal arrhythmias. JAMA 213:107-113, 1970

54. Sealy WC, Wallace AG: Surgical treatment of Wolff-Parkinson-White syndrome. J Thorac Cardiovasc Surg 68:757-770, 1974

55. Abildskov JA, Millar K, Burgess MJ: Atrial fibrillation. Am J Cardiol 28:263-267, 1971

56. Sinatra ST, Jeresatry RM: Enhanced atrioventricular conduction in atrial fibrillation after lidocaine administration. JAMA 237:1356-1357, 1977

57. Scherlag BJ, Lazzara R, Helfant RH: Differentiation of "AV junctional rhythms." Circulation 48:304-312, 1973

58. Haldemann G, Schoer H: Haemodynamic effects of transient atrioventricular dissociation in general anesthesia. Br J Anaesth 44:159-162, 1972

59. Galindo A, Wyte SR, Wetherhold JW: Junctional rhythm induced by halothane anesthesia—treatment with succinylcholine. Anesthesiology 37:261-262, 1972

60. Zipes DP, Fisch C: Premature AV junctional contractions. Arch Intern Med 128:633-635, 1971

61. Benchimol A, Desser KB: Phasic aortocoronary bypass graft blood velocity during ventricular arrhythmias in man. Am J Cardiol 40:315-318, 1977

62. Pietras RJ, Mautner R, Denes P, et al: Chronic recurrent right and left ventricular tachycardia: Comparison of clinical and hemodynamic and angiographic findings. Am J Cardiol 40:32-37, 1977

63. Cranefield PF: Ventricular fibrillation. N Engl J Med 289:732-736, 1973

64. Guedel AE, Knoefel PK: Ventricular fibrillation in anesthesia. Am J Surg 34:496-499, 1936

65. Rothfeld EL, Lipowitz M, Zucker IR, et al: Management of persistently recurring ventricular fibrillation with propranolol. JAMA 204:226-228, 1968

66. Joshpe G, Topilow A, Levitt B, et al: Recurrent ventricular fibrillation: Treatment with countershock, bretylium tosylate, and rapid cardiac pacing. NY State J Med 72:2659-2663, 1972

67. Gupta PK, Lichstein E, Chodda KD: Transient atrioventricular standstill: Etiology and management. JAMA 234:1038-1042, 1975

68. Grace WJ: Protocol for the management of arrhythmias in acute myocardial infarction. Crit Care Med 2:235-242, 1974

69. Watanabe Y, Dreifus LS: Cardiac Arrhythmias: Electrophysiologic Basis for Clinical Interpretation. New York, Grune & Stratton, 1977, pp 339-364

70. Tanaka K, Pettinger WA: Pharmacokinetics of bolus potassium injection for cardiac arrhythmias. Anesthesiology 38:587-589, 1973

71. Chipperfield B, Chipperfield JR: Magnesium and the heart. Am Heart J 93:679-682, 1977

72. Waldo AL, MacLean WAH, Karp RB, et al: Entrainment and interruption of atrial flutter with atrial pacing: Studies in man following open heart surgery. Circulation 56:737-745, 1977

73. Montoyo J, Angel J, Valle V, et al: Cardioversion of tachycardia by transesophageal atrial pacing. Am J Cardiol 32:85-90, 1973

74. Glassman E: Direct current cardioversion. Am Heart J 82:128-130, 1971

75. Bellet S: Essentials of Cardiac Arrhythmias: Diagnosis and Management. Philadelphia, WB Saunders, 1972, pp 426-436

76. Resnekov L: Present status of electroversion in the management of cardiac dysrhythmias. Circulation 47:1356-1363, 1973

77. Lown B, Kleiger R, Williams J: Cardioversion and digitalis drugs: Changed threshold to electric shock in digitalized animals. Circ Res 17:519-531, 1965

78. Usubiaga JE, Sardinas AA: Cardioversion and the anesthesiologist. Anesth Analg (Cleve) 49:818-826, 1970

79. Orko R: Anesthesia for cardioversion: Thiopentone with and without atropine premedication. Br J Anaesth 46:947-951, 1974

80. Orko R: Anesthesia for cardioversion: A comparison of diazepam, thiopental, and propranolol. Br J Anaesth 48:257-262, 1976

81. Barrett JS, Hey EB: Ventricular arrhythmias associated with the use of diazepam for cardioversion. JAMA 214:1323- 1324, 1970

82. Reier CE, Hamelberg W: Conscious analgesia and amnesia for cardioversion. JAMA 210:2052-2054, 1969

83. Budow J, Natarajan P, Kroop IG: Pulmonary edema following direct current cardioversion for atrial arrhythmias. JAMA 218:1803- 1805, 1971

84. Tacker WA, Galioto FM, Giuliani E, et al: Energy dosage for human trans-chest electrical ventricular defibrillation. N Engl J Med 290:214–215, 1974

85. Geddes LA, Tacker WA, Rosborough J, et al: The electrical dose for ventricular defibrillation with electrodes applied directly to the heart. J Thorac Cardiovasc Surg 68:593- 605, 1974

86. Pennington JE, Taylor J, Lown B: Chest thump for reverting ventricular tachycardia. N Engl J Med 283:1192- 1195, 1970

87. Hecht HH, Kossman EC, Childers RW, et al: Atrioventricular and intraventricular conduction: Revised nomenclature and concepts. Am J Cardiol 31:232- 242, 1973

88. Wynands JE: Anesthesia for patients with heart block and artificial cardiac pacemakers. Anesth Analg (Cleve) 55:626–632, 1976

89. Kastor JA: Atrioventricular block. N Engl J Med 292:462–465, 572–574, 1976

90. Rooney SM, Goldiner PL, Muss E: Relationship of RBBB and marked left axis deviation to complete heart block during anesthesia. Anesthesiology 44:64–66, 1976

91. Berg GR, Kotler MN: The significance of bilateral bundle branch block in the preoperative patient. Chest 59:62–67, 1971

92. Rorie OK, Muldoon SM, Krabill DR: Transient bundle branch block occurring during anesthesia. Anesth Analg (Cleve) 51:633–637, 1972

93. Benchimol A, Harris CL, Desser KB, et al: Resting ECG in major coronary artery disease. JAMA 224:1489- 1492, 1973

94. Blackburn H: The exercise electrocardiogram: Technological, procedural, and conceptual development. In Measurements in Exercise Electrocardiography. Springfield, Ill, CC Thomas, 1967

95. Mason RE, Likar I, Biern RO, et al: Multiple lead exercise electrocardiography. Circulation 36:517- 525, 1967

96. Dalton B: A precordial ECG lead for chest operations. Anesth Analg (Cleve) 55:740- 741, 1976

97. Robertson D, Kostuk WJ, Ahuja SP: The localization of coronary artery stenosis by 12 lead ECG response to graded exercise test. Am Heart J 91:437- 444, 1976

98. Froelicher VF, Wolthius R, Keiser N, et al: A comparison of two bipolar exercise ECG leads to lead V_5. Chest 70:611- 616, 1976

99. Fortuin NJ, Weiss JL: Exercise stress testing. Circulation 56:699- 712, 1977

100. Simonson E: ECG stress tolerance tests. Prog Cardiovasc Dis 13:269- 292, 1970

101. Noble RJ, Rothbaun DA, Knoebel SB, et al: Normalization of abnormal T waves in ischemia. Arch Intern Med 136:392- 395, 1976

102. Fortuin NJ, Freisinger GC: Exercise induced-S-T segment elements. Am J Med 49:459- 464, 1970

103. Kattus AA: Exercise ECG: Recognition of the ischemic response, false positive and negative pattern. Am J Cardiol 33:721- 731, 1976

104. Adams CW: T wave changes with inspiration. JAMA 216:1019- 1022, 1971

105. Ghani MF, Parker BM, Smith JR: Recognition of myocardial infarction after cardiac surgery and its relation to cardiopulmonary bypass. Am Heart J 88:18- 22, 1974

106. Roberts R, Henry PD, Wittereen SA, et al: Quantification of serum creatinine phosphokinase (CPK) isoenzyme activity. Am J Cardiol 33:650- 656, 1974

107. Dixon SA, Limbird LE, Roe CR, et al: Recognition of postoperative acute myocardial infarction: Application of isoenzyme techniques. Circulation 47, 48 (Suppl III):III—137- 140, 1973

108. Steinberg L, Wisneski JA, Ullyot DJ, et al: Significance of new Q waves after aortocoronary bypass surgery: Correlation with changes in ventricular wall motion. Circulation 52:1037- 1044, 1975

109. Bassan MM, Oatfield R, Hoffman I, et al: New Q waves after aortocoronary bypass surgery: Unmasking of an old infarction. N Engl J Med 290:349- 353, 1974

110. Kennedy FB, Ticzon AR, Duffy FC, et al: Disappearance of ECG pattern of inferior wall myocardial infarction after aortocoronary bypass surgery. J Thorac Cardiovasc Surg 74:585- 593, 1977

111. Righetti A, Crawford MH, O'Rourke RA, et al: Detection of perioperative myocardial damage after coronary artery bypass graft surgery. Circulation 55:173- 178, 1977

112. Muller JE, Maroko PR, Braunwald E: Precordial ECG mapping: A technique to assess the efficacy of interventions designed to limit infarct size. Circulation 57:1- 18, 1978

113. Muller JE, Maroko PR, Braunwald E: Evaluation of precordial ECG mapping as a means of assessing change in myocardial ischemic injury. Circulation 52:16- 27, 1975

114. Holland RP, Brooks H: TQ-ST segment map-

ping: critical review and analysis of current concepts. Am J Cardiol 40:110–129, 1977

115. Guyton RA, McClenothan JH, Newman GE, et al: Significance of subendocardial S-T segment elevation caused by coronary stenosis in the dog. Am J Cardiol 40:373-380, 1977

116. Hillis LD, Braunwald E: Myocardial ischemia. N Engl J Med 296:971-977, 1034-1041, 1093-1096, 1977

117. Vincent GM, Abildskov JA, Burgess MJ: Mechanism of ischemic S-T segment displacement. Circulation 56:559-565, 1977

118. Maroko PR, Kjekshus JK, Sobel BE, et al: Factors influencing infarct size following experimental coronary artery occlusion. Circulation 43:67-82, 1971

119. Bland JHL, Lowenstein E: Halothane-induced decrease in experimental myocardial ischemia in the non-failing canine heart. Anesthesiology 45:287-293, 1976

120. Hillis LD, Askenazi J, Braunwald E, et al: Use of changes in the epicardial QRS complex to assess interventions which modify the extent of myocardial necrosis following coronary artery occlusion. Circulation 54:591-598, 1976

121. Madias JE, Madias NE, Hood WB: Precordial S-T segment mapping: Effects of oxygen inhalation on ischemic injury in patients with acute myocardial infarction. Circulation 53:411-416, 1976

122. Maroko PR, Hillis LD, Muller JE, et al: Favorable effects of hyaluronidase on ECG evidence of necrosis in patients with acute myocardial infarction. N Engl J Med 296:898-904, 1977

123. Surawicz B: The disputed S-T segment mapping: Is the technique ready for wide application in practice? Am J Cardiol 40:137-140, 1977

124. Fozzard HA, Das Gupta DS: S-T segment potential and mapping: Theory and experiment. Circulation 54:533-537, 1976

125. Foerster JM, Vera Z, Janzen DA, et al: Evaluation of precordial orthogonal vectorcardiographic lead S-T segment magnitude in the assessment of myocardial ischemic injury. Circulation 55:728-732, 1977

126. Surawicz B, Lasseter KC: Effect of drugs on the ECG. Prog Cardiovasc Dis 13:26-50, 1970

127. Surawicz B: Relationship between ECG and electrolytes. Am Heart J 73:814-834, 1967

128. Burch EG, Giles TD: The importance of magnesium deficiency in cardiovascular disease. Am Heart J 94:649-657, 1977

129. Clements SD, Hurst JW: Diagnostic value of ECG abnormalities observed in subjects accidently exposed to cold. Am J Cardiol 29:729-734, 1972

130. Trevino A, Razi B, Beller BM: The characteristic ECG of accidental hypothermia. Arch Intern Med 127:470-473, 1971

131. Abbott JA, Cheitlin MD: The nonspecific camel-hump sign. JAMA 235:413-414, 1976

PART II

Disease Entities and Anesthesia

Lawrence M. Abrams, M.D.
Donn A. Chambers, M.D.

5
Preoperative Management

INTRODUCTION

Heart disease modifies the preoperative evaluation and the subsequent anesthetic management in both cardiac and noncardiac surgery. This chapter outlines the general points covered in evaluating patients with known or suspected heart disease. Detailed descriptions of the preoperative evaluations for coronary artery, valvular, and congenital lesions follow in Chapters 6, 7, and 8. Since coronary artery disease is the most common cardiac lesion encountered in both cardiac and noncardiac surgery, an abbreviated discussion of the preoperative evaluation for patients with coronary disease is included in this chapter. The second part of the chapter deals with some common medical problems associated with heart disease, emphasizing their role in modification of the anesthetic management.

BRIEF SUMMARY OF THE ESSENTIAL DATA FOR ALL PATIENTS WITH HEART DISEASE

The preoperative evaluation begins with a chart review from front to back. The heart disease is usually described by anatomic diagnosis, and the predominant symptoms, course, and complications are summarized. An effort should be made to quantitate disability resulting from heart disease in terms of reduced activity load and/or work schedule. In addition to summarizing data and complications from past evaluations and responses to past therapies, the response to current therapy should be noted. Medications and their dosages are listed, including digitalis preparations, diuretics, antiarrhythmics, antihypertensives, and any drugs taken for other conditions. The patient should be classified according to the criteria of the New York Heart Association: (1) asymptomatic; (2) symptoms with ordinary physical effort; (3) symptoms with less than ordinary effort; (4) symptoms at rest.

Data from nursing notes, vital sign charts, orders, medication schedules, and reports from the hematology, chemistry, electrocardiogram (ECG), and cardiac catheterization laboratories supplement the history and progress notes. A complete summary should contain vital sign ranges for blood pressure and heart rate, height and weight; ECG and chest x-ray report, complete blood count, electrolytes, and coagulation survey. Any abnormal studies including calcium, glucose, liver function tests and enzymes, blood urea nitrogen (BUN), and creatine levels should be noted. It is wise to confer with surgeons and cardiologists and to obtain additional consultation when questions or abnormal findings are unresolved.

A visit to the catheterization laboratory helps make familiar their special techniques and procedures. In this informal setting, one can freely discuss each parameter with the cardiologists and thus feel comfortable with the catheterization data. A review of the raw data and cineangiogram from the cardiac catheterization supplements the official report.

The patient interview should include clarification of points that are not clear from the chart and catheterization review, as well as providing reassurance and information for the patient. Progress notes, nursing notes, and business office notes may aid in indicating the patient's psychosocial profile. Time spent preoperatively reassuring the patient and explaining details should be considered part of the premedication aimed at calming the patient before surgery.

The physical examination is directed and specific. Examination of the airway is critical, since prolonged inductions by mask may precede tracheal intubation. The neck is examined for mobility, and the ease of intubation is ascertained. The neck vessels are examined for anatomic relationships, and the accessibility of the internal or external jugular vein is noted for anticipated cannulation. The pulmonary examination should include chest shape, respiratory effort and rate, and auscultation for wheezes, rales, and irregular flow. In addition to checking the heart for rate, apparent rhythm, size, murmurs, and pulsations, the S_3 and/or S_4 gallops are listened for.[1] These sounds are of low pitch and are thus heard best with the bell of the stethoscope. They are usually loudest at the apex and may be accentuated by expiration and left lateral decubitus position. Peripheral arteries are noted for pulsations and for collateral flow, especially where placement of an arterial cannula is anticipated. Carotid bruits are checked for, and a brief neurological examination, indicating mental status and local neurological deficits, is performed. Other abnormalities are pursued only if they pertain to the anesthesia.

PREOPERATIVE EVALUATION IN CORONARY ARTERY DISEASE

Coronary artery disease is now the most common indication for cardiac surgery and is the most common cardiac problem in adult patients undergoing noncardiac surgery. The following section discusses some of the preoperative considerations. Greater detail follows in Chapter 7.

History

Significant coronary artery disease usually presents with a history of chest pain or angina. Angina is a symptom of myocardial ischemia and implies a relative imbalance between oxygen supply and demand. Its most common cause is partial or sometimes complete coronary artery occlusion, but it may occur with normal coronary arteries. Angina may occur in the hypertrophied hyperdynamic heart in which oxygen demand is greatly increased or in the hypotensive patient in whom oxygen supply is deficient.

Typical angina involves pain, heaviness, or pressure in the chest, usually located retrosternally, that is related to stress or exertion and relieved by rest or nitroglycerin.[2] It rarely lasts for more than 5 minutes. The pain or discomfort may radiate to the back, arms, neck, jaws, or teeth. At times, it may occur only in one of these sites and not in the chest. Prinzmetal's angina is thought to be secondary to ischemia from spasm rather than resulting from occlusion of a coronary artery. The spasm is transient, rarely leads to infarction, is not consistently related to exertion, and is poorly responsive to rest.[3,4] Nocturnal angina may reflect increased demand on the heart from central pooling of blood from the extremities which results from reabsorption of peripheral edema when recumbent.[5] The most ominous form of angina is unstable angina. The angina either lasts for more than 5 minutes or may occur with greater frequency or with less stress than before. Although no enzyme or permanent ECG changes may occur, this angina may be a prelude to infarction.[5]

The patient should be questioned to determine as precisely as possible the stress required to produce angina. One way of doing this is to determine the number of times each day the patient experiences angina. The number of nitroglycerin tablets the patient takes is not a good indication of the frequency of angina, since some patients attempt to "save" their nitroglycerin for the more severe episodes in the mistaken belief that they will develop resistance to nitroglycerin. In addition, determining the number of steps that the patient can climb before experiencing angina may be misleading, since climbing steps may not be a part of the patient's normal routine. A simpler approach is first to determine what the normal routine of exertion was before the angina developed and then to determine at which points angina occurred and how much the patient has had to curtail those activities. This is not the same as asking if symptoms have become more frequent, since the patient may have consistently reduced activity to keep angina from increasing.

Objective data from the exercise tolerance test (ETT) may be directly applicable to the operating-room situation.[6] If the blood pressure and pulse data at the time the patient developed pain or ST depression are available, a rate-pressure product may be calculated by multiplying the systolic pressure by the heart rate. By keeping the rate pressure product below this level during induction and maintenance of anesthesia, it may be possible to prevent ischemia. Using a rate-pressure product obtained from chart data at the time of an anginal episode while in the hospital may be as useful. When only a blood pressure or a pulse was obtained the data may still be applicable.

The patient should be questioned for a history of heart failure, syncope, low-output state, or arrhythmia. It is important to determine whether these symptoms are associated with angina, are worsened by angina, or seem unrelated to angina. Association with angina may imply that the symptom is, at least in part, brought on by ischemia and is therefore potentially reversible.

Dyspnea is the most frequent symptom of congestive heart failure. When it occurs with exertion, it implies inadequate reserve for stress. Dyspnea at rest usually indicates severe cardiac decompensation. Dyspnea is a symptom of pulmonary congestion that occurs secondary to left ventricular dysfunction.[7,8] It may also result from primary pulmonary disease, however. Differentiating pulmonary from cardiac dyspnea may not be easy from the history alone; it may require pulmonary physiological or cardiac hemodynamic testing.

Orthopnea and paroxysmal nocturnal dyspnea (PND) are also symptoms of left ventricular dysfunction. Orthopnea suggests decompensation when blood pools centrally in the recumbent position and pulmonary capillary pressures rise to symptomatic levels. PND is intermittent orthopnea that occurs at night and subsides spontaneously. It may have a cardiac, pulmonary, or mixed cardiopulmonary origin. It

is possible that hypoxia and hypercarbia resulting from hypoventilation while asleep may result in myocardial decompensation leading to symptoms of increased pulmonary venous congestion.[9]

Sweating, tachycardia, and anxiety are the result of catecholamine release which may imply decreased cardiac output. Catecholamines increase peripheral resistance and heart rate. When elevated chronically as a result of low output, they also decrease renal perfusion, resulting in salt and water retention. Blood volume and left ventircular end-diastolic volume (LVEDV) increase.[10] The catecholamines may also increase the ejection fraction by increasing cardiac contractility.

When related to cardiac dysfunction, syncope, light-headedness, or dizziness may reflect low output or arrhythmia. Cerebrovascular or middle ear disease may confuse the diagnosis. Symptoms of middle ear disease frequently include the sensation that the room is spinning. Cerebrovascular disease symptoms may occur with changes in head position or may be associated with a carotid bruit. Arrhythmias may be accompanied by chest pounding or palpitations. An association with angina strongly implies a cardiac origin for these central nervous system symptoms.

Current medications should be listed, noting dosages, last dose, and patient compliance. Drugs included should be digitalis glycosides, diuretics, antihypertensives, anticoagulants including aspirin-containing medications, antiarrhythmics, and any medications taken for other medical conditions. Digitalis toxicity should always be considered when the patient has been taking these preparations (Table 5-1).[11] Symptoms include dizziness, nausea, vomiting, and visual disturbances.[12]

Critical past medical history includes history of myocardial infarction, congestive heart failure, cardiac surgery, previous catheterizations and recommendations. Actual documentation from in-hospital records is the best source of information. When such documentation is not available, it may be necessary to contact other physicians and obtain records from other hospitals.

The Physical Examination

In uncomplicated angina in which symptoms of pain are intermittent and not associated with symptoms of congestive heart failure, the

Table 5-1
Cardiac Glycoside Preparations

Agent	Gastro-intestinal Absorption	Onset of Action*	Peak Effect	Average Half-life†	Principal Metabolic Route (Excretory Pathway)	Average Digitalizing Dose Oral§	Average Digitalizing Dose Intra-venous**	Usual Daily Oral Maintenance Dose‡
Ouabain	Unreliable	5–10 min	30–120 min	21 hr	Renal; some gastrointestinal excretion	—	0.3–0.5 mg	—
Deslanoside	Unreliable	10–30 min	1–2 hr	33 hr	Renal	—	0.8 mg	—
Digoxin	60%–85%††	15–30 min	1½–5 hr	36 hr	Renal; some gastrointestinal excretion	1.25–1.5 mg	0.75–1.0 mg	0.25–0.5 mg
Digitoxin	90%–100%	25–120 min	4–12 hr	4–6 days	Hepatic‡‡ renal excretion of metabolites	0.7–1.2 mg	1.0 mg	0.1 mg
Digitalis leaf	About 40%	—	—	4–6 days	Similar to digitoxin	0.8–1.2 g	—	0.1 g

Source. Modified from Smith T: Digitalis glycosides. N Engl J Med 288:719–722, 1973.

* For intravenous dose.
† For normal subjects (prolonged by renal impairment in case of digoxin, ouabain, and probably by severe hepatic disease in case of digitoxin and digitalis leaf).
‡ Average for adult patients without renal or hepatic impairment; will vary widely among individual patients and requires close medical supervision.
§ Divided dose over 12–24 hour, at intervals of 6–8 hr.
** Given in increments for initial subcomplete digitalization, to be supplemented by further small increments as necessary.
†† For stable form of administration (may be less in malabsorption syndromes and in formulation with poor bioavailability).
‡‡ Enterohepatic cycle exists.

physical exam is frequently normal. That many patients die of an ischemic arrhythmia shortly after having a "normal" physical examination attests to the severity of coronary artery disease that may exist in the absence of physical signs or symptoms.

Subtle physical signs may precede the onset of clinical left ventricular failure. An S_3 gallop is probably caused by blood entering and distending a relatively noncompliant left ventricle after opening of the mitral valve. The S_4 corresponds to atrial contraction and is believed to represent the sound of additional atrial blood distending the left ventricle. It can occur only with effective atrial contraction. The point of maximal impulse is lateral to the midclavicular line with good consistency in cardiomegaly. The size and contractile vigor of the apical pulse roughly correspond to ventricular performance. Palpable precordial ectopic pulsations may be felt over areas of dyskinesia. Peripheral pulses reflect the vigor of heart ejection; distal capillary filling reflects the efficacy of peripheral perfusion. Poor capillary filling is a late development of heart failure and suggests an uncompensated low cardiac output state.

Fine basilar rales are a sign of increased left-sided pressures. The increased left ventricular end-diastolic pressure (LVEDP) produces increased pressure in the left atrium and from there via the pulmonary veins to the pulmonary capillaries. Depending on the balance among vascular oncotic pressure, interstitial pressure, intrapleural pressure, and intra-alveolar pressure, at some level of capillary pressure, fluid will shift from the intravascular to the extravascular space. At this point, interstitial edema will form, the patient will experience dyspnea, and rales will be present by auscultation. As the capillary pressure increases, interstitial edema will increase, and in a sitting patient, the level of rales will rise. At some point, fluid, protein, and possibly red cells will enter the alveoli, and the patient may produce red, frothy sputum. This is alveolar pulmonary edema.[7,8] In certain patients, edema will obstruct small airways, and at first, expiratory and later inspiratory wheezes will be heard.

Jugular venous distention may be an accurate index of right heart failure. The vertical height of venous distention in the external jugular vein is a close approximation of central venous pressure (CVP). The right heart frequently fails at some time after the onset of left ventricular failure. While the degree of CVP rise and right ventricular (RV) failure correlate poorly with pulmonary capillary pressure and left ventricular (LV) failure, and while RV failure frequently occurs well after the onset of LV failure, its presence is a qualitative indicator that LV failure may be present.

If examined closely, the jugular venous pulsations contain a, c, and v waves. The a wave is greatly magnified and is sometimes called a *cannon wave* when the atrium contracts simultaneously with the ventricle; it is seen in atrial flutter with block or junctional rhythm. The v wave is large in tricuspid insufficiency.

Electrocardiogram

ECG changes are most helpful when correlated with the clinical picture.[13] Diminished R-wave voltage with a preceding abnormal Q wave on the ECG suggests prior transmural infarction. In the presence of altered conduction, as in left bundle branch block or ventricular hypertrophy, however, these changes may be simulated. Ischemia correlates with ST-segment depression or, rarely, elevation, as in Prinzmetal's angina. T-wave inversion or flattening may also signal ischemia. Infarction, however, especially subendocardial infarction, may occur with any of these changes, or each of these changes may occur with no clear clinical correlation. Digitalis effect classically produces ST-segment changes. Persistent ST-segment elevation following infarction may indicate a ventricular aneurysm, while diffuse ST-segment elevation points to epicardial injury such as occurs with pericarditis.

Of equal importance to abnormal components of the ECG is the comparison of the most recent ECG with past tracings. A recent subtle voltage decline of an R wave or a relatively minor ST-segment change may not classify the tracing as markedly abnormal but may be indicative of an impending ischemic episode. When this is present, it is worthwhile to question the patient for a history of prolonged angina or symptoms suggestive of an acute or impending infarction.

Premature ventricular contractions (PVC) are usually easily diagnosed by their wide, bizarre QRS configuration and the subsequent compensatory pause. A compensatory pause exists when one PVC occurs between two normal beats, and the time interval between normal beats is exactly twice the normal R-R interval. When PVCs occur in pairs (couplets), on every other beat (bigeminy), in short or long runs (ventricular tachycardia), or on the downslope of the last normal T wave, the danger of conversion to ventricular fibrillation is greatly increased.[14] The occurrence of PVCs preoperatively, especially during cardiac catheterization, may predict their occurrence during anesthesia.

Premature atrial contractions (PAC) usually have a normal-looking QRS complex and are not followed by a compensatory pause. The PAC resets the sinoatrial node timing mechanism and therefore the R-R interval between the PAC and the next normal beat should equal the last normal R-R interval. PACs may sometimes look like PVCs if they are frequent and aberrantly conducted through a partially refractory conduction system, making detection of a compensatory pause difficult. Analysis of the first 0.04 seconds of the QRS may be helpful in distinguishing between the two. If the initial forces look like and are in the same direction as those of the normal beats, then the premature beat is probably an aberrantly conducted PAC. If the initial forces are opposite in direction to normal beats, however, it is probably a PVC.

Supraventricular dysrhythmias require classification preoperatively. Atrial fibrillation on the rhythm strip has an irregularly variable R-R interval and no clearly recognizable P waves. In atrial flutter, the atrium beats at 250 to 350 beats per minute, but ventricular response is usually less than 1:1. Tall, spiked flutter waves are usually seen in the right precordial or inferior leads. The atrium beats at 150 to 250 beats per minute in atrial tachycardia, and abnormal P waves may be seen on the ECG. In junctional rhythms the QRS is normal looking, but no preceding P wave is present on the ECG. Occasionally, the P wave is inverted shortly before or after the QRS. Digitalis is usually used to control the ventricular response to supraventricular tachyarrhythmias. Since large doses of digitalis may be required, digitalis intoxication is always a consideration. Certain rhythms, such as atrial tachycardia with block or junctional tachycardia, almost always indicate digitalis intoxication. Rapid or unstable supraventricular rhythms may be further slowed with additional digitalis or by addition of propranolol or quinidine. Digitalis should always precede

quinidine, since quinidine increases AV conduction.

Conduction blocks may be above or below the AV node. Supranodal blocks are frequently drug-related. Digitalis glycosides are the most frequently implicated drug. One common effect is an increase in the P-R interval to greater than 0.2 seconds (first-degree block). Second-degree block is characterized by some P waves not followed by a QRS and may also be a manifestation of digitalis. This block is known as Mobitz type I or Wenckebach block. Below the AV node, blocks more frequently originate from pathological anatomy rather than drug effect. As the bundle of His proceeds toward the septum, it divides into a right and left bundle. The left bundle further divides into an anterior and a posterior fascicle. Anatomic blocks may occur at any point below the AV node. With some of these blocks, it may be advisable to place a transvenous pacer prior to induction of anesthesia.

Other Laboratory Studies

Specific laboratory and x-ray findings in coronary artery disease are rare. When ischemia progresses to infarction, intracellular enzymes are released and can be measured in the plasma. While total enzyme levels may originate from multiple tissue types, isoenzymes may be very specific. The CPK-MB levels are transient and appear early, usually peaking at 24 hours and are gone by 48 hours after infarction. Cardiac LDH isoenzymes may appear at 48 hours, peak at 3 to 5 days, and persist for 10 to 14 days. On the chest x-ray, there may be cardiomegaly in subacute or chronic heart failure, evidence of left ventricular aneurysm, or signs of increased pulmonary capillary pressure such as perihilar infiltrates, peribronchial cuffing, or pleural effusions.

Suspected significant pulmonary disease should be an indication for pulmonary function tests (PFT), including arterial blood gases (ABG). When interpreting PFT and ABG, the patient's age should be considered (see Tables 5–2 and 5–3 for changes in P_{O_2} with age and for interpretation of pulmonary function tests).[15,16] Acute changes in the ABG or PFTs may be as important, if not more important, than isolated abnormal findings.

Table 5-2
Table to Aid Interpretation of Spirometry

Functional Class	Description	Obstructive*				Restrictive			
		MVV	VC	RV	FEV$_{1.0}$ %VC	MVV	VC	RV	FEV$_{1.0}$ %VC
		% of predicted				% of predicted			
Class O	Breathlessness appropriate to activity	>80	>80	80–120	>75	>80	>80	80–120	>75
Class I (minimal)	Dyspnea on rapidly climbing stairs and hills and while running	65–80	>80	<150	60–75	>80	60–80	80–120	>75
Class II (moderate)	Dyspnea with routinely climbing stairs and hills, especially during pulmonary infections	45–65	>80	150–175	40–60	>80	50–60	80±	>75
Class III (severe)	Dyspnea during walking; dyspnea at rest only with respiratory infections	30–45	↓	>200	<40	60–80	35–50	<80	>75
Class IV (very severe)	Dyspnea at rest or at least with minimal activity—talking, dressing, etc.	<30	↓↓	>200	<40	<60	<35	<80	>75

Source. Adapted from Gaensler and Wright

* Obstructed patients should be tested with a properly administered dose of bronchodilators. A positive response to bronchodilators is usually stated to have occurred if FEV$_{1.0}$ or flow rates increase by more than 10% of the initial value.

175

Table 5-3
Pulmonary Function as Related to
Age

Age (years)	V_D/V_T	$P_{(A-a)}O_2$ (mm Hg)
15–20	≥89	≤35	≤16
21–30	≥84	≤44	≤21
31–40	≥82	≤47	≤24
41–60	≥74	≤49	≤24
61–75	≥70	≤49	≤28

Source. From Mellengaard K: The alveolar-arterial oxygen difference. Acta Physiol Scand 67:10–20, 1966.

Cardiac Catheterization

Cardiac catheterization may be left-sided, right-sided, or both. Left-sided catheterization details left ventricular performance and coronary artery anatomy. Right heart catheterization is performed to detail right heart function, cardiac output and pulmonary artery pressures and to detect shunts.

Methods for left heart catheterization vary. The port of entry is usually a peripheral artery such as the brachial or femoral artery. If the brachial artery is used, subsequent radial artery pressures below the entry site may be inaccurate. From the port of entry the catheter is advanced to the aortic valve. The sequence of pressure determinations and dye injections varies, but one such sequence follows. The catheter is advanced into the left ventricle, radiopaque dye is injected, and its image and flow are recorded on motion picture film, the cineangiogram. From this ventriculogram comes information on ventricular contraction, size, and flow across the aortic and mitral valves. If either an intracardiac shunt or a problem involving the mitral valve is suspected, the catheter is advanced into the left atrium and more dye is injected. Pressures are measured in each chamber. The catheter is pulled back across the aortic valve and inserted into each coronary artery ostium for the coronary arteriograms.

In coronary artery disease with angina uncomplicated by infarction or myocardial dysfunction, all measurements are frequently normal except for the coronary arteriogram. The heart muscle is normal and free of disease; the pathology is entirely vascular.

When the heart muscle dysfunctions as a result of either intermittent ischemia, continuous ischemia, previous infarction, or muscular hypertrophy, the catheterization can help define the abnormality. From the ventriculogram, abnormal wall motion is seen. This may be classified as decreased motion (hypokinesia), absent motion (akinesia), or paradoxical motion (dyskinesia).[17,18] From measuring the difference between systolic and diastolic diameter in one plane or, better, in two planes, the ejection fraction is calculated. Ejection fractions below 50 percent reflect mildly decreased reserve, while those below 25 percent represent severe LV dysfunction (Figs. 5–1A and 5–1B).

The LVEDP measurements reflect beat-to-beat wall compliance and function. When dye is injected for the ventriculogram the blood is greatly diluted by the dye, and the oxygen concentration is reduced. Transient regional ischemia may occur in areas supplied by marginal coronary artery flow which are already borderline ischemic. Any resulting left ventricular dysfunction may be measured by a transient rise in LVEDP after injection. End-diastolic pressure rises because end-diastolic volume increases. This acute increase in volume results from the left ventricle not emptying as completely as before failure. The increased residual end-systolic volume is added to pulmonary venous return, resulting in increased end-diastolic volumes (Fig. 5–2). A normal LVEDP exists prior to the ventriculogram if there is no failure and good compliance. Ischemia both decreases compliance and reduces the ejection fraction, leaving a larger residual volume at the end of systole. A postinjection rise of 2–3 mm Hg is normal, but a rise of 5 mm Hg or more in the LVEDP is suggestive of further ischemic-induced failure. If the initial LVEDP is elevated, the heart is in compensated failure; if very high pressures exist, the heart is in decompensated failure.

ASSOCIATED DISEASES

Hypertension

Regardless of the cause, chronic hypertension leads to progressive organ degeneration when left untreated. Arteriolar smooth muscle develops increased tone, eventually hypertrophies, and interstitial edema appears. These

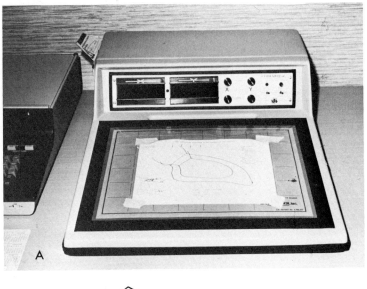

A

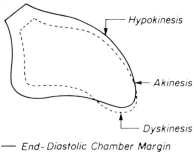

B

Fig. 5–1. (*A*) The *X-Y* plotter is shown, which is used to calculate the ejection fraction from the end-systolic and end-diastolic outlines of the heart taken from the arteriogram. (*B*) Areas of hypokinesia, dyskinesia, and akinesia are demonstrated from the ventriculogram. (Reproduced from Alderman EL: Angiographic indicators of left ventricular function. JAMA 236:1055, 1976, with permission of author and publisher.)

changes result in a smaller resting diameter of the arteriole, which by the Poisueille-Hagen formula, $R = 8nl/r^4$, increases resistance by the fourth power. Small increments of circulating catecholamines will further dramatically increase resistance. Since blood pressure is a function of resistance (BP = CO × TPR), blood pressure rises, causing the heart to work harder in order to eject its stroke volume. Left ventricular hypertrophy may result from the chronically increased blood pressure. End-organs, especially the kidneys, degenerate under this chronic pressure load, and vascular accidents

are more common and especially disastrous when they occur in the brain.

The cause of the initial arteriolar smooth muscle hypertrophy is unclear in most cases. Humoral as well as central neurological stimuli have been implicated. Humoral substances that are known to increase blood pressure include catecholamines, renin, angiotensin, vasopressin, mineralocorticoids such as aldosterone, and electrolytes (especially calcium). Since formation and metabolism of many of these substances occur in the kidneys, renal disease frequently leads to blood pressure elevations. The

PRE-ANGIO   POST-ANGIO

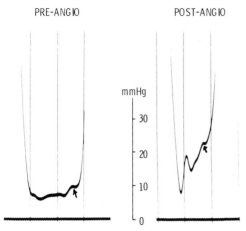

Fig. 5–2. Left ventricular pressure tracings before and after angiogram are demonstrated. The LVEDP is shown at the arrow. Prior to the angiogram the LVEDP was 10 mm Hg, and after the angiogram, it rose to 22 mm Hg.

degree to which personality and emotion contribute to the pathophysiology of hypertension is unclear.

While several antihypertensive drugs have demonstrated considerable central nervous system action, all have peripheral actions (Tables 5–4 and 5–5).[19–23] They work either by reducing preganglionic or postganglionic sympathetic stimulation, by direct arteriolar vasodilation, by producing α- or β-adrenergic blockade, or by central inhibition. Renin-angiotensin antagonists will also soon be available. The precise mode of action of the most common antihypertensives, the diuretics, is unclear, since not all patients successfully treated with diuretics have reduced plasma volumes. Reduced arteriolar interstitial edema may also play a part.

Evaluation of the hypertensive patient includes a complete history of the disease and determination of secondary end-organ changes. Information obtained should include number of years since diagnosis, severity of past blood pressure elevations, secondary complications, current and past drug programs, reasons for changing drugs, drug sensitivities or reactions, and current range of systolic and diastolic pressures. Inspection for secondary changes involves examining the ECG for hypertrophic or ischemic changes, the chest x-ray for heart enlargement, the laboratory studies for BUN and creatinine elevations, and the patient and his

history for central nervous system changes such as an old cerebrovascular accident.

Several cardiovascular changes may be evident on the physical examination. An S_3 or S_4 gallop may be present with ventricular hypertrophy. The pulses may be hyperdynamic, as may be the heart on palpation of the precordium. Blood pressure and pulse may exhibit orthostatic changes consisting of a fall in systolic pressure and an increase in heart rate upon having the patient move from the supine to the sitting position. The presence of orthostatic hypotension suggests decreased blood volume. It may be the result of overzealous diuretic therapy in the treatment of the hypertension. This patient may need crystalloid or colloid supplementation before induction of anesthesia. If the patient has taken a potassium-losing diuretic, he may be hypokalemic. A very rare cause of orthostatic changes in the hypertensive patient is a pheochromocytoma. If the eye grounds are examined with an ophthalmoscope, an approximation of end-organ arteriolar degeneration can be correlated with arteriolar changes in the retina.

At various times in the past, strong arguments were raised for stopping antihypertensive medications long before surgery. Arguments centered on interference with pressure homeostasis and maintenance in times of stress. Ample evidence now exists demonstrating an increased morbidity and mortality in inadequately or untreated hypertensives who are anesthetized.[24] Further evidence shows no adverse effects from continuing antihypertensives up to the time of surgery.[25] Acute withdrawal of certain drugs, such as propranolol and clonidine, may precipitate a crisis; in the case of propranolol, angina, ischemia, and infarction may result;[26,27] in the case of clonidine, hypertensive crisis may occur.[21] In many centers, antihypertensive drugs are now continued until the day of surgery. Propranolol and clonidine may even be given with a sip of water on the day of surgery.

Carotid and Cerebrovascular Disease

Of all the areas where peripheral artery stenosis may reduce perfusion, the brain is the most important. The anesthetic challenge, as in coronary artery disease, is one of balancing blood and oxygen supply with demand. Blood supply, as in coronary artery disease, is pres-

Table 5-4
Some Oral Antihypertensive Drugs

Drug	Frequent or Severe Adverse Effects	Some Major Interactions
Arteriolar dilators		
Hydralazine (Apresoline, Dralzine, and others)	GI disturbances, tachycardia, aggravates angina, headache and dizziness, fluid retention, nasal congestion, rashes and other allergic disorders, lupuslike syndrome	
Prazosin (Minipress)	Sudden syncope, dizziness and vertigo, palpitation, edema, dyspnea, headache, depression, drowsiness, weakness, anticholinergic effects	
Saralasin		Specific angiotensin II inhibitor
Drugs with peripheral sympathetic action		
Propranolol (Inderal)	Bradycardia, reduced exercise tolerance, congestive heart failure, GI disturbances, increased airway resistance, rare blood dyscrasias and other allergic disorders; sudden withdrawal can be dangerous	Blocks sympathetic response → hypoglycemia; blocks adrenergic bronchodilation
Reserpine (Serpasil and others)	Psychic depression, nightmares, nasal stuffiness, drowsiness, GI disturbances, bradycardia, impotence	CNS excitation and increased hypertension possible with MAO inhibitors; false-negative urinary VMA
Guanethidine (Ismelin)	Orthostatic hypotension, diarrhea, may aggravate bronchial asthma; bradycardia, inhibition of ejaculation, sodium and water retention	Effects antagonized by sympathomimetic amines, tricyclic antidepressants, and phenothiazines; enhances effect of hypoglycemic drugs; false-negative urinary VMA
Drugs with central sympathetic action		
Methyldopa (Aldomet)	Sedation, headache, and other CNS symptoms; orthostatic hypotension, impotence, bradycardia, GI disturbances, acute or chronic hepatitis,	Increases toxicity of haloperidol and lithium; effects antagonized by sympathomimetic amines; false-negative urinary VMA
Clonidine (Catapres)	Severe rebound hypertension upon sudden withdrawal, CNS reactions similar to methyldopa but more sedation and dry mouth	Effects inhibited by tricyclic antidepressants

Source. Modified from Drugs for hypertension. Med Lett 19:21, 1977.

Table 5-5
Characteristics of Diuretic Drugs

Generic Name	Brand Name	Dose	Usual Dosage	Onset of Effects	Peak Effects	Duration
Chlorothiazide	Diuril	500-mg tablet	500–1000 mg/day	1 hr	4 hr	6–12 hr
Hydrochlorothiazide	Hydro-Diuril	50-mg tablet	50–100 mg/day	2 hr	4 hr	12 hr or more
Trichloromethiazide	Metahydrin, Naqua	4-mg tablet	4–8 mg/day	2 hr	6 hr	24 hr
Chlorthalidone	Hygroton generic	100-mg tablet	100 mg/day	2 hr	6 hr	24 hr
Meralluride	Mercuhydrin	10-ml vial	0.5–0.2 ml I.M. 3 times/wk	2 hr	6–9 hr	12–24 hr
Mercaptomerin	Thiomerin	10-ml vial	0.5–0.2 ml I.M. 3 times/wk	2 hr	6–9 hr	12–24 hr
Triamterene	Dyrenium	100-mg capsule	100–300 mg/day	2 hr	6–8 hr	12–16 hr
Spironolactone	Aldactone	25-mg tablet	25 mg q.i.d.	Gradual onset	2–3 days after initiation of therapy	2–3 days after cessation of therapy
Furosemide	Lasix	40-mg	40–120 mg/day	P.O.: 1 hr I.V.: 5 min	1–2 hr 30 min	6 hr 2 hr
Ethacrynic acid	Edecrin	50-mg tablet	50–100 mg/day	P.O.: 30 min I.V.: 15 min	2 hr 45 min	6–8 hr 3 hr

Source. Modified from Frazier HS, Yager H: The clinical use of diuretics. N Engl J Med 288:246–249, 1973.

sure-dependent. Cerebral oxygen demand is independent of pressure, however. Unlike most peripheral artery beds, the brain vessels autoregulate to maintain the cerebral blood flow (CBF) at a constant level of 40–50 ml/100 gm/min.[28] The autoregulation responds to three physiological parameters: mean perfusion pressure, P_aCO_2, and P_aO_2. Cerebral blood flow remains constant with mean aortic pressures from 50 to 150 torr, while above and below these limits, flow is dependent on perfusion pressure. With blood pressure and Po_2 held constant, CBF varies directly with changes in Pco_2. Oxygen tensions cause cerebral vasodilation only at Po_2 levels below 50 torr. (Fig. 5–3).[28].

In the presence of isolated stenosis, autoregulation may increase or decrease the proportion of cerebral blood reaching the poststenotic and possibly ischemic region. With stimuli producing generalized vascular dilation, the already maximally dilated poststenotic region can dilate no further. Therefore, blood may shift to the normal vascular regions, away from the ischemic region, since the normal regions now offer less resistance to runoff (cerebral steal syndrome). Conversely, with vasoconstrictive stimuli, blood may shift to the poststenotic areas as resistance in normal areas increases (the reverse steal, or Robin Hood syndrome). Since the poststenotic areas may be ischemic, autoregulation may not be intact, and increased flow may produce regional cerebral edema, which may further impinge upon the vascular supply and increase ischemia (luxury perfusion syndrome).

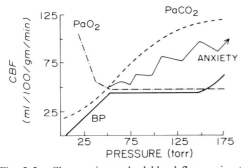

Fig. 5–3. Changes in cerebral blood flow owing to alterations in $PaCO_2$, PaO_2, and blood pressure are shown. (Reproduced from Shapiro H: The physiologic basis of neurosurgical anesthesia. 1977 Annual Refresher Course Lectures, American Society of Anesthesiology, with permission of author.)

Anesthetic agents further complicate the picture. Most intravenous agents, including morphine, thiopental, fentanyl, droperidol, and diazepam, do not change or decrease cerebral blood flow. Ketamine greatly increases CBF. Agents decreasing CBF tend to make cerebral vasculature less sensitive to Pco_2. Volatile drugs, such as halothane and ethrane, increase CBF. In addition, volatile agents abolish autoregulation to mean blood pressure in a dose-dependent manner.[28]

Vasoconstrictive and vasodilator drugs given to treat circulatory derangements may unpredictably affect cerebral blood flow. If a poststenotic vessel is nonischemic and therefore still reactive, upon administering a vasopressor the region supplied by that vessel may become ischemic. If the region past the stenosis is already ischemic and therefore unable to react to a vasopressor, then vasoconstriction in normal vessels may shunt blood to the ischemic area and luxury perfusion with resultant cerebral edema may result. While vasodilators may increase total cerebral blood flow by decreasing cerebral vascular resistance, they may shunt blood away from an ischemic region. If the poststenotic vessel is already maximally vasodilated secondary to ischemia, further ischemia may result.

In most centers, the anesthetic management of patients with known or suspected cerebrovascular disease is directed toward keeping the parameters of autoregulation as close to normal and/or preanesthetic values as possible. Mean arterial pressure is maintained close to preanesthetic pressures, Po_2 levels are kept high, and Po_2 levels are maintained at 30–40 torr.

Cerebral vascular disease should be considered whenever there is a history of stroke, syncope, light-headedness, convulsions, diabetes, hypertension, or other peripheral vascular disease. Patients with known neurological or cerebrovascular disease are considered to be at greater risk of developing one of the most common complications of cardiopulmonary bypass—neurological deficits.

Patients suspected of having cerebral vascular disease should be carefully checked for the presence of a carotid bruit. If found, surgery should be delayed until a carotid arteriogram is performed and a decision made whether to operate on the carotid artery obstruction before or at the same time as the proposed cardiac operation. This involves consultation with the appropriate surgeons and neurologists.

Lung Disease

Significant lung disease may involve one of several parenchymal, vascular, or neuromuscular changes leading to altered ventilation/perfusion (V/Q) relationships.[29] Clinically, lung disease is classified as obstructive, restrictive, or vascular.

OBSTRUCTIVE

The spectrum of obstructive disease involves acute and chronic changes of the larger bronchi, the terminal bronchioles, and the alveoli. Acute large airway disease (acute bronchitis) may include inflammation, edema, or hypersecretion. Small airways may be spastic (asthma) or edematous (bronchiolitis). Exudative alveolar diseases are infiltrative pneumonias. A history of recent cough, sputum production, cold, wheezing, or fever should prompt suspicion of an acute obstructive process. Wheezing, rales, or tachypnea may be present on the physical examination. The chest x-ray may show infiltrates or hyperinflation but is most often nondiagnostic for either small or large acute airway disease. An elevated white blood count with immature polymorphonuclear leukocytes occurs earlier and is more specific for acute infectious processes than are the x-ray changes. Similarly, pulmonary function tests, especially the arterial blood gases, demonstrate acutely decreased function before x-ray changes appear.

Whenever possible, surgery should be delayed until the acute process is treated and resolved. Antibiotics and tracheal suction may be helpful. Bronchodilators are useful when the patient's cardiac condition permits administration. Xanthine bronchodilators such as aminophylline and theophylline can, like caffeine, induce arrhythmias. Adrenergic bronchodilator receptors are β_2 while inotropic and chronotropic cardiac receptors are β_1. β-adrenergic agents such as isoproterenol affect β_1- and β_2-receptors, and therefore may induce angina by increasing heart rate and contractility. Isoetharine has more β_2 than β_1 properties and thus may be a better choice. The β-antagonist propranolol blocks both β_1- and β_2-receptors and can increase bronchoconstriction. Other β-blockers that act primarily on β_1-receptors may soon be available.[29]

Chronic airway disease is often called chronic obstructive pulmonary disease (COPD). When large airway disease is present, the hypersecretion and edema are called chronic bronchitis. Chronic destruction of parabronchial areas is bronchiectasis. Emphysema is small airway lumen collapse, especially on expiration, associated with loss of alveolar surface area. A history of chronic smoking, persistent cough, progressive dyspnea, or prolonged exposure to fumes or dust should prompt suspicion of COPD. On examination, the patient's chest may appear hyperinflated, with an increased anteroposterior diameter and lowered, less mobile diaphragms. The respiratory rate may be increased, and the expiratory phase may be prolonged and, in late stages, labored. Breath sounds may be generally decreased and dominated by rales, rhonchi, or wheezes. Typical chest x-ray findings include hyperinflation, lowered diaphragms, increased retrosternal air space on the lateral projection, and occasionally blebs or bullae. These blebs or bullae are potential sources of pneumothorax with positive pressure ventilation.

When the patient's COPD appears to be more than minimal by history and physical examination, especially when it has caused an alteration of normal daily activities, pulmonary function tests are ordered. Some PFTs can be performed at the bedside. These include the tidal volume, vital capacity, and forced expiratory time (FET). The FET is determined by having the patient take a maximal inspiration and then timing the forced complete expiration. An FET of 2 seconds or less suggests minimal disease. In most patients with COPD, a full set of PFTs should be obtained in a pulmonary function laboratory. Results of these tests allow classification of the extent of the disease (Table 5–2). An arterial blood gas should be included with the PFTs. As shown in Table 5–3, Po_2 declines with age, and the ABG must be interpreted with this in mind. Any acute change since a previous measurement should be considered as important as the current Po_2 level. Elective operations should be delayed when there is evidence of acute worsening of baseline disease, significant untreated or reversible bronchoconstriction, or inadequately treated bronchosecretions.

Preoperative medications for patients with both acute and chronic airway disease should be chosen for their minimal depression of the respiratory drive. The usefulness and desirability of drying agents such as atropine and scopolamine may be less important than the circulatory and central nervous system effects of these drugs. Even when Po_2 levels are very low on room air, oxygen should be given cautiously to a patient with obstructive lung disease. If there is evidence of CO_2 retention, the patient should be attended by personnel experienced in airway management. Chronic CO_2 retention leads to increased serum and cerebrospinal fluid (CSF) bicarbonate levels as a metabolic compensatory mechanism. Since CO_2 controls respiratory drive by varying the pH of CSF, the elevated CSF bicarbonate in these patients will prevent elevated Pco_2 from stimulating respiration and leaves only the hypoxic drive.

RESTRICTIVE LUNG DISEASE

When parenchymal or neuromuscular disease reduces tidal volumes to levels below those predicted for sex, age, and height, the patient is classified as having restrictive disease. This condition may co-exist with obstructive or vascular lung disease or may exist alone. The ratio of dead space to tidal volume ($\dot{V}_D/\dot{V}_T$) is increased. This results from a decrease in tidal volume, as absolute dead space may be increased, decreased, or unchanged. In obstructive lung disease, however, the $\dot{V}_D/\dot{V}_T$ ratio is increased as a result of an increase in dead space, while tidal volumes may be variable.

Known causes of restrictive lung disease include neuromuscular disease, chest wall or spinal deformity, pulmonary fibrosis, chronic exposure to atmospheric or environmental irritants, radiation, chronic infections, and inflammatory diseases. The patient may complain only of mild dyspnea on exertion (DOE) and tachypnea. On examination, respiration is rapid and shallow. Lung volumes are variable on the PFTs (Table 5-2) except for the tidal volume and vital capacity, which are less than predicted. Arterial Po_2 levels are less than predicted for age, but there may be no CO_2 retention. In pure restrictive disease, secretions are rarely a problem, and bronchodilation is not needed, since obstruction is absent.

PULMONARY VASCULAR DISEASE

Pulmonary vascular disease usually originates from increased pressures in the pulmonary veins, arteries, or capillaries. Pressure changes may be acute or chronic and may originate from either the heart or the lung.

Acute elevations in pulmonary vascular pressures may originate in the pulmonary veins or arteries. Elevated pulmonary venous or capillary pressures are usually secondary to acute left ventricular failure. Acute pathological change of the mitral valve, such as occurs with ruptured chordae tendineae, will also produce elevated pulmonary venous pressures. Eventually, pulmonary interstitial edema will result from the increased capillary pressures. Pulmonary compliance and $\dot{V}/\dot{Q}$ ratios will decline. Pulmonary artery pressures then rise, perhaps on a reflex basis.[30] Elevated right atrial pressures and right heart failure are usually secondary to these pulmonary events. Acute elevations in pulmonary artery pressure, such as would occur with a left-to-right shunt, may produce right ventricular failure.

With *chronic* elevations of venous pressure, such as occurs with mitral valvular disease, chronic interstitial edema leads to chronic interstitial fibrosis. As the fibrosis progresses, reversibility of the decreased $\dot{V}/\dot{Q}$ ratios and compliance become less. While pulmonary artery pressures are high and pathology can be demonstrated in the walls of the pulmonary arteries, pressures often return toward normal with correction of the mitral valvular disease. With chronic left-to-right shunts associated with elevated pulmonary artery pressures, however, the elevated pulmonary vascular resistance may not return to normal with correction of the anatomic defect.

End-stage lung disease often leads to increased pulmonary artery pressures. The mechanism may be chronic hypoxia and/or hypercarbia leading to reflex pulmonary artery vasoconstriction. The degree to which chronic fibrosis of the pulmonary arteries adds to the vascular resistance is unclear. Correction of the hypoxia and hypercarbia often leads to partial reversal of the increased resistance. However, with chronic pulmonary hypertension, right heart failure eventually develops.

Chronic pulmonary hypertension leading to right heart failure (cor pulmonale) develops insidiously. In patients with chronic heart and lung disease, it may be easily overlooked. It should be suspected whenever the patient has severe long-standing lung disease or valvular heart disease, particularly mitral valvular disease. On examination, an increase in the pulmonic component of the second heart sound (S_2P) may be heard. There may be a left parasternal lift and elevated venous pressures in the neck veins, which may be associated with a pulsating enlarged liver, peripheral edema, or ascites if right ventricular and/or tricuspid regurgitation has occurred. The chest x-ray will show an enlarged heart and chronic pulmonary parenchymal disease. The laboratory studies may show elevated bilirubin and hepatic enzymes. The Po_2 is frequently decreased, and the Pco_2 is increased.

INTRAOPERATIVE MANAGEMENT
OF LUNG DISEASE

In patients with lung disease, a variety of ventilation methods will provide acceptable blood gases and a satisfactory operative field. Positive pressure-controlled ventilation in the supine anesthetized patient results in an increased V_D/V_T ratio. This ratio also increases with age (Table 5-3). Small tidal volumes may result in hypoventilation in patients with obstructive and restrictive lung disease, since the V_D/V_T ratio is already increased. Large tidal volumes, however, increase the possibility of producing a pneumothorax. A suggested method is to ventilate with tidal volumes in the range of 8–12 ml/kg and adjust the respiratory rate until the Pco_2 is acceptable. When $\dot{V}/\dot{Q}$ derangements are so severe that adequate oxygenation cannot be achieved even with large tidal volumes, it may be beneficial to add positive end-expiratory pressure. Hyperventilation, alkalosis, and hypokalemia should be avoided in patients with lung disease on digitalis glycosides, since such patients appear to be more sensitive and prone to digitalis toxicity.[31]

Diabetes Mellitus

Managing diabetes mellitus in the operating room involves more than obtaining blood glucoses or subscribing to a cookbook scheme for giving insulin to "the diabetic." Adult-onset diabetes (AODM) differs significantly from juvenile diabetes in pathophysiology and management.

JUVENILE DIABETES

Far less common than AODM, juvenile diabetes involves a primary and absolute insulin deficiency as confirmed by radioimmunoassay.[32] While glucose levels are often elevated, daily glucose production or glucose production in response to stress appears to be normal. Consequently, juvenile diabetics rarely require more than 20–30 units of total insulin daily or 3–7 extra units for stress. This requirement closely approximates the insulin production in the normal nondiabetic. Ketoacidosis from insulin insufficiency and hypoglycemia from insulin overdose are the two major primary complications of juvenile diabetes.

Ketoacidosis occurs when there is insufficient insulin, glucose or both for metabolic requirements. Metabolism of fat instead of glucose becomes the primary source of energy; ketoacids are a by-product of fat metabolism. Hyperglycemia does not produce ketoacidosis but is instead the result of inadequate insulin to utilize available glucose.

When evaluating the juvenile diabetic, the clinical history should be assessed, enumerating the number and severity of the ketotic and/or hypoglycemic episodes. The duration of the disease should be established and the secondary complications with their severity listed. These may include retinopathy, nephropathy, peripheral neuropathy, and peripheral vascular disease. It is important to determine the patient's insulin history, including current type and dosage, past types of insulin and response, sensitivity, and history of insulin reactions. Table 5-6 lists the various insulins and their usual durations of action.[33] During the physical examination, it is frequently observed that the teeth and veins are in poor condition. Laboratory findings are evaluated for evidence of secondary complications, noting the BUN/creatinine, complete blood count, electrolytes, and of course the serum and urine glucose and ketones.

Preoperative and intraoperative management varies. Any plan that is logical and that follows the important parameters should suffice. One suggested plan is as follows. No insulin is given the morning of surgery. Using frequent serum glucose measurements as a guide, insulin therapy is titrated to the desired effect, using

Table 5-6
Insulin Preparations

| Type of Insulin | Suspension | Hours After Subcutaneous Injection | | Duration of Effect (hours) |
		Effects Begin	Maximum Action	
Regular (crystalline)	Solution	1/4	4-6	6-8
Semilente	Amorphous	1/2	4-6	12-16
Globin	Solution	2-3	6-10	12-18
NPH	Crystalline	3	8-12	18-24
Lente	30% Amorphous and 70% crystalline	3	8-12	18-28
PZI	Amorphous	3-4	14-20	24-36
Ultralente	Crystalline	3-4	16-18	30-36

Source. Santiago JV, Witztum JL: *In* Costrini NV, Thomson WM (eds): Manual of Medical Therapeutics (ed 22). Boston, Little, Brown, 1977, p. 320.

boluses of 5-7 units of regular insulin as needed to keep serum glucose between 200 and 300 mg/100 ml, in order to avoid any possibility of hypoglycemia or severe hyperglycemia. In another method, the patient is given a continuous intravenous infusion of 1-2 units of regular insulin in 50 ml of 5-10% dextrose per hour, again checking serum glucose frequently. In some cases the insulin may attach to the plastic or glass, making the actual dose given unpredictable. Glucose should be given at all times as a guard against hypoglycemia and as a source of carbohydrate. If urinary glucose measurements are used instead of serum glucose, it should be remembered that the normal renal threshold for glucose of 180 mg/100 ml may vary a great deal. Periodic serum glucoses should be obtained to confirm urinary findings. Sliding scales work better in the intensive care unit than in the operating room, where conditions change quickly and radically. Many recent studies have shown that even in ketoacidosis, intravenous administration of 5-10 units of regular insulin per hour is adequate both for the conversion of metabolism back to glucose from fat and for the reduction of hyperglycemia.[34,35]

ADULT-ONSET DIABETES

The hallmark of adult-onset diabetes is hyperglycemia. High-calorie diets and obesity appear to worsen the hyperglycemia, suggesting an exogenous factor. Various endogenous factors are also implicated, including imbalance of glucose-producing hormones, such as catecholamines, growth hormone, glucocorticoids, ACTH, glucagon, and somatostatin.[36] In contrast to juvenile diabetes, daily insulin production may be greater than in the nondiabetic.[32] In some AODM patients, endogenous insulin may not be enough to handle the increased glucose load, and they may require exogenous insulin or an oral hypoglycemic agent. In others, total insulin may be enough, but it is secreted at inappropriate times, leading to wide swings in blood glucose. This second group may present clinically with hypoglycemia, although they usually rebound quickly to normal or supranormal glucose levels.

The major complications of AODM are hyperglycemia and the hyperosmolar syndrome. Ketoacidosis is extremely rare, even in those AODM patients who have progressed to some insulin dependence, since even these patients have enough insulin to maintain glucose rather than fat metabolism. Hypoglycemia with overzealous correction of hyperglycemia is a major iatrogenic complication. Secondary complications of AODM involve the same systems as juvenile diabetes: renal system, peripheral nerves, the retina, peripheral vascular system, and especially the microvascular system. Lactic acidosis and pancreatitis are secondary iatrogenic complications in those patients using the oral agent phenformin to control their blood glucose.[37-39] Still unsettled is the issue of whether or not oral hypoglycemic agents increase the diabetic's already accelerated rate of coronary vascular atherosclerosis.

The preoperative evaluation of the patient with AODM should include a detailed history of the course and complications up to the time of surgery. If not available from the chart, the patient should be questioned for a history of hyperglycemic and hypoglycemic episodes. An attempt should be made to determine how labile or "brittle" the patient's blood sugar has been. In addition to determining whether the patient is controlled by diet, drug, or insulin, it is important to describe the effectiveness of his therapy. Table 5-7 lists commonly used oral agents and their duration of action. Note that chlorpropamide has a duration of about 60 hours and a half-life of 35 hours. Patients on this drug who fail to eat preoperatively, including those NPO for surgery, may develop hypoglycemia.[41]

It is worthwhile to check for some complications of diabetes mellitus. BUN and creatinine levels should be checked. Since coronary artery disease in these patients is only one manifestation of generalized atherosclerosis, one should assume disease to be elsewhere. A funduscopic examination may give some idea of the severity of peripheral microvascular disease.

Frequent glucose and potassium determinations should be obtained intraoperatively.

Should glucose rise to levels greater than 300 mg/100 ml, small doses of regular insulin (5–10 units I.V.) should suffice. When giving insulin, it is wise to administer dextrose intravenously to offer some protection against hypoglycemia. Serial potassium levels should be checked and potassium added to the intravenous fluids as needed to keep the serum potassium above 4 mEq/liter.

During cardiopulmonary bypass, insulin secretion may decline.[42] In the AODM patient, this may lead to significant hyperglycemia. While regular insulin is justified in this circumstance, it should be given carefully, as insulin secretion will begin again with the termination of bypass. We suggest smaller and perhaps more frequent doses of 2–6 units I.V., remembering that it takes 20 to 40 minutes for regular insulin to be maximally effective.

When serum glucose exceeds the renal threshold, which is about 180 mg/100 ml in the normal kidney, glycosuria begins. With glycosuria comes an osmotic diuresis. A patient who has had glycosuria for some time preoperatively may come to surgery with a decreased blood volume. Since sodium is lost with the water in the osmotic diuresis, there may be an absolute sodium deficit. Since free water loss is greater than sodium loss, however, the serum will have

Table 5-7
Metabolism of Antidiabetic Drugs

Drug	Metabolism	Serum Half-life (hours)	Duration (hoqrs)	Mean Effective Dose (grams)	Dose Range (grams)
Tolbutamide	Oxidized in liver; excreted in urine	4–5	6–12	1.0	0.5–2.0
Chlorpropamide	Minimally altered; primarily excreted in urine	35	60	0.25	0.1–0.5
Acetohexamide	60% reduced in liver to hydroxyhexamide (secreted by renal tubules actively)	6–8	12–24	0.50	0.25–1.5
Phenformin	Accumulates in liver and gastric juice; 95% of ^{14}C label in urine after 24 hr	35	6–8 8–14*	0.1 0.1	0.05–0.2 0.05–0.2

Source. Adapted from Shen S, Bressler R: Clinical pharmacology of oral antidiabetic agents. N Engl J Med 296:493–497, 1977.

* Time-disintegration tables.

a high concentration of sodium and a high osmolality. Therefore, treatment requires free water but also some sodium. Five percent dextrose in 0.45 percent saline offers an excellent composition to treat these derangements. Although urine output may be replaced volume for volume by intravenous fluids, a more rational approach would be to utilize hemodynamic parameters such as the pulmonary wedge pressure to guide blood volume expansion.

If the blood glucose rises rapidly to very high levels, intracellular glucose may not increase as rapidly as extracellular glucose. Cellular dehydration may result as the osmolality of the extracellular fluid draws water.[43] While this principle is used when mannitol is given to treat cerebral edema, severe cellular dehydration can be devastating. If the hyperglycemia is treated too rapidly, serum glucose may fall to levels making serum osmolality lower than cellular osmolality since by this time some glucose has entered the cell. The result may be an equally devastating cellular edema. Consequently, when very high serum glucose levels occur (greater than 500 mg/100 ml), it is best to lower the serum concentration slowly. A suggested and, in most cases, an adequate schedule would be to give from 3 to 7 units of regular insulin per hour until levels of 200–300 mg/100 ml are reached.

Renal Disease

In terms of anesthetic management, functional pathology, rather than morphological or etiologic description, is the most important information when renal disease exists. Anesthetic management of metabolic function and drug excretion or evaluation of intraoperative function depends on baseline functional status. Baseline function is defined by renal function tests.

The BUN and creatinine values remain normal as long as at least 50 percent of renal function remains. Once the BUN and creatinine values begin to rise, significant dysfunction and little reserve exist. Trends or serial BUN/creatinine determinations are more useful than single determinations, since several days may elapse after a change before a new steady-state equilibrium develops. Starvation of protein or hepatic dysfunction may yield a low baseline BUN. A rise to the normal BUN values may represent significant dysfunction in that patient,

although the creatinine will rise to an abnormal value. Similarly, a high-protein diet will give a higher baseline BUN and may slightly elevate the creatinine if animal muscle is the source of the protein.[44]

A better or more accurate assessment of renal function is a clearance test of creatinine, or inulin. An arbitrary but useful division of function using the creatinine clearance is to designate 80–130 ml/min as normal function, 50–80 ml/min as mild dysfunction, 25–50 ml/min as moderate dysfunction, and less than 25 ml/min as severe dysfunction.

Renal function tests may be abnormal secondary to nonrenal causes even with normal renal parenchyma. Circulatory derangements such as decreased blood volume or low cardiac output may lead to decreased renal perfusion and result in elevated BUN and creatinine values (prerenal azotemia). Obstruction to urine outflow also may interfere with renal function (postrenal azotemia). In both cases, renal function tests promptly return to normal with correction of the primary problem, provided that the primary problem has not itself damaged the kidneys. When renal function tests are abnormal preoperatively, adequate tests and/or consultation should be obtained to clarify the true status and, if necessary, to correct any nonrenal component to azotemia. At the bedside, evidence for low cardiac output or congestive heart failure may be evident by examination of the heart and lungs. With decreased blood volume, orthostatic changes occur in blood pressure and heart rate upon sitting up.

Salt and water excretion may not decline with progressive renal dysfunction until very late stages. The ability of the kidney to concentrate or dilute both salt and water does progressively worsen, however. Conceptually, this can be viewed as fewer and fewer normal nephrons having to handle more and more of the load until they become overloaded and can neither concentrate nor dilute effectively but instead act as passive conduits. Total excretion may not decline but does tend to become fixed. Salt and water balance become dependent on intake.[45]

Preoperative weight loss or orthostatic changes in blood pressure and heart rate may suggest that water balance has been negative. Intraoperatively, a pulmonary artery pressure catheter may serve as a guide while restoring and maintaining blood volume. Since water and sodium are lost at independent rates, the serum sodium concentration may not accurately reflect total body sodium. If dietary intake of sodium tends to be high, sodium balance may tend to be positive in renal insufficiency; in some cases, however, it may be negative. Thus, restoration of blood volume usually requires free water but may require some sodium or even normal saline. Maintenance of salt and water balance requires measuring the urinary sodium and potassium loss and replacing those ions with solutions of equivalent content.[46]

Potassium excretion also becomes progressively fixed, usually at fairly high levels. Balance tends toward the negative until very late stages, at which time excretion falls off markedly and balance becomes very positive. Consequently, in the usual patient with moderate renal dysfunction, hypokalemia rather than hyperkalemia manifests itself both preoperatively and intraoperatively. Care should be exercised in replacing this potassium deficit, since the kidneys cannot handle a large potassium load. From 5 to 20 mEq of potassium chloride in 50–100 ml of fluid should be given over several hours, and then the potassium concentration should be reassessed. A conservative approach such as this should prevent hyperkalemia.

Hydrogen ion production is dependent on metabolism and on intake of acid drugs or solutions. While acidosis is rare in renal disease except in very late stages, it will develop if hydrogen ion balance is positive. Stress, including surgery, increases endogenous hydrogen ion production. Acidic drugs, such as aspirin, increase acid load just as basic drugs, such as sodium bicarbonate, decrease the acid load.

Correction of an increased acid load in the patient with renal insufficiency is fraught with hazards. Sodium bicarbonate is a hyperosmolar solution and, if given in sufficient quantity, may produce an increase in blood volume leading to vascular overload or, if given in very large quantity, to cellular dehydration. Alkalinizing the serum will drive some potassium back into the cells, possibly leading to dangerous hypokalemia. Alkalinization also shifts calcium from the active ionized form to the inactive protein-bound form, increasing the risk of convulsions or decreased myocardial contractility in a patient who already has low calcium levels secondary to his renal disease. An acute drop in pH decreases hemoglobin oxygen affinity (Bohr effect). If the acidosis becomes persistent or chronic, RBC 2,3-DPG decreases, producing a compensatory increase in oxygen affinity. Acutely raising the pH eliminates the Bohr effect of decreased affinity almost instantly, but the increased affinity from depressed 2,3-DPG does not subside for several hours. During this time, tissue hypoxia may occur unless cardiac output is greatly increased.[47] Bicarbonate does not enter the CSF as rapidly as does CO_2. If bicarbonate levels are low in the serum and in the CSF, quickly increasing the serum levels will drive CO_2 into the CSF, paradoxically decreasing its pH. This may cause the respiratory drive to increase and, unless ventilation is controlled, will produce a respiratory alkalosis. Therefore, even though normal pH is desirable the chronically acidotic patient should be treated slowly.

The severely dysfunctioning kidney with a creatinine clearance of less than 10–15 ml/min is essentially a nonfunctioning kidney. Sodium, potassium, and water should be replaced only with measured losses or as needed to correct depleted levels. A cardiopulmonary bypass machine can adjust blood volume but functions poorly as kidney. Sodium and potassium that go in cannot easily be removed. Glucose, insulin, and bicarbonate will transiently lower serum potassium, but only dialysis will reduce total body levels.

Drugs that are totally excreted by the kidney, such as gallamine, or partially excreted, such as pancuronium or digitalis glycosides, should either not be given or be given in reduced doses as determined by the creatinine clearance. Formulas and nomograms for calculating the reduced doses use the creatinine clearance.[48,49] Acid–base balance may also play a role in renal drug clearance. Acidic drugs are reabsorbed less and therefore excreted better when ionized at a low pH. Alkaline drugs are best excreted at high pH. The critical pH is in the tubular lumen rather than in the serum, and therefore manipulation of serum pH to enhance drug excretion is only possible when the kidneys are still able to excrete an acid or an alkaline load.

Drugs potentially toxic to the kidney must also be given in reduced dosages. Antibiotics such as the aminoglycocides (gentamycin, streptomycin, and kanamycin), as well as certain fluorinated anesthetic agents (methoxyflurane, enflurane), are included in this category.

Measuring urine output in the operating room is an excellent, though limited method of monitoring renal function. In the adult, renal function is considered adequate if output is greater than 0.5–1.0 ml/kg/hr. By conventional standards, an output of less than this frequently means hypoperfusion (prerenal azotemia) to the kidneys and indicates the need for fluid or blood. In fact, dramatic changes in blood volume or renal perfusion must occur before urine output is altered.[50]

Within wide limits, urine volume is determined by antidiuretic hormone (ADH) which is regulated primarily by changes in osmolality, and secondarily by blood volume.[51] Only significantly increased or decreased blood volume can override the control of osmolality. The blood pressure, pulse, central venous pressure, or pulmonary artery wedge pressure are far more sensitive indicators of blood volume. ADH is also increased under conditions of stress such as intubation, incision, and surgery. So many factors cause ADH release that monitoring urine output alone is a poor method of following renal function, perfusion, or blood volume.

Determining the urinary sodium or the urine-to-plasma (U/P) urea or creatinine ratio is a far more sensitive method of monitoring renal function.[16] Using these tests, one can evaluate and diagnose conditions of increased or decreased urine output with great accuracy.

Prime considerations in low urine output states are prerenal azotemia, increased ADH levels, and acute tubular necrosis (ATN). In prerenal azotemia, normal nephrons actively reabsorb sodium so that very little reaches the collecting ducts. Urinary sodium concentration is less than 20 mEq/liter. Since nephron function is normal, the U/P creatinine is greater than 20. When ADH levels are increased in the presence of normal or high blood volume and cardiac output, renal perfusion is also normal. Nephrons do not maximally extract sodium, and so the urinary sodium concentration is greater than 20 mEq/liter. As in prerenal azotemia, nephron function is normal, and so U/P creatinine is also normal at greater than 20. In ATN, malfunctioning nephrons cannot extract sodium, and so urinary sodium concentration is greater than 20 mEq/liter, as in increased ADH; however, unlike increased ADH, the U/P creatinine is less than 20, since nephrons cannot concentrate creatinine.[46]

Increased plasma volume alone may not result in diuresis. A common cause of diuresis is increased osmotic load from glucose or mannitol. Thiocyanate from metabolism of sodium nitroprusside may also produce sufficient diuresis to severely dehydrate a patient.[52] The urine osmolality will be increased in each of these instances. Diabetes insipidus is characterized by low urine sodium levels when blood volume is low, while in the diuretic phase of acute tabular necrosis (ATN), the urine sodium level is elevated.

Hematologic Abnormalities

Conditions leading to abnormal or prolonged bleeding are multiple, but the abnormalities involve either the fibrin clot and its precursors or the platelets. With the onset of bleeding, the initial event in clotting is formation of the platelet plug. The fibrin clot then forms and organizes behind the platelet plug.

PLATELETS

The most commonly used parameter of platelets is the platelet count. Normal counts range between 100,000 and 300,000. Below 20,000 in the resting patient and below 50,000 in the surgical patient, spontaneous bleeding occurs. Likewise, when above 1 million, platelet embolization and spontaneous bleeding occur. Low platelet counts (thrombocytopenia) may result from decreased production owing to pathological marrow states or drugs; increased consumption, as seen during prolonged bleeding; or increased destruction as a result of diseases of the spleen or reticuloendothelial system, drugs, or extracorporeal circulation including cardiopulmonary bypass and dialysis. High platelet counts (thrombocytosis) result from increased production in patients with chronic bleeding, diseased bone marrow, or drug effects or from decreased destruction in recently splenectomized patients.

Platelet counts tell little about *platelet function*.[53] Recently produced platelets function better than old platelets do. They have a half-life of 4 days and life span of 10 days.[54] Therefore, if they are damaged, 8 to 10 days must pass before the new crop has replaced the old damaged platelets. Thus, with drugs such as aspirin, that permanently damage platelets, normal counts coexist with greatly decreased function for about 10 days after the last dose.[53] Other drugs, such as acetaminophen, depress platelet function, but their effect is transient.[55]

The quickest and most easily performed platelet function test is the bleeding time. Cessation of bleeding from small skin punctures is almost entirely dependent on the platelet plug. Other, more sophisticated tests are not always readily available or always reliable.

Platelet transfusions should be considered when there is evidence of decreased production, increased destruction or consumption, or decreased function. It is no longer customary to give platelets to every patient undergoing cardiopulmonary bypass, although extensive destruction occurs in the first 15 minutes. Instead, platelets are usually reserved for prolonged pump runs, uncontrolled bleeding, or patients with abnormalities of platelet function.

Sources of platelets include fresh whole blood or platelet packs. Fresh frozen plasma is separated from the platelet-rich layer and therefore is poor in platelets. Regular, packed, or whole blood may contain significant numbers of platelets, but they are nonfunctional, since platelets survive for only 24 to 48 hours in storage. One unit of platelets should be given per 7 kg of body weight in order to increase the count by 50,000. Platelets are usually only typed by ABO groups. Patients who have received multiple previous transfusions often develop antibodies, and HL-A-matched donors or siblings should be found.[56]

COAGULATION FACTORS

Fibrin clot formation depends on coagulation factors that are produced in the liver. While production depends on intact hepatocellular function, levels remain adequate until very late stages of liver disease. Hepatic dysfunction depresses levels of different factors unequally, and minimum levels of each factor necessary for coagulation differ. Vitamin K (Aquamephyton) is a necessary cofactor for coagulation factor production. When depressed liver function results in decreased clotting, exogenously administered vitamin K will augment endogenous factor production.

In vivo coagulation is simulated by several in vitro tests. The prothrombin time (PT) measures the extrinsic pathway, and the partial thromboplastin time (PTT) measures the intrinsic pathway of sequentially activated factors

leading to coagulation. Both pathways have a common final sequence and are dependent on calcium. Calcium is required, but increased levels do not augment coagulation. The activated clotting time (ACT) uses diatomaceous earth (Celite) to initiate the clotting sequence. It is more rapid and reproducible than the conventional Lee-White clotting time. The PT depends on the addition of thromboplastin, which simulates tissue destruction and therefore represents the extrinsic stimulus to coagulation.[57] The PTT depends on phospholipid addition, which simulates phospholipid release by platelets after they form a vascular plug and therefore represents intrinsic coagulation.[58] The ACT depends on surface activation, which triggers the intrinsic system of platelet-triggered coagulation.

Warfarin derivatives and heparin are the two most commonly used drugs that interfere with coagulation factors. Warfarin competitively inhibits vitamin K in the liver, thus depressing coagulation factor production. Its action is thus delayed by at least 12 hours and is not maximal until 36 hours. It is counteracted by supplying more vitamin K, which competitively reoccupies its receptor sites.[59] Heparin directly binds several factors including Xa, which is in the common coagulation pathway. Its action is immediate and its half-life is 1¼ to 2 hours.[60] With hypothermia the half-life is longer. Protamine competitively binds heparin and, by so doing, inactivates it. Reversal doses are 1 mg of protamine per 1 mg of heparin remaining in the circulation.

The PT is used to monitor warfarin therapy because factor VI in the extrinsic pathway has the shortest half-life of the factors, and therefore the PT responds to warfarin more quickly than does the PTT. The PTT is used to monitor heparin therapy because it corresponds to the clotting time.

If the patient has prolonged PT and PTT preoperatively and has been on warfarin-type drugs or is suspected of having liver malfunction, vitamin K (10–20 mg I.M.) should be given. It may be given intravenously, but there have been reports of hypotension and anaphylactoid reactions to intravenous administration. Although this dose may be repeated several times, failure to respond suggests that the only way to raise factor levels is to give exogenous fresh frozen plasma or fresh whole blood.

In those patients in whom anticoagulation

therapy should not be interrupted, warfarin therapy may be stopped if heparin therapy is substituted concurrently. PT and PTT levels should be maintained at 2 to 2½ times control values. Full heparinization may require 300 units/kg/day (100 units = 1 mg). It may be given by continuous intravenous infusion or intermittent intravenous or intramuscular doses at least every 2 to 4 hours. Heparin anticoagulation may be reversed by administering protamine.

See Chapter 12 for details of anticoagulation during cardiopulmonary bypass and its reversal.

The syndrome of diffuse intravascular coagulation (DIC), sometimes called a consumption coagulopathy, represents a disastrous derangement of the coagulation system. In DIC, fibrin clot formation is occurring at the same time that a separate system of fibrinolysis is dissolving clot formation. The result is a simultaneous consumption of clotting factors with diffuse uncontrolled bleeding. Sepsis and hypoperfusion are suggested etiologies, but the exact cause is unknown. Treatment involves removing the cause, which may mean antibiotic therapy or surgery, and increasing the blood volume to perfuse hypoperfused areas. The diagnosis is suspected when the PTT, PT, and platelet count are all low. Some investigators have suggested heparin therapy to prevent further consumption of clotting factors, but this therapy is not universally accepted. Most authorities would recommend giving whole blood and clotting factors in an effort to increase perfusion and restore depleted factors.[57]

Liver Disease

Liver dysfunction can be an acute process in which most hepatocytes function abnormally, or it can be a chronic disease in which large numbers of hepatocytes are slowly destroyed, but the few remaining ones have normal function. Both processes interfere with administration of an anesthetic by affecting protein and carbohydrate metabolism, drug detoxification and excretion, and salt and water metabolism.

Virtually all proteins are manufactured in the liver except for the gamma globulins. These include albumin, blood coagulation factors, lipoproteins, and various transport proteins. In late or far-advanced liver dysfunction, all these proteins are produced in less quantity.[61] Gamma globulin production in the reticuloendothelial system (RES) increases, and the globulin/albumin ratio increases.[62] Although the concentration of protein may not decline as a result of this shift, gamma globulins are more massive molecules than albumin, and there are fewer molecules per gram; thus the plasma colloid osmotic pressure may decline. Fluid shifts from the vascular space to the interstitial space. While these events are most marked in late disease, they begin at early stages. Consequently, if the CVP or pulmonary capillary wedge pressure indicate blood volume depletion, at least a portion of the replacement should be with a colloid such as plasma, whole blood, or albumin.[63]

Significant liver disease must occur before coagulation tests indicate factor deficiency. This is related to the fact that many coagulation factors require only 30 percent of normal concentrations for coagulation to proceed at normal rates.[64] Vitamin K will enhance factor production when levels are low if there is sufficient hepatocellular reserve function. If vitamin K cannot increase factor levels, exogenous coagulation factors must be given in the form of fresh frozen plasma or fresh whole blood.

Glucose is converted to glycogen in the liver. Chronic liver disease may result in decreased glycogen stores. Hypoglycemia may result if the patient is stressed, since there are reduced stores of quickly convertible carbohydrate.

Chronic drug usage or chronic liver disease causes induction of liver microsomal enzyme activity.[65] Consequently, anesthetic drugs normally metabolized by the liver, such as diazepam, pancuronium, narcotics, and the short-acting barbiturates, may be cleared from the serum more rapidly in the induced liver. Increased intravenous drug anesthetic requirements should be anticipated in any patient who has chronically taken medication, alcohol, or other drugs. Digitoxin is almost exclusively cleared by the liver, and digoxin is partially metabolized by the liver. Induction speeds their metabolism. In far-advanced liver disease, drug detoxification and metabolism is less efficient, and so those drugs metabolized by the liver must be given in greatly reduced dosages.

In far-advanced liver disease, any stress can push the patient into hepatic encephalopathy.[66] Ammonia produced by bowel bacteria when breaking down ingested protein is normally transported to the liver by the hepatoportal circulation, where it is converted to urea. With liver decompensation, inadequate conversion occurs, and blood ammonia levels rise. Any event, such as surgery or anesthesia, that causes increased catabolism can lead to hepatic encephalopathy by overcoming the marginal reserve of a barely compensated liver. In addition, hypovolemia or dehydration result in recirculation of ammonia normally excreted by the kidney and thus increased blood levels. In states of liver decompensation, no dietary or other sources of protein should be given. The need to give albumin to expand blood volume and to provide protein for hepatic recovery must be weighed against the dangers of inducing hepatic encephalopathy.

Bilirubin is the product of hemoglobin breakdown in the RES.[67] The liver conjugates the bilirubin and secretes it into the bile. Elevations of serum bilirubin suggest a block in conjugation or secretion but not necessarily a decrease in liver function. Posthepatic obstruction or sudden overproduction of bilirubin, as in hemolytic states, may be the cause. Alternatively, the patient may have a congenital defect in bilirubin excretion with normal hepatocellular function. When hepatocellular dysfunction has occurred, conjugation and secretory functions may be affected before other functions. When conjugation is inadequate, drugs normally conjugated by the liver before excretion by the kidney, such as the steroidlike drugs pancuronium and digitalis, are less efficiently excreted.

The BSP test and the rose bengal scan are tests of liver secretion and do not indicate other function. Other tests of hepatocellular function are needed to get an overall picture. The LDH, SGOT, and the alkaline phosphatase are the enzymes most often used to assess liver function.[68] These serum enzymes are nonspecific for the liver, but when all are elevated, hepatocellular destruction has usually occurred. They are not indicators of function. If active cellular destruction is not going on at the time of testing, such as in an end-stage cirrhotic liver, enzyme levels will be low despite near-absent function. Even in acute massive hepatocellular necrosis, enzyme levels will not be grossly elevated after the enzymes released from all dead hepatocytes have been cleared. In both of these end-stage conditions, however, the bilirubin, PT, and PTT will be elevated or prolonged and the BSP will be abnormal.

Changes in salt and water metabolism occur secondarily to late hepatic dysfunction.[69] Decreased blood volume as a result of fluid loss to the extravascular spaces produces prerenal azotemia. There may also be redistribution of renal blood flow from cortical to medullary nephrons. The result is sodium and water retention, sometimes referred to as the hepatorenal syndrome. These renal hemodynamic changes are further complicated by an increase in ADH that occurs with hepatic disease and by a decrease in hepatic metabolism of salt-retaining steroids such as aldosterone, thereby producing a secondary aldosteronism. The decreased perfusion may also result in increased renin release, leading to angiotensin formation and resulting in hypertension.

The elevated ADH may cause so much water retention that serum sodium measurements may show a dilutional hyponatremia. Giving diuretics in this situation will only further decrease blood volume, thereby worsening the hepatorenal syndrome. A more rational approach is free water restriction with blood volume restoration by colloid as indicated by the CVP or pulmonary capillary wedge pressure. If the CVP or wedge pressure is already high, as is sometimes the case, then volume replacement must approximate as closely as possible the volume loss.

PREOPERATIVE MEDICATIONS

One purpose of the preoperative medication is to reduce anxiety and to decrease stress on the cardiovascular system secondary to the anxiety. A thorough discussion of the anesthetic plan with the patient and his family can reduce anxiety as effectively as drugs. Included in the discussion should be a description of the intensive care unit and what the patient may expect to experience there. He should be informed if he will wake up with an endotracheal tube in place and be on a ventilator. One objective is to prevent postoperative psychosis, which is common in intensive care units.

Sedation may prevent or reduce catecholamine-induced stress on the cardiovascular system secondary to the anxiety of having a cardiac operation. The maximum sedation possible without further depression of the myocardium or respiratory drive is the objective. In the case of patients for coronary artery surgery, one recommended approach is to give morphine (0.1mg/kg), scopolamine (0.2–0.5mg), and diazepam (5–10 mg). One disadvantage to this approach is fairly well marked preinduction respiratory depression and prolonged postoperative drowsiness and confusion. Other drug combinations may be just as effective. The objective is to keep the patient's anxiety from causing an increase in afterload and heart rate secondary to

catecholamine release. Any program that achieves this end is desirable.

In the case of severe myocardial disease, drug doses should be reduced and in some cases eliminated. Myocardial depression may occur, and the patient may respond to smaller doses with decreased consciousness and respiratory drive. Whether this is a manifestation of low cardiac output or some other altered mechanism in heart disease is unclear.

REFERENCES

1. Harvey WP: Gallop sound, clicks, snaps, whoops, honks, and other sounds. *In* Hurst JW (ed): The Heart (ed 4). New York, McGraw-Hill, 1969, pp 257–262

2. Hurst JW, Logue RB, Walter PF: The clinical recognition and management of coronary atherosclerotic heart disease. *In* Hurst JW (ed): The Heart (ed 4). New York, McGraw-Hill, 1978, pp 1173–1175

3. Garfinkel H, Inglesby T, Lansing A, et al: ST segment elevation, transient left posterior hemiblock, and recurrent ventricular arrhythmias unassociated with pain. Ann Intern Med 79: 795–799, 1973

4. Endo M, Hirosawa K, Kaneko N, et al: Prinzmetal's variant angina. N Engl J Med 294:252–255, 1976

5. Hurst JW, Logue RB, Walter PF: The clinical recognition and management of coronary atherosclerotic heart disease. *In* Hurst JW (ed): The Heart (ed 4). New York, McGraw-Hill, 1978, p 1193

6. Ellestad M: Ischemic ST segment depression: Hemodynamic, electrophysiologic, and metabolic factors in its genesis. *In* Ellestad M: Stress Testing. Philadelphia, Davis, 1975, pp 227–247

7. Luz P. Shubin H, Weil M: Pulmonary edema related to changes in colloid osmotic and pulmonary artery wedge pressure in patients after acute myocardial infarction. Circulation 51: 350–357, 1975

8. Stein L, Beraud J, Cavanilles J: Development of pulmonary edema during fluid infusion in the absence of heart failure. Circulation 48:114, 1973

9. Rapaport E: Dyspnea: Pathophysiology and differential diagnosis. Prog Cardiovasc Dis 8:532–544, 1971

10. Cannon P: The kidney in heart failure. N Engl J Med 296:26–32, 1977

11. Smith T: Digitalis glycosides. N Engl J Med, 288:719–722, 1973

12. Spann JF, Hurst JW: Treatment of heart failure. *In* Hurst JW (ed): The Heart (ed 4). New York, McGraw-Hill, 1978, p 590

13. Hurst JW, Logue RB, Walter PF: The clinical recognition and management of coronary atherosclerotic heart disease. *In* Hurst JW (ed): The Heart (ed 4). New York, McGraw-Hill, 1978, pp 1159–1167

14. Rubermam W, Weinblatt E, Goldberg J, et al: Ventricular premature beats and mortality after myocardial infarction. N Engl J Med 297:750–757, 1977

15. Gaensler EA, Wright GW: Evaluation of respiratory impairment. Archives of Environ Health 12:146–189, 1966

16. Mellengaard K: The alveolar-arterial oxygen difference: Its size and components in normal man. Acta Physiol Scand 67:10–20, 1966

17. Herman M, Heinle R, Klein M, et al: Localized disorders in myocardial contraction: Asynergy and its role in congestive heart failure. N Engl J Med 277:222–232, 1967

18. Helfant R, Bodenheimer M, Bawka V: Asynergy and coronary heart disease. Ann Intern Med 87:475–482, 1977

19. Frazier HS, Yager H: The clinical use of diuretics. N Engl J Med 288:246–249, 1973

20. Drugs for hypertension. Med Lett 19(474):7–11, 1977

21. Pettinger W: Clonidine, a new antihypertensive drug. N Engl J Med 293:1179–1180, 1975

22. Lilley J, Hsu L, Stone R: Racial disparity of plasma volume in hypertensive man. Ann Intern Med 84:707–728, 1976

23. Brano E, Tarazi R, Dustan H: β-adrenergic blockade in diuretic-treated patients with essential hypertension. N Engl J Med 292:66–70, 1975

24. Prys-Roberts C: Studies of anesthesia in relation to hypertension. V: Adrenergic beta-receptor blockade. Br J Anaesth 45:671–680, 1973

25. Ominsky AJ, Wollman H: Hazards of general anesthesia in the reserpinized patient. Anesthesiology 30:443–446, 1969

26. Harrison DC, Aldermal EL: Discontinuation of propranolol therapy, cause of rebound angina pectoris and acute coronary events. Chest 69:1–2, 1976

27. Boudoulas H, Lewis R, Kates R, et al: Hypersensitivity to adrenergic stimulation after propranolol withdrawal in normal subjects. Ann Intern Med 87:433–436, 1977

28. Shapiro H: The pharmacological basis of neurosurgical anesthesia. Americal Society of Anesthesia refresher course lecture, ASA National Meeting, New Orleans, 1977, lecture 202

29. Webb-Johnson D, Andrews J: Bronchodilator therapy. N Engl J Med 297:476–482, 758–764, 1977

30. Zapol W, Snider M: Pulmonary hypertension in severe acute respiratory failure. N Engl J Med 296:476–480, 1977

31. Green L, Smith T: The use of digitalis in patients with pulmonary disease. Ann Intern Med 87:459–465, 1977

32. Genuth S: Plasma insulin and glucose profiles in 31 normal, obese, and diabetic persons. Ann Intern Med 79:812–822, 1973

33. Santiago JV, Witztum JL: Treatment of diabetes mellitus. In Costrini NV, Thomson WM (eds): Manual of Medical Therapeutics (ed 22). Boston, Little, Brown, 1977, p 320

34. Kitabchi A, Ventachalam A, Guerra S, et al: The efficacy of low dose versus conventional therapy of insulin for treatment of diabetic ketoacidosis. Ann Intern Med 84:633–638, 1976

35. Fisher J, Shashahani N, Kitabchi A: Diabetic ketoacidosis: Low dose insulin therapy by various routes. NEngl J Med 297:238–241, 1977

36. Sherwin R, Fisher M, Hendler R, et al: Glucagon and glucose regulation in normal, obese, and diabetic subjects. N Engl J Med 294:455–461, 1976

37. Misbin R: Phenformin associated lactic acidosis: Pathogenesis and treatment. Ann Intern Med 87:591–595, 1975

38. Conlay L, Lowenstein JE: Phenformin and lactic acidosis. JAMA 235:1575–1578, 1976

39. Chase H, Morgan G: Phenformin-associated pancreatitis. Ann Intern Med 87:314–315, 1977

40. Shen S, Bressler R: Clinical pharmacology of oral antidiabetic agents. N Engl J Med 296:493–497, 1977

41. Hamwi GJ: Oral hypoglycemic agents. Curr Med Digest 33:1184, 1966

42. Allison SP: Changes in insulin secretion during open heart surgery. Br J Anaesth 43:138–142, 1971

43. Axelrod L: Response of congestive heart failure to correction of hyperglycemia in the presence of diabetic nephropathy. N Engl J Med 293:1243–1245, 1975

44. Addis T, Barrett L, Poo L, et al: The relationship between protein consumption and diurnal variations of the endogenous creatinine clearance in normal individuals. J Clin Invest 30:206, 1951

45. Danovitch G, Bourgoignie J, Britcher N: Reversibility of the "salt-losing" tendency of chronic renal failure. N Engl J Med 296:14–19, 1977

46. Harrington J, Cohen J: Measurement of urinary electrolytes—indications and limitations. N Engl J Med 293:1241–1243, 1975

47. Bellingham A, Detter J, Lenfant C: The role of hemoglobin affinity for oxygen and red cell 2, 3-DPG in the management of diabetic ketoacidosis. Trans Assoc Am Physicians 83:1136120, 1970

48. Jelliffe RW: An improved method of digoxin therapy. Ann Intern Med 69:703, 1968

49. Jelliffe RW: An improved method of digitoxin therapy. Ann Intern Med 74:453, 1970

50. Schrier R, Berl T: Nonosmolar factors affecting renal water excretion. N Engl J Med 292:141–145, 81–88, 1975

51. Hays R: Antidiuretic hormone. N Engl J Med 295:659–665, 1976

52. Michenfelder J, Tinker J: Cyanide toxicity and thiosulfate protection during chronic administration of sodium nitroprusside in the dog. Anesthesiology 47:441–448, 1977

53. Weiss H: Platelet physiology and abnormalities of platelet function. N Engl J Med 293:531–541, 1975

54. Stuart M, Scott M, Oslsi F: A simple nonradioisotope technique for the determination of platelet life span. N Engl J Med 292:1310–1313, 1975

55. Genton E, Gent M, Hirsh J, et al: Platelet inhibiting drugs in the prevention of clinical thrombotic disease. N Engl J Med 293:1236–1240, 1274–1278, 1975

56. Wu K, Hook J, Thompson J, et al: Use of platelet aggregometry in selection of compatible platelet donors. N Engl J Med 292:130–133, 1975

57. Rosenberg R: Actions and interactions of antithrombin and heparin. N Engl J Med 292:146–151, 1975

58. Ginsberg M, O'Malley M: Serum factors releasing serotoxin from normal platelets: Relation to the manifestations of systemic lupus erythematous. Ann Intern Med 87:564–567, 1977

59. Stenflo J: Vitamin K: Prothrombin and delta-carboxyglutamic acid. N Engl J Med 296:624–626, 1977

60. Guffin AV, Dunbar RW, Kaplan J: Successful use of reduced dose of protamine after cardiopulmonary bypass. Anesth Analg 55:110, 1976

61. Tavil AS: The synthesis and degradation of liver-produced protein. Gut 13:225, 1972

62. Howens WP, Dickensheets J, Bierly, et al: The

half-life of I^{131} labeled normal human gamma globulin in patients with hepatic cirrhosis. J Immunol 73:256, 1954

63. Wilkinson P, Sherlock S: The effect of repeated albumin infusions in patients with cirrhosis. Lancet 2:1125, 1962

64. Bachman F, McKenna R, et al: The hemostatic mechanism after open heart surgery: Studies plasma coagulation factors and fibrinolysis in 512 patients after extra corporeal circulation. J Thorac Cardiovasc Surg 70:76, 1975

65. Gelehrter T: Enzyme induction. N Engl J Med 294:589-595, 1976

66. Sherlock S: Hepatic pre-coma and coma. *In* Sherlock S: Diseases of the Liver and Biliary System (ed 5). Oxford, Blackwell, 1975, pp 84-106

67. Sherlock S: Jaundice. *In* Sherlock S: Diseases of the Liver and Biliary System (ed 5). Oxford, Blackwell, 1975, pp 234-259

68. Sherlock S: Serum enzyme changes. *In* Sherlock S: Diseases of the Liver and Biliary System (ed 5). Oxford, Blackwell, 1975, pp 37-40

69. Sherlock S: Functional renal failure. *In* Sherlock S: Diseases of the Liver and Biliary System (ed 5). Oxford, Blackwell, 1975, pp 142-149

Donn A. Chambers, M.D.

6

Acquired Valvular Heart Disease

For the safe anesthetic management of patients with valvular heart disease, it is crucial that the anesthesiologist understand the basic pathophysiology of the patient's valvular lesion, the compensatory mechanisms the heart calls upon in dealing with this mechanical burden, and the changes that occur during anesthesia and surgery. Accordingly, after a discussion of normal valvular and ventricular function and evaluation of the patient with valvular disease, the pathophysiology of each specific valvular lesion will be analyzed and some comments made about considerations for anesthesia. Etiology and physical findings will not be emphasized, as these are summarized in many excellent sources.[1-4] Also, the discussion will be mainly concerned with abnormalities of the left side of the heart, since mitral and aortic valvular problems comprise the overwhelming majority of valvular lesions in adults.[5] The concepts set forth, however, are applicable to tricuspid and pulmonic lesions as well.

NORMAL VALVULAR AND VENTRICULAR FUNCTION

The systolic and diastolic sequence of events occurring during a normal cardiac cycle are shown in Figure 6-1. After the onset of

systole the aortic valve does not open until left ventricular systolic pressure (LVSP) exceeds aortic pressure; and it closes at the dicrotic notch of the aortic pressure tracing, when LVSP falls below aortic pressure. The mitral valve opens when left ventricular pressure (LVP) falls below the left atrial (LA) v-wave pressure. After atrial systole the LVP is transiently raised above left atrial pressure (LAP), and the mitral valve closes at this time, slightly before the onset of ventricular contraction.[5] The pressure within the left ventricle at the onset of ventricular contraction is the left ventricular end-diastolic pressure (LVEDP).

Also shown in Figure 6-1 is the change of LV volume with time during a cardiac cycle. Left ventricular end-diastolic volume (LVEDV) is the volume of the left ventricle at the onset of LV contraction; and left ventricular end-systolic volume (LVESV) is the minimal LV volume during the cardiac cycle at the end of ventricular systole.

The four phases of the cardiac cycle are shown at the bottom of Figure 6-1, but they can be better understood if LV pressure is plotted against LV volume for one cardiac cycle, as in Figure 6-2.

1. Phase 1 is the phase of diastolic filling of the ventricle, marked in the normal left ventri-

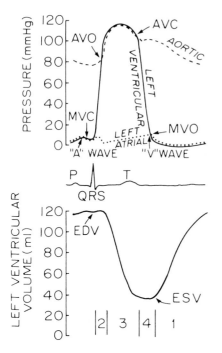

LVEDV and LVESV is the stroke volume (SV) for that cardiac cycle, normal values being 45 ± 13 ml/m². [6]

4. Phase 4 is the phase of isovolumic relaxation, during which LVP falls with negligible volume change until it is less than the LV v-wave pressure, when the mitral valve opens and the cycle begins again.

The area within the pressure-volume loop represents the net work that the left ventricle must do during that cardiac cycle. [7] Another value obtainable from such a graph is the *ejection fraction* (EF), which is defined as

$$EF = \frac{EDV - ESV}{EDV} = \frac{SV}{EDV} \qquad (6\text{-}1)$$

Normally the *systolic function of the left ventricle depends on three factors:* [8]

1. *Preload.* Rigorously, preload is defined as the end-diastolic stress on the left ventricle, [7] but it can be thought of as the end-diastolic resting fiber length, or LVEDV. Preload should not be equated with LVEDP, since

Fig. 6–1. Changes in left-sided pressures (top) and volumes (bottom) during one cardiac cycle for a normal heart. Timing is shown in reference to ECG events in center of figure. AVO = aortic valve opens. AVC = aortic valve closes. MVO = mitral valve opens. MVC = mitral valve closes. EDV = end-diastolic volume. ESV = end-systolic volume. Numbers at the bottom of figure refer to the four phases of the cardiac cycle as shown in Figure 6-2. Volume data from reference 6.

cle by a large increase in volume with little increase in pressure (and hence a high compliance or low diastolic stiffness) until end-diastole. The normal LVEDV is 70 ± 20 ml/m² of body surface area. [6]

2. Phase 2 is the phase of isovolumic contraction. There is negligible change in LV volume during this phase, but LV pressure increases rapidly until it exceeds aortic diastolic pressure and the aortic valve opens.

3. Phase 3 is that of systolic ejection, during which the left ventricle ejects blood into the aorta, decreasing its volume with a further slight increase in pressure to a peak value ("peak LVP") until the aortic valve closes. The volume remaining in the left ventricle at this time is the LVESV. The difference along the horizontal volume axis between

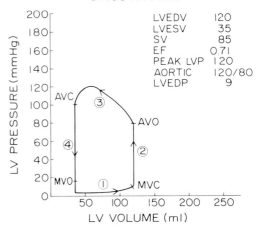

Fig. 6–2. Pressure-volume loop for the typical normal left ventricle shown in Figure 6-1. (1) Diastolic filling phase. (2) Isovolumic contraction phase. (3) Ejection phase. (4) Isovolumic relaxation phase. Valve openings and closings as in Figure 6-1. Arrow indicates sequence during cardiac cycle. For other abbreviations see text. Note that volumes are in milliliters, *not* in milliliters per square meter of body surface area.

it is the degree of stretch of LV fibers that determines the amount of work the left ventricle can do at any given level of contractility, and LVEDV and LVEDP are not linearly related. LVEDP, however, is the best indicator of preload that is currently available for clinical use.

2. *Contractility*. This is an intrinsic property of the myocardium and reflects its ability to do mechanical work at any given level of end-diastolic fiber length (preload). Contractility is increased by sympathetic β stimulation and drugs such as digitalis and is decreased by drugs such as halothane.

3. *Afterload*. Afterload is the wall stress faced by the myocardium during LV ejection[7,9,10] and therefore depends on LV size, shape, pressure, and wall thickness in a complicated way.[9] Afterload can be thought of, however, as the impedance to LV ejection, which in the absence of aortic stenosis depends on the distensibility of the large arteries and the systemic vascular resistance (SVR).[9,10] Arterial blood pressure is not a good measure of afterload, since systolic pressure depends on both stroke volume and the impedance to LV ejection.[10] Thus, a patient with a low systolic blood pressure

might have a high afterload combined with a low stroke volume. In many clinical situations, however, a high arterial systolic or diastolic blood pressure may be the only available indicator of increased impedence to LV ejection. The determinants of systolic and diastolic blood pressures are shown in Figure 6-3.

The way preload, contractility, and afterload interact to determine stroke volume can be seen in Figure 6-4. The basic concept is this: together, preload and contractility determine the total amount of work that the left ventricle can do during systole, and the afterload determines which part of this work will be done to raise intraventricular pressure during systole and which part will be devoted to fiber shortening. In other words, at the start of systole the left ventricle "knows" how much total work it can do during that systole because preload and contractility are known. The left ventricle then "finds out" how much of this work will result in decrease in its volume (and generation of stroke volume) as it encounters afterload after the onset of contraction. Loop A in Figure 6-4 is a typical pressure-volume loop for a normal left ventricle. If preload (LVEDV) is increased,

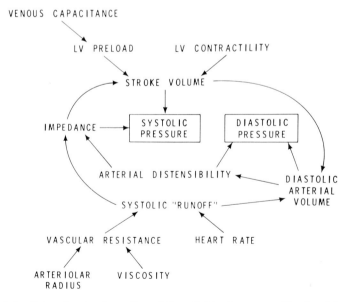

Fig. 6–3. Determinants of systolic and diastolic blood pressure. (Reprinted from Cohn JN: Blood pressure and cardiac performance. Am J Med 55:351, 1973, with permission of author and publisher.)

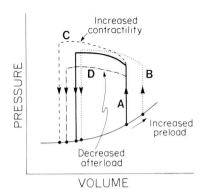

Fig. 6–4. Determinants of stroke volume. Loop A (dark solid line): pressure-volume loop for a hypothetical normal left ventricle. Loop B: loop resulting if contraction begins from a higher end-diastolic volume. Loop C: preload same as in A, but contractility is increased. Loop D: preload and contractility same as in A, but afterload is reduced.

loop B results. From a higher LVEDV, more total work is done in B (area of B > area of A), and stroke volume increases; but since both LVEDV and SV increase, the ejection fraction is relatively unaffected.

If contractility is increased with the preload unchanged (systole begins from the same LVEDV), loop C results. Again, total LV work is higher (area of C > area of A), and stroke volume is increased because the left ventricle now ejects down to a lower LVESV. The ejection fraction is increased (increased SV, unchanged LVEDV). In loop D afterload has been decreased after a contraction beginning at the same LVEDV and with the same contractility as in A. The total amount of work done by the left ventricle is unchanged (area of D = area of A), but LV volume is reduced more and LV pressure raised less. Stroke volume and ejection fraction increase.[9]

A fourth factor affecting stroke volume is *LV dyssynergy*, in which there are localized areas of the left ventricle that are hypokinetic, akinetic, or dyskinetic (bulging outward during systole). Thus, at any given level of preload, contractility, and afterload, stroke volume will be less if there is LV dyssynergy.[8] This is not found in normal ventricles but is common in patients with coronary atherosclerotic heart disease and is also implicated in the LV dysfunction associated with mitral stenosis.[11-13]

The behavior of the normal left ventricle

during *diastole* (phase 1 of the pressure-volume loop) depends on properties of ventricular relaxation, affecting early-diastolic filling; and ventricular stiffness, which affects mainly mid- and late-diastolic filling.[14] *Ventricular relaxation* is an energy-dependent process that can be altered separately from contraction and is probably dependent on the rate of sequestration of Ca^{++} by the sarcoplasmic reticulum after systole. Relaxation is enhanced by β_1 stimulation but can be impaired by heart failure, myocardial ischemia, hypercalcemia, and pacing-induced tachycardia.[14] In these conditions, therefore, early-diastolic filling can be impaired.

Ventricular stiffness (the inverse of compliance) can be increased either by disease of the LV wall, such as fibrosis after myocardial infarction, or by increased thickness of the LV wall, as occurs in the LV hypertrophy associated with aortic stenosis (AS) and aortic or mitral regurgitation (AR or MR). The amount of stiffness is greater in concentric hypertrophy (as in pure aortic stenosis) than it is in eccentric hypertrophy (as it occurs in aortic and mitral regurgitation).[14] The significance of increased LV stiffness is that a higher LVEDP will be required in the stiffer ventricle to achieve the same LVEDV (preload).

The left atrium normally serves as a reservoir during ventricular systole and a conduit during early- and mid-diastole, but it contracts near end-diastole, causing an ''a'' wave on the LAP tracing (see Fig. 6–1) and pumping an additional amount of blood into the left ventricle to raise its volume and pressure to their end-diastolic values. Normally about 20 percent of the LVEDV is provided by atrial systole.[15] The importance of LA contraction to LV filling depends on the following factors:

1. Heart rate: LA contraction is more important at higher heart rates, as diastole is shortened.[15,16]
2. P-R interval. If the P-R interval is too short (< 0.08 seconds), there will not be enough time for full transfer of blood before LV contraction begins. If it is too long (> 0.21 seconds), some blood may regurgitate back into the left atrium before LV contraction begins.[17]
3. Atrial contractility: This is increased by β stimulation and decreased by vagal stimulation.[18] The normal left atrium also obeys

Starling's law, with an increase in contractility when LAP increases.[19]

4. Ventricular stiffness: LA contraction is more crucial for adequate LV filling when stiffness is increased, as in AS.[15]

5. State of mitral valve: Although most of the energy of LA contraction may be wasted as kinetic energy of turbulent flow across a stenotic mitral valve, LA contraction may be important in preventing a late-diastolic fall-off in LV filling as the LA-to-LV pressure gradient falls.[15]

Normally the LVEDP is 0–2 mm Hg higher than the mean LAP, but in patients with stiff left ventricles, LVEDP is found to be as much as 7–9 mm Hg higher than the mean LAP.[19,20] In these patients, LA contraction allows greater LV filling without much rise in LA and pulmonary capillary pressures. If the atrial "kick" is lost in these patients, the mean LA pressure will have to rise as much as 7–9 mm Hg in order to achieve the same LVEDP (and hence LVEDV). This could result in pulmonary congestion.[18]

EVALUATION OF THE PATIENT WITH VALVULAR DISEASE

As for any patient with cardiovascular disease, there are a variety of sources of data about a patient with valvular disease, including history, physical examination, tests on arterial and venous blood, ECG, chest x-ray, echocardiogram, radionuclide scans, and cardiac catheterization. Some sources may be more useful than others for certain evaluative purposes. It is suggested that the anesthesiologist look for data to help answer the following questions about the patient with valvular disease.

What Are the Specific Valvular Lesions?

Most lesions can be diagnosed from physical examination (murmurs, rumbles, opening snaps, venous or carotid pulse abnormalities) and chest x-ray (specific chamber enlargements).[1] Echocardiography is highly specific for the diagnosis of mitral stenosis, but less so for other valvular abnormalities.[21] Cardiac catheterization can show transvalvular pressure gradients and regurgitant flows on cineangiography.

How Severe Is the Mechanical Abnormality?

As opposed to cardiac dysfunction seen in primary myocardial diseases such as coronary atherosclerotic heart disease or cardiomyopathy, valvular diseases cause a *mechanical* interference with cardiac function, with the later development of *secondary* myocardial failure. These mechanical problems are of two general types:[8]

1. Diastolic mechanical interference with ventricular filling (ventricular underloading), as seen in mitral stenosis.

2. Systolic mechanical ventricular overloading, either pressure overloading (as in aortic stenosis) or volume overloading (as in mitral or aortic regurgitation) or both.

When the left ventricle is subjected to systolic pressure or volume overloading, stroke volume tends to fall, either because of the increased afterload in pressure overloading or because of the loss of effective forward SV as a result of the regurgitant flow. When forward SV drops, three compensatory mechanisms may come into play:[8]

1. Increased sympathetic nervous system activity, which helps to maintain cardiac output by increasing heart rate and contractility via β-receptor stimulation. This mechanism is used mainly in acute states, and there is usually accompanying α-receptor stimulation, with an increase in SVR.

2. Use of the Frank-Starling principle to help maintain forward stroke volume by increasing ventricular preload (increase in LVEDV because of ventricular dilatation). The dilated left ventricle also has a geometric mechanical advantage, being able to eject a given SV with less shortening of circumferential fibers. In chronic cases, this compensatory mechanism is facilitated by renal salt and water retention. It is not used in cases of chronic pure pressure overload, such as aortic stenosis.

3. Ventricular hypertrophy: The increase in intramyocardial *tension* associated with elevated LVP in pressure overloading or LV dilatation in volume overloading leads to increased protein synthesis and eventually an increase in the thickness of the LV wall.[8] This increased thickness tends to normalize

the systolic and diastolic *stress* on the myocardium (since stress = tension ÷ wall thickness) and helps maintain SV by addition of more contracting units.[7] Pressure overloading leads to concentric hypertrophy, whereas volume overloading is followed by eccentric hypertrophy. In the latter case the LV wall thickness and mass tend to rise in direct proportion to the increase in LV size.[6,7]

All three compensatory mechanisms help to maintain stroke volume in the face of mechanical systolic overloading, but at the price of symptoms attributable to each mechanism. Increased sympathetic nervous activity causes excessive tachycardia and sweating with exercise. LV dilatation, with increase in LVEDV and LVEDP, causes symptoms of dyspnea because of the elevation of pulmonary capillary pressure. Hypertrophy and dilatation can both increase myocardial oxygen consumption ($M\dot{V}O_2$) and cause angina.[8] Unfortunately, the presence and severity of these symptoms do not give a good estimate of the severity of valvular stenosis or regurgitation. The major reason for this is that these compensatory mechanisms also occur in primary myocardial diseases in which a primary decrease in contractility causes a decrease in stroke volume and evokes the compensatory mechanisms. Thus, a patient with a relatively mild valvular abnormality could be severely dyspneic if he has coexisting unrelated myocardial disease, or he could have severe angina with only mild aortic stenosis if there is coexisting coronary atherosclerotic heart disease. To accurately predict a patient's response to anesthesia and surgery, as well as his degree of improvement after surgery corrects the mechanical abnormality, the valvular problem and myocardial contractility must be evaluated separately.

Quantitating the Severity of Valvular Stenosis

Although a small pressure gradient must exist across a heart valve for there to be flow across it, normal atrioventricular and semilunar valves are able to accommodate normal cardiac output (this flow occurring during diastole for atrioventricular valves and during systole for semilunar valves) without a significant transvalvular pressure gradient being detectable at cardiac catheterization. For example, the normal aortic valve gradient is 2–4 mm Hg[22–24] (see Fig. 6–1). As a valve becomes stenotic, with a decrease in its effective cross-sectional area for blood flow, flow becomes turbulent and is proportional to the square root of the pressure gradient.[23] Because of this relationship there must be a 50 percent reduction in valve area before a significant transvalvular pressure gradient is detectable at catheterization.[24]

Figure 6–5 shows the relations between flow, valve area, and pressure gradient for the aortic valve. As the valve area gets progressively smaller, the curve of flow versus the pressure gradient becomes flatter, so that it takes progressively greater increments in gradient in order to force the same flow across the valve.[22,23] Therefore, as stenosis worsens, a pressure gradient develops first only during states of increased flow such as exercise, anxiety, anemia, and pregnancy.[24,25] With still worse stenosis, a significant gradient develops at rest; and with very severe stenosis, the pressure gradient needed to maintain even normal resting flow may be unacceptably high, with a resultant drop in resting cardiac output.

Thus, both pressure gradient *and* flow must be measured at catheterization in order to assess valvular stenosis accurately. If cardiac output is low during catheterization, the measured transvalvular pressure gradient may be misleadingly low, leading to underestimation of the severity of stenosis if cardiac output is not measured also. If a valve is both stenotic and regurgitant, the total flow across it is the sum of forward and regurgitant flow; therefore, the gradient across such a valve must be higher for any given valve area. Since the amount of regurgitant flow is difficult to quantitate, the area of such a valve can be determined with less accuracy.[22,24] Practically, the valve areas are calculated from the following formulas:[22]

$$\text{Mitral valve area (cm}^2\text{)} = \frac{\text{mitral valve flow}}{31 \sqrt{\text{mean mitral valve gradient}}} \quad (6\text{-}2)$$

where mitral valve flow =

$$\frac{\text{cardiac output in ml/min}}{\text{diastolic filling period in sec/min}}$$

$$\text{Aortic valve area (cm}^2\text{)} = \frac{\text{aortic valve flow}}{44.5 \sqrt{\text{mean aortic valve gradient}}} \quad (6\text{-}3)$$

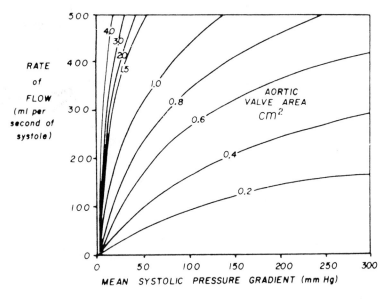

Fig. 6–5. Relation between valve area, flow rate across valve and mean trans-valvular systolic pressure gradient for the aortic valve. (Reprinted from Schlant RC: In Hurst JW (ed): The Heart (ed 4). New York, McGraw-Hill, 1978, pp 965–981. Copyright 1978. Used with permission of author, editor, and the McGraw-Hill Book Company.)

where aortic valve flow =

$$\frac{\text{cardiac output in ml/min}}{\text{systolic ejection period in sec/min}}$$

Or, dividing by heart rate,

$$\text{aortic valve flow} = \frac{\text{stroke volume in ml}}{\text{duration of ejection in sec}}$$

Quantitating the Severity of Valvular Regurgitation

Judging the severity of regurgitation is more difficult and less precise than quantitating the degree of stenosis. Many clinical signs and non-invasive techniques are *not* reliable indicators of the severity of regurgitation. Among these are the intensity of the regurgitant murmur,[26] pulse pressure or aortic diastolic pressure in aortic regurgitation,[26-28] the size of the chamber into which regurgitation takes place,[27-29,110] and echocardiography[21] (except in severe cases, such as aortic regurgitation with premature mitral valve closure[30]).

Certain measurements at catheterization can give a somewhat better idea of the amount of regurgitation. The size of the v wave in the LAP or pulmonary capillary wedge pressure

(PCWP) tracing is not necessarily related to the degree of mitral regurgitation,[31] because for a given amount of MR the size of the v wave depends on the size and compliance of the left atrial-pulmonary venous system. In a given patient, however, the size of the v wave does correlate directly with the degree of regurgitation changing as a result of acute changes in afterload.[9] The severity of MR can also be estimated by simultaneous indicator dilution curves made from sampling in the left atrium and a systemic artery after LV injection. This technique is thought to be less accurate than cineangiographic methods.

A *qualitative* estimate of the severity of regurgitation can be made by visual examination of cineangiograms after injecting contrast material into the chamber just beyond the incompetent valve (e.g., into the aorta in AR, or into the left ventricle in MR).[24] Regurgitation is usually graded as "one-plus...three-plus," etc. This method tends to overestimate the severity of aortic regurgitation, for example, in patients with small left ventricles, reduced ejection fraction, or coexisting aortic or mitral stenosis.[6]

The most accurate assessment of the severity of regurgitation is made by calculating *total* stroke volume from measurements of LVEDV and LVESV on cineangiogram and comparing this with the *forward* stroke volume calculated from cardiac output and heart rate.[6,7] The *re-gurgitant* stroke volume per beat can then be calculated as the difference between total SV and forward SV. Then the *regurgitant fraction* (RF), the best index of severity of regurgitation, is determined by

$$RF = \frac{\text{regurgitant SV}}{\text{total SV}} \qquad (6\text{-}4)$$
$$= \frac{\text{total SV} - \text{forward SV}}{\text{total SV}}$$

What Is the Functional Status of the Myocardium?

It has been found that myocardial contractility is decreased in both acute and chronic pressure and volume overloading and that this decrease in muscle performance in the face of systolic mechanical overloading usually worsens with time and is responsible for clinical deterioration in these patients, despite the compensatory mechanisms noted above.[7,8,26,32] *Acute* pressure overloading, such as results from increased impedance to LV ejection, is associated with a greater depression of contractility than is acute volume overloading, such as from aortic or mitral regurgitation. In *chronic* states, however, contractility per unit muscle mass is more depressed in volume overloading (chronic AR and MR) than in pressure overloading (chronic aortic stenosis). Also, the reversibility of the decreased contractility is thought to be less after correction of the mechanical abnormality in volume overloading than in pressure overloading.[8] Early degrees of decline in contractility will result in impaired LV performance (decreased stroke volume) only during stress such as exercise. Eventually, however, contractility falls below a critical level, so that in order to maintain a normal stroke volume even at rest the LV must dilate further (thus increasing its preload by the use of its Frank-Starling reserve) and call on increased activity of the sympathetic nervous system to help bolster its output by increasing contractility and heart rate. This critical level of depressed contractility for resting LV failure to occur is lower for aortic stenosis than for chronic aortic or mitral regurgitation.[8] In other words, myocardial contractility must, in gen-

eral, be depressed to a greater extent in aortic stenosis than in AR or MR for the development of resting LV failure.

Once contractility has reached this critical level of depression, the terminal course of some patients with pressure or volume overloading may be determined by changes in afterload. If impedance to ejection is increased, a *normal* left ventricle responds by transiently dilating (increasing preload) slightly to maintain stroke volume in the face of the increased afterload (see Fig. 6–4). Within a few cardiac cycles, however, there is an intrinsic increase in contractility which allows the left ventricle to maintain its SV now from its previous lower level of EDV (EF is unchanged).[10] In contrast, an *abnormal* left ventricle responds to an increase in afterload by acute dilatation (use of Frank-Starling reserve) but no intrinsic increase in contractility. Thus, LVEDV rises and remains elevated with an attendent rise in LVEDP, and SV is unchanged or falls (EF is decreased). Such a ventricle is said to be functioning on the "flat part" of its ventricular function curve, such that an increase in preload is not followed by an increase in SV.[10,33] Thus, in a left ventricle with critically depressed contractility, an increase in impedance to ejection may result in a fall in SV despite LV dilation, which can precipitate a vicious cycle of compensatory sympathetic vasoconstriction, further increase in impedance to ejection, further decrease in forward SV, and so on.[10] This may be especially operative in patients with mitral or aortic regurgitation and account for their rapid terminal deterioration.[34]

The clinical course of a patient with pressure or volume overloading would typically progress as follows:

1. New York Heart Association (NYHA) functional class I: Despite the mechanical abnormality and a minimal decrease in contractility, normal cardiac output is maintained at rest and during exercise without increase in PCWP.
2. NYHA class II: Contractility is worsened, but cardiac output is maintained through compensatory dilatation and/or hypertrophy, with acute LV dilatation and increased filling pressures (LVEDP, LAP, PCWP) necessary only during exercise.
3. NYHA class III: Contractility is further diminished, with a normal cardiac output

during usual activity being maintained by increased filling pressures and symptoms of pulmonary congestion.

4. NYHA class IV: Contractility is critically decreased, so that cardiac output may not be maintained at rest despite high filling pressures (with dyspnea); therefore, symptoms and signs of low cardiac output may now appear: fatigue, weakness, cachexia, mental confusion, oliguria.[8]

Positive inotropic agents such as digitalis may modify this course by augmenting the myocardial contractility, thereby sparing somewhat the use of dilation and hypertrophy as compensatory mechanisms. Chronic oral vasodilator therapy in valvular regurgitation may achieve similar sparing by reducing the impedance to LV ejection.[35] Despite the typical course noted above, a patient's symptoms are not a reliable indicator of myocardial contractility.[7] As noted before, symptoms depend on the severity of the mechanical overload and the extent of depression of contractility (either secondary to the mechanical abnormality or due to coexisting primary myocardial disease). Thus, contractility must be assessed independently.

The most accurate measures of contractility are *isovolumic phase indices,* such as peak-measured contractile element velocity (V_{pm}) or extrapolated maximum contractile element velocity (V_{max}), and *ejection phase indices,* such as circumferential fiber shortening rate (V_{cf}). Most studies of contractility in valvular heart disease are based on these indices, but they are not generally available clinically.[8]

LVEDP is *not* a good index of contractility for several reasons.[7] First, although a failing left ventricle dilates to help bolster its stroke volume, LVEDV itself is not a good indicator of contractility; for example, in aortic or mitral regurgitation, LVEDV is dependent on the severity of regurgitation as well as the contractility.[36] Second, LVEDP is not linearly related to LVEDV, their relationship being dependent on LV diastolic stiffness. In patients with aortic stenosis and increased LV stiffness, LVEDP can be greatly increased with only a minor decrease in contractility.[8,24,37] On the other hand, LVEDP can be normal in patients with decreased contractility, if LV stiffness is decreased or if blood volume is low.[38]

Systolic time intervals can give some infor-mation about contractility. The ratio of preejection period to LV ejection time (PEP/LVET) has been found to correlate inversely with contractility in coronary atherosclerotic heart disease and cardiomyopathies, but it is less accurate in valvular disease because of the mechanical abnormalities.[24] Nevertheless, PEP/LVET reflects diminished LV pump performance in mitral stenosis when PEP/LVET ≥ 0.44, in mitral regurgitation when PEP/LVET > 0.50, and in aortic stenosis or aortic regurgitation when the ratio returns to normal (0.35 ± 0.04) after being depressed during the compensated phases of these diseases.[39]

Although the *ejection fraction* (EF) depends on preload and afterload as well as contractility in acute situations,[7] in chronic valvular disease the EF, as measured by cineangiographic,[6,7,24] echocardiographic,[40] or radioisotopic[24] methods, has been shown to reflect myocardial function in general and correlate with measures of muscle performance and prognosis with corrective surgery.[7,10,36] Ejection fraction will be discussed more fully under specific valvular lesions, but in general, it tends to be well preserved in the normal or low-normal range (normal 0.67 ± 0.08, 1 S.D.) until LV failure develops.[26] For most valvular lesions a resting EF of less than 0.50 indicates significant impairment of myocardial contractility, especially if systemic vascular resistance is normal or low at the time of measurement.[11,27,37,41] If EF is normal at rest but falls significantly with angiotensin infusion, decreased contractility exists but is less severe than in cases where resting EF is subnormal.[11,42]

Are There Abnormalities in Left Ventricular Diastolic Function?

Left ventricular diastolic function should also be assessed in patients with valvular heart disease, including intrinsic problems with LV filling such as mitral stenosis and increased LV diastolic stiffness and extrinsic problems such as arrhythmias and blood volume. Ventricular stiffness is important in that it determines the relation between LVEDV and LVEDP, the slope of phase 1 in Figure 6–2, and the importance of LA contraction to LV filling.[14,18,19] Arrhythmias can affect LV filling by the loss of the atrial "kick" and the decreased diastolic filling period in tachyarrhythmias. Blood volume should be evaluated as in any other patient for surgery. Although blood volume is usually elevated in patients with valvular disease coming to surgery,[43] it may be excessively low or high, especially in emergency situations when fluid or drug therapy has been acutely rendered.

What Is the Status of the Pulmonary Circulation and Right Ventricle?

Patients with chronic pulmonary venous hypertension secondary to mitral valve or, less commonly, aortic valve disease may develop chronic intimal fibroelastosis in pulmonary venules and arterioles which tends to strengthen these vessel walls.[44] However, such chronic pulmonary venous and secondary pulmonary arterial hypertension can cause the following:

1. A chronic increase in pulmonary extravascular water with changes in lung mechanics.[45]
2. Redistribution of blood flow to less dependent regions of the lungs, with a change in the normal distribution of V/Q ratios.[46]
3. Noncompliant pulmonary vessels, so that these patients are unable to accommodate relatively small increases in blood volume.[46]
4. A secondary increase in pulmonary vascular resistance, which increases mean pulmonary artery pressure (PAP) still more.[47]
5. Chronic right ventricular (RV) pressure overload with RV hypertrophy and eventually RV failure.

Patients with these changes are more likely to have RV failure and therefore LV underloading postoperatively. They may show significant discrepancies between PA diastolic and PCW pressures[46,47] and may have hemodynamic deterioration if pulmonary vascular resistance is increased further intraoperatively or postoperatively.[47,48] LV dysfunction secondary to RV hypertrophy or RV failure may occur.[12,49] For these and other reasons, evaluation of the pulmonary circulation and right ventricle is important, especially in patients with mitral valve disease. Optimally, this will be done with right heart catheterization and determination of RA, RV, PA, and PCW pressures, calculation of pulmonary vascular resistance and a search for tricuspid regurgitation.

What Is the Status of the Coronary Circulation?

Angina may occur in valvular disease despite normal coronary arteries, secondary to both problems with subendocardial flow and an increase in myocardial oxygen consumption. This is especially characteristic of aortic stenosis with or without aortic regurgitation.[8] However, coronary atherosclerotic heart disease may also occur in patients with valvular disease, with the same age- and sex-related frequency as in the general population,[50] and, if present, may increase the operative mortality of valve replacement.[50,51] The patient with angina who is about to undergo valvular surgery should have preoperative coronary arteriography to determine the presence and severity of coronary disease, both in evaluation for possible concomitant aortocoronary bypass and so that the anesthesiologist can be more aware of possible myocardial oxygen supply–demand problems intraoperatively. Also, evidence of previous myocardial infarction should be sought, including dead zones on ECG (although apparent anteroseptal dead zones can occur in ECGs of patients with aortic stenosis with normal coronaries) and localized dyssynergic areas on LV cineangiogram which may also compromise LV pump function.[37]

SPECIFIC VALVULAR LESIONS

Mitral Stenosis

Mitral stenosis is a chronic disorder that is almost always rheumatic in etiology, with progressive thickening of the mitral valve leaflets, fusion of their commissures, and shortening and fusion of the chordae tendineae, so that there is a progressive diminution in the effective orifice area for blood flow from the left atrium to the left ventricle.[5,25]

PATHOPHYSIOLOGY

Left Ventricular Diastolic Underloading. The major problem in mitral stenosis is mechanical inhibition of LV diastolic filling secondary to the progressive decrease in mitral valve area (MVA).[8] As shown in Figure 6-6, as the MVA decreases from its normal value of 4–6 cm² in adults, either flow through the valve must de-

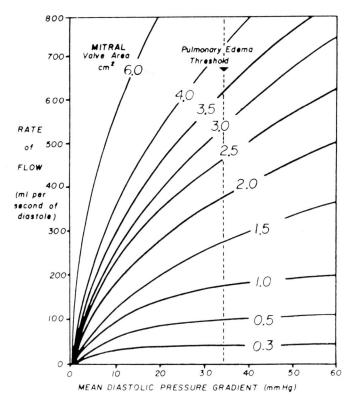

Fig. 6–6. Relation between valve area, flow rate across valve, and mean trans-valvular diastolic pressure gradient for the mitral valve. (Reprinted from Schlant RC: In Hurst JW (ed): The Heart (ed 4). New York, McGraw-Hill, 1978, pp 965–981. Copyright 1978. Used with permission of author, editor, and the McGraw-Hill Book Company.)

crease, resulting in a drop in cardiac output, or the pressure gradient across the valve must increase to maintain the same cardiac output. Except in rare patients,[52] cardiac output tends to be maintained until the terminal stages of the disease, but at the expense of an increase in the pressure gradient from left atrium to left ventricle. Since there is a limit to how far the LVEDP (and hence the LVEDV) can fall before there is a drop in cardiac output because of the Frank-Starling relationship,[53] cardiac output is maintained in mitral stenosis primarily by an increase in LAP and hence PCWP.[26]

The usual progression of rheumatic mitral stenosis is shown in Figure 6–7. The MVA must usually fall to below 2.6 cm² before there is a significant obstruction to flow and clinical symptoms ensue; this process usually takes 20 years from the episode of acute rheumatic fever.[25] Pa-

tients with mild clinical mitral stenosis, with MVA of 1.5–2.5 cm², are asymptomatic at rest but develop symptoms of pulmonary congestion during exercise. They are able to maintain a normal resting cardiac output without an increase in mean LAP; however, exercise demands a higher output to meet the increased tissue demands for oxygen. As demonstrated in Figure 6–6 this increase in flow through the mitral valve is made possible by an increase in LAP and hence in PCWP, resulting in net filtration at the pulmonary capillaries and the symptom of dyspnea. In general, these patients are only mildly disabled unless there are complicating conditions demanding higher cardiac output even at rest, such as anemia, fever, pregnancy, or hyperthyroidism.[26]

Moderate mitral stenosis occurs over the next 10 years or so as MVA declines to the

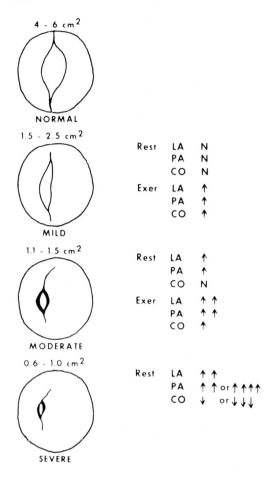

patients is usually decreased, secondary to an increased pulmonary vascular resistance (PVR) with RV dysfunction or failure. An MVA of 0.3–0.4 cm² is the smallest area found compatible with life.[25,26]

Left Ventricular Dysfunction. The left ventricular pressure-volume loop from a typical patient with moderate mitral stenosis is shown in Figure 6–8. Despite the impediment to diastolic filling imposed by the stenotic mitral valve, LVEDV is in the normal range in about 85 percent of these patients and is only mildly reduced in the remaining 15 percent (normal 70 ± 20 ml/m², 1 S.D.).[6] A high LVEDV in patients with presumably pure mitral stenosis should imply the presence of MR, AR, or primary myocardial disease.[6] LV mass is normal. As can be seen from the figure, the shape of the loop is normal, but its area is reduced slightly, consistent with a mild decrease in net LV work. Most patients with moderate mitral stenosis also have a stroke volume in the low-normal range resulting in a normal ejection fraction. Patients with severe disease may still have a normal EF, because SV and LVEDV are both reduced slightly.[6,13,54]

About 33 percent of patients with mitral stenosis have an EF below normal (normal 0.67 ± 0.08, 1 S.D.), however, and about 15 percent

Fig. 6–7. Relative changes in left atrial (LA) and pulmonary arterial (PA) pressures and cardiac output (CO) at rest and during exercise with progressive narrowing of the mitral valve orifice in mitral stenosis. (Reprinted from Rapaport E: Natural history of aortic and mitral valve disease. Am J Cardiol 35:221, 1971, with permission of author and publisher.)

range of 1.1–1.5 cm².[25] Now, even at rest, an elevated LAP is necessary to maintain cardiac output in the low-normal range. With minimal exercise, output can still increase, but at the expense of a severe increase in LA, PCW, and PA pressures. These patients have severe dyspnea on exertion and usually experience orthopnea and paroxysmal nocturnal dyspnea.[25,26]

When the mitral valve is narrowed to less than 1.0 cm² (severe mitral stenosis, Fig. 6–7), a mean LAP of 25 mm Hg is necessary to maintain even a minimally adequate resting cardiac output. In fact, resting cardiac output in these

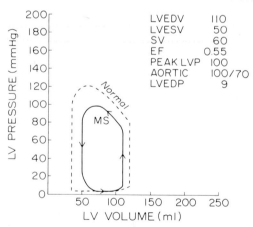

Fig. 6–8. Left ventricular pressure-volume loop for a typical patient with pure mitral stenosis. Dashed line shows pressure-volume loop for a normal left ventricle for comparison. Volume data are average values from reference 6. Note that volumes are in milliliters, *not* in milliliters per square meter of body surface area.

have an EF of less than 0.40.[6] Also, several patients with mitral stenosis have been found to have an *elevated* LVEDP either at rest or during exercise,[55,56] which is associated with an apparent decrease in LV compliance.[55] These findings, plus the clinical observation that several patients with pure mitral stenosis fail to increase their cardiac output as much as expected after corrective surgery, suggested the possibility that LV function was abnormal in these patients.

Although indices of myocardial contractility are normal in pure mitral stenosis,[57] even in patients with reduced ejection fractions, LV cineangiograms have shown that many, if not most, patients with moderate-to-severe mitral stenosis have abnormal contraction patterns marked by hypokinesis or akinesis of the posterobasal area.[6,11–13] At autopsy, chordae tendineae of the posterior mitral valve leaflet are found fused into a single rigid columnar structure, and the posterobasal part of the left ventricle is found drawn toward the mitral valve annulus and is nearly immobile.[13,58] Mitral stenosis patients with lower ejection fractions have more severe posterobasal contraction abnormalities.[11] This nearly immobile segment of the LV wall could help explain the failure of LV function to improve with digitalis therapy in patients with mitral stenosis in sinus rhythm[26,59] and might account in part for the decrease in LV compliance seen in some patients.[55] Some patients with mitral stenosis are also found to have contraction abnormalities of the anterolateral LV wall similar to those seen in patients with RV hypertrophy from other causes, which raises speculation that RV dysfunction may affect LV synergy in some patients.[12]

As mentioned, *digitalis* has not been shown to produce demonstrable benefit at rest or during exercise in patients with mitral stenosis in sinus rhythm, but digitalis does improve LV filling in patients with atrial fibrillation by prolonging diastole.[26] *Isoproterenol* infusion at 1 μg/min does increase cardiac output in patients with mitral stenosis, but intrapulmonary shunting also increases, suggesting that isoproterenol causes preferential perfusion of nonventilated lung areas.[60] *Propranolol,* given to patients with moderate mitral stenosis in sinus rhythm, causes a decrease in heart rate, PAP, PCWP, and mitral valve gradient and causes no change in LVEDP. There is a mild decrease in cardiac output, however.[61]

Role of the Left Atrium. Although patients with mild mitral stenosis may have a significant gradient across the mitral valve only during the rapid filling periods in early diastole and after atrial contraction, those with moderate and severe mitral stenosis have a pressure gradient throughout diastole.[26] In these patients the *rate* of LV filling may be normal or only slightly decreased, and the left ventricle may fill to a low-normal LVEDV as long as diastole is long enough, but this is accomplished at the price of a high LAP.[13,15] Tachycardia, as occurs during exercise, can severely lower LV filling and SV because of the shortened filling phase, and this explains why patients with severe mitral stenosis may be unable to raise their cardiac output with exercise despite a large increase in LAP.[26,62,63]

In most patients with mitral stenosis, the presence of a properly timed atrial contraction has been shown to significantly improve LV filling, although it is less crucial than in patients with aortic stenosis.[15] At a given heart rate, changing from atrial pacing to ventricular pacing (or from *sequential* atrial and ventricular pacing to *simultaneous* atrial and ventricular pacing, as could occur in a junctional rhythm) results in a 22 percent decrease in diastolic flow per beat in patients with moderate-to-severe mitral stenosis.[63] Similarly, in studies where P-R interval is varied, a P-R interval of 0.14 to 0.20 is found to be optimal, and changing from a P-R interval of zero (no preceding atrial systole) to a P-R interval in this range leads to a 24 percent increase in diastolic flow per beat (and cardiac output).[64]

There is evidence that properly timed LA contraction may have a greater effect on cardiac output in patients with mild mitral stenosis than in patients with moderate or severe mitral stenosis.[26] This may result from a greater loss of energy because of turbulent flow across the severely stenotic valve or because of dilatation and impaired contractility of the left atrium as the disease progresses. The atrial myocardium is damaged by the rheumatic process,[5] and the height of the LA "a" wave has been found to decrease as the disease progresses.[24]

In patients with severe mitral stenosis, atrial fibrillation is the rule, and the stroke volume varies directly with the length of the preceding diastolic filling period. If the ventricular rate is uncontrolled, LV filling is severely impaired, and digitalis exerts its beneficial effect in mitral stenosis by slowing the ventricular response to atrial fibrillation.[26,59] Patients with mitral stenosis and atrial fibrillation tend to have lower cardiac outputs than patients with mitral stenosis in sinus rhythm at similar heart rates.[26]

Role of the Peripheral Circulation. An increase in systemic and pulmonary vascular resistance induced by *angiotensin* infusion in patients with mitral stenosis leads to an increase in PAP, PCWP, and LVEDP, with a fall in cardiac output.[11] In contrast, *norepinephrine* infusion causes no change in cardiac output, perhaps because of its positive inotropic effect.[60] It appears that patients with mitral stenosis are less able than normal people to adjust to an acute increase in impedance to LV ejection, possibly because of their abnormal LV function or because the limitation in LV filling may impair the ventricle's ability to use the Frank-Starling mechanism (increased preload) to normalize its stroke volume in the face of increased afterload.

Reduction in SVR by *sodium nitroprusside* at 30–80 μg/min has been found to decrease PAP, PCWP, and LVEDP, with no change in cardiac output in patients with mitral stenosis. The heart rate increases, however, suggesting reflex sympathetic discharge in an effort to maintain SV at the reduced LVEDP.[11] Administration of *nitroglycerin* (0.4 mg sublingually) to patients with mitral stenosis has been found to decrease PAP, PCWP, and LVEDP, with SV falling only if PCWP falls to 12 mm Hg or less.[53,65] Hence, vasodilators in patients with mitral stenosis can reduce pulmonary artery and pulmonary capillary pressures, but because of the gradient across the mitral valve, LVEDP and LVEDV may fall to levels low enough to cause a decrease in SV, limiting the effectiveness of the vasodilators.[11,65]

Pulmonary Circulation and Right Ventricle. As the mitral valve becomes mildly stenotic and the mean LAP rises slightly, pulmonary venous pressure rises, causing an increase in pulmonary blood volume.[26] With the increase in PCWP, PAP rises in order to maintain the perfusion pressure and blood flow across the pulmonary circulation. Some capillaries in the less dependent parts of the lung (zones I and II) may open, permitting more flow to these areas and actually decreasing pulmonary vascular resistance. Lung

mechanics are unchanged.[46] With more severe stenosis, pulmonary extravascular water (PEVW) begins to increase as LAP rises still further. PEVW has been found to correlate with the levels of LAP in patients with mitral and aortic valve disease, being increased in 50 percent of patients with LAP of 12–25 mm Hg and in 100 percent of patients with LAP greater than 25 mm Hg.[45] With this interstitial edema, which occurs at first only during exercise, lung compliance and gas flow rates begin to decrease, and patients are more symptomatic (NYHA class II).[46]

With chronic and progressively increased pulmonary venous pressures, intimal fibroelastosis begins and progresses in proportion to the duration and severity of the pulmonary venous hypertension, involving both pulmonary arteries and pulmonary veins. Although these vascular changes tend to strengthen the walls of these vessels, their lumens are not narrowed.[44] Their compliance decreases, allowing high LAPs to be more efficiently transmitted backward into the pulmonary artery and resulting in greater pressure overloading of the right ventricle and RV hypertrophy.

As the MVA becomes critical (about 1.0 cm^2) with LAP chronically greater than 25 mm Hg even at rest, there may be a sharp increase in PVR secondary to pulmonary arteriolar constriction.[26,47] This is greatest in dependent lung areas and causes a further shift of blood flow toward less dependent areas. The increase in PVR may cause a mild decrease in PCWP, and pulmonary blood volume often decreases, but these beneficial effects occur at the price of increased RV pressure overloading. PCWP nevertheless remains high enough to cause more marked changes in lung mechanics, and dyspnea now occurs on mild exertion or at rest (NYHA classes II to IV).[46] At this point the patient has two sites of obstruction to blood flow: the mitral valve and the pulmonary arteriole. Resting cardiac output falls. If RV failure occurs, it falls further, and the dilated right ventricle may mildly interfere with LV systolic and diastolic function.[8,12] Tricuspid regurgitation may occur secondary to RV dilatation, with further decrease in cardiac output, signs of peripheral venous congestion, and atrial fibrillation if this has not occurred earlier.[26]

Such pulmonary vascular changes can occur in any patient with an increased LAP and are seen commonly in patients with mitral regurgitation or combined mitral stenosis and mitral regurgitation. They are less common in aortic valve disease, since LAP tends to be lower until the terminal phase of the disease.

Effects of Mitral Valve Replacement. In most patients with mitral stenosis or mitral regurgitation, after surgical correction the elevated PVR falls quickly in association with the surgically induced fall in LAP, the PVR falling to approximately one-half its preoperative value during the first two postoperative days and returning to normal by the eighth postoperative day.[66] This is in contrast to patients with intracardiac left-to-right shunts whose PVR usually remains elevated even after surgical correction.[29,67] Preoperative infusion of pulmonary vasodilators, such as acetylcholine or tolazoline, during right heart catheterization may transiently lower PVR and help determine the role active (and reversible) vasoconstriction plays in its elevation. Perioperative mortality is higher in patients with mitral stenosis who have an elevated PVR, both for valve replacement and for closed valvulotomy.[66]

Mitral valve prostheses have an average valve area of 2.1–2.6 cm^2 and an average trans-prosthesis diastolic pressure gradient of about 4–7 mm Hg at normal cardiac outputs.[68] Despite this persistent small gradient, LAP falls to normal levels within 24 hours after correction of mitral stenosis.[66] In general, cardiac output increases progressively during the first 2 postoperative days. Since pulmonary hypertension is secondary to both the increase in LAP and the increase in PVR, pulmonary artery pressures are decreased on the first postoperative day.[66] Functional tricuspid regurgitation usually resolves with the abolishment of the RV pressure overload.[29,69]

ANESTHETIC CONSIDERATIONS

1. There is some controversy about premedication in patients with mitral stenosis. On the one hand, excessive preoperative anxiety with tachycardia could decrease the diastolic filling period with resultant increase in mitral valve gradient and PCWP. This possibility would argue for the use of heavy premedication in these patients. On the other hand, heavy premedication can be deleterious, resulting in a further increase in alveolar-to-arterial Po$_2$ gradient and possibly lowering cardiac output slightly. A compromise solution may be to order light premedication but take extra care in the preoperative visit to gain the patient's confidence and allay any anxiety. Scopolamine is probably preferable to atropine as an anticholinergic in these patients, as it is less likely to cause tachycardia and has sedative and amnesic effects.[70] If the patient is taking digoxin for control of the ventricular response to atrial fibrillation, this should usually be continued up to the time of operation; and if the ventricular response is high when the patient arrives for surgery, consideration should be given to administering a small supplemental dose.

2. Monitoring PA and PCWP pressures with a balloon-tipped, flow-directed catheter (Swan-Ganz) can be important, especially in those patients with very high PVR preoperatively. With catheters having double lumens, right atrial pressures can be monitored as well, and pulmonary and systemic vascular resistances can be calculated if cardiac output is measured by the thermodilution technique. Even without output measurement, PVR can be assumed to be increased if there is a gradient between PA diastolic and PCW pressures.[47] Such catheters may be more difficult to "float" into position in patients with mitral stenosis (or mitral regurgitation) because of the often-present atrial fibrillation, pulmonary hypertension, tricuspid regurgitation, and reduced RV stroke volume.

3. Regardless of whether PCWP or LAP is monitored after cardiopulmonary bypass for mitral valve surgery in these patients, it should be remembered there may still be a small gradient across the mitral valve, either secondary to unsuccessful commissurotomy or as a result of intrinsic mild obstruction to flow posed by the mitral valve prosthesis (average gradient, 4–7 mm Hg).[68] Therefore, in patients with atrial fibrillation, the mean LAP will slightly overestimate LVEDP. In patients in sinus rhythm after bypass, the mean LAP will closely approximate the value of the LVEDP instead of being 0–4 mm Hg lower.

4. Patients with mitral valve disease often have decreased compliance of the pulmonary vessels because of existing overdistention of the pulmonary veins and intimal fibroelastosis. Pulmonary venous and PCW pressures will then rise more with a given increase in blood volume. Thus, patients with mitral stenosis can be very susceptible to fluid overload,[46] either exogenous or attendant to a shift of blood centrally from head-down positioning or peripheral vasoconstriction. The latter commonly occurs with sympathetic stimulation from surgery and endotracheal intubation.

5. Tachycardia is to be avoided if possible for reasons mentioned above. Drugs that tend to produce tachycardia, such as ketamine, pancuronium, and gallamine, should be used with caution; but in some patients with severely depressed cardiac output, such agents may be preferred to drugs with ganglionic-blocking properties, such as curare. Metocurine may be the muscle relaxant of choice in patients with mitral stenosis, since it has no vagolytic action and only mild ganglionic-blocking effects.[71] Inhalational agents such as halothane and enflurane may be dangerous in patients with severely decreased resting cardiac output, but in patients with less severe stenosis, these agents can be beneficial in blunting the sympathetic response to intubation and surgery[72,73] and in decreasing pulmonary vascular resistance.[74] Mean LAP can increase, however, perhaps secondary to a rise in LVEDP because of myocardial depression.[74] If tachycardia does occur intraoperatively, it should be treated aggressively. Sinus tachycardia or an acute increase in the ventricular response to atrial fibrillation can be treated with agents such as halothane, a rapidly acting glycoside, or small (0.25–0.50 mg) intravenous doses of propranolol.[61] If atrial fibrillation occurs before bypass in a patient previously in sinus rhythm, direct-current countershock may be indicated if the ventricular response is high.

6. Nitrous oxide (N_2O), when added to morphine anesthesia before the surgical incision, causes an increase in PVR and SVR.[47,48] In some patients with right ventric-ular dysfunction the resultant increase in PAP could cause acute RV failure.[47,48] After surgical stimulation begins, there are large increases in SVR and PVR;[75] and if N_2O is added to morphine anesthesia at this time, its myocardial depressant effect may predominate.[76]

7. Although PVR usually decreases rapidly after surgical correction of mitral stenosis or mitral regurgitation,[66] other perioperative events such as hypoxemia, hypercarbia, acidosis, hypothermia, endogenous angiotensin effects, and release or administration of catecholamines with α-adrenergic agonist effects may help keep PVR elevated postoperatively. Also, if LAP exceeds 25 mm Hg postoperatively, PVR is likely to increase.[47] Such persistence of an elevated PVR may cause RV failure and the low-output syndrome, so that these causes should be avoided if possible. If PVR does remain elevated and is associated with clinical deterioration, the use of vasodilators such as sodium nitroprusside or phentolamine can lead to afterload reduction for the right ventricle and marked hemodynamic improvement.[47] Such therapy can be monitored by calculation of PVR from measurements of PAP, PCWP, and cardiac output; by following the gradient between PA diastolic pressure and PCWP; or by merely keeping the mean PAP less than 30, as this has been found to minimize PVR.[47]

8. Preoperatively, patients with mitral stenosis usually have decreased lung compliance, increased airway resistance, elevated alveolar-arterial oxygen gradient, and an increased work of breathing.[26,44] These abnormalities will affect the management of their ventilation while under anesthesia, especially the minimum inspired oxygen concentration they can tolerate. Postoperatively, the oxygen cost of breathing may be quite high, with total O_2 consumption being 25 percent higher for spontaneous than for controlled ventilation,[77] and not returning to normal for 2 to 3 weeks.[78] The postoperative O_2 cost of breathing is inversely proportional to the preoperative vital capacity.[77] Lung compliance is diminished even further after surgery. Also, patients having mitral valve replacement

(MVR) have significant depression of their CO_2 response curve during the first 24 hours after anesthesia with morphine (1–2 mg/kg)[79] possibly because they have lower rates of urinary morphine excretion than do patients having aortocoronary bypass surgery.[80] The dead-space-to-tidal-volume ratio (V_D/V_T) may be persistently high for days after MVR.[79] For all these reasons, it is advisable to use controlled mechanical ventilation for at least the first night after MVR.

9. The low-output syndrome, characterized by decreased total cardiac output, oliguria, peripheral vasoconstriction, and restlessness or mental confusion, occurs rather commonly after correction of mitral stenosis. It is more likely to occur in patients who preoperatively have decreased cardiac output, atrial fibrillation, pulmonary hypertension, combined mitral stenosis and mitral regurgitation, surgically uncorrected aortic valve disease, or a history of previous mitral valve surgery.[81] Full cardiac monitoring, with measurement of PAP and cardiac output, and calculation of PVR and SVR are helpful if not crucial in diagnosing the etiology (arrhythmias, LV failure, RV failure, hypovolemia) so that appropriate therapy can be given. Isoproterenol can be a very useful drug in treating RV or LV failure in this setting, as it also reduces PVR and SVR.

10. The syndrome of transverse midventricular disruption has recently been noted, occurring in elderly patients with mitral stenosis usually 1 to 4 days after MVR.[82] It is manifested by pump failure or LV rupture with exsanguination. The exact etiology is unknown, but transverse tears are found in the wall of the left ventricle, raising speculation that the problem may be caused by increased diastolic tension on the LV wall after surgical dissection of the mitral subvalvular apparatus. Thus, it is suggested that preload (LVEDV) be kept intentionally lower in such elderly mitral stenosis patients after cardiopulmonary bypass and that adequate cardiac output be achieved with inotropic agents or afterload reduction.

11. Patients undergoing MV surgery are prone to arrhythmias, especially supraventricular, in the postoperative period. Also, not uncommonly, they may have atrioventricular conduction disturbances secondary to surgical trauma, necessitating ventricular or sequential atrial and ventricular pacing.

Mitral Regurgitation

In contrast to mitral stenosis, which is a chronic valvular disorder nearly always rheumatic in origin, pure mitral regurgitation may be either acute or chronic and may be caused by abnormalities of the valve, subvalvular apparatus, left ventricle, and cardiac skeleton. Roberts has recently written an excellent review of the anatomy of the mitral valve and the pathology of the disorders that cause it to function abnormally.[5]

PATHOPHYSIOLOGY

Left Ventricular Systolic Volume Overloading. The basic hemodynamic problem in MR is a decrease in forward (effective) stroke volume because part of the total left ventricular SV is regurgitated through an incompetant mitral valve into the left atrium. The amount of regurgitation per systolic stroke depends on the size of the regurgitant orifice, the duration of LV ejection, and the pressure gradient between the left ventricle and the left atrium; this, in turn, depends on the contractile function of the left ventricle, the compliance of the left atrium and pulmonary veins, and the impedance to forward LV ejection into the aorta. The mitral valve may not be incompetent throughout systole. In MR associated with papillary muscle dysfunction, regurgitation often occurs during only part of systole; MR associated with asymmetric septal hypertrophy or the mitral valve prolapse syndrome is usually confined to late systole.[5] On the other hand, MR secondary to rupture of chordae tendineae and MR into large, compliant left atria occur throughout systole and may even continue into the phase of isovolumic relaxation.[29] In general, a regurgitant fraction (RF) of 0.3 or less indicates mild MR, and a RF of 0.3–0.6 indicates moderate MR. Patients with a RF greater than 0.6 have severe MR.[27]

Because regurgitation is occurring in a low-resistance pathway parallel to the systemic circuit, the total impedance to LV ejection is actually decreased in MR.[83,84] Therefore, at a given level of preload (LVEDV), the left ventricle is better able to reduce its wall tension during ejection so that more of its contractile activity can be used for fiber shortening and less for tension (intraventricular pressure) development.[84] Thus, MR leads to a greater reduction in LV volume during systole and to a lower peak LVSP from a given level of preload.[26,29] Since myocardial oxygen consumption is related to LV wall tension, heart rate, and contractility, and since fiber shortening itself consumes little oxygen,[10,29] the energy costs of MR are modest. In fact, myocardial oxygen consumption does not change significantly when acute MR is induced experimentally in dogs.[29,84,85] There may be a modest increase in O_2 consumption in acute MR in humans because of compensatory tachycardia and increased contractility, and in chronic MR because of compensatory hypertrophy.[6] However, energy requirements of MR per unit of external work done are less than those of aortic regurgitation or aortic stenosis; and angina in patients with MR is rare in the absence of coexisting coronary disease.[85]

Compensatory mechanisms in response to the diminished forward stroke volume in MR differ, depending on whether the MR is acute or chronic.

Acute Mitral Regurgitation. The most common causes of acute MR are rupture of chordae tendineae secondary to endocarditis, papillary muscle dysfunction secondary to myocardial ischemia in patients with coronary atherosclerotic heart disease, and papillary muscle rupture in the presence of acute myocardial infarction.[5] Rupture of one head of a papillary muscle leads to severe MR, but rupture of an entire papillary muscle trunk is usually incompatible with survival.[78,91] In MR associated with papillary muscle disease, surgical replacement of the mitral valve is likely to be beneficial only in those cases where MR is severe and associated with a relatively normal-sized left ventricle.[29]

The LV pressure-volume loop of a typical patient with severe acute MR secondary to ruptured chordae tendineae is shown in Figure 6–9. In response to the acute decrease in forward SV, there is compensatory sympathetic stimulation with tachycardia and increased contractility, and compensatory use of the ventricle's Frank-Starling reserve with LV dilatation. As can be seen from the figure, the LVEDV is increased in acute MR (average 142 ml/m² as compared with a normal LVEDV of 70 ± 20 ml/

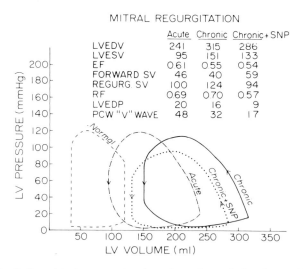

MITRAL REGURGITATION

	Acute	Chronic	Chronic+SNP
LVEDV	241	315	286
LVESV	95	151	133
EF	0.61	0.55	0.54
FORWARD SV	46	40	59
REGURG SV	100	124	94
RF	0.69	0.70	0.57
LVEDP	20	16	9
PCW "V" WAVE	48	32	17

Fig. 6–9. Left ventricular pressure-volume loops for typical patients with acute and chronic pure mitral regurgitation, showing changes with sodium nitroprusside (SNP) therapy in chronic MR. Loop for a normal left ventricle is shown for comparison. Values shown represent averages of data from references 6, 86, 90, and 34. Note that volumes are in milliliters, *not* in milliliters per square meter of body surface area.

m²), as are the LVESV and total SV.[86] The forward (effective) SV is less than normal (27 ml/m² versus the normal of 45 ml/m²), however, because of the large regurgitant fraction (69 percent of each total SV is regurgitated into the left atrium)[86] Ejection fraction is normal (0.61) in this patient, although this would not be the case when MR occurs acutely in diseased left ventricles.[87] LVEDP is elevated, both because the left ventricle is on a steep part of its compliance curve in late diastole and probably partly because of the confining effects of the pericardium.[14] Despite the compensatory mechanisms, the resting cardiac output is reduced (mean cardiac index, 2.3 liter/min/m² in this case).[86]

Figure 6-9 also shows how LV systolic dynamics are changed in acute and chronic MR. There is no isovolumic contraction period (period 2 in Fig. 6-2) because the early reflux into the left atrium allows the left ventricle to begin reducing its volume as soon as contraction begins.[6] The entire loop appears more horizontal than normal because of the large total SV, and the peak in LVSP tends to occur earlier than normal.[83] Finally, the period of isovolumic relaxation (period 4 in Figure 6-2) is shortened because LV filling begins as soon as LVP drops below the left atrial v-wave pressure, which is much greater than normal (PCWP v is 48 versus normal upper limit of 15).[6,24]

Acute mitral regurgitation occurs into smaller and less distensible left atria than does chronic MR,[88] and LVEDP tends to be higher[88] so that mean LAP, LA v-wave pressure, and pulmonary venous pressure are higher,[26] with resultant pulmonary congestion, PA hypertension, and acute RV failure.[26] Indeed, papillary muscle dysfunction in patients with myocardial ischemia secondary to coronary atherosclerotic heart disease can cause devastatingly severe MR with acute pulmonary edema, resolving with nitrate therapy.[89]

Chronic Mitral Regurgitation. In chronic MR there is further LV dilatation, compensatory eccentric hypertrophy, and less use of the sympathetic nervous system as a compensatory measure. Because of the Laplace relationship (tension = pressure × radius), LV *tension* rises with progressive LV dilatation. In chronic MR, however, the LV hypertrophies such that wall tension is not increased when expressed per unit of wall thickness; in other words, LV *stress* is

normal.[41] The isovolumic contraction period is nonexistent because of early emptying into the left atrium, and this early systolic reduction in LV wall tension helps minimize the increase in myocardial O_2 consumption in chronic MR. Also, the left ventricle becomes more spherical than normal (major/minor axis 1.44 as compared with a normal of 1.92), and this change in geometry allows a greater total stroke volume to be ejected with relatively less fiber shortening.[41]

A pressure-volume loop for the left ventricle in a typical patient with chronic MR is shown in Figure 6-9. LVEDV is still larger than in acute MR, 185 ml/m² in one study as compared with 142 ml/m² in acute MR.[86] LVESV and total SV are increased.[6,34,41,86] The regurgitant fraction of 0.70 indicates that this patient has severe MR, as the range of RFs in chronic symptomatic MR is usually 0.4-0.7.[6,41,86,90] Since the LVEDV and total SV usually increase in direct proportion in chronic MR, ejection fraction is in the normal range in 75 percent of these patients. The low-normal EF in this patient (0.55) probably indicates reduced myocardial contractility and may explain why the forward SV is no greater than in the patient with acute MR.[6,86]

As indicated in the figure, LVEDP tends to be lower in chronic MR than in acute MR and may be normal despite a higher LVEDV, indicating a decrease in diastolic LV stiffness, although this may still be greater than in the normal ventricle.[14,26] The lower LVEDP and the larger, more distensible left atria seen in chronic MR[86,88] result in lower mean LAP, LA v-wave, and pulmonary venous pressure, at least until the terminal stages of the disease.[26,86]

Left Ventricular Contractility. In acute MR, left ventricular contractility is normal or may be supranormal secondary to sympathetic nervous system stimulation,[26,83] unless the MR is secondary to or associated with LV myocardial disease.[26] Thus, in rupture of chordae tendineae the clinical course depends mainly on the severity of the regurgitation (RF), previous LV contractility, and the degree of increase in LAP.[26]

However, most patients with chronic MR show a variably progressive decrease in myocardial contractility; although total contractility may be normal secondary to eccentric hypertrophy, contractility *per unit of muscle mass* decreases.[8,26,41] Mild-to-moderate reduction in

LV contractile ability can be well tolerated in chronic MR without marked increases in mean LAP,[26] although the left ventricle must compensate for this diminished contractility by further dilatation in order to put out the same total SV. Thus, EF falls. Eventually, however, contractility reaches a depressed point at which resting LV failure occurs, with further dilatation and no increase in total SV (EF falls further). At this point, LVEDP and mean LAP rise,[8,26] and the LV may be critically sensitive to even small changes in impedance to aortic ejection such as increased systemic vascular resistance.[10]

As mentioned, because of the lower LV afterload that occurs in MR, ejection fraction in these patients probably overestimates the true contractile state.[6] In acute MR in dogs, EF was found to increase above normal, although isovolumic-phase measures of contractility (V_{max}) remained normal.[83,84] Hence, a low-normal EF in patients with MR should be taken as evidence of reduced contractility,[6,26] unless SVR is significantly increased at the time of measurement of EF. An EF of less than 0.50 in the setting of MR and normal SVR means severely reduced contractility, which is unlikely to be reversible after mitral valve replacement, at least acutely.[8,91] If a patient with MR has a low or low-normal EF despite digitalis therapy at the time of measurement, then the inotropic support of this drug will quite likely be needed after MVR.

In patients with MR secondary to papillary muscle disease, the EF tends to be lower, even acutely, averaging 0.41 in one study.[87] This is most likely due to the coexisting LV myocardial disease (primary decrease in LV contractility), as well as to the high SVR found in these patients with coronary disease.[87] These factors probably explain why such patients have very large LVEDVs (average 238 ml/m²), since in any patient with MR the LVEDV depends on both the severity of regurgitation (RF) and the adequacy of LV contractility.[87,92]

Role of the Left Atrium. In MR, for a given regurgitant SV the pressure-volume characteristics of the left atrium and pulmonary veins will determine the degree of elevation of LAP and PCWP and therefore the severity of pulmonary edema, pulmonary artery hypertension, and RV pressure overloading.[29] There is a spectrum of disease in MR depending on the size and distensibiliy of the left atrium.[29,31] The two extremes of this spectrum are shown in Figure 6-10.

At one end of the spectrum (top part of Fig. 6-10) the left atrium is normal or slightly increased in size and is relatively noncompliant because of early atrial hypertrophy.[5,29,31] This pattern is characteristic of acute MR, such as occurs from ruptured chordae or ruptured papillary muscle head. Mean LAP is greatly increased; there are large regurgitant v waves on LA and PCW pressure tracings; sinus rhythm is usually maintained; intimal fibroelastosis begins in the pulmonary vessels; and there is pulmonary hypertension with RV pressure overloading.[29] Surgical replacement of the mitral valve is most beneficial in this group, with rapid return of PA pressures to normal postoperatively.[29,31]

At the other extreme (bottom part of Fig. 6-10) are patients with chronic MR into very large, compliant left atria that microscopically show replacement of LA muscle with fibrous tissue, possibly secondary to rheumatic involvement of the LA walls. These patients tend to have normal LAP, atrial fibrillation, little pulmonary vascular disease, and mild or absent RV hypertrophy. MVR in these patients leads to an increase in forward cardiac output.[5,29,31]

Most patients with chronic MR fall between the extremes of the spectrum, with moderate increases in LA size and pressure and in the incidence of atrial fibrillation and severity of pulmonary vascular changes.[20]

Unless there is coexisting mitral stenosis, patients with MR are less dependent on a properly timed LA contraction for adequate LV filling than are patients with mitral or aortic stenosis. Conversion from atrial fibrillation to sinus rhythm causes little change in cardiac output in pure MR.[8] Because of the large LA "v" waves in most patients, there is an increased pressure gradient for early diastolic filling.

Role of the Peripheral Circulation. Since the left ventricle in MR can eject into either of two paths, the absolute sizes of regurgitant and forward stroke volumes for a given total SV (and therefore the RF) will depend on the relative impedance that each path offers to ejection. Impedance to ejection into the aorta is determined by the SVR and the compliance characteristics of the large arteries.[10] Thus, it is not surprising that changes in arterial impedance in-

THE SYNDROME OF MITRAL REGURGITATION

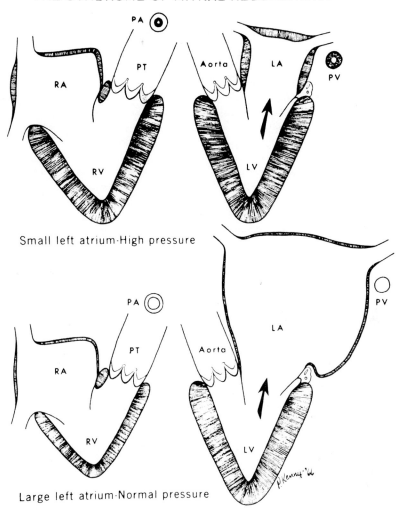

Fig. 6–10. The extremes of the syndrome of mitral regurgitation discussed in the text. Top: MR into small, hypertrophied LA results in pulmonary vascular changes and RV hypertrophy. Bottom: MR into large, thin-walled LA results in little or no change in pulmonary vessels or RV. (Reprinted from Roberts WC, Perloff JK: Mitral valvular disease. Ann Intern Med 77:939, 1972, with permission of author and publisher.)

duced by drugs or the sympathetic nervous system can have marked effects on forward and regurgitant flows at any given level of LVEDV (preload) and contractility.

When SVR is increased in patients with MR by *angiotensin, methoxamine,* or the combination of *norepinephrine and β-adrenergic blockade,* a 20 mm Hg increase in mean arterial pressure is followed by a 50 percent increase in LAP, a 120 percent rise in regurgitant flow, and a 16

percent fall in forward flow.[93] Infusion of *norepinephrine without β-blockade* leads to the same increase in mean LAP but no changes in forward or regurgitant flows.[93] This suggests that the β-adrenergic-mediated improvement in LV contractility offsets the α-adrenergic effects on arterial impedance. Such β effects may be especially important in patients with MR secondary to LV dilatation, as the better contractility will allow the left ventricle to function with a smaller systolic volume, thus improving mitral valve competence.[26]

Many patients with severe acute or chronic MR have elevated SVR at rest.[34,87,90] In these patients with MR secondary to valvular[34,90] or subvalvular[87] abnormalities, infusion of *sodium nitroprusside* intravenously at 15–30 μg/min is followed by marked hemodynamic improvement. Oral therapy with the vasodilator prazosin appears to achieve similar hemodynamic results.[35]

Changes in LV volumes and pressures with sodium nitroprusside therapy in chronic MR are shown in Figure 6–9. In these patients, LVEDV tends to decrease slightly, although changes in total SV and EF are not significant. There is a significant increase in forward SV, however, and reduction in regurgitant SV and RF. Heart rate does not increase; in fact, it decreases in the patients with the highest control LVEDPs. Thus, cardiac index rises in association with falls in mean LAP, LA v-wave pressure, and LVEDP.[34,87,90]

Such changes in PCWP and LVP before and after sodium nitroprusside therapy are shown in Figure 6–11 for a patient with MR secondary to papillary muscle dysfunction. In such patients, sodium nitroprusside may have other beneficial effects besides reduction in arterial impedance. It may also improve mitral valve competence by decreasing LV size slightly and by improving papillary muscle function secondary to reduced myocardial ischemia.[87]

Vasodilator treatment in patients with acute MR secondary to acute myocardial infarction with papillary muscle dysfunction can allow mitral valve replacement to be deferred until the acute phase of the infarction, associated with a high surgical mortality, is over.[94,95] Similarly, vasodilator therapy in patients with acute MR secondary to ruptured chordae from acute endocarditis may allow MVR to be postponed until a full course of antibiotics is given.

Nitroglycerin has slightly different effects than sodium nitroprusside in patients with MR. A dose of 0.6 mg sublingually reduces the LVEDV and apparently decreases the regurgitant SV, although forward SV and cardiac index are unchanged.[96]

This difference between nitroglycerin and sodium nitroprusside may be related to the more marked effect of nitroglycerin on preload (venodilation) than on afterload (arteriolar dilation).[9] Nitroglycerin may be more beneficial in MR as a result of papillary dysfunction or LV dilation than in MR secondary to valvular abnormalities because of the greater beneficial effects that improvement of myocardial ischemia and reduction in LV size would have in the former patients.

Combined Mitral Stenosis and Regurgitation. Patients with *pure* MR may have a LA-to-LV pressure gradient across the mitral valve during early- to mid-diastole, disappearing in late-diastole if the heart rate is slow enough.[26] For any given degree of severity of MR the presence of even mild mitral stenosis will increase the mean LAP considerably. Conversely, for any given reduced mitral valve area, the presence of even mild MR will significantly increase the gradient across the mitral valve and hence the LAP because of the increased flow that must cross the mitral valve (see Fig. 6–6).[26] Severe mitral stenosis is incompatible with a significant amount of MR, because the increased mitral valve flow required by such a mixed lesion would require a LAP greater than the 25–35 mm Hg "ceiling" on chronic LAP elevation imposed by the Starling balance of oncotic and hydrostatic pressures at the pulmonary capillary.[26]

Patients with combined mitral stenosis and mitral regurgitation do not fit into the spectrum of pure MR noted above. They tend to have large left atria, atrial fibrillation, and pulmonary vascular changes with pulmonary hypertension and RV pressure overloading. LV volumes tend to be intermediate between those of pure mitral regurgitation and those of pure mitral stenosis, LVEDV averaging 101 ml/m² with a SV of 60 ml/m² and a normal EF.[6]

Effects of Mitral Valve Replacement. The major effect of MVR is cessation of regurgitant flow, so that forward SV now equals total SV. Despite the mild residual diastolic gradient across the mitral valve prosthesis (4–7 mm Hg),[68] LAP and pulmonary vascular pressures fall significantly on the first postoperative day, and cardiac output rises.[66] A competent mitral valve prosthesis now prevents LV ejection into the low-resistance LA pathway, however, so that impedance to LV ejection increases markedly, especially in the first few hours after bypass when SVR is increased. If, in addition, myocardial contractility is further impaired by effects of cardiopulmonary bypass, ischemia, or cardioplegic drugs used during bypass, LV failure can occur in the early postoperative period.

ANESTHETIC CONSIDERATIONS

1. A pulmonary artery catheter can be very helpful in monitoring hemodynamic events in patients with MR, especially one that allows measurement of CVP, PAP, PCWP, and thermodilution cardiac output. In the prebypass period it can show relative changes in the severity of regurgitation as reflected in changes in PCWP v-wave magnitude (see Fig. 6–11), and it can help determine whether a given change in blood pressure has been caused by changes in cardiac output or SVR. After bypass, it offers advantages over a LA catheter in allowing measurement of cardiac output, mixed venous Po_2, PA pressures, and calculation of SVR and PVR. In the postoperative period, monitoring PA pressures can indicate whether a drop in LAP (PCWP) is due to hypovolemia or RV failure, and it can be used to monitor the effectiveness of treatment for increased PVR.

2. The presence of an atrial "kick" is less important in patients with MR than in those with mitral or aortic stenosis. Loss of sinus rhythm is not catastrophic, and tachycardia is better tolerated. After MVR the atrial "kick" may be more important for adequate LV filling at acceptable LA pressures.

3. Volatile anesthetics such as halothane and enflurane, while decreasing SVR to a mild extent, are severe depressants of myocardial contractility.[98] Since patients with acute MR are dependent on sympathetic nervous β effects to help the left ventricle cope with an acute volume load, and since patients with chronic MR already have depressed contractility, the negative inotropic effects of volatile agents may more than offset the mild decrease in arterial impedance and result in a fall in forward SV.

4. Nitrous oxide, when added in 50–60 percent concentrations to morphine analgesia in patients before surgical stimulation, has been found to increase SVR[99] and PVR.[48] If N_2O is added *after* the surgical incision, there is no further increase in SVR,[48] and its myocardial depressant effects[76] seem to predominate. It is possible that some patients with severe MR and pulmonary hypertension could experience RV failure owing to

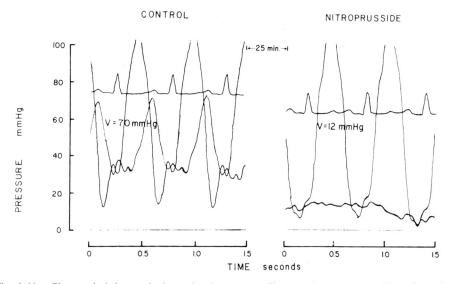

Fig. 6–11. Changes in left ventricular and pulmonary capillary wedge pressures with sodium nitroprusside therapy in a patient with mitral regurgitation resulting from papillary muscle disease. Note the fall in LVEDP, disappearance of abnormal PCW v waves, and unchanged heart rate. (Reprinted from Chatterjee K et al: Circulation 48:648, 1973, with permission of the author and the American Heart Association, Inc.)

the further mild increase in PVR or worsened LV failure owing to an increase in SVR if N_2O is added before the incision.

5. In patients with MR or AR undergoing morphine/N_2O anesthesia, surgical stimulation (sternotomy) has been shown to lead to great increases in SVR and PVR, with a fall in forward SV and cardiac index and a rise in PCWP, PAP, and CVP. Despite these changes, mean arterial pressure often rises misleadingly. After infusion of sodium nitroprusside (10–90 μg/min), these parameters all return to preincision levels.[75] It therefore appears that, at least in patients with MR or AR, the α-adrenergic effect of sympathetic stimulation during this period overcomes the potentially beneficial β-adrenergic effects. It would seem logical that drugs with mainly arteriolar-dilating properties, such as sodium nitroprusside or phentolamine,[9] would have advantages in this situation over drugs with mainly venodilating properties (such as nitroglycerin[9]) or significant ganglionic-blocking actions (such as trimethaphan) or complicating myocardial depressant effects (such as halothane or enflurane).

6. It is hard to predict the optimal LV filling pressure (PCWP or LAP) that will be needed after cardiopulmonary bypass and MVR. A patient with acute MR occurring in a normal left ventricle may need a relatively low LAP for adequate cardiac output once the mechanical overload is corrected. On the other hand, a patient with chronic MR and critically reduced preoperative LV contractility will probably need a rather high LAP after MVR. It is often possible during emergence from bypass to get an idea of the LAP or PCWP below which blood pressure or cardiac output seems to drop precipitously. This amounts to finding the "shoulder" of the steep part of a Starling curve. Then the LAP or PCWP can be kept a few millimeters of mercury above this point. It should be remembered that vasodilator or inotropic therapy will lower the filling pressure necessary to achieve a given cardiac output. Also it should be remembered that LVEDP reflects preload better than either LAP or PCWP does, and the relation between these will depend on the pressure gradient across the mitral valve prosthesis,[68]

the stiffness of the left ventricle, and the presence or absence of the atrial "kick."

7. The hypocontractile left ventricle in chronic MR is able to continue functioning in part because of the low impedance to ejection. After MVR, with the low-resistance pathway into the left atrium blocked by a competent mitral valve prosthesis, the left ventricle may not be able to eject effectively against even a normal arterial impedance,[100] much less against the elevated SVR occurring during anesthesia and surgery[75] (although the lowered blood viscosity immediately after bypass may transiently attenuate the effect of arteriolar constriction). Hence, afterload reduction (with vasodilators and/or intra-aortic balloon counterpulsation) or inotropic support or both will frequently be needed in addition to adequate preload to provide adequate SV (and cardiac output) after MVR.

8. As in patients with mitral stenosis, the PVR in patients with MR or combined MR and MS falls after MVR if it was initially elevated.[66] However, many factors can raise PVR in the postoperative period, and RV failure should be part of the differential diagnosis of the low-output syndrome. Also as in mitral stenosis, patients with MR are prone to supraventricular arrhythmias postoperatively, especially those patients who preoperatively have large, fibrillating left atria.

Aortic Stenosis

Aortic stenosis is a chronic disorder that, when isolated, is usually secondary to acquired changes in a congenitally malformed valve (bicuspid, unicuspid, or tricuspid with leaflets of unequal size).[25,101] If aortic stenosis occurs in a patient secondary to rheumatic disease, it is highly likely that the mitral valve will also be abnormal.[101]

PATHOPHYSIOLOGY

Left Ventricular Systolic Pressure Overloading. The basic hemodynamic problem that results as the aortic valve narrows from its normal area of 2.6–3.5 cm^2 can be understood by referring to Figure 6–5. The ejection of a normal SV of about 80 ml within a normal systolic ejection time of 0.25–0.32 seconds (dependent on heart rate) demands a flow rate of about 250 ml per systolic second across the aortic valve. A person with a normal aortic valve area (AVA) can accomplish this flow rate with a very small pressure gradient from left ventricle to aorta. Indeed, the normal mean systolic gradient is only 2–4 mm Hg.[22] As the AVA becomes smaller, however, such flow rates can be achieved only by increasingly large pressure gradients across the valve. For example, to achieve even a low-normal SV of 65 ml (equivalent to a flow rate of about 200 ml/sec across the valve) in a patient with an AVA of 0.4 cm[2] would demand a gradient of 130 mm Hg across the valve, requiring an LV systolic pressure of about 220 mm Hg if the aortic systolic pressure is to be as high as 90. To increase this SV back to the normal of 80 ml would now necessitate a pressure gradient of 200 mm Hg, which the LV might not be able to achieve,[22] since the upper limit of LVSP seems to be about 260 mm Hg or, rarely, as high as 300 mm Hg.[25,26]

Another way of thinking about aortic stenosis is to rearrange Equation 6–3:

$$SV = 44.5 \times AVA \times \sqrt{\text{mean gradient}} \times (\text{duration of ejection}) \qquad (6\text{-}5)$$

As the AVA decreases, SV must fall unless either the mean LV-to-aorta pressure gradient increases or the duration of ejection per beat increases or both. Maintenance of SV is accomplished mainly by increasing the LVSP, and hence the transvalvular gradient. This increased afterload on the left ventricle (higher LV wall *tension* as a result of increased intraventricular pressure) is a potent stimulus for protein synthesis.[8] This results in concentric hypertrophy of the LV wall, which tends to normalize the wall *stress* on the left ventricle, since stress equals tension per unit of wall thickness.[7,102] The hypertrophied left ventricle is able to generate high intraventricular pressure because of the increased total force of contraction. The velocity of fiber shortening is reduced, however, leading to a prolonged systolic upstroke time and duration of ejection.[20]

An increased duration of ejection allows a given SV to be ejected at a lower flow rate across the aortic valve.[26] During exercise, however, the duration of ejection falls as heart rate increases, as in normal subjects. Because the peak LVSP is limited, the mean gradient may not increase, so the SV falls as heart rate increases. For this reason, cardiac output may not rise during exercise in patients with severe aortic stenosis.[20]

Thus the major compensatory mechanism in aortic stenosis is concentric hypertrophy, the degree of hypertrophy being proportional to the mean pressure gradient across the valve.[103] Since there is little or no use of Frank-Starling compensation (dilatation) in these patients until LV failure occurs, LV volumes tend to be normal, as seen in Figure 6–12.[6,8,26] Only about 10 percent of patients with aortic stenosis have a LVEDV above the normal range.[6] EF is normal or even high-normal unless LV failure is present.[6] The LV pressure-volume loop is elongated vertically because of the high LV systolic pressures, but isovolumic contraction and relaxation periods are maintained.[6] The diastolic part of the loop shows reduced compliance (increased stiffness), with a greater-than-normal LV diastolic pressure necessary for any given diastolic volume.[14] The area of the loop is increased, reflecting the fact that LV external work is usually about two times normal in pure aortic stenosis,[22] although the effective work available to the circulation is only a fraction of that.

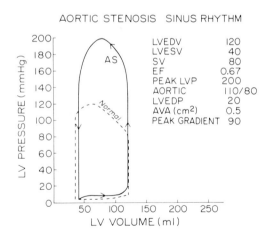

AORTIC STENOSIS   SINUS RHYTHM

LVEDV	120
LVESV	40
SV	80
EF	0.67
PEAK LVP	200
AORTIC	110/80
LVEDP	20
AVA (cm2)	0.5
PEAK GRADIENT	90

Fig. 6–12. Left ventricular pressure-volume loop for a typical patient with severe pure aortic stenosis. Loop for a normal left ventricle is shown for comparison. Volume data from ref. 6. AVA = aortic valve area. Note that volumes are in milliliters, *not* in milliliters per square meter of body surface area.

The aortic valve must be narrowed to about 25 percent of its normal area before there is significant obstruction to flow across it.[26] The AVA usually must decrease to 0.5–0.7 cm^2 before pure aortic stenosis is associated with the three major symptoms of angina, syncope, and dyspnea, although these symptoms usually occur at greater valve areas if there is associated AR, mitral valve disease, or coronary disease.[26] Although a patient with even severe aortic stenosis can be asymptomatic (in contrast to the patient with severe mitral stenosis[25]), he is a candidate for sudden death.[25,101] Once one or more of these symptoms has appeared, the average survival rate is less than 5 years.[25,101]

Patients with *mild* (AVA index greater than 0.8 cm^2/m^2) or *moderate* (AVA index 0.5–0.8 cm^2/m^2) aortic stenosis have normal cardiac output, SV, LVEDP, and PVR, although calculated LV systolic work is increased in patients with mild aortic stenosis and is even higher in patients with moderate stenosis.[20] Patients with *severe* aortic stenosis (AVA index less than 0.5 cm^2/m^2), however, may have significantly decreased resting cardiac output and SV and increased LVEDP and PVR.[20] Interestingly, the LV systolic work is lower in this group than in patients with moderate stenosis, consistent with the finding of decreased contractility in many of the patients with severe stenosis.[20]

Left Ventricular Contractility. Patients with mild or moderate aortic stenosis are generally asymptomatic except with severe exercise[26] and are usually found to have normal myocardial contractility.[103] Although the left ventricle in severe aortic stenosis and in older patients with moderate stenosis is able to generate high LV systolic pressures,[103] it usually demonstrates decreased contractility per unit of muscle mass, as measured by V_{max} and V_{pm}.[8,26,103] Even though patients with severe compensated aortic stenosis have a high resting LVEDP,[20] their LAP and PCWP are normal at rest. Mild-to-moderate exercise may necessitate some use of Frank-Starling reserve, however, if SV is to be maintained despite a shorter duration of ejection. Thus, there may be a transient increase in LVEDV, LVEDP, and LAP, with symptoms of pulmonary congestion.[26]

With time, contractility decreases further in most patients with severe aortic stenosis, perhaps in part as a result of functional and structural changes from long-term relative coronary insufficiency.[37] This decline, although not necessarily continuous, is thought to be responsible for the clinical deterioration of patients with severe aortic stenosis. Once contractility per unit of muscle mass decreases below a critical level, resting LV failure supervenes. Here, there is resting use of dilatation to help generate a high enough LVSP in the face of reduced contractility. Even with the higher preload (LVEDV), however, SV does not rise to its previous level, so EF decreases. At the higher LVEDV, LVEDP rises as do LAP, PCWP, and PAP.[8,26,37]

Therefore, even among patients with severe aortic stenosis (AVA index less than 0.5 cm^2/m^2), there is a clinical spectrum of compensated or decompensated LV dysfunction, depending on the level of myocardial contractility per unit of LV muscle mass. Even nonfailing ventricles in severe aortic stenosis usually have a high resting LVEDP because of increased diastolic stiffness, and so increased LVEDP is not necessarily a sign of LV failure.[26] However, an EF of less than 0.5 in severe aortic stenosis has been found to be associated with reduced resting cardiac index, increased LVEDV with further rise in LVEDP, high pulmonary artery pressures, and decreased fiber shortening rate.[37] Thus, when EF is low in severe aortic stenosis, it strongly suggests a critically diminished LV contractility with resort to resting use of Frank-Starling preload reserve (increased LVEDV without increase in SV). When the EF is low in a patient with only moderate aortic stenosis (AVA index 0.5–0.8 cm^2/m^2), this should suggest the possibility of significant aortic regurgitation or coexisting primary myocardial disease unless the patient is elderly.[103]

Digitalis is helpful in patients with aortic stenosis and reduced contractility because of its positive inotropic effects. In patients with LV failure, digoxin can improve contractility enough to spare the use of compensatory dilatation, so that it may actually decrease myocardial oxygen consumption by reducing LV size.[8] On the other hand, *propranolol*, when given to patients with severe aortic stenosis, has been found to cause increased LVEDV, decreased cardiac output, and decreased rate of fiber shortening, implying that in these patients there is some reliance on endogenous β stimulation to maintain compensation.[104] The decrease in fiber shortening rate is found to persist even if a propranolol-induced fall in heart rate is prevented by atropine.[105]

Role of the Left Atrium.   As the valve area decreases in aortic stenosis with resulting increase in LV concentric hypertrophy, LV diastolic stiffness increases in proportion to the increase in wall thickness (stiffness per unit of wall thickness remaining nearly normal).[14,26] Thus, for any given level of LV volume during diastole, a greater-than-normal LV diastolic pressure is necessary. Because the LA-to-LV pressure gradient would then be lower during early- and mid-diastole, the rate of *passive* LV filling is lower in patients with aortic stenosis than in normal subjects.[15]

On the other hand, the late-diastolic atrial contraction (*active* filling) contributes more toward LV filling in aortic stenosis patients than in normal subjects. Atrial systole in patients with moderate-to-severe aortic stenosis is found to contribute about 30 percent of the total LVEDV, as compared to 20 percent in normal ventricles;[15] and the atrial contraction in aortic stenosis doubles the rate of LV filling, whereas active filling rate is no greater than passive filling rate in normal subjects and in patients with mitral stenosis.[15] A P-R interval of 0.10–0.15 is found to achieve the optimal filling in most patients with moderate-to-severe aortic stenosis[106] and RV pacing leads to decreased LV systolic pressure and SV.[106]

For these reasons, the presence of a properly timed LA contraction can be crucial in patients with aortic stenosis to ensure the attainment of an adequate LVEDV for the generation of the needed LVSP. This is especially true at high heart rates, where time for passive diastolic filling is reduced.[15] The onset of atrial fibrillation in a patient with severe aortic stenosis can be a catastrophic event.[14,26]

Despite the increased diastolic stiffness, a significant increase in mean LAP occurs only very late in the course of aortic stenosis, and significant pulmonary hypertension or pulmonary vascular disease is unusual in patients with pure aortic stenosis, in contrast to patients with mitral valve disease.[26] This is largely because the LA contraction in aortic stenosis is causing a large increase in LVEDP (an *instantaneous* pressure), but the LA "a" wave does not raise *mean* LAP very much. So LVEDP is higher than mean LAP in patients with aortic stenosis

in sinus rhythm.[19] In fact, the difference between LVEDP and mean LAP is proportional to the severity of the stenosis.[20] Thus, in patients with mild stenosis, LVEDP is found to be 1 mm Hg higher than mean LAP, which is no different than their normal relationship. In moderate aortic stenosis, this difference averages 4.4 mm Hg; and in severe stenosis, the difference is 7.4 mm Hg.[20]

Role of the Peripheral Circulation.   In severe aortic stenosis the afterload on the left ventricle is affected to only a minor extent by changes in systemic arterial impedance (determined by SVR and the distensibility of large arteries) because of the huge impedance at the aortic valve itself. SV can be significantly affected, however, especially in patients with LV failure who have already maximally utilized their Frank/Starling preload reserve and therefore cannot increase LVEDV on a beat-to-beat basis.[37]

Angiotensin-induced vasoconstriction is followed by a slight increase in LVEDP and little change in SV in patients with moderate-to-severe aortic stenosis and good LV function;[26,107] in patients with poor LV function, however, angiotensin leads to a reduction in SV and a large increase in LVEDP.[26] By increasing arterial impedance to LV ejection, angiotensin tends to reduce the LV-to-aorta pressure gradient. Apparently, patients with good LV contractility respond to this by a transient increase in LVEDV (and LVEDP), thereby generating a greater LVSP so that the transvalvular gradient is returned to its previous level and SV remains the same. Patients with very severe aortic stenosis and/or decreased contractility may already be generating the maximum possible LVSP, however, so that the gradient must fall with an increase in arterial impedance, despite further LV dilatation.

A *decrease* in arterial impedance might be expected to raise the LV-to-aorta pressure gradient and thus increase SV. Stroke volume, however, could only increase in proportion to the square root of the higher pressure gradient (see Equation 6–5). Hence, mean arterial pressure could decrease, with hypoperfusion of the brain (with syncope) and coronary arteries (with myocardial ischemia and further LV dysfunction).

Angina Pectoris. Although coronary atherosclerotic heart disease occurs in aortic stenosis patients with the same frequency and severity as in the general population,[26] the presence of angina pectoris in a patient with aortic stenosis does not indicate the presence of coronary atherosclerotic heart disease.[50,51] Myocardial ischemia occurs in patients with aortic stenosis and normal coronary arteries because of both increased myocardial O_2 consumption and decreased subendocardial perfusion. Left ventricular O_2 consumption is far more dependent on the pressure generated by the left ventricle than on the SV ejected, as fiber shortening consumes little energy.[10] In aortic stenosis, myocardial oxygen consumption rises in direct proportion to the amount of hypertropy, so that O_2 consumption per gram of LV myocardium remains normal.[102]

Although resting total coronary blood flow also increases in proportion to the extent of LV hypertrophy in aortic stenosis so that flow per gram of myocardium is normal,[102] much of the extra flow may be redistributed to *subepicardial* areas. Many factors in aortic stenosis hinder delivery of O_2 to the *subendocardium.* The coronary arteries may be chronically maximally dilated in an effort to supply the hypertrophied LV myocardium, which may have a lower-than-normal density of capillaries with resultant greater diffusion distance from capillary to mitochondrion.[26] If the coronaries *are* maximally dilated, then subendocardial perfusion, which occurs only in diastole because of the high LV systolic pressures, becomes dependent on only two factors:

1. The driving pressure for subendocardial flow. This is is usually decreased in aortic stenosis because of the relatively low coronary diastolic pressure and the high LV diastolic pressure which can impede flow to the subendocardium.[10,102,108]
2. Duration of diastole. Although tachycardia is not dangerous in normal subjects because the coronary arteries can dilate to maintain flow, further coronary artery dilatation may be impossible in severe aortic stenosis. In this case, tachycardia can lower subendocardial flow because of the fall in duration of diastole.[26,108] In fact, 50 percent of aortic stenosis patients in one study who underwent atrial pacing to rates of 120 to 140

beats per minute exhibited a switch from net myocardial lactate extraction to net lactate production, indicating myocardial ischemia.[102]

Nitroglycerin may or may not relieve angina in patients with aortic stenosis and normal coronaries. In patients with moderate-to-severe stenosis, administration of 0.4–0.6 mg sublingually lowers the tension-time index consistently, secondary to decreased LVSP, diminished duration of ejection, and probably a reduction in LV size. Aortic diastolic pressure also decreases,[109] however, so that, in a given patient, the net effect of nitroglycerin may depend on a variety of factors, such as control LV and aortic pressures, LV volume, and whether the coronaries are already maximally dilated.

It may be that myocardial ischemia is the reason for the apparent upper limit on attainable LV systolic pressure. Above a LVSP of about 260 mm Hg, myocardial O_2 consumption may increase far more than O_2 supply, and the resultant subendocardial ischemia and LV dysfunction might prevent the LV from generating a higher LVSP.

Aortic Stenosis with Other Valvular Lesions. In combined aortic stenosis and aortic regurgitation there can be significant regurgitant flow (2–5 liters/min) through even small regurgitant orifices because of the relatively high diastolic pressure gradient from aorta to left ventricle.[22,26] This regurgitant flow in turn leads to increased forward flow across the stenotic aortic valve, so that for a given AVA the left ventricle must generate a higher LVSP than would be necessary in pure aortic stenosis of equal severity. Because of the regurgitant flow, LVEDV increases, the average value being about 130 ml/m². LV diastolic and systolic tension increase greatly, so that hypertrophy and LV mass are greater than in pure aortic stenosis.[6] The external work done by the left ventricle is often four times normal,[22] although only a small part of this work is actually responsible for forward blood flow. For these reasons, symptoms of pulmonary congestion and myocardial ischemia occur at a larger AVA than in pure aortic stenosis.[26] In fact, the critical valve area for severe stenosis is approximately 0.9 cm²/m² when significant aortic regurgitation is present, as opposed to about 0.5 cm²/m² for pure aortic stenosis.[22]

When aortic stenosis occurs with mitral stenosis, the latter tends to predominate hemodynamically and to be responsible for the major clinical signs and symptoms. The limitation of flow through the mitral valve limits the flow across the aortic valve, so that a smaller aortic valve pressure gradient is needed for a given degree of aortic stenosis, although cardiac output is also lower. Thus, there tends to be minimal increase in LV systolic and diastolic pressures, so that there is little or no compensatory hypertrophy.[22,26]

The presence of aortic stenosis can cause severe regurgitation across even a mildly incompetent mitral valve because the high LVSP creates a large pressure gradient for MR. Surgical relief of aortic stenosis usually is followed by a dramatic decrease in MR.[26] This combination is not rare and may occur even when the stenosis is not rheumatic in origin. In aortic stenosis occurring in a congenitally malformed valve, there is nearly always associated fibrosis and atrophy of the posteromedial papillary muscle, so subvalvular MR can occur.[5]

Effects of Aortic Valve Replacement. Aortic valve replacement (or commisurotomy in younger patients) removes the afterload on the hypertrophied left ventricle, so that now the same SV can be ejected with a much smaller LV systolic pressure. Thus, LVEDP decreases, and cardiac index increases if it was depressed preoperatively.[101] The lower LVEDP allows a fall in pulmonary capillary pressure. The ratio of myocardial oxygen supply to demand increases because of the fall in systolic and diastolic LV wall tension and the slight increase in diastolic coronary perfusion pressure.

The average aortic valve prosthesis area is 1.3–2.0 cm².[68] The systolic pressure gradient across the aortic valve is not entirely eliminated by aortic valve replacement (AVR), as the aortic valve prostheses have a residual gradient that ranges from about 7 to 19 mm Hg.[68] There may be a mild decrease in LV contractility immediately after AVR, possibly owing to myocardial effects of cardiopulmonary bypass, and this may persist at least for the first 4 postoperative days.[97] However, even the failing left ventricle in pure aortic stenosis will improve remarkably in its function postoperatively because of the reduction in afterload, which is now determined by the impedance of the arterial system.

Patients with combined aortic stenosis and coronary atherosclerotic heart disease may have higher operative mortality than patients with stenosis alone (mortality as high as 10 to 14 percent in the former group in reported studies, whether aortocoronary bypass surgery is done or not,[50,51] although recent experience at Emory University Hospital has shown much lower mortality). Patients with aortic stenosis and massive hypertrophy have been shown to have a higher surgical mortality.[102]

ANESTHETIC CONSIDERATIONS

1. Premedication should probably be light in patients with severe aortic stenosis with LV failure, since venodilation could lower LVEDV enough to cause a significant decrease in LVSP and SV, especially if the patient's blood volume is low secondary to diuretic therapy and preoperative fasting. Also, the hypoxemia often occurring after heavy premedication could reduce O_2 delivery to the myocardium and cause angina.

2. If angina occurs in a patient with aortic stenosis before induction of anesthesia, supplemental O_2 therapy should be the first consideration. Nitroglycerin is less consistently effective in relieving subendocardial ischemia in these patients than in patients with pure coronary atherosclerotic heart disease[109] and can even be potentially harmful owing to its reduction of aortic diastolic pressure.[109] If angina occurs and there is evidence of high LVEDP (such as rales on chest exam), then nitroglycerin may be more likely to help than if the angina occurs in association with sinus tachycardia or supraventricular arrhythmia.

3. Monitoring lateral precordial ECG leads such as V_5 during anesthesia in patients with aortic stenosis can help detect the onset of subendocardial ischemia. Although a pulmonary artery catheter can add information about LV preload in these patients, its insertion can pose significant hazards. Patients with aortic stenosis are prone to ventricular arrhythmias,[101] and the onset of ventricular tachycardia during insertion of a pulmonary artery catheter in a patient with critical aortic stenosis could be a catastrophic event, possibly leading to a vicious cycle of ischemia and LV dysfunction.

Since patients with pure aortic stenosis generally do quite well after aortic valve surgery, a LAP catheter can suffice for after-bypass monitoring in most cases. For these reasons, the decision for PA catheterization should not be made lightly.

4. If PCWP is monitored, or when LAP is monitored after bypass, it should be remembered that because of the increased diastolic LV stiffness, in sinus rhythm the mean LAP underestimates the LVEDP by about 1–7 mm Hg, depending on the stiffness of the left ventricle.[20] The true LVEDP can in fact be better estimated by the height of the "a" wave in the LAP or PCWP tracing. If the atrial "kick" is lost, however, the mean LAP will be equal to or higher than the LVEDP, especially during junctional rhythm or ventricular pacing when giant "a" waves may result from atrial contraction against a closed mitral valve and raise the mean LAP misleadingly. After AVR the LV diastolic stiffness is probably unchanged,[91] so that a relatively high LVEDP may still be needed for optimal LV filling.

5. Morphine sulfate (0.5–1.0 mg/kg) has been found to be well tolerated in patients with aortic stenosis, especially those in whom resting SVR is increased. In these patients, morphine leads to reductions in SVR and PAP and increases in SV and cardiac output.[43] In contrast, a volatile anesthetic such as halothane or enflurane would seem a poor choice for the patient with severe stenosis. These drugs not only severely depress contractility with resultant decrease in LVSP and SV[98] but also depress sinoatrial node automaticity, in many cases causing a junctional rhythm to emerge with loss of the atrial "kick."

6. In patients with severe aortic stenosis the preservation of sinus rhythm is of utmost importance, since the left ventricle is vitally dependent on a properly timed atrial systole to achieve an adequate LVEDV. Although arrhythmias are common during endotracheal intubation, normal sinus rhythm is in most jeopardy during insertion of the right atrial cannula(e) before bypass. It is advisable to correct conditions such as hypokalemia that may predispose to arrhythmias (especially in patients taking digitalis) as soon as possible. If a supraventricular tachycardia does occur, it should be treated aggressively, usually by direct-current cardioversion, even if bypass is about to begin.

7. Even sinus tachycardia may not be well tolerated by patients with aortic stenosis for long periods because of the increase in myocardial O_2 consumption and decrease in the time available for diastolic subendocardial flow.[70,102,108] If sinus tachycardia is severe and persistent, and especially if it is associated with ST depression in lead V_5 of the ECG (or angina if the patient is awake), it may be treated gingerly with small (starting with 0.25 mg) intravenous doses of propranolol. Overdose of propranolol can be equally devastating, since these patients may be somewhat dependent on endogenous β stimulation to maintain SV, especially in the face of the increase in SVR that occurs after surgical stimulation begins.[75] Severe bradycardia is also harmful in that SV may be relatively fixed by the "ceiling" on LVSP, so that cardiac output will fall if heart rate decreases. Persistence of heart rates of less than 45 should probably be treated at first with atropine, unless the surgical incision is just about to be made.

8. Because patients with severe aortic stenosis may already be generating their maximum possible LVSP, acute increases in arterial impedance associated with surgical stimulation during morphine/N_2O anesthesia[75] may decrease the gradient for flow across the aortic valve, resulting in a fall in SV. Volatile anesthetic agents can attenuate this sympathetic response,[110] but they can also depress the ability of the left ventricle to deal with it. If *marked* hemodynamic deterioration ensues in association with surgical stimulation, a *cautious* trial of vasodilator therapy, using sodium nitroprusside or phentolamine, may be begun.

Aortic Regurgitation

In contrast to aortic stenosis, aortic regurgitation may be either acute, usually secondary to infective endocarditis, trauma, or aortic aneurysm; or chronic, resulting from rheumatic disease, hypertension, syphilis, or less common causes.[26,28]

PATHOPHYSIOLOGY

Left Ventricular Systolic Volume Overloading. The basic hemodynamic problem in AR is a decrease in effective (net forward) SV because of diastolic regurgitation of part of the total SV from the aorta back into the left ventricle. The amount of regurgitation can vary from a short, insignificant "whiff" in early-diastole, to 75 to 80 percent of the total SV [a regurgitant fraction (RF) of 0.75–0.80].[25,26] The determinants of the regurgitant volume are as follows:

1. The valve area for regurgitation, usually less than the calculated AVA for forward flow.[22]
2. The mean diastolic pressure gradient from aorta to LV which depends on a variety of factors including diastolic arterial blood volume, distensibility of the large arteries, LVESV, and diastolic stiffness of the LV (see Fig. 6–3)[10,22]; and
3. The duration of diastole, which is related inversely to heart rate.[22,111]

Thus the amount of regurgitation will be increased by high SVR, low LV diastolic stiffness, and bradycardia and will be decreased by the opposite changes.

Calculation of the regurgitant fraction (see Equation 6–4) gives the best estimation of the severity of AR. Patients with a RF of less than 0.10 have trivial AR, with regurgitant flows less than 1 liter/min. Patients with a RF of 0.10–0.40 have mild AR, with regurgitant flows of about 1–3 liters/min. A RF of 0.40–0.60 usually indicates moderate AR, with total regurgitant flows of about 3–6 liters/min. Patients with a RF greater than 0.60 have severe AR, with regurgitant flows usually above 6 liters/min.[6,27,111]

The influence of the duration of diastole on the amount of regurgitant flow is revealed by studies in which patients with moderate-to-severe AR underwent right atrial pacing to increase heart rate from a mean of 70 to 100 beats per minute.[111] This resulted in a fall in RF from 0.59 to 0.51 and no significant change in forward SV, so that cardiac output increased 40 percent with a fall in LVEDV and LVEDP.[111] On the other hand, bradycardia can lead to a longer duration of diastole, more regurgitation per beat, and a higher LVEDV and LVEDP. This is consistent with the clinical observation that patients with AR often tolerate exercise well but may develop symptoms of pulmonary congestion at rest.[111] Thus, LVEDP in patients with AR is affected by LV diastolic stiffness and systolic function (which determines the LVESV), as well as by the severity of the regurgitation.[42,111]

There is a mild decrease in impedance to LV ejection in aortic regurgitation because the lowered aortic diastolic pressure and volume allow LV ejection to begin at a lower LV systolic pressure[83] (shortened isovolumic contraction phase). However, because the aorta offers greater impedance to LV ejection than does the left atrium, left ventricular wall tension is not reduced as much in AR as it is in MR.[29] As a result, the left ventricle in AR resorts to greater use of dilatation and hypertrophy as compensatory mechanisms for the drop in forward SV.[8,27] Thus, myocardial O_2 consumption increases in AR. This factor, along with the decrease in aortic diastolic pressure, can cause subendocardial ischemia and angina even in patients with normal coronary arteries,[26] although this occurs less commonly than in aortic stenosis,[28,111] and only in severe aortic regurgitation.[25] In contrast to the usual relationship, tachycardia in AR can actually improve subendocardial flow, as the increase in aortic diastolic pressure can outweigh the decrease in duration of diastole.[108] In fact, when patients with AR underwent atrial pacing to heart rates of 120 to 140 beats per minute, none exhibited myocardial ischemia as estimated by myocardial lactate extraction measurements, whereas 50 percent of aortic stenosis patients did show evidence of ischemia with atrial pacing.[102]

Acute Aortic Regurgitation. In acute AR, a systolic volume overload is imposed on an unprepared left ventricle.[30] Immediate compensation for the decrease in net forward SV is provided by acute dilatation, with increase in preload (LVEDV), and sympathetic nervous system stimulation, with resulting tachycardia and positive inotropic effects.[8] Since there is now a significant amount of *regurgitant* volume per beat, the *total* SV increases in an effort to minimize the fall in *forward* SV. The LV accomplishes this increase in total SV, *not* by more complete emptying from the same LVEDV (which would increase the EF), but by increasing LVEDV with the EF essentially unchanged.[30,112] In addition, the SVR may increase in acute AR via baroreceptor reflexes,[112] which tends to uphold aortic diastolic pressure.

A left ventricular pressure-volume loop from a typical patient with acute AR is shown in Figure 6-13. The RF of 0.60 indicates that this is severe AR, with 60 percent of every total SV regurgitated back from the aorta to the left ventricle. To maintain the net forward SV in the low-normal range, the LVEDV and total SV are increased, with a normal EF, and cardiac output is maintained by tachycardia. The isovolumic contraction phase (phase 2 in Fig. 6-2) is much shorter than normal because of both the elevation in LVEDP and the decrease in aortic diastolic pressure.[6] The isovolumic relaxation phase (phase 4 in Fig. 6-2) is nonexistent because the regurgitant flow begins to fill the left ventricle as soon as the active state of contraction is over.[6] The left ventricle is on a very steep part of its compliance curve (phase 1 in Fig. 6-2), so that the LV diastolic pressure increases greatly for each small change in volume. The area of the loop is increased, reflecting the greater net work per stroke that the left ventricle can do because of its dilatation and sympathetic inotropic support.

If acute AR is very severe, many patients will have equalization of LV pressure and aortic pressure in the latter part of diastole ("diastasis").[30] If this occurs the mitral valve will close prematurely, well before the onset of LV contraction. LV filling from the left atrium can then occur only during a limited part of diastole, and forward flow is severely reduced. Early mitral valve closure in severe AR can be diagnosed by echocardiography.[21,30]

Chronic Aortic Regurgitation. With time and worsened severity of AR, both LVEDV and total SV tend to increase further in direct proportion to the magnitude of the regurgitant volume, at least until LV failure occurs.[6] This use of the Frank-Starling relationship (LV dilatation) to increase total SV is one of the major compensatory mechanisms in chronic AR.[8] The dilated left ventricle in chronic AR also enjoys a geometric mechanical advantage, as was the case in MR, the more spherical shape allowing a greater SV with relatively less circumferential fiber shortening.[7,102] The increase in LV wall *tension* that occurs when the left ventricle dilates is a potent stimulus for eccentric hypertro-

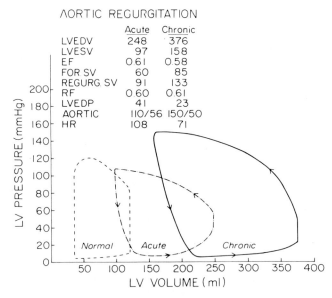

Fig. 6–13. Left ventricular pressure-volume loops for typical patients with acute and chronic pure aortic regurgitation, with a loop for a normal left ventricle shown for comparison. HR = heart rate. Otherwise abbreviations same as in previous figures and as explained in text. Values shown represent averages of data from references 6, 30, 111, 113, and 115. Note that volumes are in milliliters, *not* in milliliters per square meter of body surface area.

phy. As in MR, hypertrophy in chronic AR tends to keep the LV wall *stress* (tension per unit of wall thickness) relatively normal,[102] so that the amount of hypertrophy is proportional to the amount of dilatation.[7] The LV mass is higher in pure aortic regurgitation and in combined aortic stenosis and aortic regurgitation than it is in pure aortic stenosis,[6] and this contributes to the increase in myocardial oxygen consumption seen in chronic AR. However, coronary blood flow and LV oxygen consumption both increase in proportion to the amount of hypertrophy in chronic AR (as in aortic stenosis), so that the blood flow and O_2 consumption per gram of LV myocardium remain normal.[102]

Figure 6–13 shows the LV pressure-volume loop for a typical patient with chronic AR. The LVEDV has been increased greatly by further LV dilatation, and the left ventricle can now eject a much larger total SV with an unchanged EF, so that despite the severe regurgitation (RF = 0.61), the forward SV is now normal, and cardiac output can be maintained at a lower heart rate. The extra dilatation and hypertrophy allow the left ventricle to greatly increase its net external work (area of the loop is about four times normal), generating higher peak LV pressure. The diastolic stiffness of this greatly enlarged left ventricle is less than in acute AR, allowing LVEDP to be slightly lower despite the increase in LVEDV.[14,25,26] As in acute AR, the isovolumic contraction phase is shortened, and the isovolumic relaxation phase is eliminated.[6]

The mean LVEDV in chronic AR is 197 ml/m², with the EF in the low-normal range (average 0.55).[6]

Left Ventricular Contractility. Patients with mild, moderate, or even severe AR can remain virtually asymptomatic, except for mild dyspnea, for many years, unless there is a co-existing primary myocardial disease. Despite dilatation and hypertrophy, LVEDP and therefore LAP and PCWP remain essentially normal.[25,26] Eventually, however, LV contractility per unit of muscle mass begins to decrease in patients with severe AR,[8] so that the left ventricle must dilate further to keep the total SV from falling. Thus the LVEDV and LVEDP increase without an increase in total SV (EF falls). Because of the effect of tachycardia in AR, some patients at this stage may be more symptomatic at rest than during exercise.[111] Finally, contrac-

tility may decline to a critical point at which the total SV falls despite a further increase in LVEDV, with EF decreasing still further.[26] LVEDP, LAP, and PCWP rise, with resting dyspnea, and resting cardiac output falls. Compensatory sympathetic stimulation may now increase SVR and set into action a terminal vicious cycle of decreased net forward flow and further increase in impedance to LV ejection. Thus the usual course in chronic AR is one of years without symptoms, with rapid deterioration once LV failure sets in.[25,28]

Ejection fraction is maintained in the normal range in AR until LV failure develops.[6,26,42] A finding of an EF of less than 0.5 in the presence of a normal SVR indicates a severe degree of impairment of LV contractility. It has been suggested that patients with AR and normal resting ejection fractions who respond to angiotensin infusion with a significant fall in EF have a lesser degree of impairment of contractility.[42]

Role of the Peripheral Circulation. Many patients with chronic AR have a mild chronic peripheral vasodilation, which may help maintain LV forward stroke volume by reducing impedance to LV ejection and the diastolic pressure gradient for regurgitation.[25,26]

When SVR is increased by *methoxamine* in patients with isolated AR, there is a decrease in net forward SV, a fall in heart rate, no significant change in LVEDV, but great increases in LVEDP and mean LAP.[113] In contrast, *norepinephrine* infusion leads to great increases in PCWP but no decline in net forward SV, suggesting that its positive inotropic (β) effects allow the left ventricle to increase its total SV enough to keep net forward SV from falling even in the presence of increased afterload.[114] *Isoproterenol* infusion, by decreasing SVR and increasing contractility, causes an increase in net forward SV from a smaller LVEDV and LVEDP.[113]

When SVR is decreased by *sodium nitroprusside* in patients with acute or chronic severe AR, the response depends on the existing SVR and LV function. In patients with decreased forward SV and elevated resting LVEDP, sodium nitroprusside infusion leads to a reduction in RF, an increase in forward SV, a decrease in LVEDV and LVEDP, and no change in heart rate.[115,116] On the other hand, in patients with normal resting LVEDP, infusion of sodium nitroprusside will decrease it and cause a decrease or no change in forward SV and no consistent change in RF.[115] In all patients with AR, sodium nitroprusside causes a decrease in LV volumes that can reduce myocardial oxygen consumption and improve the supply-to-demand ratio of myocardial O_2[115] unless aortic diastolic pressure drops too far.

Thus, vasodilators are not as uniformly beneficial in AR as they are in MR.[115] The patients with AR most likely to benefit from vasodilator therapy are those with reduced forward cardiac output, decreased EF, increased LVEDP, and elevated SVR.[115] Patients with acute severe AR are likely to improve with afterload reduction, since they usually meet most of these criteria even though EF is normal. Isosorbide dinitrate has been shown to produce hemodynamic improvement in this setting.[9] In patients with acute AR secondary to endocarditis, vasodilator therapy may allow aortic valve replacement to be postponed until a full course of antibiotic therapy has been given.[9]

Role of the Left Atrium. The presence of a properly timed atrial contraction appears to be less crucial in assuring adequate LV filling in AR than it is in aortic or mitral stenosis. In chronic AR, left ventricular diastolic stiffness is only minimally increased,[14] so that a significant LA-to-LV pressure gradient may be present in early- and mid-diastole, allowing effective *passive* LV filling. In acute AR the acutely dilated left ventricle is less compliant during diastole, potentially increasing the importance of the atrial "kick." If diastasis (equalization of LV and aortic diastolic pressures) occurs with premature closure of the mitral valve, however, the period of passive filling will be shortened, and the left atrium may contract against a closed mitral valve. In this situation, sodium nitroprusside therapy will stop the premature mitral valve closure as a result of its effect in decreasing regurgitant flow.[116] In this way, sodium nitroprusside can aid forward filling of the left ventricle by allowing the left atrium to contract while the mitral valve is open.

Early closure of the mitral valve in severe AR serves some useful purposes, however. It poses a barrier against regurgitation from the aorta to the left atrium and thus protects the pulmonary capillary bed from the high LV pressures late in diastole. It also allows the left ventricle to achieve a greater LVEDV from a given amount of regurgitant flow, thereby increasing its preload as an aid in ejecting the necessary large total SV.[26,112,117]

When the mitral valve is regurgitant in a patient with AR, the high LV diastolic pressures are transmitted directly back to the pulmonary capillaries and LV preload drops. Thus, when MR is superimposed on AR, forward SV has been found to fall further, along with a fall in LVEDP and a large increase in LAP.[112] The usual causes of this combination are (1) AR with ruptured chordae tendineae, (2) rheumatic disease of both valves, and (3) AR with functional MR secondary to LV dilatation.[5,117] In the last case, replacement of the aortic valve alone is usually sufficient.[117]

Effects of Aortic Valve Replacement. Aortic valve replacement stops regurgitant flow through the valve, so that now the effective (net forward) SV is equal to the total SV ejected by the left ventricle. The left ventricle may now achieve a normal cardiac output with a vastly reduced SV, so that use of its Frank-Starling preload reserve decreases. The LV diastolic pressure-volume curve is unchanged, but the resting end-diastolic position of the left ventricle on the curve is shifted down postoperatively.[91] Often, this results acutely in a more marked decrease in LVEDP than in LVEDV.[91] With the fall in LV volumes, any preoperative functional MR is markedly diminished or abolished.[117] In addition, LV systolic tension drops, causing a decrease in myocardial O_2 consumption, and this change, along with an increase in aortic diastolic pressure,[91] causes an improvement in the ratio of myocardial O_2 supply to demand.

LV contractility may be slightly further depressed soon after AVR. One study in patients who had predominant AR preoperatively showed a decrease in EF and circumferential fiber shortening rate at 1 week after AVR, although LVEDV had decreased significantly by that time.[118] At 4 months after AVR the indices of contractility had returned to their preoperative values, and at 18 months, contractility was greater than preoperatively, despite further mild decrease in LVEDV and evidence of regression of eccentric hypertrophy.[118] Another study using systolic time intervals showed a decrease in LV contractility 4 hours postoperatively that persisted at least until the fourth postoperative day.[97] This early decline in LV function after AVR may, in part, result from myocardial effects of cardiopulmonary bypass, ischemic periods during valve replacement, or residual effects of cardioplegic drugs used during bypass.[97] The effect of this apparent early postoperative decrease in contractility can be exacerbated by the increase in impedance to LV ejection that occurs when the AR is abolished, especially in the first few hours after bypass when SVR is increased.[97] The effect of the mild (7–19 mm Hg) gradient across the aortic valve prosthesis is probably minimal.[68]

ANESTHETIC CONSIDERATIONS

1. Light premedication is preferable for patients with severe AR, as these patients usually tolerate tachycardia rather well[111] but are sometimes exquisitely sensitive to vasodilation.[70] Also, the hypoxemia associated with heavy premedication can be harmful to a left ventricle that is already marginal in terms of O_2 supply and demand.[110]

2. Monitoring a lateral precordial ECG lead (V_5) intraoperatively for signs of subendocardial ischemia is advisable. Use of pulmonary artery catheter for PAP and PCWP monitoring is very helpful in these patients, as this may allow measurement of left-sided pressures and cardiac output and calculation of SVR and PVR. This can be especially important in the early hours after AVR. It should be remembered that in patients with severe AR and diastasis with premature mitral valve closure, the PCWP may significantly underestimate the LVEDP.[30]

3. Bradycardia is poorly tolerated in patients with AR and should be prevented, if possible, with atropine and/or the use of vagolytic muscle relaxants such as pancuronium or gallamine. Should significant bradycardia occur, treatment with atropine or small doses of β-adrenergic agonists, or atrial pacing if the chest is open, is indicated.

4. Volatile anesthetic agents such as halothane or enflurane can be hazardous in AR because of their negative inotropic effects on ventricles whose contractility is already reduced. Nitrous oxide-narcotic anesthesia is

better tolerated, but the increase in SVR and PVR occurring after the onset of surgery with this technique can lead to an increase in PCWP and a decrease in forward cardiac output.[75] Sodium nitroprusside in small doses by intravenous infusion (10–90 μg/min) can reverse these effects, resulting in an increase in forward cardiac output and a decrease in PCWP by reducing SVR and PVR to preincision levels.[75] Patients with AR can be exquisitely sensitive to vasodilators, however, and the hemodynamic situation can deteriorate rapidly if aortic diastolic pressure drops enough to decrease coronary perfusion significantly.[70] After AVR, vasodilation may be important because of the increased impedance to LV ejection and is relatively safer because of the higher aortic diastolic pressure.

5. As in MR, it is difficult to predict the optimal LV filling pressure that will be needed after cardiopulmonary bypass. Patients having AVR for acute AR will likely have relatively normal LV contractility and diastolic properties and will need normal LVEDPs after the mechanical overload is corrected. In contrast, patients with chronic severe AR and reduced LV contractility may need somewhat higher filling pressures. The postbypass period is marked by complex changes in a number of variables, including residual effects of cardioplegic drugs, abnormal serum ionized calcium concentration, acid–base abnormalities, severe afterload changes, changes in blood viscosity, arrhythmias, transient conduction system abnormalities, and administration of multiple drugs with cardiovascular effects. For this reason, it is desirable to initially choose a level of LAP or PCWP that is likely to be above the "shoulder" of the steep part of the patient's ventricular function curve, say 15 mm Hg, and yet not be high enough to cause interstitial edema at the pulmonary capillary. With subsequent preload changes, one can determine the level of LAP below which blood pressure or cardiac output seem to fall rapidly, and the LAP can be kept a few millimeters of mercury above this level. It should be remembered that the optimal level of LAP or PCWP will have to be slightly higher if there is nonsinus rhythm

and can be relatively lower if normal sinus rhythm is present or if inotropic agents or vasodilators are being given.

Asymmetric Septal Hypertrophy

Idiopathic hypertrophic subaortic stenosis, once thought to be a rare disease causing symptoms similar to those of aortic stenosis, is now considered to represent one extreme of the disease spectrum of the disorder known as asymmetric septal hypertrophy (ASH).[119] ASH is defined as a type of cardiomyopathy in which every patient is found (usually by echocardiography) to have disproportionate hypertrophy of the intraventricular septum when compared to the thickness of the LV posterobasal free wall. The hypertrophied septum contains bizarrely shaped, disorganized myocardial cells with decreased efficiency of development of contractile force so that the contractility of involved areas of myocardium is decreased.[119]

ASH is a relatively common autosomal dominant inherited disorder with a wide variety of clinical and hemodynamic manifestations. Most patients are probably completely asymptomatic throughout their lives, but several de-

velop symptoms after variable periods of time. Basically, the disease spectrum seems to be determined by the distribution of abnormal myocardial tissue and response of the normal myocardium to it.[119] As illustrated in Figure 6–14, there are two main categories within the spectrum: nonobstructive ASH and obstructive ASH.

NONOBSTRUCTIVE ASYMMETRIC SEPTAL HYPERTROPHY

In nonobstructive asymmetric septal hypertrophy, a patient's symptoms depend on how much of the LV free wall is also involved by abnormal myocardial cells. If the LV free wall is largely normal, as shown on the left side of Figure 6–14, the patient is usually asymptomatic, often a relative of a patient with more severe disease, and ASH is diagnosed only by screening echocardiography. If, on the other hand, the LV free wall is involved with abnormal myocardial cells to a significant extent, as seen in the middle illustration in Figure 6–14, symptoms of dyspnea, chest pain, syncope, and fatigue are usually present. These patients have normal LV volumes but greatly increased LV diastolic stiffness, so that a high LVEDP is

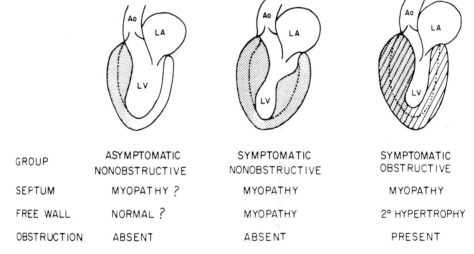

GROUP	ASYMPTOMATIC NONOBSTRUCTIVE	SYMPTOMATIC NONOBSTRUCTIVE	SYMPTOMATIC OBSTRUCTIVE
SEPTUM	MYOPATHY ?	MYOPATHY	MYOPATHY
FREE WALL	NORMAL ?	MYOPATHY	2° HYPERTROPHY
OBSTRUCTION	ABSENT	ABSENT	PRESENT

Fig. 6–14. The spectrum of asymmetric septal hypertrophy. Far left: representation of the LV of an asymptomatic patient with nonobstructive ASH. Middle: LV of a symptomatic patient with nonobstructive ASH. Far right: LV of a symptomatic patient with obstructive ASH. Heavily stippled areas show the distribution of abnormal myocardial cells. Parallel lines represent areas of secondary LV hypertrophy. (Reprinted from Epstein SE (moderator): Asymmetric septal hypertrophy. Ann Intern Med 81:650, 1974, with permission of author and publisher.)

needed for adequate LV filling, and the presence of an atrial "kick" is often of crucial importance. Motion of the mitral valve is normal.[119] The chest pain is usually ischemic in origin, even if the coronary arteries are normal, secondary to the abnormal myocardial hypertrophy.[119]

Anesthesia for patients with nonobstructive disease can be guided by the anesthesiologist's assessment of the severity of the disease. Adequate monitoring of the left-sided filling pressures may be necessary in severely symptomatic patients undergoing major procedures. Maintaining an adequate blood volume is important for LV filling, but these patients can be very sensitive to fluid overload. Arrhythmias can remove the atrial "kick" and result in decreased stroke volume. Tachycardia can cause myocardial ischemia, but ischemia occurring at normal heart rates may respond to nitroglycerin. Volatile agents such as halothane and enflurane have the disadvantages of further reducing myocardial contractility and suppressing the sinoatrial node with resultant junctional rhythm.

OBSTRUCTIVE ASYMMETRIC SEPTAL HYPERTROPHY

Of more unique interest is the obstructive disease, otherwise known as hypertrophic obstructive cardiomyopathy[120] or idiopathic hypertrophic subaortic stenosis (IHSS).[121] In this disease the septum is greatly hypertrophied with bizarrely shaped myocardial cells, but the LV free wall, although hypertrophied, contains no abnormal cells, as shown in the far-right illustration in Figure 6–14. The LV free wall in obstructive ASH hypertrophies in response to high intraventricular pressure, just as the entire LV myocardium does in valvular aortic stenosis.[119] The anterior leaflet of the mitral valve is also abnormal. It is positioned close to the septum and thickened, with an endocardial fibrotic plaque covering the surfaces of leaflet and septum that face each other.[5,119] During early systole, there is rapid ejection from the left ventricle into the aorta.[5,119,122] This rapid flow of blood past the anterior leaflet is thought to push (or pull by a Venturi effect) it away from its closed position to a position within the LV outflow tract, which it obstructs in mid- to late-systole.[5,119]

The symptoms of patients with obstructive ASH are secondary to their LV outflow tract obstruction, the increased diastolic stiffness of their hypertrophied myocardium, and the re-

sulting increase in myocardial oxygen consumption. Dyspnea occurs in about 75 percent of patients, syncope in 25 percent, and angina in about 50 percent.[123] Unfortunately, there is also a significant incidence of sudden death, the risk of which is not predictable by the severity of the patient's other symptoms or the severity of his outflow obstruction.[123] Sudden death in these patients may be related in part to the high incidence of conduction problems, usually left anterior fascicular block or left bundle branch block.[124] Symptoms have been noted to develop in association with the onset of LV outflow tract obstruction and are generally progressive,[123,125] although not inevitably so.[119] Left ventricular volumes in obstructive ASH tend to be normal[119,126] or slightly elevated,[120] but as in the nonobstructive form, LV diastolic stiffness is greatly increased,[119,120] so that LVEDP is elevated in about 70 percent of patients.[120] The left atrium is often dilated[119] and hypertrophic, generating large LA "a" waves in an effort to fill the noncompliant LV chamber.[120] Although the ejection fraction is normal in most patients,[120,126] those with severe obstruction may eventually develop resting LV failure, with LV dilation and evidence of reduced contractility (decreased EF and fiber shortening rate).[125] At this point LVEDP rises further, and pulmonary capillary and pulmonary artery pressures are elevated at rest.[124]

The unique feature of obstructive ASH is the dynamic nature of the systolic pressure gradient across the subvalvular part of the LV outflow tract. In *valvular aortic stenosis* the orifice area is constant throughout systole, so that the pattern of blood flow into the aorta is normal and a pressure gradient across the valve is present throughout ejection.[122] In *obstructive ASH*, on the other hand, the dimensions of the outflow tract are not fixed, varying with changes in LV volume during ejection.[121] Thus, there is a high flow rate in early systole; in fact, about 80 percent of the total SV is ejected during the first half of systole, compared to 55–60 percent in the normal person.[122] As outflow obstruction appears and worsens in mid- to late-systole, a pressure gradient from the left ventricle to the aorta arises, flow decreases, and the calculated outflow tract orifice gets progressively smaller.[122] The average peak gradient for patients with symptomatic IHSS is 85 mm Hg.[119]

Not all patients with symptomatic obstructive ASH have a resting pressure gradient. In other patients a gradient may be provoked by certain maneuvers. Even in patients with resting gradients the magnitude of the gradient can vary greatly from minute to minute, even within the same catheterization procedure.[121] The three main determinants of the severity of the outflow obstruction (and pressure gradient) are arterial pressure, LV volume, and LV ejection velocity.[119]

Interventions that tend to decrease arterial pressure or LV volume and increase LV ejection velocity will worsen a resting gradient or provoke a gradient in a patient in whom it was not present at rest.[119,122] Thus, *hypovolemia* or the *Valsalva maneuver* will lower venous return, LV volume, and arterial pressure, increasing LV ejection velocity by baroreceptor reflexes. The pressure gradient increases. *Digitalis, calcium chloride,* and *isoproterenol* increase the gradient by increasing LV contractility, although isoproterenol also reduces arterial pressure. Vasodilators, such as *nitroglycerin* and *amyl nitrite,* increase the gradient by reducing arterial pressure and LV volume and may increase LV ejection velocity reflexively. When nitroglycerin is given to a patient with IHSS, not only does arterial pressure decrease, but LV systolic pressure actually increases.[119]

Interventions that tend to increase arterial pressure and LV volume and decrease LV ejection velocity will lessen or abolish the LV-to-aorta pressure gradient.[119,122] Expanding the *blood volume* will reduce the gradient. Vasoconstrictors, such as *phenylephrine* and *methoxamine,* will increase arterial pressure and LV volume, reduce the gradient, and actually decrease LV systolic pressure. *Propranolol* will decrease LV ejection velocity if sympathetic tone is high, such as during exercise or anxiety, thereby reducing the gradient.[127] This is the basis for long-term medical therapy of symptomatic patients with propranolol, which in most patients results in symptomatic improvement.[127,128] Propranolol probably does not influence the progression of the disease, however, and many patients become refractory to it.[127]

Patients with severe symptoms that do not respond to propranolol are candidates for ventriculomyotomy and myomectomy, in which a vertical trough about 10–12 mm in depth is cut into the most prominent part of the septal bulge.[119,124] This results in a great reduction in or elimination of the pressure gradient, reduction in LVEDP and pulmonary vascular changes, and symptomatic improvement.[124] Because of the location of the atrioventricular conduction system near the area of dissection, however, there is an extremely high incidence of conduction problems (mainly left bundle branch block) postoperatively.[124]

Mitral regurgitation occurs quite commonly in obstructive ASH as a result of abnormal systolic motion of the thickened anterior mitral leaflet.[5,119,124] Its severity does not seem to be related to the magnitude of the pressure gradient or LV systolic pressure, but it occurs in late-systole after the development of the gradient.[129] Pharmacologic interventions affect the MR in IHSS in opposite ways from isolated MR. For example, vasodilators worsen the MR in IHSS, and vasoconstrictors lessen it.[129] Ventriculomyotomy will abolish this secondary MR or reduce it to trivial levels in most cases.[124,129]

Anesthetic management of these patients is based on efforts to reduce the outflow tract gradient or minimize its increase during surgery. A pulmonary artery catheter is important, as the PCWP may give the only information obtainable about LV volume. LV preload must be kept from falling or even be maintained at a slightly elevated level, as this has been shown to reduce the outflow tract gradient.[124] High mean airway pressure should probably be avoided if possible, as this can reduce venous return and therefore LV volume. Because of the diastolic stiffness of the hypertrophied LV, the maintenance of a properly timed presystolic atrial contraction is important, and arrhythmias are poorly tolerated. Even sinus tachycardia can be a problem, since LV volume falls as a result of the reduced diastolic filling period, LV ejection velocity increases, and subendocardial ischemia may be detectable in the lateral precordial ECG leads. Intravenous propranolol in 0.25–0.50 mg boluses or halothane is logical treatment for this situation.

Since blood pressure is related to both cardiac output and arterial impedance (see Fig. 6-3), patients with *valvular* disease can have a normal or even high cardiac output in association with a slightly low arterial pressure if vascular resistance is low. Indeed, afterload reduction with vasodilators can markedly improve forward flow, especially in patients with MR and in many with AR. The situation is more complicated in IHSS, where vasodilators are harmful.[119,122] Although cardiac output should be measured whenever possible, if intraoperative hypotension develops, the output is probably low and the outflow-tract gradient high. The first thought for therapy should be to increase intravascular volume, and the second thought should be the administration of vasoconstrictors such as phenylephrine.

Halothane is a good choice for an anesthetic agent in patients with obstructive ASH because it depresses myocardial contractility and has been shown to decrease the outflow-tract gradient.[121,124] Thus, in these patients, the decrease in contractility may not lead to a reduction in cardiac output. Enflurane and isoflurane may be slightly less preferred because of their greater vasodilatory effects.[98] When using any of these drugs the ECG should be watched closely for the onset of junctional rhythm, and the drug concentration should be quickly reduced if this occurs. In patients on propranolol therapy, a nitrous oxide and narcotic technique can be equally well tolerated, since the sympathetic stimulation during surgery will have predominately α-adrenergic effects, which are beneficial in these patients.[75]

Tricuspid Regurgitation

Tricuspid regurgitation (TR) may occur either in isolated form or in association with other valvular lesions, including tricuspid stenosis. Until recently, isolated pure TR was a rare disease caused by chest trauma, right-sided endocarditis, the carcinoid syndrome, and congenital abnormalities such as Ebstein's anomaly.[130] This has become more common with the rising incidence of tricuspid endocarditis secondary to intravenous drug abuse.[131] Far more commonly, however, TR occurs in association with or as a hemodynamic consequence of diseases of the mitral and aortic valves.[1,26,132]

ISOLATED TRICUSPID
REGURGITATION

Since the architectural design of the right ventricle is appropriate for the ejection of large volumes of blood with minimal amounts of fiber shortening, the RV volume overload imposed by isolated pure TR is remarkably well tolerated.[130] The high compliance of the right atrium and

venae cavae cause minimal increase in right atrial pressure, even in the face of large regurgitant volumes,[26] and the right ventricle increases its total SV by dilatation so that forward SV remains the same. Even total removal of the tricuspid valve, as in addicts with pseudomonas endocarditis, can in fact be tolerated in most patients for years, the only hemodynamic change being an increase in mean RAP. With total valvulectomy, however, some patients do develop RV failure with increased RVEDP and decreased cardiac output.[131]

Venous return is inversely proportional to the RAP. Thus the forward flow in the venae cavae normally reaches its peak in early systole as a result of the descent of the tricuspid valve toward the apex of the heart, and during early diastole as a result of rapid RV filling from the right atrium. In TR, systolic flow in the venae-cavae is backward, and all forward flow is in diastole.[130] Hepatic pulsations and jugular venous v waves are sometimes detectable in severe TR.[1,132] During a normal inspiration the more negative intrapleural pressure causes RAP to fall in relation to systemic venous pressure, resulting in a transient increase in venous return, better RV filling, and increased regurgitant volume. Thus the murmur of TR can increase during inspiration.[1]

Although a pure RV volume overload secondary to TR is relatively benign, the addition of a RV *pressure* overload changes the picture greatly.[130] In patients with TR, increased impedance to forward RV ejection, as in LV failure or high pulmonary vascular resistance, will often lead to RV failure.[26] This causes increased regurgitant volume through the tricuspid valve, decreased forward flow, LV underloading, and low cardiac output. There is some evidence that the combination of RV pressure and volume overloading can also affect the LV filling by, in effect, increasing LV diastolic stiffness.[49] In some cases, the combination of RV failure and LV underloading can cause RAP to be significantly higher than LAP, with right-to-left shunting through a patent foramen ovale.[26]

TRICUSPID REGURGITATION
COMBINED WITH OTHER
LESIONS

In some cases of multiple valve disease, TR occurs as a result of the rheumatic process; in this case, tricuspid stenosis is also almost invariably present.[1] More commonly, TR occurs late in mitral or aortic disease as a consequence of LV failure, pulmonary hypertension, and RV pressure overloading. Since the RV is structurally unsuited to deal with a sudden or prolonged pressure load,[130] RV failure often occurs with dilatation, abnormal tension on the tricuspid chordae tendineae, and functional TR.[133] As noted earlier, when this occurs, cardiac output falls significantly, but symptoms of pulmonary congestion are often reduced.[26] The severity of TR in this setting has been found to be proportional to the pulmonary vascular resistance, PAP, and RVEDP.[132]

Purely functional TR is usually greatly reduced after correction of the left-sided valvular lesion and subsequent reduction in PAP and RV volume.[69] Since the in-hospital mortality increases for multiple valve surgery,[133] it is important to try to ascertain whether the TR in a patient with mitral or aortic disease is purely functional or the result of anatomic disease of the tricuspid valve. Demonstration of significant tricuspid stenosis is an accepted sign that the valve will need repair or replacement at operation.[69,132] This can be difficult, however, even during right-heart catheterization, since diastolic gradients across the tricuspid valve may be small and occur only during part of diastole.[1,60] If PAP is only modestly increased but there are signs of severe TR, then surgical correction of the TR is more likely to be necessary.[1] Often a decision cannot be made until the tricuspid valve is examined at surgery.[69,133]

Anesthetic considerations will be similar whether the patient's TR is isolated or associated with left-sided valvular lesions; in the latter case, however, considerations for management of the mitral or aortic lesion should take precedence. High mean airway pressures secondary to positive-pressure ventilation will decrease venous return, as could excessive venodilation. Blood volume and CVP may have to be kept high in order to assure adequate RV forward output for LV filling. Events or therapies known to increase pulmonary vascular resistance should be avoided, such as hypoxemia, hypercarbia, acidosis, and α-adrenergic agonists. Nitrous oxide is a weak pulmonary vasoconstrictor and could increase the TR,[48] as could the α effect of sympathetic stimulation during surgery under morphine/N_2O anesthesia.[75] In the latter case, vasodilator therapy may improve RV for-

ward output by decreasing pulmonary vascular resistance. Halothane may be better tolerated because of its pulmonary vasodilating effects.[74]

REFERENCES

1. Crawley SI, Morris DC, Silverman BD: Clinical recognition and medical management of rheumatic heart disease and other acquired valvular disease. B. Valvular heart disease. In Hurst JW (ed): The Heart (ed 4). New York, McGraw-Hill, 1978, pp 992–1080

2. Reichek N, Shelburne JC, Perloff JK: Clinical aspects of rheumatic valvular disease. Prog Cardiovasc Dis 15:491, 1973

3. Hultgren HN, Hancock EW, Cohn EK: Auscultation in mitral and tricuspid valvular disease. Prog Cardovasc Dis 10:298, 1968

4. Perloff JK: Clinical recognition of aortic stenosis. Prog Cardiovasc Dis 10:323, 1968

5. Roberts WC, Perloff JK: Mitral valvular disease. Ann Intern Med 77:939, 1972

6. Dodge HT, Kennedy JW, Petersen JL: Quantitative angiocardiographic methods in the evaluation of valvular heart disease. In Sonnenblick E, Lesh M (eds): Valvular Heart Disease. New York, Grune & Stratton, 1974, pp 85–107.

7. Rackley CE, Hood WP: Quantitative angiographic evaluation and pathophysiologic mechanisms in valvular heart disease. Prog Cardiovasc Dis 15:427, 1973

8. Mason DT: Regulation of cardiac performance in clinical heart disease. In Mason DT: Congestive Heart Failure. New York, Yorke Medical Books, 1976, pp 111–128.

9. Chatterjee K, Parmley WW: The role of vasodilator therapy in heart failure. Prog Cardiovasc Dis 19:301, 1977

10. Cohn JN: Blood pressure and cardiac performance. Am J Med 55:351, 1973

11. Bolen JL, Lopes MG, Harrison DC, et al: Analysis of left ventricular function in response to afterload changes in patients with mitral stenosis. Circulation 52:894, 1975

12. Curry GC, Elliott LP, Ramsey HW: Quantitative left ventricular angiographic findings in mitral stenosis. Ao J Cardiol 29:621, 1972

13. Heller SJ, Carleton RA: Abnormal left ventricular contraction in patients with mitral stenosis. Circulation 42:1099, 1970

14. Grossman W, McLaurin LP: Diastolic properties of the left ventricle. Ann Intern Med 84:316, 1976

15. Stott DK, Marpole D, Bristow JD: The role of atrial transport in aortic and mitral stenosis. Circulation 41:1031, 1970

16. Sarnoff SJ, Brockman SK, Gilmore JP, et al: Regulation of ventricular contraction: Influence of cardiac sympathetic and vagal nerve stimulation on atrial and ventricular dynamics. Circ Res 8:1108, 1960

17. Jochim K: The contribution of the auricles to ventricular filling in complete heart block. Am J Physiol 122:639, 1938

18. Mitchell JH, Gilmore JP, Sarnoff SJ: The transport function of the atrium. Am J Cardiol 9:237, 1962

19. Braunwald E, Frahm CJ: Studies on Starling's law of the heart. IV. Observation on the hemodynamic function of the left atrium in man. Circulation 24:633, 1961

20. Lee SJK: Hemodynamic changes at rest and during exercise in patients with aortic stenosis of varying severity. Am Heart J 79:318, 1970

21. Parisi AF, Tow DE, Felix WR, et al: Non-invasive cardiac diagnosis. N Engl J Med 296:316, 1977

22. Gorlin R, McMillan IKR, Medd WE, et al: Dynamics of the circulation in aortic valvular diseases. Am J Med 18:855, 1955

23. Gorlin R, Gorlin SG: Hydraulic formula for calculation of the area of the stenotic mitral valve, other cardiac valves and central circulatory shunt. Am Heart J 41:1, 1951

24. Mason DT, Miller RR, Berman DS, et al: Cardiac catheterization in the clinical assessment of heart disease and ventricular performance. In Mason DT: Congestive Heart Failure. New York, Yorke Medical Books, 1976, pp 225–271

25. Rapaport E: Natural history of aortic and mitral valve disease. Am J Cardiol 35:221, 1975

26. Schlant RC, Nutter DO: Heart failure in valvular heart disease. Medicine 50:421, 1971

27. Tyrell MG, Ellison RC, Hugenholtz PC, et al: Correlation of degree of left ventricular volume overload with clinical course in aortic and mitral regurgitation. Br Heart J 32:683, 1970

28. Goldschlager N, Pfeifer J, Cohn K, et al: The natural history of aortic regurgitation. Am J Med 54:577, 1973

29. Braunwald E: Mitral regurgitation. N Engl J Med 281:425, 1969

30. Mann T, McLaurin L, Grossman W, et al: Assessing the hemodynamic severity of acute aortic regurgitation due to infective endocarditis. N Engl J Med 293:108, 1975

31. Braunwald E, Arve WC: Syndrome of severe mitral regurgitation with normal left atrial pressure. Circulation 27:29, 1963

32. Scheuer J: Ventricular dysfunction associated with valvular heart disease. Am J Cardiol 30:445, 1972

33. Ross J, Braunwald E: The study of left ventricular function in man by increasing resistance to ventricular ejection with angiotensin. Circulation 29:739, 1964

34. Harshaw CW, Grossman W, Munro AB, et al: Reduced systemic vascular resistance as therapy for severe mitral regurgitation therapy for severe mitral regurgitation of valvular origin. Ann Intern Med 83:312, 1975

35. Miller RR, Awan NA, Maxwell KS, et al: Sustained reduction of cardiac impedance and preload in congestive heart failure with the antihypertensive vasodilator prazosin. N Engl J Med 297:303, 1977

36. Miller GAH, Kirklin JW, Swan HJC: Myocardial function and left ventricular volumes in acquired valvular insufficiency. Circulation 31:374, 1965

37. Liedtke AJ: Determinants of cardiac performance in severe aortic stenosis. Chest 69:192, 1976

38. Braunwald E, Ross J: Editorial: Ventricular end-diastolic pressure: Appraisal of its value in the recognition of ventricular failure in man. Am J Med 34:147, 1963

39. Weissler AM: Systolic time intervals. N Engl J Med 296:321, 1977

40. DeMarie AN, Neumann AL, Mason DT: Echographic evaluation of cardiac function. In Mason DT: Congestive Heart Failure. New York, Yorke Medical Books, 1976, pp 191–224

41. Eckberg DL, Gault JH, Bouchard RL, et al: Mechanics of left ventricular contraction in severe mitral regurgitation. Circulation 47:1252, 1973

42. Bolen JL, Holloway EL, Zener JC, et al: Evaluation of left ventricular function in patients with aortic regurgitation using afterload stress. Circulation 53:132, 1976

43. Lowenstein E: Cardiovascular responses to large doses of intravenous morphine in man. N Engl J Med 281:1389, 1969

44. Hutchins GM, Ostrow PT: The pathogenesis of the two forms of hypertensive pulmonary vascular disease. Am Heart J 92:797, 1976

45. McCredie RM: Measurement of pulmonary edema in valvular heart disease. Circulation 36:381, 1967

46. Laver MB, Hallowell P, Goldblatt A: Pulmonary dysfunction secondary to heart disease: Aspects relevant to anesthesia and surgery. Anesthesiology 33:161, 1970

47. Lappas DG: Pulmonary circulation in patients with cardiac disease. Lecture at McGill University Annual Review Course in Anaesthesia, May 26, 1977

48. Lappas DG: Left ventricular performance and pulmonary circulation following addition of nitrous oxide to morphine during coronary artery surgery. Anesthesiology 43:61, 1975

49. Kelly DT, Spotnitz HM, Beiser GD, et al: Effects of chronic right ventricular volume and pressure loading on left ventricular performance. Circulation 44:403, 1971

50. Hancock EW: Aortic stenosis, angina pectoris, and coronary artery disease. Am Heart J 93:382, 1977

51. Berndt TB, Hancock EW, Shumway NE, et al: Aortic valve replacement with and without coronary artery bypass surgery. Circulation 50:967, 1974

52. Carman GH, Lange RL: Variant hemodynamic patterns in mitral stenosis. Circulation 24:712, 1961

53. Christensson B, Gustafson A, Westling H, et al: Hemodynamic effects of nitroglycerin in patients with mitral valvular disease. Br Heart J 30:822, 1968

54. Curry CL, Behar VS, McIntoch HD, et al: Atrial contraction in mitral stenosis. Circulation 40 (suppl III): III—64, 1969

55. Feigenbaum H, Campbell RW, Wunsch CM, et al: Evaluation of the left ventricle in patients with mitral stenosis. Circulation 34:462, 1966

56. Kasalicky J, Hurych J, Widimsky J, et al: Left heart hemodynamics at rest and during exercise in patients with mitral stenosis. Br Heart J 30:188, 1968

57. Ahmed SS, Regan TJ, Fiore JJ, et al: The state of the left ventricular myocardium in mitral stenosis. Am Heart J 94:28, 1977

58. Grant RP: Architectronics of the heart. Am Heart J 46:405, 1953

59. Beiser GD, Epstein SE, Stampfer M, et al: Studies on digitalis. XVII. Effects of ouabain on the hemodynamic response to exercise in patients with mitral stenosis in normal sinus rhythm. N Engl J Med 278:131, 1968

60. Sanders CA, Harthorne JW, Heitman H, et al: Effect of vasopressor administration on blood gas exchange in mitral disease. Clin Res 13:351, 1965

61. Meister SG, Engel TR, Feiton GS: Propranolol in mitral stenosis during sinus rhythm. Am Heart J 94:685, 1977

62. Arani DT, Carlton RA: The deleterious role of tachycardia in mitral stenosis. Circulation 36:511, 1967

63. Thompson ME, Shaver JA, Leon EF: Effect of tachycardia on atrial transport in mitral stenosis. Am Heart J 94:297, 1977

64. Heidenreich FP, Thompson ME, Shaver JA: Left atrial transport in mitral stenosis. Circulation 50:545, 1969

65. Rothbaum DA, Dillon JC, Feigenbaum H: Hemodynamic effects of nitroglycerin in patients with mitral stenosis, abstracted. Circulation 47 (suppl IV): IV–209, 1973

66. Dalen JE: Early reduction of pulmonary vascular resistance after mitral valve replacement. N Engl J Med 277:387, 1966

67. Braunwald E, Braunwald NS, Ross J, et al: Effects of mitral valve replacement on pulmonary vascular dynamics of patients with pulmonary hypertension. N Engl J Med 273:509, 1965

68. Lefrak E, Grunkemeier G, Lambert L, et al: Analysis of current heart valve prostheses. Presented at the annual meeting of the American Heart Association, November 1977

69. Braunwald NS, Ross J, Morrow AG: Conservative management of tricuspid regurgitation in patients undergoing mitral valve replacement. Circulation 35(suppl I):I—63, 1967

70. Thomas SJ: Acquired valvular disease and anesthesia. ASA Annual Refresher Course Lectures, #132, 1976

71. Savarese JJ, Hassan HA, Antonio RP: The clinical pharmacology of metocurine: Dimethyltubocurarine revisited. Anesthesiology 47:277, 1977

72. Sorensen MB, Jocobsen E: Pulmonary hemodynamics during induction of anesthesia. Anesthesiology 47:381, 1977

73. Stoelting RK: Circulatory changes during direct laryngoscopy and tracheal intubation. Anesthesiology 47:381, 1977

74. Stoelting RK, Reis RR, Longnecker DE: Hemodynamic responses to nitrous oxide-halothane and halothane in patients with vavular heart disease. Anesthesiology 37:430, 1972

75. Faltas AN, Hoar PF, Stone JG: Nitroprusside therapy for cardiac failure during valve replacement. Presented at the ASA Annual Meeting, New Orleans, October 18, 1977

76. Price HL: Myocardial depression by nitrous oxide and its reversal by calcium. Anesthesiology 44:211, 1976

77. Wilson RS, Sullivan SF, Malm JR, et al: The oxygen cost of breathing following anesthesia and cardiac surgery. Anesthesiology 39:387, 1973

78. Hand BR, Malm JR, Bowman FO, et al: The effects of anesthesia and cardiac bypass on pulmonary compliance in man. Bull NY Acad Med 46:23, 1970

79. Bedford RF, Wollman H: Postoperative respiratory effects of morphine and halothane anesthesia: A study in patients undergoing cardiac surgery. Anesthesiology 43:1, 1975

80. Stanley TH, Lathrop GD: Urinary excretion of morphine after valvular and coronary-artery surgery. Anesthesiology 46:166, 1977

81. Litwak RS, Silvay J, Gadboys HL, et al: Factors associated with operative risk in mitral valve replacement. Am J Cardiol 23:335, 1969

82. Cobbs BW: Personal communication
83. Urschel CW, Covell JW, Sonnenblick EH, et al: Myocardial mechanics in aortic and mitral valvular regurgitation: Concept of instantaneous impedance as determinant of performance of intact heart. J Clin Invest 47:867, 1968
84. Urschel CW, Covell JW, Graham TP, et al: Effects on acute valvular regurgitation on the oxygen consumption of the canine heart. Circ Res 23:33, 1968
85. Braunwald E, Welch GH, Sarnoff SJ: Hemodynamic effects of quantitatively varied experimental mitral regurgitation. Circ Res 5:539, 1957
86. Baxley WA: Hemodynamics in ruptured chordae tendineae and chronic rheumatic mitral regurgitation. Circulation 48:1288, 1973
87. Chatterjee K, Parmley WW, Swan HJC, et al: Beneficial effects of vasodilator agents in severe mitral regurgitation due to dysfunction of subvalvular apparatus. Circulation 48:684, 1973
88. Kennedy JW, Baxley WA, Dodge HT: Hemodynamics of ruptured chordae tendineae, abstracted. Circulation 34(suppl III):III—142, 1966
89. Brody W, Criley JM: Intermittent severe mitral regurgitation. N Engl J Med 283:673, 1970
90. Goodman DJ, Rossen RM, Holloway EL, et al: Effect of nitroprusside on left ventricular dynamics in mitral regurgitation. Circulation 50:1025, 1974
91. Gault JH, Covell JW, Braunwald E, et al: Left ventricular performance following correction of free aortic regurgitation. Circulation 42:773, 1970
92. Sandler H, Dodge HT, Hay RE, et al: Quantitation of valvular insufficiency in man by angiocardiography. Am Heart J 65:501, 1963
93. Jose AD, Taylor RR, Bernstein L: The influence of arterial pressure on mitral incompetence in man. J Clin Invest 43:2094, 1964
94. Buckley MJ, Mundth ED, Daggett WM, et al: Surgical therapy for early complications of myocardial infarction. Surgery 70:814, 1971
95. Cohen LS, Morrow AE, Braunwald NS, et al: Severe mitral regurgitation following acute myocardial infarction and ruptured papillary muscle: Hemodynamic findings and results of mitral valve replacement in four patients. Circulation 39(suppl II)II—87, 1967
96. Sniderman AD, Marpole DGF, Palmer WH, et al: Response of left ventricle to nitroglycerin in patients with and without mitral regurgitation. Br Heart J 36:357, 1974
97. Seabra-Gomes R, Sutton R, Parker DJ: Left ventricular function after aortic valve replacement. Br Heart J 38:491, 1976

98. Stevens WC: Anesthetic management. Anesth Analg 55:622, 1976
99. Stoelting RK, Gibbs PS: Hemodynamic effects of morphine and morphine-nitrous oxide in valvular heart disease and coronary artery disease. Anesthesiology 38:45, 1973
100. Brown DR, Starek P: Sodium nitroprusside-induced improvement in cardiac function in association with left ventricular dilatation. Anesthesiology 41:521, 1974
101. Morrow A: Obstruction to left ventricular outflow: Current concepts of management and operative treatment. Ann Intern Med 69:1255, 1968
102. Trenouth RS, Phelps NC, Neill WA: Determinants of left ventricular hypertrophy and oxygen supply in chronic aortic valve disease. Circulation 53:644, 1976
103. Simon H, Krayenbuehl HP, Rutishauser W, et al: The contractile state of the left ventricular myocardium in aortic stenosis. Am Heart J 79:587, 1970
104. Hamer J, Fleming J: Effect of propranolol on left ventricular work in aortic stenosis. Br Heart J 29:871, 1967
105. Hamer J, Fleming J: Action of propranolol on left ventricular contraction in aortic stenosis when a fall in heart rate is prevented by atropine. Br Heart J 31:670, 1969
106. Kroetz FW, Leonard JJ, Shaver JA, et al: The effect of atrial contraction on left ventricular performance in valvular aortic stenosis. Circulation 35:852, 1967
107. Perloff JK, Binnion P, Caulfield WH, et al: The use of angiotensin in the assessment of left ventricular function in fixed orifice aortic stenosis. Circulation 35:347, 1967
108. Vincent WR, Buckberg ED, Hoffman JIE: Left ventricular subendocardial ischemia in severe valvular and supravalvular aortic stenosis. A common mechanism. Circulation 49:326, 1974
109. Perloff JG, Ronan JA, deLeon AC: The effect of nitroglycerin on left ventricular wall tension in fixed orifice aortic stenosis. Circulation 32:204, 1965
110. Lowenstein E, Bland JHL: Anesthesia for cardiac surgery. In Norman JC: Cardiac Surgery. New York, Appleton-Century-Crofts, 1972, pp 75-102
111. Judge TP, Kennedy JW, Bennett LJ, et al: Quantitative hemodynamic effects of heart rate in aortic regurgitation. Circulation 44:355, 1971
112. Welch GH, Braunwald E, Sarnoff SJ: Hemodynamic effects of quantitatively varied experimental aortic regurgitation. Circ Res 5:546, 1957
113. Klosten FE, Bristow JD, Lewis RP, et al: Phar-

macodynamic studies in aortic regurgitation. Am J Cardiol 19:644, 1967

114. Regan TJ, Defazio V, Binak K, et al: Norepinephrine-induced pulmonary congestion in patients with aortic valve regurgitation. J Clin Invest 38:1564, 1959

115. Bolen JL, Alderman EL: Hemodynamic consequences of afterload reduction in patients with chronic aortic regurgitation. Circulation 53:879, 1976

116. Pepine CJ, Nichols WW, Curry RC, et al: Reversal of premature mitral valve closure by nitroprusside infusion in severe aortic insufficiency: Beat-to-beat pressure-flow and echocardiographic relationships. Am J Cardiol 37:161, 1976

117. Shine KI, DeSanctis RW, Sanders CA, et al: Combined aortic and mitral incompetence: Clinical features in surgical management. Am Heart J 76:728, 1968

118. Schuler G, Reghetti A, Hardarson T, et al: Serial studies on ventricular function following valve replacement for volume overload. Circulation 53, 54 (suppl II):II—104, 1976

119. Epstein SE (moderator): Asymmetric septal hypertrophy. Ann Intern Med 81:650, 1974

120. Goodwin JF: Congestive and hypertrophic cardiomyopathies. Lancet 1:731, 1970

121. Braunwald E: Idiopathic hypertrophic subaortic stenosis. I. A description of the disease based on an analysis of 64 patients. Circulation 30 (suppl IV):IV—3, 1964

122. Pierce GE, Morrow AG, Braunwald E: Idiopathic hypertrophic subaortic stenosis. II. Intraoperative studies of the mechanism of obstruction and its hemodynamic consequences. Circulation 30 (suppl IV):IV—152, 1964

123. Shah PM, Adelman AG, Wigle ED, et al: The natural (and unnatural) history of hypertrophic obstructive cardiomyopathy. Circ Res 34, 35 (suppl II):II—179, 1974

124. Morrow AG, Reitz BA, Epstein SE, et al: Operative treatment in hypertrophic subaortic stenosis. Circulation 52:88, 1975

125. Williams RG, Ellison RC, Nadas AS: Development of left ventricular outflow obstruction in idiopathic hypertrophic subaortic stenosis. Report of a case. N Engl J Med 288:868, 1973

126. Weiss MB, Ellis K, Sciacca RR: Myocardial blood flow in congestive and hypertrophic cardiomyopathy. Circulation 54:484, 1976

127. Stenson RE, Flamm MD, Harrison DC, et al: Hypertrophic subaortic stenosis. Clinical and hemodynamic effects of long-term propranolol therapy. Am J Cardiol 31:763, 1973

128. Shah DM, Gramiak R, Adelman AG, et al: Echocardiographic assessment of the effects of surgery and propranolol on the dynamics of outflow obstruction in hypertrophic subaortic stenosis. Circulation 45:516, 1972

129. Wigle ED, Adelman AG, Auger P, et al: Mitral regurgitation in muscular subaortic stenosis. Am J Cardiol 24:698, 1969

130. Ohn AJ, Segal BL: Isolated tricuspid insufficiency: Clinical features, diagnosis, and management. Prog Cardiovasc Dis 9:166, 1966

131. Robin E, Thoms NW, Arbulu A: Hemodynamic consequences of total removal of the tricuspid valve without prosthetic replacement. Am J Cardiol 35:481, 1975

132. Hansing CE, Rowe GG: Tricuspid insufficiency: A study of hemodynamics and pathogenesis. Circulation 45:793, 1972

133. Carpentier A, Deloche A, Hanania G: Surgical management of acquired tricuspid valve disease. J Thorac Cardiovasc Surg 67:53, 1974

134. Schlant RC: Altered cardiovascular function of rheumatic heart disease and other acquired valvular disease. In Hurst JW (ed): The Heart (ed 4). New York, McGraw-Hill, 1978, pp 965–981.

John L. Waller, M.D.
Joel A. Kaplan, M.D.
Ellis L. Jones, M.D.

7
Anesthesia for Coronary Revascularization

Coronary artery disease (CAD) is the most common serious medical problem in the United States today. Almost 700,000 patients die each year from ischemic heart disease and its complications.[1]

Of the approximately 1.3 million patients who have a myocardial infarction, at least one-third die within 1 month of this insult. The number of Americans suffering from congestive heart failure secondary to ischemic myocardial damage is vast. Cooper states that CAD is, for all ages and both sexes, "the primary factor limiting activities, the principle diagnosis on most hospital discharge sheets, the largest single cause of days spent in the hospital, and the primary reason for patients seeking advice from their physicians."[2] The dollar cost to society of this health care, plus resultant disability payments and lost income, is staggering. It is estimated that if the premature deaths of all individuals who die of myocardial infarction before age 65 *in any one calendar year* could be prevented and their lives remain productive, 2.6 billion dollars would be added to our gross national product.[2]

Recent data indicate a slight decline in deaths related to ischemic heart disease during the years 1971 through 1977.[3] The reasons for reversal of the former trend toward increasing numbers of coronary deaths are not clear, but they may be related to increased public awareness of and attention to coronary risk factors. (Table 7-1).[4]

While prevention offers the only real opportunity to avoid the ravages of coronary artery disease, the required changes in smoking, exercise, diet, and stress patterns are so extreme that large percentages of the general population are not likely to adhere to them in the near future. Without widespread, effective preventive programs, therapy of existing CAD will continue to be necessary.

The history of attempts to intervene surgically in coronary artery disease is at least 60 years old. Surgical sympathectomy had been reported as helpful in treating angina pectoris before 1920. During the 1930s and 1940s, various attempts to create collateral blood supply involved abrading epicardium and pericardium or placing vascularized pedicles on the epicardium. Retrograde coronary vein perfusion enjoyed some popularity in the 1950s, and myocardial implantation of the internal mammary artery (Vineberg's procedure) was utilized in the 1960s.[5]

With direct visualization of the coronary arterial tree made possible by the development of selective cine coronary arteriography by Sones and Shirey in 1962, Favaloro performed the first reported saphenous vein aortocoronary

Table 7-1
Risk Factors for Coronary Atherosclerotic Heart
Disease

1. Nonmodifiable risk factors
    a. Age
    b. Sex
    c. Familial history of premature atherosclerosis
2. Modifiable risk factors
    a. Major
        1. Elevated serum lipid levels (cholesterol and triglyceride)
        2. Habitual diet high in total calories, total fats, saturated fats,
           cholesterol, refined carbohydrates, salt
        3. Hypertension
        4. Cigarette smoking
        5. Carbohydrate intolerance
        6. Obesity
    b. Minor
        1. Oral contraceptives
        2. Sedentary living
        3. Personality type
        4. Psychosocial tensions
        5. Miscellaneous

bypass in 1967.[6] Surgeons in other centers rapidly followed his lead, to the extent that coronary revascularization has become one of the most frequently performed surgical procedures in the United States. Although exact figures are not available, it is estimated that more than 70,000 bypass procedures are performed each year in this country.[5] In the past decade, it is estimated that more than 400,000 patients have undergone aortocoronary artery bypass procedures.[7]

Although controversies regarding indications for and results of these procedures continue, this number is expected to continue growing rapidly during the next several years. Since this growth will involve more and more anesthesia personnel in the care of patients with CAD, greater familiarity with the principles governing proper management of such patients will be required. It is safe to predict that as anesthesiologists and surgeons gain further experience with coronary revascularization, better and better results will be demanded of them. Just as anesthetic practices that once represented the standard of care (e.g., use of in-circle vaporizers for inhalational agents) are now viewed as inadequate, so attention to indices of myocardial oxygenation during coronary artery surgery (multi-

lead ECG monitoring, quantitation of hemodynamic state) are readily becoming the standard of practice. Thus, this chapter attempts to bring into focus those considerations in preoperative and intraoperative evaluation and management that contribute to optimal care of the patient undergoing coronary revascularization surgery.

PREOPERATIVE EVALUATION

The importance of the anesthesiologist's personal preoperative visit with the patient is, in many cases, underestimated. Few surgical procedures invoke as much preoperative anxiety in patients as does surgery involving the heart. Thus the opportunities for allaying anxiety are perhaps greater here than prior to procedures perceived as less life-threatening. A calm and unhurried explanation of normal procedures, such as introducing vascular cannulae following local anesthetic infiltration, breathing oxygen during the induction, the intensive care unit experience (particularly the endotracheal tube and its temporary prevention of speaking), and the competence and willingness of the intensive care unit staff to understand needs and relieve pain result in a much calmer patient being brought to the operating room. Such calmness is of more than psychological import, since anxiety and its associated release of endogenous catecholamines may produce increases in both heart rate and systolic blood pressure, with a resultant net increase in myocardial oxygen demand.[8] It is not rare for these anxiety-produced changes to result in angina attacks, which are hazardous events in the preinduction period. Thus, in addition to being what some anesthesia personnel dismiss as a "social visit," the preoperative visit serves a most vital physiological function for these patients.

Including the patient's family in this preoperative discussion can provide for their understanding of the expected proceedings and secure their aid in lessening the patient's anxiety. Most frequently, as the family's understanding of the procedures increases, the patient's anxiety decreases.

We feel, then, that prime emphasis on a calm, unhurried, and understanding preoperative visit with the patient is entirely warranted.

History

The goals of an anesthesiologist obtaining a history from a patient scheduled for coronary bypass surgery are threefold:

1. To understand the type and extent of the patient's cardiac disease, the manner in which it affects the patient, and the limitations it imposes.
2. To understand the effects of the heart disease on other body systems and, conversely, the effects of other systemic diseases upon the cardiovascular system.
3. To explore and understand the impact of the contemplated surgery and anesthesia on items 1 and 2 (above).

When evaluating patients for potential cardiac surgery, it is imperative that the cardiac disease be considered *first*. This is true because the severity of the heart disease dictates the relative importance of coexisting disease states. For example, a patient who has been maintained until the time of preoperative evaluation on sodium warfarin would be an inappropriate candidate for totally elective surgery, and would properly have his surgical procedure postponed until adequate correction of the hemostatic de-

fect could be carried out. Should this same patient present with preinfarction angina unresponsive to maximal medical therapy, however, coronary revascularization might well be carried out immediately despite the increased bleeding difficulty that might be encountered.

ANGINA PECTORIS

In evaluating a patients cardiac status, two interrelated but separate aspects of heart function must be considered individually. These are (1) the myocardial oxygen supply/demand relationship; and (2) function of the heart as a pump. Whereas myocardial oxygen deprivation may impair pumping action, electrocardiographic evidence of myocardial ischemia may be present without symptoms of pump failure.

Tissue oxygen deprivation has been called ischemia or hypoxia. These terms are not synonymous. Braunwald defines *ischemia* as oxygen deprivation secondary to *reduced perfusion*, and *hypoxia* as reduced oxygen supply despite *adequate perfusion*.[1]

Anesthesia in patients with coronary artery disease must interfere as little as possible with myocardial metabolism in order to reduce the incidence of perioperative myocardial infarctions. There is a delicate balance between myocardial oxygen supply and myocardial oxygen demand that must be preserved during anesthesia (Fig. 7-1).

Myocardial oxygen supply should not be decreased or myocardial oxygen demand increased. Hypotension, tachycardia, hypoxemia, anemia, or an increase in blood viscosity will all tend to decrease myocardial oxygen supply. The other side of the balance, increase of myocardial oxygen demand, has not been recognized as being as important until recently. The four main factors that increase myocardial oxygen demand are (1) hypertension (increased afterload), (2) increased heart volume (increased preload), (3) tachycardia, and (4) increased contractility. These factors must also be taken into account and controlled by the anesthetic technique.

Ischemic chest discomfort in patients with coronary atherosclerosis is broadly divided into two categories according to its duration—brief chest discomfort lasting 2 to 15 minutes and prolonged chest discomfort lasting longer. Brief chest discomfort associated with myocardial ischemia is termed *angina pectoris,* literally translated "strangling in the chest."[9] Described by

MYOCARDIAL O$_2$ BALANCE

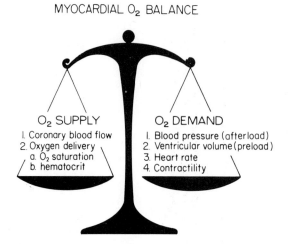

Fig. 7–1. The myocardial oxygen balance is demonstrated. The two sides of the balance are the oxygen supply and the oxygen demand; the factors that affect them are shown.

William Heberden in 1768, this symptom accounts for the largest proportion of patients scheduled for myocardial revascularization. Angina pectoris is termed ''stable'' when it has not changed in frequency, duration, time of appearance, or precipitating factors during the preceding 60 days. Stable angina may be mild (of brief duration, not markedly interfering with the patients life-style) or disabling (occurring at less than usual daily activity level but not at rest).[10]

Unstable angina describes a whole group of syndromes varying in some fashion from the above definition.[10] Patients whose angina is of recent onset or progressive, who may or may not experience pain at rest and who may or may not have had previous episodes compatible with myocardial ischemia, all fit into this broad category. The terms ''preinfarction syndrome,'' ''preinfarction angina,'' and ''intermediate coronary syndrome'' have been used to describe some or all of the subsets included here. These patients all have angina, the characteristics of which exceed those of stable angina, but lack serum enzyme evidence of myocardial damage.

A widely used and more narrow definition of unstable angina was established by the multi-institutional myocardial infarct research unit (MIRU) study, which limits the definition to the following criteria:[5]

1. Anginal pain lasting longer than 30 minutes within 7 days of the current hospitalization.

2. Documented electrocardiographic ST-T-wave changes of myocardial ischemia associated with at least one episode of ischemic pain during the period of hospitalization.

3. No evidence of progression to actual myocardial infarction by electrocardiographic or serum enzyme changes.

A third type of angina was first described in 1959 by Prinzmetal.[11] Now termed Prinzmetal's angina, or variant angina, it differs from classic angina in that chest pain occurs at rest or with ordinary exercise but not during vigorous exertion. Also unusual is the fact that ST-segment *elevation* occurs in the ECG during pain, returning to normal with cessation of the pain. Ventricular dysrhythmias are common during these episodes. Coronary artery spasm is clearly involved in the etiology of Prinzmetal's syndrome and may occur in the presence of angiographically normal coronary arteries or in the presence of fixed coronary obstructions.[12] Surgical therapy in this condition is generally reserved for those patients with demonstrable fixed intracoronary lesions.

Once the nature of the patient's ischemic symptoms is understood, the issue of ventricular function may be approached. It is easy to understand that the patient who has three-pillow orthopnea, gives a history of peripheral edema, and takes a digitalis preparation daily has impaired ventricular function. The patient's symptoms can be graded according to the New York Heart Association's (NYHA) classification (Table 7-2).[13] It may be more difficult to elicit from the history indications of transient episodes of left ventricular failure. Transient episodes of myocardial ischemia can cause episodic left ventricular failure.[1] Should the patient give such a history, more extensive intraoperative hemodynamic monitoring may be indicated to allow prompt detection and treatment of any such episodes. Shortness of breath following the onset of angina, angina decubitus, nocturnal angina, and paroxysmal nocturnal dyspnea suggest episodic ventricular failure ("ischemic left ventricular paralysis").

A chronic history of ventricular dysfunction is more common in the patient who has previously sustained one or more myocardial infarctions. Such symptoms as dyspnea on exertion, orthopnea, dyspnea at rest, and peripheral edema are consistent with chronic failure. Noting whether or not the patient takes a digitalis preparation is a helpful but sometimes misleading index of past or continued heart failure. Some patients are placed on digoxin for "heart trouble" without ever having had episodes of heart failure.

Cardiac catheterization provides quantitative, objective data regarding ventricular function. Nonetheless, catheterization may not reflect the severity of ventricular dysfunction. For example, a patient who has been at bed rest in the hospital, has been receiving large doses of diuretics, and has had salt intake vigorously restricted for several days may be hypovolemic when coming to the catheterization laboratory. In this volume-contracted state, left ventricular end-diastolic pressure may be "normal," failing to reflect high end-diastolic pressure that may be present after the patient receives adequate

fluids to allow stability during anesthetic induction. Conversely, a patient who comes to the catheterization laboratory in a very anxious state may have increased myocardial oxygen demand on the basis of his own output of catecholamines, adversely affecting the myocardial oxygen supply/demand ratio and causing transient ventricular dysfunction. For these reasons, it is important to have solid *historical* information from the patient to understand whether physical activity, emotional stress, or changes in body position provoke symptoms of heart failure.

Resting Electrocardiogram

While evaluation of the resting electrocardiogram is essential before anesthetizing patients with major coronary artery disease, it is important to understand that the resting ECG does not predict the extent of coronary artery disease. Benchimol and colleagues reported that 17 of 106 patients, 3 of whom had a total obstruction of a major coronary artery, had normal electrocardiograms.[14] When abnormalities do appear, however, they may dictate further preoperative therapy. Should changes suggestive of electrolyte disturbances appear, these may be investigated and properly treated prior to surgery. Changes consistent with acute ischemia suggest the need for additional medical therapy or immediate surgery, and changes compatible with acute myocardial infarction may dictate postponement of surgery or emergency revascularization, depending on the circumstances. It is useful to bear in mind any long-standing electrocardiographic abnormalities as well. Q waves observed following completion of cardiopulmonary bypass are of no concern if they were also present on the preoperative ECG, but they may suggest the need to reinstitute bypass and explore a surgical anastomosis if they are new. The same may be said for a number of other ECG abnormalities, including conduction disturbances and dysrhythmias.

Exercise Electrocardiography

Since 1908, when Einthoven recorded electrocardiographic changes after "running a staircase," cardiologists have been aware that exercise electrocardiographic examination often

Table 7-2
New York Heart Association
Classification

Class 1	Heart disease, no symptoms
Class 2	Comfortable at rest, symptoms with ordinary activity
Class 3	Comfortable at rest, symptoms with minimal activity
Class 4	Symptoms at rest

yields information in addition to that found in the resting ECG.[15] Extensive evaluation of the exercise tolerance test has been made, and both its usefulness and its inherent risks have been well described.

Bruce and Irving list four currently accepted purposes of exercise testing:[16]

1. Detection of latent coronary artery disease
2. Evaluation of established coronary artery disease
3. Evaluation of surgical or medical therapy
4. Monitoring of physical training programs

It is contraindicated in subjects with the following problems:

1. Acute myocardial infarction
2. Unstable angina pectoris
3. Acute illness of any system
4. Locomotor or neurological disability
5. Toxicity from cardiovascular drugs

Widespread use of exercise testing is based on the fact that it provides information regarding changes in rhythm, conduction, ventricular repolarization, heart rate, and blood pressure noninvasively and at relatively low cost.[17] Often neglected and sometimes of particular importance is documenting the correlation of any of these changes with the onset of angina. For example, while it has not been shown that anginal threshold during exercise tolerance testing is identical to the threshold for ischemic changes occurring during the induction of anesthesia, many cardiac anesthesiologists feel that knowledge of the heart rate and systolic blood pressure at which chest discomfort or electrocardiographic changes of ischemia first occurred can be quite helpful. This impression is supported by Robinson's observation that angina was provoked at a constant rate-pressure product in a given patient regardless of the various physical or emotional stresses triggering the attack.[18]

Of exercise tests in common usage, the Master's two-step test is a simple one that is supported by many years of clinical usage.[19] The number of steps taken during this test are adjusted for age and weight. The newer treadmill tests have the advantage of requiring predictable energy outputs throughout their course and higher expenditures of energy at maximal loads

than does the step test. The multistage tests involve uninterrupted treadmill exercise, with graduated increases in the tilt of the treadmill and the walking or running speed. Designated stages I, II, III, and so on last 3 minutes each and are adjusted each subsequent 3 minutes to increase the speed and percent grade until the completion of the test. In stage I, the subject walks at 1.7 miles per hour up a 10 percent grade, whereas he walks 4.2 miles per hour up a 16 percent grade in stage IV. A well-trained marathon runner may tolerate these graded exercise increases for as long as 21 minutes, but a patient with severe cardiac disease (NYHA class IV) may not last as long as 15 seconds.[16] It is our feeling that the exercise tolerance test, when viewed together with the patient's history and cardiac catheterization data, is an important part of preoperative evaluation for coronary artery surgery. It must be remembered, however, that a positive exercise test is reported either when severe ST-segment changes occur on the ECG or when the patient complains of angina pectoris. The rate-pressure product (RPP) usually reported is that present at the maximum exercise—*maximum RPP*. This is different from the RPP at which ischemic ECG changes *first occur*. Robinson found that patients with coronary artery disease developed angina at a RPP of about 22,000 during exercise testing.[18] He did not report the RPP at which the ECG *first* demonstrated ischemia. This information can be very useful to the anesthesiologist.

Cardiac Catheterization

Coronary arteriography and left ventriculography provide an enormous amount of objective data regarding the extent of coronary atherosclerosis and left ventricular performance. Since 1958, when Sones first performed selective coronary arteriography, this procedure has become the standard to which other methods of diagnosing coronary artery disease are compared.[20] Likewise, the ability of left ventriculography to observe performance of separate portions of the left ventricular wall provides the clinician with more specific understanding of ventricular performance than is available from hemodynamic pressure and flow measurements. A basic understanding of the performance of cardiac catheterization and interpretation of its results greatly expands the anesthesiologist's understanding of such patient's disease and facilitates prediction of the patient's response to the stresses of anesthesia and surgery.

Left Ventricular Function

Cineangiography utilizing 35-mm film or rapid-change, large-film techniques is available. Left anterior oblique (LAO) and right anterior oblique (RAO) views of the left ventricle are most commonly utilized. The ejection fraction (end-diastolic volume minus end-systolic volume divided by end-diastolic volume) is a useful quantitative measurement of ventricular function. Single-plane and biplane methods are used. Good correlations between these two methods have been reported in patients with valvular heart disease and a uniform contractile pattern.[21] This may not be true in patients with coronary artery disease and abnormal ventricular wall motion. According to King and Douglas, the single-plane RAO ventriculogram frequently underestimates left ventricular contraction because it visualizes those segments of the left ventricle most commonly involved in myocardial infarction.[22] Regardless of the method used, a normally contracting ventricle will eject at least 55 percent of end-diastolic volume with each beat. Ejection fractions between 0.40 and 0.55 are most common in patients with a history of a single previous myocardial infarction and are compatible with reasonable cardiac function without symptoms of heart failure. When the ejection fraction is between 0.25 and 0.40, most patients experience some symptoms with exertion but may well be asymptomatic at rest (NYHA class III). When the ejection fraction is less than 0.25, most patients are symptomatic at rest (NYHA class IV).[23]

Resting left ventricular end-diastolic pressure (LVEDP) is another indicator of ventricular function. Rapidly altered by factors such as bed rest, fluid restriction, and drug therapy, its normal value is ≤ 12 mm Hg. While the degree of elevation above this value does not always correlate with the degree of ventricular dysfunction, levels above 18 mm Hg usually imply poor ventricular performance.[23] A large increase in LVEDP after contrast injection during ventriculography may indicate poor ventricular response to stress.

Analysis of segmental ventricular wall motion abnormalities has become extremely im-

portant when planning coronary surgery. Recent advances have been made in predicting which portions of the left ventricle should respond favorably to revascularization. Dumesnil and colleagues demonstrated that nitroglycerin causes improvement in segmental wall motion of hypokinetic segments but not of dyskinetic or akinetic regions.[24] McAnulty et al. demonstrated that when nitroglycerin improved segmental wall motion, ejection fraction increased by an average of one-third.[25] Other methods reported to aid in identification of reversible wall motion abnormalities include the use of inotropic agents and postextrasystolic potentiation. Response to these interventions has been shown to correlate with improvement in contraction of the involved segments following coronary bypass surgery.[22]

Two newer noninvasive methods of measuring heart performance are echocardiography and radionuclide imaging. Echocardiography uses reflected ultrasound to study the location and motion of cardiac structures. It can be used to determine approximate systolic and diastolic volumes and the ejection fraction. Analysis of segmental ventricular wall motion is also possible. Radionuclide imaging requires intravenous injection of a gamma-emitting radiopharmaceutical and its detection in the body by a camera that transmits the picture or image to a display system. Information thus obtained can be used to calculate the ejection fraction and segmental or global performance of the left and right ventricles. Comparison of scans done at rest and during exercise can detect reversible wall motion abnormalities, as well as demonstrating wall motion abnormalities occurring only with exercise-induced ischemia.[26] Such noninvasive techniques offer enormous potential for real-time hemodynamic monitoring and are expected to enjoy more widespread application in the future.

Cardiac output may also be determined in the catheterization laboratory by the Fick, dye-dilution, or thermodilution methods, used singly or in combination. The cardiac index (cardiac output divided by body surface area) provides another useful parameter of cardiac performance. While a normal resting cardiac index of 3 liters/min/m² in no way guarantees acceptable ventricular performance in response to stress or exercise, a cardiac index below 2.0 liters/min/m² is an ominous sign, often associated with severe cardiac decompensation.

Coronary Arteriography

The coronary arteriogram not only provides objective mapping of the coronary anatomy but also identifies the location and severity of obstruction lesions. It also provides information regarding the size and condition of vessels distal to these lesions and aids evaluation of their functional importance by allowing observation of the mass and location of myocardium that they serve. Appreciation of the three-dimensional spatial relationships among the coronary arteries is necessary to understand the two-dimensional image produced on film.

There are several important pieces of information the anesthesiologist should obtain from the coronary arteriogram. While this information is most frequently available from the catheterization report, these reports may be unavailable at times (particularly prior to urgent night or weekend surgery). Thus, it behooves the diligent cardiac anesthesiologist to have some knowledge of the criteria involved in diagnosis based on coronary arteriograms. While some catheterization laboratories grade stenotic lesions according to the percentage of diameter reduction, the American Heart Association has recently recommended that the estimated reduction in cross-sectional area be reported. With this method, a 50-percent diameter reduction is equivalent to a 75 percent cross-sectional reduction; and a 75 percent diameter reduction is equal to a 90 percent reduction in cross-sectional area.[22] While the percentage of reduction in cross-sectional diameter determines the relative reduction in blood flow in any given artery, the absolute size of the distal vessel determines the feasibility of bypass grafting. A distal vessel lumen diameter of less than 1.5 mm ordinarily makes surgical anastomosis very difficult.

When evaluating coronary arteriograms, it is well to keep in mind the anatomy of the blood supply to certain special areas of the heart. In humans, the right coronary artery supplies the sinus node in about 55 percent of patients, while the left circumflex artery supplies the sinus node in the other 45 percent.[27] Although collateral circulation to the sinus node is present, the major portion of blood is supplied from a single artery. As the largest atrial artery, the sinus node artery also supplies a major portion of the atrial myocardium and interatrial septum. Occlusions of this artery lead to sinus node infarc-

tion and atrial rhythm disturbances. Proximal stenosis of the right or circumflex artery giving rise to the sinus node artery seems to be associated with a high incidence of atrial rhythm disturbances upon venous cannulation at the time of surgery.

Blood supply to the atrioventricular (AV) node is provided by the right coronary artery in 90 percent of human beings and by the circumflex branch of the left coronary artery in the remaining 10 percent.[27] For this reason, third-degree heart block may complicate posterior myocardial infarctions. AV nodal ischemia may be transient, since its collateral supply is more adequate than that of the sinus node. Thus, when patients with a history of prior posterior myocardial infarction complicated by AV block requiring temporary pacing undergo revascularization, transient recurrence of third-degree heart block is not rare.

The papillary muscles of the left ventricle are of vital functional significance. The anterior papillary muscle is almost always supplied by branches of the left coronary artery, while the posterior muscle usually receives blood flow from both left and right coronary artery branches. In both instances, collateral supply is relatively good, so that occlusion of a single major coronary artery does not usually cause infarction of a papillary muscle. Severe ischemia may produce papillary muscle dysfunction, however, leading to mitral insufficiency. Such mitral regurgitation may be intermittent and may appear only during the worst episodes of ischemia. Prompt treatment of the ischemia usually results in rapid reversal of the mitral incompetence.

In general, the more extensive a patient's coronary artery disease, the less he is able to tolerate unfavorable alterations in the myocardial oxygen supply/demand ratio. This fact is best illustrated by the patient with high-grade obstructive disease of the left main coronary artery. Since it supplies blood to a large portion of the left ventricle, significant obstruction in this vessel places large areas of the myocardium in substantial jeopardy. Such patients tolerate episodes of myocardial ischemia poorly, and meticulous attention to all factors influencing myocardial homeostasis is required for their successful management. Perhaps the most hazardous anatomic combination of lesions is total proximal obstruction of the right coronary artery in combination with high-grade left main coronary artery stenosis. Another extremely dangerous combination of lesions that may be overlooked by the anesthesiologist is the so-called left main equivalent. Anatomically, this refers to high-grade proximal obstructions of the two branches of the left main coronary artery, the left anterior descending, and the circumflex coronary arteries. This combination is particularly significant in the 10 percent of patients in whom the circumflex artery branches to form one or more posterior descending arteries[27] (see Fig. 7–2).

Additional useful bits of information from the catheterization laboratory include, both as positive and negative findings, the occurrence of ischemia, rhythm or conduction disturbances, and transient episodes of heart failure during catheterization. If any of these have occurred, the precipitating stress should be identified with a view toward avoiding similar problems intraoperatively.

From a combined analysis of the patient's specific cardiac history and catheterization data, the skeleton of a developing anesthetic management plan may be constructed by dividing patients roughly into two categories—those with *good left ventricular function* and those with *poor left ventricular function* (Table 7–3). Typically, the patient scheduled for coronary bypass surgery who has good ventricular function gives a history of angina as his primary problem. Systemic arterial hypertension is frequently an as-sociated problem. Since the patient's left ventricle functions well as a pump, his history will not reveal symptoms typical of congestive heart failure (orthopnea, paroxysmal nocturnal dyspnea, nocturnal angina, etc.). Cardiac catheterization data from such a patient usually reveals a normal left ventricular ejection fraction (0.55 or more), normal left ventricular end-diastolic pressure (LVEDP = 12 mm Hg or less), normal left ventricular segmental wall motion, and a normal cardiac index (2.5–3.0 liters/min/m²).

By contrast, a patient typical of those with poor left ventricular function frequently gives a history of one or more previous myocardial infarctions and describes some or all of the signs and symptoms of congestive heart failure. Catheterization data in such a patient might show a left ventricular ejection fraction of 0.40 or less, a LVEDP of more than 18 mm Hg, abnormal left ventricular wall motion, and a cardiac index below normal.

Obviously, many patients fit into a group between the two described here, having only intermittent symptoms of congestive heart failure and little functional impairment in day-to-day activities. These two general categorizations of patients nevertheless provide a useful frame of reference, because anesthetic management of patients who clearly fit one or the other of these groups may be profoundly different. A detailed discussion of anesthetic management is covered later in this chapter.

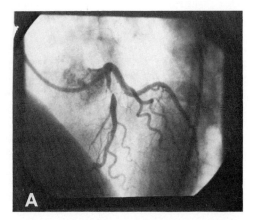 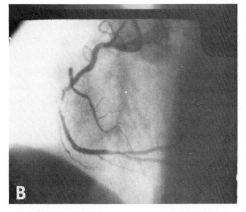

Fig. 7–2. Coronary arteriograms in the left anterior oblique view are shown in 2 patients with severe obstructive disease. (A) A 95 percent obstruction of the left anterior descending coronary artery. (B) A 95 percent obstruction of the right coronary artery.

Table 7-3
Two Groups of Coronary Artery Patients

Group A
  Patients with coronary artery disease and good left ventricular function
  a. History
    1. Angina as the primary problem
    2. Hypertension and obesity frequently associated
    3. No symptoms of congestive heart failure
  b. Catheterization
    1. Ejection fraction greater than 0.55
    2. LVEDP less than 12 mm Hg
    3. No areas of ventricular dyskinesia
    4. Normal cardiac output
Group B
  Patients with coronary artery disease and poor left ventricular function
  a. History
    1. Multiple myocardial infarctions
    2. Signs and symptoms of congestive heart failure
  b. Catheterization
    1. Ejection fraction less than 0.40
    2. LVEDP greater than 18 mm Hg
    3. Multiple areas of ventricular dyskinesia
    4. Decreased cardiac output

Other Organ-System Disorders

Although particular attention is paid to the cardiovascular system in evaluating patients prior to coronary artery surgery, it would be inappropriate to evaluate other body systems less thoroughly. Such evaluation may properly ask the questions: (1) Is the cardiac lesion so grave that correctable disorders of other systems should be ignored and emergency surgery carried out? (2) Are other system disorders likely to adversely affect the outcome of the contemplated cardiac procedure, and if so, is the cardiac disorder sufficiently stable to warrant postponement of surgery, allowing other problems to be resolved or brought under optimum control? With these questions in mind, further systematic evaluation of the patient may proceed.

RESPIRATORY SYSTEM

Evaluation of the respiratory system is an extremely important part of the preoperative workup. Respiratory dysfunction impinges directly on the homeostatic abilities of the heart. Many events during cardiovascular surgery may contribute to further pulmonary insult. Cardio-

pulmonary bypass, hemodilution and volume support with crystalloid solutions, hypothermia, and postoperative cardiac dysfunction are among the factors predisposing to respiratory insufficiency in patients with previously *normal* lungs. Underlying lung disease added to these unavoidable stresses greatly increases the likelihood of postoperative respiratory failure. Therefore, identification and adequate preoperative treatment of underlying lung disease is important.

Patients with significant acute respiratory tract infections should have their surgery postponed pending adequate treatment and resolution of their infectious process, cardiac stability permitting. But acute processes represent only a small portion of the significant pulmonary disorders found during preoperative evaluation.

Chronic obstructive pulmonary disease (COPD) accounts for the major share of preoperative pulmonary dysfunction encountered in patients coming for coronary artery surgery. Methods of preoperative evaluation and management of these patients vary widely from institution to institution but are in general directed to (1) hydration, expectoration, and chest therapy; (2) antibiotic therapy for any acute exacerbation of chronic bronchitis; and (3) cautious use of bronchodilators. If bronchodilators are used, extreme caution must be employed, as these agents all possess positive inotropic and chronotropic properties that may produce increased myocardial oxygen demand and trigger angina or infarction.

Although some centers have routinely recommended preoperative arterial blood gas measurement and complete pulmonary function testing, we feel that these examinations usually are not indicated in patients without evidence of lung disease. In patients who do have such evidence, however, these tests may indicate whether or not the lung disease is significant enough to warrant treatment. Table 7–4 lists our current indications for partial spirometric and arterial blood gas examinations.

INFECTIOUS DISEASES

Since the reticuloendothelial system functions poorly in the postcardiopulmonary bypass period, patients at this time are unusually susceptible to infection. Preexisting bacterial infection can often progress unchecked and become overwhelming. Unless emergency surgery is absolutely mandatory, adequate preoperative treatment is essential.

Even in patients without existing infectious diseases, wound contamination from normal skin flora is a threat during this period of decreased bodily defense mechanisms. For this reason, many surgical groups prophylactically administer antibiotics effective against ordinary skin bacteria. When initiated preoperatively, such therapy has been shown to decrease this incidence of wound infection.[28]

COAGULATION DISORDERS

Preoperative screening for coagulation abnormalities is imperative for all patients scheduled to undergo cardiopulmonary bypass. The prothrombin time (PT), partial thromboplastin time (PTT), platelet count, and the bleeding time are the tests routinely employed at Emory University Hospital. Abnormal results from any of these tests should trigger a search for the underlying cause, under the guidance of a consultant hematologist. The approach to the patient receiving anticoagulant drugs is discussed in Chapter 5.

PERIPHERAL VASCULAR DISEASE

The coexistence of severe coronary artery and peripheral vascular obstructive disease is

Table 7-4
Preoperative Indications for Specific Respiratory Evaluations

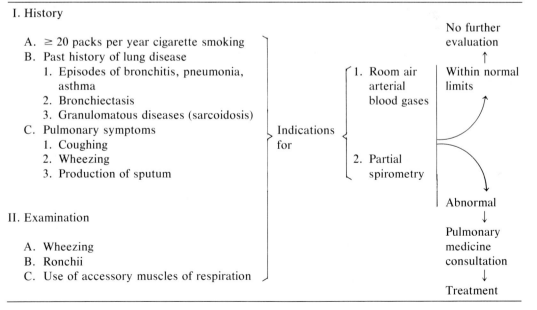

I. History

  A. ≥ 20 packs per year cigarette smoking
  B. Past history of lung disease
    1. Episodes of bronchitis, pneumonia, asthma
    2. Bronchiectasis
    3. Granulomatous diseases (sarcoidosis)
  C. Pulmonary symptoms
    1. Coughing
    2. Wheezing
    3. Production of sputum

II. Examination

  A. Wheezing
  B. Ronchii
  C. Use of accessory muscles of respiration

Indications for: 1. Room air arterial blood gases / 2. Partial spirometry

Within normal limits → No further evaluation

Abnormal → Pulmonary medicine consultation → Treatment

common. Significant extracranial carotid arterial stenosis was found in 5.6 percent of 874 consecutive candidates for coronary artery bypass.[29] This group of patients should be considered to be at high risk for neurological deficits following cardiopulmonary bypass.

There is general agreement that symptomatic or asymptomatic carotid bruits require evaluation.[30] In some centers, all patients with carotid bruits undergo selective carotid arteriography. In other centers, ophthalmodynometric measurements are utilized as the primary screening method, with carotid arteriography reserved for those whose ophthalmodynometric findings suggest hemodynamically significant lesions. Whatever the screening method, there is general agreement that hemodynamically significant, surgically accessible carotid lesions need surgical correction prior to instituting nonpulsatile cardiopulmonary bypass. Whether carotid surgery should be performed as a separate operative procedure or at the same time as coronary bypass surgery is not yet clearly established. In patients with stable coronary artery disease, it is our practice to undertake carotid surgery first, returning later for coronary revascularization. When this is not possible, as in patients who have unstable angina pectoris and severe carotid obstructive disease, both procedures are performed at a single operative setting. If the carotid surgery is undertaken as an initial separate procedure, it is essential that the patient be adequately monitored and properly anesthetized to avoid production of myocardial ischemia and possible infarction.

Occasionally patients with old, stable cerebrovascular accidents (CVA) present as candidates for coronary artery surgery. Although this group of patients is at increased risk of additional cerebral insult, an old CVA does not in itself contraindicate surgery.

Aortoiliac disease represents another threat to coronary bypass patients, especially those with poor left ventricular function. Should the intra-aortic balloon pump (IABP) be required to allow discontinuation of cardiopulmonary bypass, the presence of severe aortoiliac occlusive disease could make balloon insertion difficult or impossible.[31] Thus, we feel that angiographic views of this region should be obtained during cardiac catheterization in patients with poor ventricular function. Such an evaluation represents very little, if any, additional risk to the

patient. Severe disease in the iliac region might well contraindicate surgery in patients with an extremely high likelihood for the need for the IABP. On the other hand, knowledge that the disease was limited primarily to one iliofemoral region would be extremely valuable in the event balloon insertion was required.

Renal vascular disease represents another instance in which nonpulsatile cardiopulmonary bypass presents increased risk of vital organ ischemia. In addition, intraoperative control of the blood pressure is often more difficult in patients with significant renal artery lesions. Therefore, it may be wise to perform aortography preoperatively in patients with abdominal bruits. Whereas renal revascularization generally does not need to be carried out before coronary artery bypass, advance knowledge of significant renal artery disease might prompt consideration of additional measures to ensure adequate renal protection during bypass (see below).

RENAL DYSFUNCTION

Blood urea nitrogen (BUN) and serum creatinine levels are routinely measured preoperatively in coronary revascularization candidates to provide an index of renal function. Patients without historical evidence of renal disease who demonstrate marked increases in these laboratory values have their functional capacity quantified by measurement of creatinine clearance. Although coronary revascularization has been successfully performed on patients with no renal function who are maintained on chronic hemodialysis, marked decreases in renal function require the anesthesiologist to pay closer attention than usual to urine quality and quantity intraoperatively.[32] This is especially true during cardiopulmonary bypass. A recently developed addition to the standard roller-pump bypass circuit is the pulsatile assist device (PAD).[33] Marginal renal reserve in patients may represent one of the indications for the use of the PAD.

THYROID DISORDERS

Patients with thyroid hypofunction may occasionally present as candidates for coronary revascularization. Myxedema in these patients may be iatrogenic, since thyroid ablation was once a popular treatment for intractable angina pectoris.[34] Since small amounts of thyroid supplementation may result in exacerbations of angina, most of these patients must be anesthetized with little or no preoperative thyroid replacement. This may be done safely, and we do not feel that myxedema is a contraindication to coronary bypass surgery.[34]

PREOPERATIVE DRUG THERAPY

Medical management of myocardial ischemia improves myocardial oxygenation primarily by reducing myocardial oxygen demand rather than by increasing coronary blood flow. Nitrates remain the backbone of treatment of angina pectoris. Recently, β-adrenergic blockers have been added to the armamentarium. The hemodynamic effects of propranolol and nitroglycerin are such that each counteracts the oxygen-wasting properties of the other. Table 7–5 summarizes the effects of propranolol and nitroglycerin on the major determinants of myocardial oxygen consumption (MVO_2).

Nitrates

Sublingually administered nitroglycerin is the mainstay of drug therapy in the symptomic treatment of angina pectoris.[25] Its continued use for over a century attests to its remarkable efficacy. The drug's favorable effect on myocardial oxygen balance in patients with angina results principally from its venodilator effect causing a reduction in ventricular filling pressures, ventricular volume, and thereby wall tension (preload reduction). It may improve the endocardial-to-epicardial blood flow ratio through coronary artery dilation and resultant increased collateral blood flow.[35]

Because of the relatively brief duration of action of sublingually administered nitroglycerin, other nitrate drugs with more prolonged effects have come into clinical usage. Isosorbide dinitrate, pentaerythritol tetranitrate, and erytherityl tetranitrate are the long-acting nitrates in common use. While the time course of these may differ, their important pharmacologic effects appear to be identical to those of nitroglycerin.[36] The duration of action of long-acting nitrates is the subject of controversy in the literature. Reichek feels, however, that these preparations are effective in producing, for at least 1 hour, enhanced exercise tolerance in patients with stable angina and can be shown to improve the resting hemodynamics for up to 2 hours.[37]

Cutaneous administration of nitroglycerin ointment has recently been reinvestigated as a novel approach to prolonging nitrate effects. Although viewed with skepticism by most clinicians when first described in the 1950s, there is good theoretical basis from industrial toxicity studies to expect reliable and rapid percutaneous absorption of nitroglycerin. One group of patients was able to markedly prolong exercise duration 1 hour after such cutaneous application. This effect persisted for 3 hours.[38]

More recent investigations have demonstrated a reduction in the determinants of myocardial oxygen consumption for at least 4 hours in resting patients after administration of large-dose (20 mg) oral isosorbide dinitrate or nitroglycerin ointment (12.5–40 mg) in patients with regional left ventricular dysfunction. Sustained improvement of wall motion in left ventricular segments showing abnormally small excursion was also demonstrated following either drug.[39] It is our practice to continue nitrates up to surgery and to apply nitroglycerin ointment at the time of premedication.

Beta-Adrenergic Blockers

According to Logue, propranolol is "second only to nitroglycerin in its effectiveness in

Table 7-5

Determinants of MVO_2	Propranolol	Nitroglycerin
I. Wall tension		
a. Ventricular volume (preload)	↑	↓
b. Systolic pressure (afterload)	↓	↓
II. Contractility	↓	↑ (Reflex)
III. Heart rate	↓	↑ (Reflex)

the management of angina.''[35] Propranolol produces decreases in the three major determinants of myocardial oxygen consumption: (1) heart rate, (2) systolic blood pressure, and (3) the force and rate of myocardial contraction. Its antiarrhythmic properties also protect against atrial or ventricular arrhythmias. Oxygen delivery to tissues may also be facilitated by the action of propranolol which shifts the oxyhemoglobin dissociation curve to the right, increasing the P_{50}.[40]

The pharmacokinetics of propranolol have been studied extensively by Shand and others.[41,42] The half-life of propranolol in humans is 3.4 to 6 hours after discontinuation of chronic oral administration. Propranolol disappears from the plasma and atria within 24 to 48 hours when given in doses ranging from 20 to 240 mg/day. Plasma and heart concentrations have been found to fall at about the same rate, thus negating the concept of a long-lasting pool of the drug in the myocardium. Faulkner showed that both the chronotropic and inotropic responses return to normal within 24 to 48 hours after discontinuing doses of 30 to 240 mg/day.[43] Because of its known cardiac depressant action, Viljoen and co-workers, in 1972, recommended that propranolol be discontinued 2 weeks before cardiac surgery.[44] Their recommendation was based on a series of only 5 patients in whom difficulty was encountered during complex coronary artery surgery. This 2-week withdrawal period is

inconsistent with recent studies of the drug's metabolism and duration of action. Also, in many patients, especially those with unstable angina pectoris, withdrawal of propranolol for any extended period may produce an exacerbation of symptoms and may even lead to acute myocardial infarction.[45] We recently reported a series of 169 consecutive patients undergoing cardiac operations.[46] Of these, 82 percent had received propranolol to within 2 weeks of the operation, while 52 percent received the drug to within 48 hours of surgery. The incidence of hypotension and bradycardia was found to be no different in the patients taking propranolol than in those not taking the drug (Fig. 7–3). Based on this study and others that have recently appeared in the literature, we now recommend continuing propranolol up until the time of surgery.[47,48] In those patients who are stable, propranolol may be gradually tapered during the 48 hours prior to surgery, whereas in those patients who are unstable, it should be continued at its full dose (Table 7–6). It is our current practice to administer the last dose of propranolol at 10:00 P.M. the night prior to surgery for 8:00 A.M. operations. For operations later in the day, the last dose of propranolol is given at 8:00 A.M.

The anesthesiologist should be aware that the patient is taking propranolol and plan his anesthetic management accordingly. Hypotension during anesthesia should be treated by the

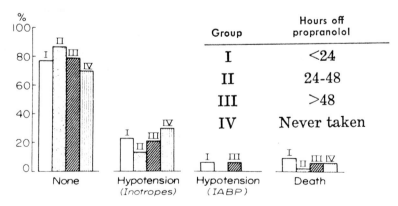

COMPLICATIONS *AFTER* CARDIOPULMONARY BYPASS

Group	Hours off propranolol
I	<24
II	24-48
III	>48
IV	Never taken

Fig. 7–3. Results of our studies on patients taking propranolol and undergoing coronary artery surgery are demonstrated. There was no difference in the incidence of complications between the four groups of patients. (Reproduced from Kaplan JA: Propranolol and cardiac surgery: A problem for the anesthesiologist? Anesth Analg 54:571, 1975, with permission of the author and publisher.)

Table 7-6
Recommended Propranolol
Management

Patients with	Management
Unstable angina	Maintain full dose until surgery
Stable angina	Taper gradually to < 160 mg/day, or maintain full dose
IHSS or TOF	Maintain full dose

Note: Do not abruptly discontinue propranolol
    preoperatively.
Key: IHSS = idiopathic hypertrophic
    subaortic stenosis
    TOF = tetrology of Fallot

usual methods, including decreasing the depth
of general anesthesia, increasing intravenous
fluid administration, altering surgical manipulation, and repositioning of the patient. In rare
instances it may be necessary to administer atropine for bradycardia or isoproterenol, glucagon,
calcium chloride, or digitalis to counteract the
β blockade.

Digitalis

The use of digitalis preparations in the immediate preoperative period remains a subject
of some controversy. In some centers, digitalis
preparations are routinely discontinued one half-
life (36 hours for digoxin, 5 days for digitoxin)
before the contemplated surgery. These groups
are likely to cite the high (20 percent) incidence
of some sign of digitalis intoxication in hospitalized patients taking digitalis preparations,[49]
the possible increase in serum digoxin levels
following cardiopulmonary bypass,[50] and the apparent lack of the ability of digitalis preparations
to increase maximum inotropic effects beyond
those produced by shorter-acting catecholamine
agents.[51] Those groups favoring administration
of digoxin the day prior to surgery are likely to
cite the success of frequent monitoring of potassium levels and aggressive replacement of
potassium in markedly reducing the perioperative incidence of digitalis-associated dysrhythmias, and the apparent efficacy of digoxin in
reducing the incidence of supraventricular arrhythmias in the postoperative period, even in
patients with no history of heart failure.[52]

Whatever the preoperative discontinuation
schedule of the digitalis preparation, perioperative problems with digitalis intoxication do not
present a major problem if the anesthesiologist
pays attention to well-described factors that predispose to this problem. Although wide individual variations occur, the following factors are
known to influence sensitivity to cardiac glycosides: electrolyte balance (potassium, magnesium, calcium), status of tissue oxidation,
acid–base balance, renal function, thyroid function, autonomic nervous system tone, concomitant drug therapy, and type and severity of underlying heart disease.[53]

Diuretics

Diuretic drugs enjoy wide usage in the management of two conditions frequently found in
patients with coronary artery disease: essential
hypertension and congestive heart failure.

In the hypertensive patient, the diuretic
(most frequently a thiazide) may be the sole drug
needed or may be used in combination with
other antihypertensive agents. A decrease in
plasma volume, found both in patients with essential hypertension and in those with coronary
artery disease, may be exacerbated by diuretic
therapy.[55,56] Such patients may require judicious
volume expansion prior to anesthetic induction.

Patients receiving diuretics for the management of their congestive heart failure may
also manifest signs of hypovolemia and require
volume supplementation prior to anesthetic induction. The sodium and potassium depletion
resulting from diuretic therapy may be present
in both groups of patients.[57,58] The same rule
that anesthesiologists are applying to a wide variety of drugs applies to the diuretics: drugs
needed to maintain a patient's homeostasis
should be continued until shortly before the time
of operation.

ANESTHETIC MANAGEMENT

Anesthetic management of patients
undergoing coronary revascularization should
ideally accomplish two things: (1) patient comfort should be provided for, and (2) the deli-
cately balanced myocardial oxygen supply/de-
mand ratio should be maintained or improved.
It is usually possible, utilizing currently avail-

able monitors and anesthetic techniques to achieve both goals simultaneously.

Little information is available regarding the effects of various anesthetic drugs, either singly or in combination, on *regional* oxygen balance in the normal *or* ischemic myocardium. For this reason, most centers now select anesthetic techniques aimed at preserving *total* myocardial oxygen supply while minimizing *total* myocardial oxygen consumption (MVO_2). To successfully achieve this goal, the anesthesiologist must be thoroughly familiar with the physiological mechanisms controlling this delicate oxygen supply/demand relationship (Fig. 7–1). The primary determinants of myocardial oxygen supply are:

1. Coronary blood flow
2. Available oxygen in arterial blood

Oxygen content of the arterial blood depends on the presence of a normal amount and type of hemoglobin containing normal amounts of 2,3-DPG, a normal pH, and a normal Pa_{CO_2}. Total coronary blood flow is primarily determined by total coronary artery resistance and coronary perfusion pressure (diastolic aortic pressure—LVEDP). Factors moderating coronary resistance include coronary artery disease, extravascular compression of intramyocardial blood vessels, blood viscosity, and a host of metabolic, neurohumoral, and drug influences on coronary arterial resistance.[59]

In the normal heart, regional myocardial blood flow is controlled through a feedback mechanism causing local dilation of small coronary artery branches in response to minute decreases in oxygen tension. This same vasodilator autoregulatory mechanism operates in diseased coronary arteries but, depending on the severity of the proximal obstructing lesion, may not be successful in restoring segmental flow. Should ischemia develop intraoperatively, manipulations of hemoglobin concentration, acid-base status, and temperature rarely cause significant increases in oxygen supply, since these parameters are usually maintained within satisfactory limits during surgery. Artificial increases in aortic pressure produced by expansion of intravascular volume (preload) or peripheral arteriolar constriction (afterload) may well increase coronary blood flow. But since such changes themselves cause increased myocardial oxygen consumption, favorable alterations of the myocardial oxygen supply/demand ratio may

not result. Additional ischemia may in fact be produced. On the other hand, various anesthetic and pharmacologic manipulations may rapidly produce favorable changes in myocardial oxygen supply/demand ratio by reducing oxygen *demand*.

The three primary determinants of myocardial oxygen demand are as follows:[60]

1. Ventricular wall tension (influenced by ventricular systolic pressure and end-diastolic volume)
2. Heart rate
3. Contractility

Since Rohde demonstrated in 1912 that myocardial oxygen consumption varies directly with the heart rate multiplied by peak developed pressure, extensive investigation into the relative effects of pressure, stroke volume, and heart rate on oxygen consumption has been carried out.[61] Braunwald has reviewed the history of these investigations and provides an excellent summary of their conclusions.[60] Briefly, his findings include the following:

1. Rohde's observations that the rate-pressure product correlates directly with myocardial oxygen consumption are confirmed.
2. There is also a close relationship between the tension-time index (integrated area beneath the left ventricular pressure curve per minute) and myocardial oxygen consumption.
3. The contractile state of the heart, reflected in the maximal velocity of isotonic shortening, is also a major myocardial oxygen consumption determinant.
4. The oxygen cost of "pressure work" is far greater than that of "flow work."

Knowledge of these basic physiological principles, together with understanding of the patient's pathophysiologic state, permits intelligent application of appropriate monitoring techniques to the patient and allows favorable alteration of the oxygen supply/demand ratio by soundly based pharmacologic and anesthetic interventions.

Monitoring

The term "monitoring" is derived from the Latin verb *monere*, which means "to warn." An ideal device to monitor patients with ischemic heart disease should continuously provide real-time measurements of tissue oxygenation, perfusion, and metabolism in all regions of the heart, especially in those vulnerable to ischemia. Such an "early warning" system would allow rapid detection of developing oxygen deprivation at a cellular level, identify its location, and provide instantaneous information as to the success or failure of therapy to correct it. Since such a device is not available, we utilize a variety of monitors yielding indirect information. The goal of monitoring is to detect and correct trends that may lead to trouble, hopefully allowing its avoidance. Failing this, monitoring should detect developing trouble early, provide information about the nature of the problem, and allow immediate corrective action to be taken.

ELECTROCARDIOGRAPHIC MONITORING

The electrocardiogram serves both of these monitoring functions. Automated heart rate counters triggered from the ECG signal warn of increased heart rate, with its associated oxygen cost. ECG monitoring also is the classic noninvasive method of detecting myocardial ischemia.

When the premedicated patient arrives in the operating room, he is transferred to the operating table and immediately connected to electrocardiographic leads. We routinely employ a five-wire system that permits lead selection among leads I, II, III, AVR, AVL, AVF, and a precordial lead (V_5).[62] Signals derived from this system are fed to two ECG preamplifiers and displayed on separate simultaneous oscilloscope channels.

It has long been recognized that multiple-lead electrocardiography is important in diagnosing ischemia during stress testing. The graded ECG exercise test is routinely used by cardiologists to diagnose coronary artery disease. Blackburn showed that 89 pecent of the ST-segment information contained in the conventional 12-lead exercise ECG is found in lead V_5.[63] Mason showed that in 56 patients with ST-segment changes, leads V_4 and V_6 were the most useful and lead I the least informative.[64] In a study of 100 patients, Redwood demonstrated that the left lateral leads (I, AVL, V_3 to V_6) had ten times more positive tests than the vertical leads (II, III, AVF).[65] Finally, Robertson has demonstrated that in most cases the location of

the ST-segment changes correlates with arteriographic localization of the patient's coronary artery disease.[66]

Although multiple-lead ECG monitoring provides the best currently available method of detecting perioperative myocardial ischemia, it is not a perfect method, and its limitations should be pointed out. ST-segment changes monitored from skin electrodes are nonspecific indicators of ischemia, particularly in connection with coronary artery surgery.[67] Manipulation of the heart or thermal and electrolyte changes intraoperatively may markedly alter the electrocardiographic pattern.[68] The measured voltage of the ECG complex and portion of the myocardium monitored by precordial lead are altered by the act of opening the chest, so that one is, in fact, monitoring a "different" V-lead after the sternal retractor is in place.[69] Despite these limitations, simultaneous lead II and V_5 monitoring, together with other monitoring methods to be discussed, provide adequate information to permit avoidance of ischemia in most patients and prompt treatment of those who develop ischemic changes. The precision of the ECG can be greatly increased by using a calibrated write-out. This allows precise determination of the magnitude of any apparent ST-segment changes that may occur.

The electrocardiogram is standardized, with 1 mv equaling 10 mm. We consider 1 mm horizontal or downsloping ST-segment depression from baseline a significant sign of myocardial ischemia. We routinely obtain a full seven-lead calibrated tracing when the patient arrives in the operating room. This tracing is repeated at the conclusion of cardiopulmonary bypass. Gross differences between prebypass and postbypass tracings may suggest a problem with graft function which, if present, may be readily corrected before chest closure.

HEMODYNAMIC MONITORING

In addition to electrocardiographic monitoring, all patients have direct arterial and central venous pressure catheters inserted. Two important varieties of information are obtainable from hemodynamic measurements. Performance of the heart as a pump may be evaluated, and inferences as to total myocardial oxygen supply and demand may be made (myocardial ischemia indices.) Since the anesthetic induction period is often accompanied by marked hemodynamic changes, we feel it is important to have monitoring lines placed prior to induction using local anesthetic infiltration.

The percutaneous approach to the radial artery is the most commonly employed route for establishing an in-dwelling arterial line. Under the following circumstances, however, it is generally wise to avoid radial artery cannulation:

1. Below a previous brachial artery cutdown, since pressure gradients frequently occur across these potential arterial narrowings, especially in association with hypothermia.
2. When ipsilateral subclavian artery stenosis is known (or suspected from unequal upper extremity blood pressure measurement).
3. When the presence of collateral ulnar artery circulation cannot be determined with Allen's test or by demonstrating palmar arch flow during radial artery compression by Doppler ultrasound techniques.

If neither radial artery is suitable for cannulation, the femoral artery may be used. Adequacy of the palpated pulse, previous arteriograms (if any), and the potential use of femoral arterial perfusion or possible insertion of the intra-aortic balloon pump must all be considered in selecting a femoral artery monitoring site. A 5½-inch, 18-gauge catheter-over-needle unit usually causes minimal trauma and provides excellent pressure tracings. A spring-tip J-guide wire may be employed if the cannula does not pass freely up the femoral artery.

Other arterial cannulation sites may be employed if necessary. The dorsalis pedis artery usually is not difficult to cannulate. The posterior tibial and superficial temporal arteries may be technically more difficult to puncture but may be important for monitoring in unusual circumstances.

The possibility that pressure monitored from peripheral arteries might not actually reflect central aortic pressure should be kept in mind, particularly at the conclusion of cardiopulmonary bypass, when the patient may be cold and vasoconstricted. Many experienced surgeons are able to estimate aortic pressure quite accurately by direct palpation. If this estimate varies greatly from arterial pressure monitored peripherally, a sterile tubing may be used to connect the arterial transducer to a needle inserted directly into the aortic arch.

Central venous pressure (CVP) is a useful parameter that should be monitored in all patients undergoing coronary bypass surgery. It is just as important to understand what CVP measurements do not indicate as to know what they do indicate. When the catheter tip is correctly placed (in the superior vena cava), CVP indicates right heart filling pressure and approximates cerebral venous pressure. Since net cerebral perfusion pressure is equal to the difference between arterial and venous pressure within the head, significant *increases* in cerebral venous pressure may produce critical drops in cerebral perfusion pressure that are just as significant as those produced by marked decreases in arterial pressure. Increases in venous pressure may be noted immediately from the CVP monitor, and the surgeon can be notified of the sudden change. Corrective action usually involves repositioning of the superior vena cava cannula which returns blood to the pump, relieving cannula drainage obstructions caused by twists or extrinsic compression, or repositioning of packs, retractors, or surgical assistants' hands.

The CVP does not give any direct indication of left heart filling pressure. It can be used as a crude estimate of left-sided pressures. In patients with normal cardiac function, changes in right heart filling pressure (CVP) parallel changes in left heart filling pressure. In the presence of left ventricular dysfunction, left heart filling pressure may be greatly different from CVP, and changes in one pressure may not be parallel to changes in the other.[70] For this reason, direct or indirect measurement of left heart filling pressure is warranted in patients with known or suspected left ventricular dysfunction.

Measurements of Myocardial Oxygen Demand

RATE-PRESSURE PRODUCT (RPP)

RPP = systolic blood pressure × heart rate

Robinson demonstrated that during exercise stress testing, most patients with coronary artery disease experience angina at RPP = 22,000.[18] Loeb has recently shown that at similar RPPs, the stress of tachycardia resulted in more myocardial ischemia than did the stress of hypertension.[71]

We use the RPP intraoperatively as a guide to myocardial oxygen demand in patients with coronary artery disease, and attempt to keep it below the patient's preoperative maximum RPP while in the hospital. A multiplier circuit has been added to our monitoring equipment in order to continuously display the RPP on a digital readout. We keep this below 12,000, if possible (Fig. 7-4).

TRIPLE INDEX (TI)

TI = systole pressure × heart rate × PCWP

The triple index adds a third factor causing increases in the myocardial oxygen demand. We keep this below 150,000. An occasional patient will show a large increase in the PCWP before the blood pressure or heart rate, and increase in the TI before the RPP.

TENSION-TIME INDEX (TTI)

The tension-time index is the product of the heart rate multiplied by the area under the systolic portion of the aortic pressure curve. Sarnoff showed a close relationship between the TTI and myocardial oxygen demand in the dog; others, however, have not found this to correlate as well as the RPP.[72]

ENDOCARDIAL VIABILITY RATIO (EVR)

The endocardial viability ratio was proposed by Hoffman and Buckberg in 1974 to measure subendocardial ischemia.[73] It compares the ratio of the myocardial oxygen supply to the oxygen demand.

$$EVR = \frac{DPTI}{TTI} = \frac{oxygen\ supply}{oxygen\ demand}$$

where

DPTI = diastolic pressure time index

TTI = tension-time index

The EVR may be derived by planimetry, that is, by measuring the areas under the systolic and diastolic portions of the arterial pressure tracing. More conveniently it can be calculated by Phillip's formula:[74]

$$EVR = \frac{DPTI}{TTI} = \frac{(\overline{DP} - (PCWP) \times T_D)}{\overline{SP} \times T_s}$$

where

$\overline{DP}$ = mean systemic diastolic pressure

PCWP = pulmonary capillary wedge pressure

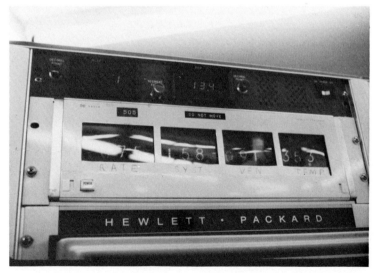

Fig. 7-4. Our rate-pressure product meter is demonstrated on the top center row of digital readouts. It works as a multiplier circuit. The number 13.4 is multiplied by 100 to give a rate-pressure product of 13,400.

$\overline{SP}$ = mean systemic arterial pressure

T_D = diastolic time

T_s = systolic time

A normal EVR is 1.0 or greater. When the EVR < 0.7 subendocardial ischemia may occur. This ischemia is associated with a decrease in the endocardial/epicardial blood flow ratio.

Relationship of Hemodynamic and Electrocardiographic Monitoring of Myocardial Ischemia

A recent study of 21 patients undergoing coronary artery revascularization was undertaken at Emory University Hospital to evaluate the frequency of ST-segment changes in lead V_5 versus lead II and to compare these ECG findings with changes in oxygen supply and demand.[75]

ECG recordings of leads II and V_5 and hemodynamic measurements were made in each patient. Two indirect indices of myocardial oxygen demand were calculated for all patients:

1. Rate-pressure product (RPP) = systolic blood pressure (SBP) × heart rate (HR)
2. Tension-time index (TTI) = SBP × HR x left ventricular ejection time

Additional measurements were made in 5 pa-

tients with Swan-Ganz catheters:

1. Endocardial viability ratio (EVR) = diastolic pressure-time index/tension-time index
2. Coronary perfusion pressure (CPP) = diastolic blood pressure (DBP) − pulmonary capillary wedge pressure (PCWP)
3. Triple index = SBP × HR × PCWP.

Eight patients had normal ST segments through out the study (group I), 11 patients had ST changes only in V_5, and 2 patients had ischemic changes in both V_5 and lead II (group II). No patient had changes only in lead II. Five patients had maximum ST-segment changes at the time of cannulation, 3 had changes upon skin incision, 2 each upon intubation and sternotomy, and 1 while awake. Only 1 patient with left main coronary artery disease had ischemia associated with a decreased oxygen supply (BP 70/45). In none of the other patients was the minimum DBP or CPP associated with ECG changes. These 12 patients, however, had ST changes when oxygen demand was increased. The maximum heart rate and RPP were significantly higher in patients with ischemic changes on the ECG (Table 7-7). Heart rates above 90 beats per minute appeared to be the most detrimental factor, and ischemic changes appeared in all patients with a RPP over 12,000 mm Hg × beats per minute. The maximum TTI and mini-

Table 7-7

	Group I (N = 8)	Group II (N = 13)
Maximum HR (beats per minute)	77 ± 4	92 ± 5[†]
Maximum SBP (torr)	146 ± 7	146 ± 6
Maximum RPP (mm Hg × beats per minute)	11,048 ± 285	13,466 ± 938[†]
Maximum TTI (mm Hg/sec/min)	3,722 ± 158	3,836 ± 266
Minimum DBP (torr)	56 ± 2	56 ± 2
Minimum CPP (torr)[‡]	52, 48	51, 50, 45
Minimum EVR[‡]	.89, .88	.94, .70, .67

[†] $P < .05$ as compared to group I by student's T test.

[‡] Individual values shown for the 5 patients with Swan-Ganz catheters.

[*] Mean values ± 1 S.E.

mum EVR did not correspond to the ECG changes. The triple index was markedly elevated in only 1 patient, who had a PCWP of 26 torr.

A recent study by Gobel confirms our findings.[72] He studied indices of myocardial ischemia (myocardial oxygen consumption, coronary blood flow, RPP, heart rate, and TTI) during exercise testing in patients with ischemic heart disease. The myocardial oxygen consumption correlated well with the heart rate ($r = .79$) and RPP ($r = .83$). Including the ejection period (TTI) did not improve the correlation ($r = .80$).

Good Left Ventricular Function Group

As mentioned earlier, patients may be divided into two different categories on the basis of left ventricular function (Table 7-3). It is important to remember that patients with coronary artery disease who have good ventricular function have just that—*good ventricular function!* If the anesthetic is managed in such a way that the balance between myocardial oxygen supply and demand is maintained, these patients generally respond to anesthesia in a manner similar to patients undergoing routine noncardiac operations. If, on the other hand, the oxygen balance is upset either through marked decreases in oxygen supply (severe hypotension) or through increases in oxygen demand (hypertension, tachycardia), the resulting ischemia can produce severe, acute left ventricular dysfunction. For these reasons the anesthetic care of the patient with good ventricular function seeks to produce an anesthetic state sufficiently profound to assure maximal attenuation of reflex responses to anesthetic and surgical manipulations and maintain adequate arterial pressure. Thereby maintenance of adequate myocardial blood flow is possible.

In practice, these goals are accomplished in a variety of ways. No single anesthetic technique has been shown to be superior to others. We frequently use diazepam in 5-mg increments or thiopental in 50–100-mg increments for induction of anesthesia. Morphine and diazepam may also be used together in alternate 5-mg increments. Droperidol is used by some to produce loss of consciousness, and fentanyl is often substituted for morphine as the analgesic component.

Although the pharmacologic effects of these drugs are familiar to most anesthesiologists, it seems pertinent to focus on those effects important to the patient with coronary artery disease.

Diazepam (Valium) is a nonbarbiturate benzodiazepine tranquilizer. It has been shown to cause coronary artery dilatation in patients with coronary artery disease and in normal subjects.[76] Diazepam also decreases the LVEDP, while producing little alteration in other hemodynamic parameters in patients with elevated filling pressures.[77] For these reasons, it has been advocated as an induction agent in patients with coronary artery disease or marginal cardiovascular reserve.[78] Other studies of diazepam in humans and in animals, however, suggest that diazepam may produce increases in systemic vascular resistance, heart rate, and LVEDP, while decreasing arterial pressure and stroke volume.[79,80] Liu et al. have shown that in dogs that had received prior large doses of fentanyl, the hemodynamic effects of small doses (0.5 mg/kg) and large doses (1 mg/kg) of diazepam produced directionally opposite effects.[81] While the lower dose produced little hemodynamic change, the larger dose was associated with significant depression of myocardial contractility, stroke volume, and arterial pressure. The degree to which endogenous catecholamines affect these results is not clear. On balance, clinical use of diazepam usually results in minimal alterations in hemodynamics. Since we rarely employ total doses greater than 20 mg of diazepam in any short time period, the myocardial depressant effects observed by some authors may have been avoided.

Thiopental (Pentothal), a short-acting thiobarbiturate, enjoys perhaps the widest usage of any drug for induction of anesthesia. It has long been known that thiopental has myocardial depressant properties.[82] Becker and Tonnesen have recently shown that in healthy human volunteers, administering an anesthetizing barbiturate concentration (ABC) that is equivalent to minimal alveolar concentration (MAC) for inhalation anesthetics produced decreases in myocardial contractility, cardiac output, stroke volume, and blood pressure.[83] When compared with published results for 0.8 MAC of halothane and 0.8 MAC of enflurane, thiopental caused less depression of myocardial function.[83]

The myocardial depressant properties of thiopental may be extremely useful intraoperatively in preventing and in treating hypertensive episodes. Its judicious, controlled use may make adequate blood pressure control easier, keeping oxygen demand from increasing excessively. Because a bolus dose of thiopental is rapidly cleared from the circulation, the effects of intraoperative stimuli, such as endotracheal intubation, skin incision, or sternotomy, may be reduced by administering a bolus of thiopental just prior to the anticipated stimulus.

Droperidol, a butyrophenone tranquilizer, causes decreased arterial pressure through vasodilator effects produced by α-adrenergic receptor blockade.[84] As with any vasodilator substance, droperidol causes venodilation, producing venous pooling with a resultant decreased ventricular filling pressure (preload). Similar changes are frequently observed during anesthetic induction when utilizing other agents that do not have specific vasodilator effects. This is often ascribed to the effect that loss of consciousness may have on peripheral vascular tone. If the patient has been anxious while awake, as many patients are when coming for major surgical procedures, endogenous catecholamine levels are elevated. The resultant vasoconstriction produced by the catecholamines may be reduced with the loss of consciousness, resulting in arterial dilation, venodilation, and a decreased blood pressure. All anesthesiologists are familiar with this pattern, which is usually treated by placing the patient in the Trendelenberg position and expanding intravascular volume. We attempt to avoid the use of vasoconstrictors at this time, since it is easy to "overshoot," producing increased afterload and myocardial work.

The pharmacologic effects of the narcotics have been extensively studied and are discussed in Chapter 1. Their use as sole induction and maintenance agents for coronary revascularization operations has been largely abandoned because production of adequate anesthesia and amnesia for the operation is not reliable, even with very high doses. These drugs, nonetheless, have minimal myocardial depressant properties, and their use may markedly reduce the requirement for other anesthetic agents.

After the patient loses consciousness, nitrous oxide/oxygen in a 50:50 ratio is added, and muscle relaxation is produced. In these patients with good left ventricular function, a volatile anesthetic agent may also be added at this time prior to any major stimulus. Either enflurane or halothane may de administered by mask to attain an adequate depth of anesthesia prior to endotracheal intubation.

The two desired effects of nitrous oxide are (1) to further deepen the anesthetic level, and (2) to produce depression of left ventricular performance.[85] Both of these effects aid in preventing untoward increases in heart rate and blood pressure during the next anticipated stimulus—laryngoscopy and endotracheal spray with 4 percent lidocaine. This laryngotracheal anesthetic has been shown by Denlinger to partially attenuate the increases in blood pressure and heart rate that occur during laryngoscopy and intubation.[86]

Prior to laryngoscopy, muscle relaxation is produced with succinylcholine, pancuronium, or d-tubocurarine. The hemodynamic effects of these drugs should be considered prior to selecting one for administration. Succinylcholine appears to cause minimal changes in parameters that affect the myocardial oxygen supply/demand ratio.[87] This drug has been widely employed, in bolus or infusion form, during coronary artery surgery. Pancuronium has become popular, since it is a long-acting drug without the hypotensive effects commonly encountered with d-tubocurarine. It may, on the other hand, have the undesirable effects of producing tachycardia and increased myocardial oxygen consumption in patients with coronary artery disease.[88,89] Supraventricular tachyarrhythmias are very poorly tolerated by these patients and lead to ST-segment changes on the ECG.[90] Such tachyarrhythmias, which apparently can be triggered by a vagolytic effect of pancuronium, are virtually eliminated in patients maintained on propranolol therapy until the time of operation.[91] d-Tubocurarine produces vasodilation through the mechanisms of histamine release and ganglionic blockade.[92] Although this property has been responsible for much unwanted hypotension, it can be used to advantage in hypertensive patients. Zaidan et al. have recently described the use of dimethyl tubocurarine (Metocurine) to provide muscle relaxation in a small group of patients undergoing coronary revascularization.[93] Metocurine produced a remarkably stable hemodynamic response. Blood pressure, heart rate, and central venous pressure remained unchanged, while a slight drop in peripheral resistance was compensated for by an increase in cardiac output. This drug may prove to be the relaxant of choice in patients with coronary artery disease, especially those patients not maintained on propranolol.

At some point during the induction sequence, it is helpful to perform a series of co-ordinated maneuvers representing increasing increments of stimulation to the patient. For example, just after consciousness is lost, hemodynamic response to the insertion of a urethral catheter may be observed. If the patient is inadequately anesthetized, increases in heart rate, blood pressure, and filling pressure may be produced. This stimulus is sufficiently mild, so that such increases in the indices of myocardial oxygen consumption are usually slight in degree and short-lived. The presence of a positive hemodynamic response indicates the need for additional anesthesia. The absence of such a response indicates readiness to proceed to the next gradation of stimulus without the need for additional anesthetic drugs. Next in the line of increasing stimuli is insertion of the oropharyngeal airway. In patients who are receiving a narcotic as a part of the induction technique, the airway is usually well tolerated early in the induction period. At about the same time, it is possible to begin a surgical scrub of the patients. If the scrub solution is cold and/or the scrub is forcefully performed, significant hemodynamic changes may be noted. Once muscle relaxation has been obtained, laryngoscopy and spraying the trachea with 4 percent lidocaine are the next stimuli. In some centers, the intravenous route for lidocaine administration is preferred. We employ the intratracheal route for lidocaine administration because it has been shown to be more effective in attenuating the response to subsequent tracheal intubation.[94] In addition, this gives us yet another indication of the adequacy of the depth of anesthesia by providing a stimulus only slightly less potent than the most powerful one in the anesthetic induction sequence—placement of a cuffed endotracheal tube. As with the preceding stimuli, a significant response can generally be treated by increasing the anesthetic depth. Since laryngoscopy is such a potent stimulus, however, and may produce hypertension, tachycardia, and resultant ischemia in the coronary patient, the addition of a vasodilator or propranolol at this point may be necessary.

After placement of the endotracheal tube,

the level of stimulation to the patient, and thus the anesthetic requirement, abruptly decreases. This may be a good time to employ one of a number of maneuvers designed to prevent *hypotension* during the next few relatively unstimulated minutes: (1) reducing the dose or discontinuing the administration of inhalation agents or vasodilators; (2) administering additional intravenous fluid; (3) tilting the patient into a slightly head-down position; or (4) using small doses of relatively mild cardiotonic or vasopressor drugs. It is good policy to first attempt the milder and less potentially hazardous modes of therapy. As the blood pressure just after intubation is generally not low, simple anticipation of the coming sequence of events usually allows the use of correct maneuvers to prevent hypotension prior to its development.

Skin incision by the surgeon represents a powerful stimulus and again calls for "deepening" the anesthetic. The potent inhalation anesthetics are particularly useful at this time, not only because they provide controllable and rapidly reversible myocardial depression but also because they appear to be more effective than the narcotics in suppressing catecholamine and renin production.[95] The pharmacology of the inhalation agents is discussed in detail in Chapter 1.

There appear to be important differences among the potent inhalational anesthetics with respect to their interaction with β-adrenergic blocking agents. Since large numbers of patients coming to coronary surgery are receiving propranolol, these differences are important to consider. Saner has shown that in dogs anesthetized with methoxyflurane or trichlorethylene, administration of practolol in association with hemorrhage produced almost irreversible shock.[96] This is in contrast to other experiments in dogs, which showed that the myocardial depressant effects of halothane and propranolol were additive. Discontinuing halothane produced prompt reversal of that portion of the myocardial depression produced originally by halothane.[97,98] In a similar dog model, a 3 percent inspired concentration of enflurane (Ethrane) was found to be intermediate between methoxyflurane and halothane in its degree of interaction with propranolol.[99] Some synergistic effect was noted, and the dogs did not respond as well to the discontinuance of enflurane as they had when halothane was discontinued. It should be stressed that these studies were performed in animals and that direct extrapolation of these results to patients may produce incorrect conclusions. Many centers (including Emory) employ enflurane as part of the anesthetic technique for coronary bypass surgery, and no reports of unusual problems with hypotension or myocardial failure have been presented. Methoxyflurane currently enjoys only limited use during coronary surgery. A number of factors, including its potential nephrotoxicity and its remarkable synergistic interaction with propranolol in dogs may be responsible (Table 7–8).

The greatest surgical stimulus occurs during the period from the skin incision through the stenotomy, and the maximum amounts of anesthetic agent will generally be needed at this time. During this phase of intense stimulation, myocardial ischemia resulting from increased oxygen demand is a common occurrence and can be a real threat to the patient's welfare. When deep general anesthesia fails to control blood pressure and heart rate adequately, therapy with vasodilators and β-blocking drugs should be used in a rational manner (Table 7–9). Mild hypotension (systolic blood pressure = 90–100 mm Hg) associated with a low normal heart rate is usually well tolerated in patients with coronary artery disease; however, the opposite extremes are less well tolerated. Although the rate-pressure product at which ischemia develops is different for each patient, we find that values above 12,000 to 15,000 are frequently associated with detectable ischemic changes on the electrocardiogram.[75] It should be emphasized that these numbers are merely a guide. Some patients will develop ischemic changes with a RPP of less than 12,000, while some show no ST-segment changes with a RPP greater than 18,000.

Vasodilator drugs are used to treat hyper-

Table 7-8

Anesthetic Interactions with Beta-blocking Drugs

Drug	Interaction
Methoxyflurane	Synergistic
Trichlorethylene	Synergistic
Enflurane (3%—dogs)	Synergistic?
Halothane	Additive
Morphine	Additive

Table 7-9

Therapeutic Interventions for ST-Segment Depression

Associated with	Treatment
1. ↑ BP	a. Deepen anesthesia
	b. Vasodilator
	Nitroglycerin, 20–200 μg/min I.V.
	Sodium nitroprusside, 10–100 μg/min I.V.
2. ↑ HR	a. Deepen anesthesia
	b. Propranolol, 0.25–2 mg I.V.
3. ↑ PCWP or ↑ CVP	a. Vasodilator (as above)
	b. Lighten anesthesia
	c. Restrict fluids
	d. Diuretics or inotropes
4. ↓ BP	a. Lighten anesthesia
	b. Volume/ Trendelenberg's position
	c. Phenylephrine, 50–100 μg I.V. or Ephedrine, 5–10 mg I.V.

tension (increased RPP) in patients who are thought to be adequately anesthetized. Nitroglycerin (50–100 μg/ml) or sodium nitroprusside (50–100 μg/ml) by intravenous infusion is the usual choice. We employ nitroglycerin as our first-line vasodilator to provide adequate blood pressure control.[100] Nitroglycerin's potential advantages include the following:

1. It has stood the test of time as effective therapy for myocardial ischemia.
2. There is no known toxicity in humans.
3. In commonly employed concentrations it is a milder drug and has less tendency to cause "overshoot" hypotension.
4. It is not thought to produce an "intracoronary steal" as reported with nitroprusside.[100–102]

We use nitroglycerin for the following indications:

1. Hypertension with a systolic blood pressure

20 percent above the highest recorded preoperative values.

2. Pulmonary capillary wedge pressure > 18 torr
3. Rate-pressure product $> 12,000$
4. Triple index (systolic blood pressure × heart rate × pulmonary capillary wedge pressure) $> 150,000$
5. Ischemic ST-segment changes on the electrocardiogram
6. Prinzmetal's angina

We have studied 20 patients during coronary artery surgery who became hypertensive with morphine, diazepam, nitrous oxide, and enflurane anesthesia. Nitroglycerin was administered at a mean dose of 80 μg/min (1 μg/kg/min), with a range of 32–128 μg/min. This produced a decrease in mean arterial pressure, central venous pressure, pulmonary capillary wedge pressure, mean pulmonary artery pressure, total peripheral resistance, pulmonary vascular resistance, and left ventricular stroke work index. The heart rate, cardiac index, and stroke index remain unchanged. Myocardial oxygen demand was decreased as measured by the rate-pressure product and tension-time index. Also, the endocardial viability ratio was increased, and 50 percent of the patients had significant improvement of their ST-segment depression on the electrocardiogram.[100]

Since nitroglycerin has less peripheral arterial effects than nitroprusside does, it may prove inadequate in managing severe hypertension in occasional patients. When this is true, we discontinue nitroglycerin and begin infusing nitroprusside. For nitroglycerin, infusion rates of 20–200 μg/min are commonly employed. Sodium nitroprusside in dosages as small as 10 μg/min can produce remarkable decreases in blood pressure. A dosage of 100 μg/min, in addition to an adequate background of anesthesia, usually provides adequate control of hypertension.[103] These are only approximate figures, and clinical situations may dictate the use of several times these concentrations and infusion rates. Curiously, it may be necessary to infuse additional volume to the patient while controlling the hypertension with a vasodilator.[103] Since these agents reduce preload as well as afterload, reflex tachycardia may result. This can be overcome by infusing volume to increase the filling pressure to an optimal level.

If the heart rate is rapid enough to produce myocardial ischemia (increased RPP), the depth of anesthesia is increased, and propranolol is administered in increments of 0.25–0.5 mg until adequate rate control is achieved. It is rare that such control requires more than a total of 2 mg of propranolol (Table 7–10).

Prevention of supraventricular tachyarrhythmias is important because they are poorly tolerated by the patient with coronary artery disease. A rapid heart rate leads to decreased coronary blood flow (resulting from inadequate diastolic filling time) and increased oxygen demand. Myocardial ischemia is frequently observed on the ECG shortly after the onset of such a rhythm disturbance. While surgical manipulation of the atrium and light anesthesia are the most common causes of this problem, the effects of all factors predisposing to the development of such rhythm disturbances are additive. Low serum potassium levels, hypovolemia, or hypervolemia, as well as several previously described pathological coronary anatomy patterns, enter into this problem.

In the patient with good ventricular func-

Table 7-10

Indications for intravenous propranolol during surgery
1. ST changes of ischemia associated with tachycardia
2. Atrial tachyarrhythmias > 120 per minute
3. Recurrent ventricular arrhythmias

Relative contraindications to propranolol
1. Cardiac failure
2. Chronic obstructive pulmonary disease

Guidelines for intravenous propranolol
1. Doses of 0.25–0.5 mg 1 to 2 minutes
2. Total dose, 2–3 mg

tion, the CVP can provide a rough index of vascular volume status. Once the pericardium is open, further estimates of heart function and volume status may be made by directly observing the heart. It is particularly important to become familiar with estimating cardiac performance and volume status by visual inspection. When the traction stitches applied to the pericardium are pulled taut, the heart is partially lifted out of the chest cavity. Partial kinking of the great veins may result, creating an artificial gradient between the superior vena caval and right atrial pressures. Since CVP catheters are generally placed in the superior vena cava, the CVP may be higher than the right atrial pressure as a result of this mechanical obstruction. Therefore, it is important to be able to recognize that if the CVP reading is elevated but the right atrium totally collapses with each heart beat, the CVP does not reflect the true filling pressure of the right heart. Patients who have normal atrial volumes seem better able to tolerate placement of the large venous cannulae (inserted via the right atrium into the inferior and superior venae cavae) than do hypovolemic patients.

Overdistention of the heart will produce myocardial ischemia by increasing ventricular wall tension. In patients with good left ventricular function, the CVP can be used to estimate the left ventricular filling pressure (LVFP). If ischemia occurs in association with an elevated CVP, a vasodilator such as nitroglycerin will frequently reduce the CVP (and the LVFP) and correct the ischemia. It must always be kept in mind, however, that the LVFP may become severely elevated without an observable change in the CVP.[104] Deep anesthesia with agents causing myocardial depression may produce elevated ventricular filling pressures. This ventricular dysfunction may be corrected by lightening the anesthetic.

Although a great deal of attention is paid to the prevention, detection, and control of myocardial ischemia during the prebypass period, other monitored parameters are not ignored. Frequent arterial blood samples are drawn for blood gas analysis, and ventilation is adjusted to produce normal Pa_{CO_2}. It is particularly important that the patient not be overventilated, since alkalosis not only decreases coronary artery blood flow but also impairs oxygen transfer to tissues by shifting the hemoglobin-oxygen dissociation curve to the left.[105,106] Adequate oxygenation is assured. Urine output is observed and, if inadequate, is treated *first* by ruling out mechanical problems, such as catheter kinking. If the catheter is patent, additional fluids or diuretics should be administered, or cardiac output should be increased.

Serum electrolytes, especially potassium, are important to monitor during the prebypass period. Even in patients who are not receiving digitalis preparations, it is our impression that hypokalemia is associated with a relatively high incidence of supraventricular rhythm disturbances during transatrial placement of caval cannulae. Particularly in patients maintained on diuretics preoperatively, elevation of serum potassium levels from low-normal (3.8 mEq/liter) to mid-normal (4.2 mEq/liter) seems to reduce the incidence of arrhythmias during cardiac manipulation.

Poor Left Ventricular Function Group

A significant number of patients undergoing myocardial revascularization have poor left ventricular function secondary to ischemic muscle damage. These patients usually have a history of previous myocardial infarctions and symptoms of congestive heart failure. Cardiac catheterization often demonstrates a depressed ejection fraction, an elevated LVEDP, and multiple areas of ventricular wall motion abnormalities (Table 7–3).

In patients with poor left ventricular function we most often induce anesthesia with morphine and diazepam in 5-mg increments. Morphine is the primary anesthetic in these patients, and the total dose is usually 0.5–1.5 mg/kg.[107] In those patients who tolerate it, 10 to 50 percent nitrous oxide is added for amnesia. In these sicker patients, however, nitrous oxide may act as more of a myocardial depressant and may not be tolerated by the cardiovascular system.[108] Pancuronium bromide is used as the muscle relaxant, since it stimulates the myocardium. Hypertension is less of a problem in these patients. Enflurane and halothane usually are not used in this group of patients, since these drugs may produce further myocardial depression. An adequate level of general anesthesia can be obtained in most cases using drugs that cause minimal cardiovascular depression, in a manner similar to the management of patients with valvular heart disease.

Stanley has recently shown that large doses of fentanyl can be used to anesthetize patients who have minimal cardiovascular reserve.[109] Doses as large as 100 μg/kg of fentanyl had minimal effects on blood pressure, filling pressure, and cardiac output. Fentanyl may have an advantage over morphine because it produces less venodilation. Addition of nitrous oxide to the fentanyl anesthetic produces decreases in blood pressure and cardiac output similar to those seen when nitrous oxide is added to a morphine anesthetic.

Part of the increased safety in the management of all patients has resulted from the use of sophisticated modern monitoring techniques. In patients with poor left ventricular function, a 7-Fr thermal dilution Swan-Ganz catheter is placed via the right internal jugular vein and positioned in the pulmonary artery (Table 7–11). It is important to be able to watch the pulmonary artery and pulmonary capillary wedge pressures, as well as the central venous pressure, in these patients. Thermal dilution cardiac output measurements are made at frequent intervals to monitor the status of the cardiovascular system. Using these monitoring techniques, it is possible to use the Starling curve to follow their cardiovascular function and response to therapeutic interventions. Therapy can be directed at either preload, afterload, or myocardial contractility. The use of the Starling curve is especially indicated in patients requiring either the intra-aortic balloon, vasodilators, or inotropic infusions (Chapter 3).

If hypertension occurs in these patients, it is frequently associated with an elevation in the PCWP.[103] This situation is aggressively treated with a vasodilator, since both ischemia and left ventricular failure may be produced. A typical patient's response to nitroglycerin is shown in Figure 7–5.[100] If left ventricular failure occurs, a drug that reduces afterload (nitroprusside or phentolamine) or a positive inotropic drug (CaCl$_2$ or dopamine) can be used to increase cardiac output and decrease the PCWP.

Nitroprusside and phentolamine are the preferred vasodilator drugs for patients with a low-output syndrome. They reduce afterload more than they reduce the preload, leading to an increase in cardiac output. Nitroglycerin frequently has the opposite effect, that is, a larger reduction in preload. All three drugs reduce pulmonary pressures; there is some evidence, however, that phentolamine may be the vasodilator most effective in the pulmonary circulation.

Hypotension is a more common occurrence in these patients than in those with good ventricular function. It is managed by decreasing the depth of anesthesia, including discontinuing nitrous oxide (amnesia can be supplied by giving scopolamine if desired). Further therapy depends on the cause of the hypotension. If the PCWP is low, volume is administered, and the patient is tilted into a head-down position. If hypotension is associated with bradycardia, atropine or ephedrine in small incremental doses

Table 7-11

Indications for Insertion of a Swan-Ganz
Catheter in Coronary Revascularization
Patients

1. LVEDP greater than 18 mm Hg
2. Ejection fraction less than 0.4
3. Significant abnormality of left ventricular wall motion
4. Recent myocardial infarction (within 3 months)
5. Postmyocardial infarction complications
   a. Ventricular septal defect
   b. Left ventricular aneurysm
   c. Mitral regurgitation (papillary muscle dysfunction)
   d. History of congestive heart failure or pulmonary edema
6. Associated mitral, aortic, or tricuspid valve lesions*

*Note: Not in tricuspid stenosis

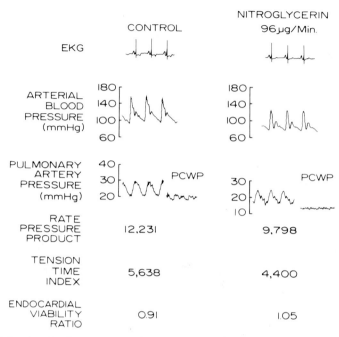

Fig. 7–5. A patient's response to nitroglycerin is demonstrated. The patient was undergoing coronary revascularization and when he became hypertensive developed an elevated wedge pressure. (Reproduced from Kaplan JA: Nitroglycerin infusion during coronary artery surgery. Anesthesiology 45:14, 1976, with permission of the author and publishers.)

is administered. Phenylephrine in 50–100-μg doses is used if the hypotension is due to peripheral vasodilation (decreased peripheral vascular resistance with an increased cardiac output). Positive inotropic drugs, such as calcium, digitalis, ephedrine, dopamine, or epinephrine, are used, with or without vasodilators, for varying degrees of heart failure.

A rapid heart rate can be just as detrimental to these patients as to those with good left ventricular function. Small incremental doses of propranolol are particularly useful in controlling and treating these supraventricular dysrhythmias. Propranolol, in small doses, is well tolerated by most patients, even those with relatively poor left ventricular function. It may be used: (1) as a primary mode of therapy, either to cause conversion to normal sinus rhythm or to slow the rate of a supraventricular tachycardia; (2) to provide rhythm stability and reduce the chance of recurrent dysrhythmias; or (3) prior to an attempt to cardiovert resistant dysrhythmias.

Electrocardioversion is the most rapidly ef-

fective method of converting rhythm disturbances that occur during atrial cannulation. Employing sterile internal defibrillator paddles, a current of 5 joules is applied directly to the atria. This is done immediately if hypotension accompanies the dysrhythmia. Attention is simultaneously given to determining what factors predisposed to the development of the dysrhythmia. If the patient is hypovolemic, volume is rapidly infused. Since the aortic cannula is generally in place at this time, the perfusionist can rapidly administer 100-ml increments of the priming solution from the cardiopulmonary bypass circuit. Hypervolemia is readily handled by allowing volume loss of 50–100 ml into the pericardium from the atriotomy site just prior to cannula insertion, or by vasodilator infusion.

Our recent experience at Emory University Hospital demonstrates that patients with severe left ventricular dysfunction can undergo coronary artery bypass grafting with good results.[110] Between October 1973 and June 1977, 188 patients were studied who had poor left ventricular function. An ejection fraction of less than 0.35 was present in 67 patients and 24 patients had ejection fractions of less than 0.20. A LVEDP greater than 20 mm Hg was present in 59 patients, unstable angina in 87 patients, congestive heart failure in 20 patients, and a previous myocardial infarction in 62 patients. Only 12 percent of the patients had normal segmental wall motion by angiography.

All the principles mentioned above were used in the management of these patients. There were 4 hospital deaths in the group (2.1 percent) and a perioperative infarction rate of 10 percent. Twenty percent of the patients required inotropic support after bypass, and 8 percent needed the intra-aortic balloon in the perioperative period. Follow-up at 16.5 months showed that 77 percent of the patients were free of angina, 17 percent had decreased angina, and 6 percent were worse or unchanged.

Kennedy et al. recently performed a comprehensive task analysis of the anesthetist's activities during coronary revascularization.[111] Time-lapse cinematography was used to record all activities. They found that 8 to 22 percent of the anesthetist's time was spent scanning the area, 11 to 22 percent observing the patient, 10 to 17 percent mixing or administering drugs, 8 to 17 percent observing monitors, 7 to 16 percent preparing the patient for anesthesia and transfer, and 10 to 15 percent recording data. The time spent looking away from the patient or surgical field was 28 to 33 percent of the total time. An automated monitoring and recording system which would allow the anesthetist to apportion more of his time to direct patient care would be useful in these high-risk patients.

MANAGEMENT OF CARDIOPULMONARY BYPASS FOR CORONARY ARTERY SURGERY

This section focuses on aspects of cardiopulmonary bypass (CPB) that are unique for the coronary patient. For a complete discussion of CPB, see Chapter 12.

All anesthetic administration is discontinued as cardiopulmonary bypass is begun. The patient remains asleep from residual nitrous oxide, enflurane or halothane, narcotics, tranquilizers, and scopolamine. Once an adequate total perfusion is established, ventilation is discontinued, 5 to 10 cm of static positive airway pressure is maintained, and any further anesthetic is administered by intravenous or "inhalational" routes through the oxygenator system.

In patients with good left ventricular function who have received minimal doses of morphine and diazepam, enflurane or halothane is administered after an adequate perfusion has been established. These are provided to the pump oxygenator via a calibrated vaporizer. The concentration that maintains the lightest possible level of anesthesia compatible with a perfusion pressure between 60 and 100 torr is used. Hypotension during bypass is managed by discontinuing the anesthetic drug, increasing the pump flow, and/or giving 100 μg of phenylephrine. Hypertension (blood pressure greater than 100 torr) is managed by increasing the anesthetic concentration and, if needed, by adding either nitroglycerin, nitroprusside, phentolamine (0.5–1.0 mg), or chlorpromazine (1–2 mg).

Potent inhalation agents should be discontinued 15 minutes before terminating cardiopulmonary bypass to remove their negative inotropic effects. If sedation is needed, diazepam (2.5–5 mg) or scopolamine (0.2 mg) can be given intravenously.

Patients with poor left ventricular function who have received large doses of morphine and diazepam rarely require enflurane or halothane during bypass. If they become vasoconstricted, however, with a mean arterial blood pressure greater than 100 torr, enflurane, halothane or a vasodilator drug may be used to produce vasodilation.

A variety of techniques are used by cardiac surgeons to protect the myocardium while performing coronary revascularization. The heart must be immobilized to permit operation. This may be accomplished by: (1) inducing ventricular fibrillation, either electrically or by systemic or local hypothermia; or (2) producing anoxic arrest by cross-clamping the ascending aorta to interrupt coronary blood flow.

Which method or combination of methods provides the most acceptable myocardial preservation is the subject of much debate. We will dwell briefly on some contrasts among these methods and their variations, as anesthetic management may need to be altered to fit prevailing surgical methodology. During ventricular fibrillation, coronary blood flow can be maintained to some degree. The nondistended fibrillating heart uses considerable oxygen, approximately 80 percent of that used by the beating heart of an individual at rest.[112] Even with coronary flow maintained, subendocardial perfusion is often compromised, and ischemia can result. Systemic and topical hypothermia produce additional reductions in MVO$_2$, but the threat of subendocardial ischemia persists. Fibrillation maintained by an electrical device rather than by hypothermia is associated with a greater amount of subendocardial ischemia.[113]

Some surgeons perform the proximal vein graft anastamoses to the aorta prior to CPB, utilizing a partially occluding aortic clamp to allow anastomosis. This maneuver effectively narrows the ascending aorta, mechanically increasing left ventricular afterload. While not generally hazardous to patients with good ventricular function, it can produce sudden, profound ventricular failure in patients with poor left ventricular function. Should this occur, vasodilators can be effective in treating this failure. In extreme situations, the surgeon may need to remove the aortic clamp and reapply it to include a smaller "bite" of the aorta within its jaws.

Ischemic arrest by aortic cross-clamping is another method of immobilizing the heart during coronary surgery. Although this method produces *anoxia* rather than ischemia, the addition of systemic and myocardial hypothermia and intracoronary cardioplegic solutions can reduce MVO$_2$ to very low levels in the decompressed heart.[114] (See Chapter 12).

Miller surveyed 400 cardiac surgeons to determine the surgical techniques they were using in 1975.[115] Ninety-four percent of the surgeons were using disposable bubble oxygenators, while only 6 percent routinely used a membrane oxygenator during coronary artery bypass graft (CABG) surgery. The majority of surgeons (87 percent) used anoxic arrest of the heart during distal coronary artery anastomosis. However, 11 percent used ventricular fibrillation, and 0.3 percent kept the heart beating on bypass. The techniques used to minimize myocardial injury during anoxic arrest were systemic hypothermia (86 percent), profound topical hypothermia (55 percent), potassium-induced cardioplegia (6 percent), and systemic steroids (38 percent). Since this survey was completed in 1975, many more surgeons are now using cardioplegia, and fewer are allowing the heart to remain in fibrillation.

Miller found that 39 percent of the surgeons were performing the proximal aortic anastomoses prior to CPB.

On completion of coronary artery revascularization, the patient is rewarmed to 37°C, and the heart is defibrillated with 10-40 watt-sec if spontaneous defibrillation does not occur. Blood samples are taken to ensure that the pH is normal and that the serum potassium level is between 4 and 4.5 mEq/liter. If large amounts of potassium cardioplegic solution are used, it may be necessary to administer NaHCO$_3$, CaCl$_2$, or 50 percent glucose and insulin to reestablish electrical conduction and myocardial function.

The surgeon carefully removes any air from the cardiac chambers, and the aortic root is vented. The left ventricular sump is removed from the right superior pulmonary vein, and a left atrial line is placed through this pulmonary vein in patients with poor left ventricular function. In patients with bradycardia or heart block, atrial or ventricular pacemaker wires are inserted.

The pump flow is gradually reduced while observing the heart, arterial and venous pressure, and ECG. All seven leads of the ECG are recorded and examined. Adequacy of volume is judged by the central venous pressure in patients with good left ventricular function or by either the left atrial pressure or pulmonary capillary wedge pressure in patients with poor left ventricular function.

Usually, bypass is easily discontinued over a 5- to 15-minute period of time. After cardiopulmonary bypass, anesthesia is used as required. Nitrous oxide is usually adequate in 20 to 50 percent concentrations, but enflurane or halothane may be added if blood pressure is stable in patients with good left ventricular function. The transition to the intensive care unit can be eased by continuing this anesthetic until just before moving and at that time adding a small dose of morphine (2-5 mg). Monitoring of the blood pressure and the electrocardiogram is continued during the transfer to the intensive care unit, and the patient is ventilated with 100 percent oxygen.

In patients with poor left ventricular function, an inotropic agent will occasionally be required to support function while cardiopulmonary bypass is discontinued. Calcium chloride (500-1000 mg) is a preferred drug, since cardiopulmonary bypass is associated with a decrease in ionized calcium. If calcium does not produce an adequate result, then either a dopamine infusion (5–10 μg/kg/min) or an epinephrine infusion (4–8 μg/min) is begun. The choice between these two agents depends on the blood pressure, heart rate, cardiac rhythm, urine output, and peripheral perfusion. In those patients with a severe low-output state after bypass, a positive inotropic drug is used along with a vasodilator (nitroglycerin or nitroprusside) to decrease the left ventricular wall tension (preload and afterload). If this is unsuccessful, then an intra-aortic counterpulsation balloon is employed. These patients must be sedated with drugs such as morphine that do not further depress the heart (see Chapters 12 and 13).

In the postanesthetic period, hypertension is again a major problem in patients with good left ventricular function.[116,117] Morphine and nitroglycerin are used to control this in most patients, and diazoxide, nitroprusside, phentolamine or chlorpromazine is used in resistant patients. The patients are usually mechanically ventilated via the endotracheal tube until the next morning, using either assisted ventilation or intermittent mandatory ventilation with positive end-expiratory pressure as required. The majority of patients are extubated the next morning after meeting the criteria of normal arterial blood gas values and minute ventilation, a vital capacity greater than 15 ml/kg, and an inspiratory force of greater than −25 cm H_2O.

Recently, many patients with good left ventricular function have been extubated within 6 hours of surgery.[118] We have found this to be safe and strongly appreciated by these otherwise healthy patients. Prior to extubation, the patients are awake and alert; meet the usual respiratory criteria for extubation, including adequate blood gases; are not bleeding more than 100 ml/hr; are normothermic; and are receiving no cardiac drugs.

SPECIAL PROBLEMS

Prinzmetal's Angina (Variant Angina)

In Prinzmetal's angina pain occurs with the patient at rest or during ordinary activity. It is not produced by vigorous exertion. During an attack, the ECG shows ST-segment elevation.[11]

This syndrome is thought to be caused by coronary artery spasm. Variant angina with a normal coronary arteriogram is treated medically with nitrates, since it has been shown that nitroglycerin promptly relieves the attacks. Patients have a varied response to propranolol, with some improving, while others get more frequent attacks.[119] Alpha-blocking agents are also effective in some patients.

Coronary revascularization is performed only in those patients who also have a fixed obstructive lesion. Reported surgical results have not been as good as in patients with classic angina pectoris, however. Weiner reported surgical results in 18 patients.[119A] Nine patients improved (50 percent), while 5 were unchanged (28 percent) and 4 died (22 percent). Four of the 18 patients had perioperative infarctions.

We manage these patients using the same techniques discussed earlier in this chapter. The one significant difference is the continuous use of intravenous nitroglycerin throughout the surgical procedure and the immediate postoperative period. This technique has seemed to help prevent attacks during surgery and has helped smooth the operative course.

Left Main Coronary Artery Disease

Left main coronary artery disease is the one form of coronary artery disease in which CABG has definitely been shown to be of benefit. Surgery will prolong the life of most of these patients. About 15 percent of patients with symptomatic coronary artery disease have significant obstruction of the left main coronary artery (LMCA). These patients frequently have severe myocardial ischemia, with very unstable angina, marked ST-segment changes with exertion, and left ventricular "paralysis" (acute heart failure) with pain.

Some authors have claimed that these patients are at greatly increased risk during CABG, especially during the anesthetic induction.[120] Cooper has even recommended the prophylactic preoperative insertion of the intra-aortic balloon in these patients.[121] We do not believe this is indicated.

These patients must be managed very carefully during anesthesia and surgery, since the margin for error is smaller than in other patients, and the entire left ventricle is potentially in jeopardy. In the past 30 months, we have operated on 101 patients with left main coronary artery disease.[122] The hospital mortality was 2 percent, and the perioperative infarction rate was only 3 percent. The intra-aortic balloon was used in only 1 patient before bypass (Chapter 13).

The following principles can be used in the care of these patients:

Surgical
1. Standard saphenous vein bypasses.
2. Infrequent use of the internal mammary artery for coronary revascularization.
3. Good myocardial preservation combining systemic hypothermia (28°C) with hypothermic, hyperkalemic, hyperosmolar cardioplegic solution. The myocardial temperature should be maintained between 15° and 18°C.
4. Infrequent use of the intra-aortic balloon—needed in about 4 percent of our left main coronary artery disease patients after bypass.

Anesthetic
1. Avoid increases in oxygen demand and treat them aggressively if they do occur.

$$RPP > 12,000$$

   (a) ↑ BP—intravenous nitroglycerin
   (b) ↑ HR—propranolol

2. Avoid decreases in blood pressure, which are very poorly tolerated by these patients.

   (a) Systolic BP < 90 mm Hg ⎤ phenylephrine
   (b) Mean BP < 65 mm Hg ⎦

3. Monitor V_5 ECG lead for ST-segment changes.
4. Monitor the RPP continuously.
5. Measure the PCWP frequently during surgery, looking for signs of left ventricular failure—maintain the PCWP at 12–15 mm Hg or less. Increase the dose of nitroglycerin if the PCWP starts rising.
6. Maintain propranolol at full dose in the preoperative period. It may be necessary to *increase* the dose prior to surgery.

Recent Myocardial Infarction

There is considerable controversy regarding the best management of patients with persistent or recurrent chest pain following an acute myocardial infarction. Medical treatment has been associated with a high mortality. Counterpulsation with the IABP has been used to manage some of these patients.[123] Historically, CABG in these patients has been attended by a high mortality.[124] As a result of the advances in CABG, several groups, including our own, have recently taken a cautious approach in redefining those patients at greatest risk and operating upon those with the greatest potential for preservation of life.

In the past 2 years, we have operated upon 35 patients with resistant chest pain shortly after an acute infarction (within 30 days).[125] Ten patients had surgery within 24 hours of infarction; 9 patients, within 1 to 7 days; and 16 patients 8 to 30 days after the infarct. Transmural infarctions were present in 16 patients and subendocardial infarctions in 19 patients. The mean ejection fraction was 0.43, and wall motion abnormalities were present in 27 patients. Four patients had left main coronary artery disease, and 28 patients had obstruction of the left anterior descending coronary artery. The operative and anesthetic techniques used were identical to those described above for left main coronary artery disease. There were no hospital deaths in this group of patients. Inotropic drugs were required in 14 percent of patients, lidocaine in 14 percent, and the IABP in 20 percent. There were no late deaths in a 10-month period. Although it may be argued that more persistent medical therapy might have been effective in controlling pain, arrhythmias, and reduced cardiac output, our present opinion is that total revascularization can be accomplished safely and offers the best chance of minimizing myocardial damage in selected patients.

Complicated Myocardial Infarctions

Included in this definition are patients who develop an acute ventricular septal defect (VSD), mitral regurgitation (MR), and/or cardiogenic shock (CS). In most cases, we have tried not to operate on these patients while they are in CS. Invasive hemodynamic monitoring is used to guide maximal medical therapy with afterload—reducing agents, inotropes, antiarrhythmics, and the IABP. Nitroprusside has been shown to improve these patients significantly by decreasing left-to-right shunting or mitral regurgitation and by reducing preload and afterload.[126,127]

Almost all of these patients have the IABP used during surgery. The anesthetic technique involves extensive monitoring, continued medical therapy, and coordination of the hemodynamic effects of the cardiac drugs and IABP with the anesthetic agents used for patients with poor left ventricular function.[107] Even in the best reported series, these patients still have a mortality approaching 50 percent.[128] If the patients can be stabilized preoperatively for days to weeks utilizing medical therapy, then the surgical results are much better.

In patients with a VSD, it should be remembered that right and left ventricular cardiac outputs are markedly different. Cardiac outputs measured by using the Swan-Ganz catheter and the thermal dilution technique are those of the right ventricle. The amount of the left-to-right shunt and the left heart cardiac output can be calculated from the measured oxygen contents of systemic arterial, right atrial, and pulmonary artery blood.[129]

Combined Coronary and Valvular Heart Disease

Coronary artery disease is frequently found during the evaluation of patients with valvular heart disease. Angiographic studies have demonstrated significant CAD in over 25 percent of patients with aortic valve disease.[130] Because of the younger age of patients with mitral valve disease, associated CAD appears to be less common. In addition, acute mitral regurgitation or papillary muscle dysfunction occurs with myocardial infarctions in older patients. When a correctable coronary artery lesion is diagnosed preoperatively, surgical treatment includes CABG along with valve replacement or repair.

Loop reported a series of 50 patients who had combined procedures.[131] Aortic valve replacement and CABG were performed in 29 patients with 2 hospital deaths. Mitral valve operations with CABG were reported in 21 patients with 2 hospital deaths. The etiology was related to rheumatic heart disease in 14 patients and to ischemic papillary muscle dysfunction in 7. The overall 8 percent operative mortality compares favorably with the risk of valve surgery alone.

Patients with tight aortic stenosis (gradient >80 mm Hg) and CAD present an anesthetic challenge. Myocardial ischemia results from coronary obstruction as well as left ventricular hypertrophy, both contributing causes of increased myocardial oxygen demand. Further increases in oxygen demand must be prevented. Vasodilators can be very useful in these patients to control blood pressure and PCWP, but they must be used *very cautiously* to avoid severe peripheral vasodilation with its attendant hypotension.

Nitroprusside is very useful in patients with aortic or mitral insufficiency. It has been shown to increase cardiac output and reduce mitral regurgitation.[126] The coronary perfusion pressure must be maintained at adequate levels, however. Patients with chronic mitral regurgitation resulting from rheumatic heart disease are usually easier to manage than those with acute mitral insufficiency secondary to ischemic heart disease.

Combined Carotid and Coronary Artery Disease

Atherosclerosis is a generalized disease, and therefore it is to be expected that a significant number of patients will have disease of both the carotid and coronary arteries. Mehigan reported that 12 percent of 874 consecutive patients for CABG had either an asymptomatic carotid bruit (63 patients), a symptomatic carotid bruit (37 patients), or a positive history of a transient ischemic attack or stroke (5 patients).[29] Abnormal arteriograms were found in 49 of the 874 patients (5.6 percent).

We believe that all patients with a carotid bruit or a strongly positive neurological history should have carotid angiography before undergoing CABG. If a significant lesion is discovered, a decision has to be made as to how to approach the coexistent disease.

We agree with Mehigan that patients with relatively stable angina should have the carotid surgery first as a separate operative procedure. This requires good anesthetic management to avoid myocardial ischemia and/or cardiovascular dysfunction. The same monitoring and anesthetic principles should be used as if the patient were having CABG. At the same time, the cerebral circulation needs to be protected. Therefore, we try to maintain the blood pressure in the patient's upper normal range and the

Paco$_2$ between 30 and 35 torr. An internal shunt is used in all cases. Thiopental and steroids can be used to help prevent cerebral ischemic damage. In addition, we ensure that a perfusionist is available in the unlikely event that coronary revascularization would have to be performed as an urgent procedure. Neither in Mehigan's study nor in our experience has this eventuality occurred.

In poor-risk or unstable coronary patients, we perform both operations in a combined procedure. The carotid endarterectomy is performed first in an effort to allow maximal cerebral perfusion on cardiopulmonary bypass. This is followed by a standard coronary artery procedure. Fortunately, maintaining a normal blood pressure and Paco$_2$ is good for both circulations, and the principles of anesthesia for CABG suffice for the combined procedure.

Endocrine or Metabolic Problems

Diabetes mellitus is frequently present in patients with CAD. Dortimer has recently shown that their CAD is no more diffuse or inoperable than in nondiabetic patients.[132] Previously, it has been shown that there is no difference in either the operative or late mortality rates between diabetic and control patients.[133] Postoperative infections were shown to be more common in diabetic patients; therefore, sterile techniques should be strictly maintained.

Blood sugar measurements are made along with each arterial blood gas analysis during surgery. The blood sugar is maintained between 100 and 300 mg/100 ml by administering approximately 100 ml/hr of 5 percent dextrose in water and intermittent doses (5 units) of regular insulin. The arterial pH and serum K$^+$ levels are also monitored closely in these patients. NaHCO$_3$ and KCl administration is guided by these values.

Surgical or medical ablation of the thyroid gland is an old treatment for patients with severe angina pectoris. Therefore, patients with severe CAD and untreated myxedema present for coronary revascularization.[34] At Emory, over 200 patients have had thyroid ablations for intractable angina; 52 of these patients have undergone cardiac catheterization, and in the past 18 months, 6 patients have had CABG. These patients have all been severely hypothyroid at the

time of surgery, since preoperative thyroid replacement therapy increased their angina. In addition, they were taking propranolol to further decrease their oxygen demands. Much to our surprise, these patients have tolerated anesthesia with morphine, diazepam, nitrous oxide, and pancuronium quite well. While the patient is on cardiopulmonary bypass, we have begun thyroid replacement therapy intravenously with 50 μg of *l*-thyroxine. Within 15 minutes, a dramatic increase in cardiac activity has been observed. Paine et al. reported on 4 patients with CAD and myxedema who also had good surgical results.[34]

Coronary revascularization is now also being reported in selected patients with chronic renal failure who are maintained on hemodialysis.[134–136] The authors feel that CABG can be successfully performed in this group of patients with minimally increased operative risk. The patients have been vigorously dialyzed prior to surgery and in the immediate postoperative period in order to maintain normal fluid and electrolyte balance. Posner has reviewed the anesthetic considerations in patients with renal failure undergoing cardiopulmonary bypass.[137] The problems include protecting the arteriovenous fistula, cannulating previously used arteries and veins, maintaining fluid and electrolyte balance, correcting anemia, altering the response to anesthetic agents, managing hypertension, and treating coagulopathies.

PROTECTION OF THE ISCHEMIC MYOCARDIUM

Research in cardiac metabolism over the past decade has resulted in new techniques to protect the ischemic myocardium. The key concept is that at the time of a myocardial infarction there is a central zone of necrotic tissue that is surrounded by a zone of "jeopardized" myocardium.[138] The jeopardized myocardium, which is also called the "twilight zone," is *reversibly* damaged by the initial ischemia. It may either become necrotic tissue if the ischemia progresses or recover if the ischemia is reversed. Survival of this tissue depends on the balance between coronary blood flow (nutrient and oxygen supply) and myocardial oxygen and energy consumption.[139] Pharmacologic and mechanical interventions may alter this delicate balance.

Studies by Hillis, Maroko, and Braunwald have identified interventions that increase or decrease myocardial injury after coronary-artery occlusion in animals.[140] They have also performed similar studies in patients with acute myocardial infarctions. A summary of these studies is included in their recent review article on myocardial ischemia.[1]

Hillis and Braunwald state that myocardial injury may be *increased* by the following factors:

1. Increasing myocardial oxygen demand with isoproterenol, glucagon, tachycardia, or fever;
2. Decreasing myocardial oxygen supply either directly (hypoxia or anemia) or indirectly (hypotension and reduced coronary perfusion pressure with hemorrhage or possibly with nitroprusside);[101] or
3. Decreasing substrate availability (hypoglycemia).

Myocardial injury may be *reduced* by:

1. Decreasing myocardial oxygen demand with propranolol, nitroglycerin, aortic counterpulsation, or digitalis in the failing heart;
2. Increasing myocardial oxygen supply either directly (coronary revascularization) or indirectly (aortic counterpulsation, elevated coronary perfusion pressure, or mannitol);
3. Increasing anaerobic metabolism with glucose, insulin, and potassium mixtures; or
4. Decreasing autolysis with corticosteroids.

THE VALUE OF CORONARY BYPASS SURGERY

Despite a decade of experience with CABG, indications for its use and benefits from it are still highly controversial. This controversy has been stirred anew by the results of the Veterans Administration's preliminary data on stable angina[141] and the NIH study of unstable angina.[142] Preston has written a highly critical textbook asking, "Is coronary artery surgery in the best interest of the patient?"[143] He examines the therapeutic decision-making process with respect to the effect of psychological and placebo factors, economic incentives, professional needs of physicians, and emotional needs of patients.

The controversy is most clearly stated in two recent articles from the Baylor College of Medicine. McIntosh (cardiologist) states that the controversy persists because of a lack of adequately controlled studies.[7] He says that "available data in the literature do not indicate that initial symptomatic improvement necessarily persists, or that myocardial infarction, arrhythmias, or congestive heart failure will be prevented, or that life will be prolonged in the vast majority of operated patients."

However, Debakey (surgeon) feels that the indications for CABG are well established.[144] He states that "the insistence on the use of prospective randomized studies for the evaluation of surgical diagnostic and therapeutic techniques reflects a naive obsession with this research tool."

We believe that the data available support the view that CABG is needed to relieve angina in some patients.[145] Also, there is adequate evidence that coronary revascularization prolongs life in carefully selected subsets of patients. These subsets include patients with left main coronary artery disease and double or triple vessel disease.[146] Results in patients with single vessel disease are still pending.

With the present state of the art in 1978, we believe that both medical and surgical therapy have a place in managing patients with severe coronary artery disease. But while medical treatment with nitrates and β-blocking drugs produces beneficial results by decreasing myocardial oxygen demand, coronary artery surgery produces its beneficial results by directly increasing coronary blood flow.

REFERENCES

1. Hillis LD, Braunwald E: Myocardial ischemia. N Engl J Med 296:971, 1977
2. Norman JC (ed): (Foreword) Coronary artery medical and surgical concepts and controversies. New York, Appleton-Century-Crofts, 1975
3. Rogers DE, Blendon RJ: The changing American health scene—sometimes things get better. JAMA 237:1710, 1977
4. DiGirolamo M, Schlant RC: Etiology of coronary atherosclerosis. *In* Hurst JW, Logue RB (eds): The Heart (ed 4). New York, McGraw-Hill, 1978, pp 1103–1121
5. Akins CW, Mundth ED, Austen WG: Coronary artery surgery: The state of the art. *In* Nyhus LM (ed): Surgery Annual—1977. New York, Appleton-Century-Crofts, 1977, pp 251–318

6. Favaloro RG: Saphenous vein autograft replacement of severe segmental coronary artery occlusion: Operation technique. Ann Thorac Surg 5:334, 1968

7. McIntosh, HD, Garcia JA: The first decade of aortocoronary bypass grafting, 1967–1977—Review. Circulation 57:405, 1978

8. Epstein SE, Redwood DR, Goldstein RE, et al: Angina pectoris: Pathophysiology, evaluation and treatment. Ann Intern Med 75:263, 1971

9. Hurst JW, Logue RB, Walter PF: The clinical recognition and management of coronary atherosclerotic heart disease. In Hurst JW, Logue RB (eds): The Heart (ed 4). New York, McGraw-Hill, 1978, pp 1156–1290

10. Hurst JW, King SB: Definitions and classification of coronary atherosclerotic heart disease. In Hurst JW, Logue RB (eds): The Heart (ed 4). New York, McGraw-Hill, 1978, pp 1094–1102

11. Prinzmetal M, Kennamer R, Merliss R, et al: Angina pectoris I. A variant form of angina pectoris. Am J Med 27:235, 1959

12. Higgins CB, Wexler L, Silverman JF, et al: Clinical and arteriographic features of Prinzmetal's variant angina: documentation and etiologic factors. Am J Cardiol 37:831, 1976

13. Criteria Committee of the New York Heart Association, Inc: Diseases of the Heart and Blood Vessels (Nomenclature and Criteria for Diagnosis) (ed 6). Boston, Little, Brown, 1964

14. Benchimol A, Harris CL, Desser KB, et al: Resting electrocardiogram in major coronary artery disease. JAMA 224:1489, 1973

15. Einthoven W: Weiters über des elektrokardiogram. Arch Ges Phisiol Menschen Thiere 122:517, 1908

16. Bruce RA, Irving JB: Exercise electrocardiography. In Hurst JW, Logue RB (eds), The Heart (ed 4). New York, McGraw-Hill, 1978, pp 336–348

17. Ellestad MH: Stress Testing—Principles and Practice. Philadelphia, F. A. Davis, 1975, p 36

18. Robinson BF: Relation of heart rate and systolic blood pressure to the onset of pain in angina pectoris. Circulation 35: 1073, 1967

19. Master AM: The two-step exercise electrocardiogram: A test for coronary insufficiency. Ann Intern Med 32:842, 1950

20. Sones FM, Jr, Shirey EK: Cine coronary arteriography. Mod Concepts Cardiovasc Dis 31:735, 1962

21. Greene DG, Carlisle R, Grant C, et al: Estimation of left ventricular volume by one-plane cineangiography. Circulation 35:61, 1967

22. Shuford WH, Hurst JW: Fluoroscopic examination of the heart and great vessels. In Hurst JW, Logue RB (eds): The Heart (ed 4). New York, McGraw-Hill, 1978, pp 378–381

23. Alderman EL: Angiographic indicators of left ventricular function. JAMA 236:1055, 1976

24. Dumesnil JG, Ritman EL, George DP, et al: Regional left ventricular wall dynamics before and after sublingual administration of nitroglycerin. Am J Cardiol 36:419, 1975

25. McAnulty JH, Hattenhaur MT, Rösch J, et al: Improvement in left ventricular wall motion following nitroglycerin. Circulation 51:140, 1975

26. Wexler LF, Pohost GM: Hemodynamic monitoring: Noninvasive techniques. Anesthesiology 45:156, 1976

27. James TN: Anatomy of the coronary arteries and veins. In Hurst JW, Logue RB (eds): The Heart (ed 4). New York, McGraw-Hill, 1978, pp 32–47

28. Goldmann DA, Hopkins CC, Karchmer AW, et al: Cephalothin prophylaxis in cardiac valve surgery: A prospective, double-blind comparison of two-day and six-day regimens. J Thorac Cardiovasc Surg 93:470, 1977

29. Mehigan JT, Burch WS, Pipkin RD, et al: A planned approach to coexistant cerebrovascular disease in coronary artery bypass candidates. Arch Surg 112:1403, 1977

30. Reis RL, Hannah H III: Management of patients with coexistent coronary artery and peripheral vascular disease. J Thorac Cardiovasc Surg 73:909, 1977

31. McCabe JC, Abel RM, Subramanian VA, et al: Complications of intra-aortic balloon insertion and counterpulsation. Circulation 57:770, 1978

32. Crawford FA Jr, Selby JH Jr, Bower JD, et al: Coronary revascularization in patients maintained on chronic hemodialysis. Circulation 56:684, 1977

33. Bregman D, Bailin M, Bowman FO, et al: A pulsatile assist device (PAD) for use during cardiopulmonary bypass. Ann Thorac Surg 24:574, 1977

34. Paine TD, Rogers WJ, Baxley WA, et al: Coronary arterial surgery in patients with incapacitating angina pecotris and myxedema. Am J Cardiol 40:226, 1977

35. Logue RB, King SB, Douglas JS: A practical approach to coronary artery disease, with special reference to coronary bypass surgery. In Harvey WP (ed): Current Problems in Cardiology, vol. 1. Chicago, Year Book Medical Publishers, 1976

36. Reichek N: Long-acting nitrates in the treatment of angina pectoris. JAMA 236:1399, 1976

37. Davidov M, Mroczek W: The effect of nitroglycerin ointment on exercise capacity in patients with angina pectoris. Presented at American

College of Pharmacology Meeting, Washington, D.C., April 1977

38. Reichek N, Goldstein RE, Redwood DR, et al: Sustained effects of nitroglycerin ointment in patients with angina pectoris. Circulation 50:348, 1974

39. Hardarson T, Henning H, O'Rourke RA: Prolonged salutary effects of isosorbide dinitrate and nitroglycerin ointment on regional left ventricular function. Am J Cardiol 40:90, 1977

40. Schrumpf JD, Sheps DS, Wolfson S, et al: Altered hemoglobin-oxygen affinity with long-term propranolol therapy in patients with coronary artery disease. Am J Cardiol 40:76, 1977

41. Nies AS, Shand DG: Clinical pharmacology of propranolol. Circulation 52:6, 1975

42. Evans GH, Shand DG: The disposition of propranolol. Independent variation in steady state circulatory drug concentration and half-life as a result of plasma binding in man. Clin Pharmacol Ther 14:494, 1973

43. Faulkner SL, Hopkins JT, Boerth RC, et al: Time required for complete recovery from chronic propranolol therapy. N Engl J Med 289:607, 1973

44. Viljoen JF, Estafanous FG, Kellner GA: Propranolol and cardiac surgery. J Thorac Cardiovasc Surg 64:826, 1972

45. Pantano JA, Lee Y: Abrupt propranolol withdrawal and myocardial contractility. Arch Intern Med 136:867, 1976

46. Kaplan JA, Dunbar RW, Bland JW, et al: Propranolol and cardiac surgery: A problem for the anesthesiologists? Anesth Analg 54:571, 1975

47. Jones EL, Kaplan JA, Dorney ER, et al: Propranolol therapy in patients undergoing myocardial revascularization. Am J Cardiol 38:696, 1976

48. Romagnoli A, Keats AS: Plasma and atrial propranolol after preoperative withdrawal. Circulation 52:1123, 1975

49. Beller GA, Smith TW, Abelmann WH: Digitalis intoxication: A prospective clinical study with serum level correlations. N Engl J Med 284:989, 1971

50. Coltart DJ, Chamberlain DA, Howard MR, et al: Effect of cardiopulmonary bypass on plasma digoxin concentrations. Br Heart J 33:334, 1971

51. Beiser GD, Epstein SE, Goldstein RE, et al: Comparison of the peak inotropic effects of a catecholamine and a digitalis glycoside in the intact canine heart. Circulation 42:805, 1970

52. Johnson LW, Dickstein RA, Fruehan CT, et al: Prophylactic digitalization for coronary artery bypass surgery. Circulation 53:819, 1976

53. Smith TW, Haber E: Digitalis (first of four parts). N Engl J Med 289:945, 1973

54. Smith TW, Haber E: Digitalis (third of four parts). N Engl J Med 289:1063, 1973

55. Tarazi RC, Frohlich ED, Dustan HP: Plasma volume in men with essential hypertension. N Engl J Med 278:762, 1968

56. Cohn LH, Moore FD, Collins JJ: Intrinsic plasma volume deficits in patients with coronary artery disease. Arch Surg 108:57, 1974

57. Spann JF, Hurst JW: Treatment of heart failure. In Hurst JW, Logue RB (eds): The Heart (ed 4). New York, McGraw-Hill, 1978, pp 580–606

58. Gunnells JC Jr, Orgain ES, McGuffin WL: Treatment of systemic hypertension. In Hurst JW, Logue RB (eds): The Heart (ed 4). New York, McGraw-Hill, 1978, pp 1435–1455

59. Gorlin R, Herman MV: Physiology of the coronary circulation. In Hurst JW, Logue RB (eds): The Heart (ed 4). New York, McGraw-Hill, 1978, pp 101–107

60. Braunwald E: Control of myocardial oxygen consumption. Am J Cardiol 27:416, 1971

61. Rohde E: Über den einfluss der mechanischen bendinungen auf die tatigkeit und den sauerstoffverbruche der warmblutenherzens. Naunyn-Schmiedenberg Arch Exp Pathol Pharmacol 68:401, 1912

62. Kaplan JA, King SB: The precordial electrocardiographic lead (V_5) in patients who have coronary artery disease. Anesthesiology 45:570, 1976

63. Blackburn H, Taylor HL, Okamoto N, et al: The exercise electrocardiogram: a systematic comparison of chest lead configurations employed for monitoring during exercise. In Karlomen M (ed): Physical Activity and the Heart. Springfield, Ill, Charles C Thomas, 1966

64. Mason RE, Likar I, Biern RO, et al: Multiple lead exercise electrocardiography. Circulation 36:517, 1967

65. Redwood DR, Epstein SE: Use and limitations of stress testing in the evaluation of ischemic heart disease. Circulation 46:1115, 1972

66. Robertson D, Kostuk WT, Ahuja SP: The localization of coronary artery stenosis by 12-lead ECG response to graded exercise test. Am Heart J 91:437, 1976

67. Reves JG, Samuelson PN, Younes HJ, et al: Anesthetic considerations for coronary artery surgery. Anesthesiol Rev, pp 19–31, August 1977

68. Gilbert CA: Temperature and humidity, radiation, underwater environment, hyperbaric oxygen, and the cardiovascular system. In Hurst JW, Logue RB (eds), The Heart (ed 4). New York, McGraw-Hill, 1978, pp 1829–1836

69. Lowenstein E: Personal communication, 1977

70. Swan HJC: Central venous pressure monitoring

is an outmoded procedure of limited practical value. *In* Ingelfinger FJ, Ebert RV, Finland M, et al (eds): Controversy in Internal Medicine II. Philadelphia, WB Saunders, 1974, pp 185–193

71. Loeb HS, Saudye A, Croke RP et al: Effects of pharmacologically-induced hypertension on myocardial ischemia and coronary hemodynamics in patients with fixed coronary obstruction. Circulation 57:41, 1978

72. Gobel FL, Nordstrom LA, Nelson RR, et al: The rate-pressure product as an index of myocardial oxygen consumption during exercise in patients with angina pectoris. Circulation 57:549, 1978

73. Hoffman JIE, Buckberg GD: Regional myocardial ischemia—causes, prediction and prevention. Vasc Surg 8:115, 1974

74. Philips PA, Marty AT, Miyamoto AM, et al: A clinical method for detecting subendocardial ischemia after cardiopulmonary bypass. J Thorac Cardiovasc Surg 69:30, 1975

75. Kaplan JA, Jones EL: Monitoring of myocardial ischemia during coronary artery surgery, abstracted. Presented at the American Society of Anesthesiologists, annual meeting, 1977, pp 507, 508

76. Ikram H, Rubin AP, Jewkes RF: Effect of diazepam on myocardial blood flow of patients with and without coronary artery disease. Br Heart J 35:626, 1973

77. Côté P, Campeau L, Bourassa MG: Therapeutic implications of diazepam in patients with elevated left ventricular filling pressure. Am Heart J 91:747, 1976

78. Knapp RB, Dubow HS: Diazepam as an induction agent for patients with cardiopulmonary disease. South Med J 63:1451, 1970

79. Jenkinson JL, Macrae WR, Scott DB, et al: Haemodynamic effects of diazepam used as a sedative for oral surgery. Br J Anaesth 46:294, 1974

80. Bianco JA, Shanahan EA, Ostheimer GW, et al: Cardiovascular effects of diazepam. J Thorac Cardiovasc Surg 62:125, 1971

81. Liu WS, Bidwai AV, Stanley TH, et al: The cardiovascular effects of diazepam and pancuronium during fentanyl and oxygen anesthesia. Can Anaesth Soc J 23:395, 1976

82. Dundee JW: Thiopentone and Other Thiobarbiturates. Edinburgh and London, Churchill-Livingstone, 1956

83. Becker KE, Tonnesen AS, et al: Cardiovascular effects of plasma levels of thiopental necessary for anesthesia. Anesthesiology 49:197, 1978

84. Whitwam JG, Russell WJ: The acute cardio-

vascular changes and adrenergic blockade by droperidol in man. Br J Anaesth 43:581, 1971

85. McDermott RW, Stanley TH: The cardiovascular effects of low concentrations of nitrous oxide during morphine anesthesia. Anesthesiology 44:89, 1974

86. Denlinger JK, Ellison N, Ominsky AJ: Effects of intratracheal lidocaine on circulatory response to tracheal intubation. Anesthesiology 41:409, 1974

87. Williams CH, Deutsch S, Linde HW, et al: Effects of intravenously administered succinylcholine on cardiac rate, rhythm, and arterial blood pressure in anesthetized man. Anesthesiology 22:947, 1961

88. Kelman GR, Kennedy BR: Cardiovascular effects of pancuronium in man. Br J Anaesth 43:355, 1971

89. Miller RD, Eger EI II, Stevens WC, et al: Pancuronium-induced tachycardia in relation to alveolar halothane, dose of pancuronium, and prior atropine. Anesthesiology 42:352, 1975

90. Anderson EF, Rosenthal MH: Pancuronium bromide and tachyarrhythmias. Crit Care Med 3:13, 1975

91. Slogoff S, Keats AS, Ott E: Preoperative propranolol therapy and aortocoronary bypass operation. JAMA 240:1487, 1978

92. McCullough LS, Reier CE, Delaunois AL, et al: The effect of *d*-tubocurarine on spontaneous post-ganglionic sympathetic activity and his tamine release. Anesthesiology 33:328, 1970

93. Zaidan J, Philbin PM, Antonio R, et al: Hemodynamic effects of metocurine in patients with coronary artery disease receiving propranolol. Anesth Analg 56:255, 1977

94. Denlinger JK, Messner JT, D'Orazio DJ, et al: Effect of intravenous lidocaine on circulatory response to tracheal intubation. Anesth Rev, Feb 1976, 13

95. Stanley TH, Isern-Amaral J, Lathrop GD: The effects of morphine and halothane anaesthesia on urine norepinephrine during and after coronary artery surgery. Can Anaesth Soc J 22:478, 1975

96. Saner CA, Foëx P, Roberts JG, et al: Methoxyflurane and practolol: A dangerous combination? Br J Anaesth 47:1025, 1975

97. Roberts JG, Foëx P, Clarke TNS, et al: Haemodynamic interactions of high-dose propranolol pre-treatment and anaesthesia in the dog. I: Halothane dose-response studies. Br J Anaesth 48:315, 1976

98. Slogoff S, Keats AS, Hibbs CW, et al: Failure of general anesthesia to potentiate propranolol activity. Anesthesiology 47:504, 1977

99. Horan BF, Prys-Roberts C, Hamilton WK, et al: Haemodynamic responses to enflurane anaesthesia and hypovolaemia in the dog, and their modification by propranolol. Br J Anaesth 49:1189, 1977

100. Kaplan JA, Dunbar RW, Jones EL: Nitroglycerin infusion during coronary artery surgery. Anesthesiology 45:14, 1976

101. Chiariello M, Gold HK, Leinbach RC, et al: Comparison between the effects of nitroprusside and nitroglycerin on ischemic injury during acute myocardial infarction. Circulation 54:766, 1976

102. Mann T, Cohn PF, Holman BL, et al: Effect of nitroprusside on regional myocardial blood flow in coronary artery disease: results in 25 patients and comparison with nitroglycerin. Circulation 57:732, 1978

103. Lappas DG, Lowenstein E, Waller J, et al: Hemodynamic effects of nitroprusside infusion during coronary artery operation in man. Circulation 54 (suppl III):4, 1976

104. Forrester JS, Diamond G, McHugh TJ, et al: Filling pressures in the right and left sides of the heart in acute myocardial infarction: A reappraisal of central venous pressure monitoring. N Engl J Med 285:190, 1971

105. Vance JP, Brown DM, Smith G: The effects of hypocapnia on myocardial blood flow and metabolism. Br J Anaesth 45:455, 1973

106. Neill WA, Hattenhauer M: Impairment of myocardial O_2 supply due to hyperventilation. Circulation 52:854, 1975

107. Kaplan JA: Anesthesia for patients with coronary artery disease. Surgical Rounds, p 46, January 1978

108. Lappas DG, Buckley MJ, Laver MB, et al: Left ventricular performance and pulmonary circulation following addition of nitrous oxide to morphine during coronary artery surgery. Anesthesiology 38:394, 1973

109. Stanley TH: Anesthetic requirements and cardiovascular effects of fentanyl-oxygen and fentanyl-diazepam-oxygen anesthesia in man. Anesth Analg 57:411, 1978

110. Jones EL, Craver JM, Kaplan JA, et al: Criteria for operability and reduction of surgical mortality in patients with severe left ventricular ischemia and dysfunction. Ann Thorac Surg 25:413, 1978

111. Kennedy PJ, Feingold A, Wiener EL, et al: Analysis of tasks and human factors in anesthesia for coronary-artery bypass. Anesth Analg 55:374, 1976

112. Hottenrott CE, Towers B, Kurkji HJ, et al: The hazard of ventricular fibrillation in hypertrophied ventricles during cardiopulmonary bypass. J Thorac Cardiovasc Surg 66:742, 1973

113. Reis RL, Cohn LH, Morrow AG: Effects of induced ventricular fibrillation on ventricular performance and cardiac metabolism. Circulation 36 (suppl I):234, 1967

114. Iyengar SRK, Ramchand S, Charrette EJP, et al: Anoxic cardiac arrest: An experimental and clinical study of its effects. J Thorac Cardiovasc Surg 66:722, 1973

115. Miller DW Jr, Hessel EA, Winterscheid LC, et al: Current practice of coronary artery bypass surgery. J Thorac Cardiovasc Surg 73:75, 1977

116. Roberts AJ, Niarchos AP, Subramanian VA, et al: Systemic hypertension associated with coronary artery bypass surgery. J Thorac Cardiovasc Surg 74:846, 1977

117. Taylor KM, Morton IJ, Brown JJ, et al: Hypertension and the renin-angiotensin system following open-heart surgery. J Thorac Cardiovasc Surg 74:840, 1977

118. Prakash O, Jonson B, Meij S, et al: Criteria for early extubation after intracardiac surgery in adults. Anesth Analg 56:703, 1977

119. Selzer A, Langston M, Ruggeroli C, et al: Clinical syndrome of variant angina with normal coronary arteriogram. N Engl J Med 295:1343, 1976

119A. Wiener L, Kasparian H, Duca PR, et al: Spectrum of coronary arterial spasm. Clinical, angiographic and myocardial metabolic experience in 29 cases. Am J Cardiol 38:945, 1976

120. Garcia JM, Mispireth LA, Smyth NPD: Surgical management of life-threatening coronary artery disease. J Thorac Cardiovasc Surg 72:593, 1976

121. Cooper GN, Singh AK, Vargas LL, et al: Preoperative intra-aortic balloon assist in high risk revascularization patients. Am J Surg 133:463, 1977

122. Jones EL, Craver JM, Kaplan JA, et al: Left main coronary artery disease: Patient selection and intra-operative management as a guide to reduction of surgical mortality (manuscript in preparation)

123. Gold HK, Leinbach RC, Buckley MJ, et al: Refractory angina pectoris: Follow-up after intraaortic balloon pumping and surgery. Circulation 54 (suppl III):41, 1976

124. Dawson JT, Hall RJ, Hallman GL, et al: Mortality in patients undergoing coronary artery bypass surgery after myocardial infarction. Am J Cardiol 33:483, 1974

125. Jones EL, Douglas JS, Craver JM, et al: Results of coronary revascularization in patients with recent myocardial infarction. J Thorac Cardiovasc Surg 76:545, 1978

126. Chatterjee K, Parmley WW, Swan HJC, et al: Beneficial effects of vasodilator agents in severe mitral regurgitation due to dysfunction of sub-valvular apparatus. Circulation 48:684, 1973

127. Forrester JS, Diamond G, Chatterjee K, et al: Medical therapy of acute myocardial infarction by application of hemodynamic subsets (first of two parts). N Engl J Med 295:1356, 1976

128. Mundth ED, Buckley MJ, Daggett WM, et al: Intra-aortic balloon pump assistance and early surgery in cardiogenic shock. Adv Cardiol 15:159, 1975

129. Franch RL: Cardiac catheterization. In Hurst JW, Logue RB (eds): The Heart (ed 4). New York, McGraw-Hill, 1978, pp 479–501

130. Coleman EH, Soloff LA: Incidence of significant coronary artery disease in rheumatic valvular heart disease. Am J Cardiol 25:401, 1970

131. Loop FD, Favaloro RG, Shirey EK, et al: Surgery for combined valvular and coronary heart disease. JAMA 220:372, 1972

132. Dortimer AC, Prakash NS, Shiroff RA, et al: Diffuse coronary artery disease in diabetic patients—fact or fiction? Circulation 57:133, 1978

133. Chychota NN, Gau GT, Pluth JR, et al: Myocardial revascularization—comparison of operability and surgical results in diabetic and nondiabetic patients. J Thorac Cardiovasc Surg 65:856, 1973

134. Lansing AM, Masri ZH, Karalakulasingam R, et al: Angina during hemodialysis. JAMA 232:736, 1975

135. Siegel MS, Norfleet EA, Gitelman HJ: Coronary artery bypass surgery in a patient receiving hemodialysis. Arch Intern Med 137:83, 1977

136. Sakurai H, Ackad A, Friedman HS, et al: Aorta-coronary bypass graft surgery in a patient on home hemodialysis. Clin Nephrol 2:208, 1974

137. Posner MA, Reves JG, Lell WA: Aortic valve replacement in a hemodialysis-dependent patient: Anesthetic considerations-a case report. Anesth Analg 54:24, 1975

138. Sobel BE, Shell WE: Jeopardized, blighted and necrotic myocardium. Circulation 47:215, 1973

139. Kones RJ, Phillips JH: Prevention of heart cell death. South Med J 69:422, 1976

140. Braunwald E, Maroko PR: Protection of the ischemic myocardium. In Braunwald E (ed): The Myocardium: Failure and Infarction. New York, HP Publishing, 1974, pp 329–342

141. Murphy ML, Hultgren HN, Detre K, et al: Treatement of chronic stable angina: A preliminary report of survival data of the randomized veterans administration cooperative study. N Engl J Med 297:621, 1977

142. Hutter AM Jr, Russell RO Jr, Resnekov L, et al: Unstable angina pectoris—national randomized study of surgical vs. medical therapy: Results in 1, 2, and 3 vessel disease, abstracted. Circulation 56 (suppl III):60, 1977

143. Preston TA: Coronary Artery Surgery: A Critical Review. New York, Raven Press, 1977

144. Debakey ME, Lawrie GM: Aortocoronary-artery bypass—assessment after 13 years. JAMA 239:837, 1978

145. Hurst JW, King SB III, Logue BL, et al: The value of coronary bypass surgery. Am J Cardiol 42:308, 1978

146. Takaro T, Hultgren HN, Lipton MJ, et al: The VA cooperative randomized study of surgery for coronary arterial occlusive disease, II. Subgroup with significant left main lesions. Circulation 54 (suppl III):107, 1976

James W. Bland, Jr., M.D.
Willis H. Williams, M.D.

8
Anesthesia for Treatment of Congenital Heart Defects

Malformations of the heart and vascular system are among the most clinically significant yet treatable anomalies of the human newborn. Some form of congenital heart disease occurs in 1 of every 123 live births (an incidence of 0.8 percent).[1-3] Each year in the United States 32,000 infants are born with significant cardiac abnormalities. These numbers assume even more importance when one considers that over 50 percent of these babies will die before their first birthday and at least 30 percent will die before the age of 1 month if they are not treated. Early recognition, precise anatomic diagnosis, and promptly instituted medical and surgical treatment are essential if this ominous natural history is to be altered. In an environment of high-quality medical care, salvage of more than 90 percent of these infants can be anticipated.[4]

HISTORICAL BACKGROUND

Remarkable progress has been made during the past 25 years in the closely allied disciplines of pediatric cardiology, cardiovascular surgery, anesthesiology, and intensive care. Tables 8-1 and 8-2 list some of the important therapeutic and diagnostic modalities routinely used in the care of infants and children with congenital heart defects.

Successful surgical treatment of congenital heart disease began in 1938 when Gross and Hubbard reported the first survivor of ligation of a patent ductus arteriosus.[5] In the mid-1940s the surgical efforts of Blalock and Taussig,[6] Potts,[7] and Brock[8] provided palliation for infants and children with tetralogy of Fallot, pulmonary atresia, tricuspid atresia, and related forms of cyanotic congenital heart disease. Coarctation of the aorta was successfully repaired in 1945 by Gross[9] in Boston and by Crafoord[10] in Sweden. In the mid-1950s, Lillehei successfully closed ventricular septal defects in children using controlled cross-circulation, with the mother serving as the source of oxygenated blood for perfusion of the child.[11,12] Lewis and Taufic successfully corrected atrial septal defects using only circulatory arrest with surface-induced total-body hypothermia.[13]

History's most significant cardiovascular surgical innovation occurred in 1953, when John H. Gibbon, Jr., demonstrated the first use of a "heart-lung machine" in the laboratory and then employed this new membrane oxygenator and pump for cardiopulmonary bypass in the successful closure of an atrial septal defect in a young patient.[14] The pump oxygenator with its many modifications has since been employed for circulatory support during correction of thousands of congenital heart defects.

The evolution of a safe technique for prolonged extracorporeal support of the circulation made possible many dramatic extensions of surgical technique. In 1964, Mustard, of the Hospital for Sick Children in Toronto, described his now time-tested operation for the redirection of venous blood within the atria using a pericardial patch, thus making possible a physiological,

Table 8-1
Diagnostic Techniques in Congenital Heart
Disease

History
Physical examination
Chest x-rays
Electrocardiogram
Fluroscopy
  Image Intensification
    Cine recording
    Videotape recording
Vectorcardiogram
Phonocardiogram
Echocardiogram
  Sector (two-dimensional) echocardiogram
  Apex cardiogram
  Computerized axial tomography
  Radionuclear techniques
    Myocardial imaging
    Ventilation-perfusion scanning
    Radionuclide angiography
Isotopic measurement of intracardiac shunting
Microchemical blood gas measurements
Continuous blood gas measurement
Exercise stress testing
  Treadmill
  Bicycle ergometry
Ambulatory ECG Recording
  Self-contained recorder
  Telemetry
Measurement of cardiac output
  Thermodilution
  Green dye dilution
  Impedance
  Fick principle (oxygen consumption)
Bedside hemodynamic assessment with flow-di-
rected balloon-tipped catheter (Swan-Ganz)
Bedside determination of intracardiac shunts
  Green dye dilution
  Thermodilution
  Radionuclear techniques
Cardiac catheterization
  Pressure measurement
  Anatomic course of catheter passage
  Oxygen measurements
  Cineangiography
  Pharmacologic responses
  Exercise responses
  Responses to inspired oxygen
  Coronary arteriography (selective)

Table 8-2
Useful Medical Adjuncts in the Surgical
Management of Congenital Heart Disease

Systemic and pulmonary vasodilator medica-
tions
  Nitroglycerin
  Sodium nitroprusside
  Tolazoline hydrochloride
Inotropic medications
  Digitalis
  Dopamine
  Isoproterenol
  Epinephrine
  Calcium chloride
Beta-blocking medications
  Propranolol
Pharmacologic maintenance of a patent ductus
arteriosus
  Prostaglandins
Pharmacologic closure of a patent ductus arter-
iosus
  Prostaglandin synthetase inhibitors: aspirin,
    indomethacin
Potent diuretics
  Furosemide
  Ethacrynic acid
Potent antibiotics for treatment of endocarditis
Antiarrhythmic medications
Antihypertensive medications
Parenteral hyperalimentation
Direct blood level determinations of cardiovas-
cular medications
Prolonged ventilatory support of the infant
Miniaturized pacing systems
  Atrial
  Ventricular demand
  Atrioventricular synchronous
  P-wave synchronous
Rashkind balloon atrioseptostomy

although not anatomic, correction of transposition of the great arteries.[15] The 1960s seemed a
decade of almost limitless surgical imagination.
William F. Bernhard, of the Children's Hospital
Medical Center, Boston, utilized hyperbaric operating conditions of 3 or more atmospheres to
carry out aortic valvotomies and pulmonary valvotomies, systemic-arterial-to-pulmonary-arterial anastomoses, and atrial septectomies during
brief periods of inflow occlusion and circulatory

arrest in severely hypoxemic infants.[16,17] Survival rates were exceptionally good.

Dillard, Merendino, and associates in Seattle,[18,19] Sir Brian Barrett-Boyes in New Zealand,[20] and the Kyoto group in Japan[21] developed the combined techniques of surface-induced deep hypothermia supplemented by further core-cooling to about 16°C on cardiopulmonary bypass, repair of complex defects during a period of circulatory arrest of at least 1 full hour, and rewarming to normothermia on cardiopulmonary bypass. This technique greatly facilitated the ease, accuracy, and safety of operations in tiny infants by eliminating blood, tubing, and cardiac motion from the operative field and shortened the duration of cardiopulmonary bypass. This technique still enjoys widespread popularity for operations performed during the first year of life, and it stimulated interest in one-stage totally corrective operations in infancy rather than mere palliation.

In 1969, Rastelli and his colleagues at the Mayo Clinic described techniques for repair of transposition of the great arteries associated with a ventricular septal defect and pulmonary stenosis using a valve-containing aortic homograft to connect the right ventricle to the pulmonary artery.[22] The techniques developed by Rastelli have been extended to the treatment of many complex forms of right and left ventricular outflow tract obstruction and malposition of the great arteries using, in most cases, tightly woven Dacron fabric conduits containing porcine gluteraldehyde-preserved stent-mounted aortic valves.[23] Although unsolved problems remain, Appendix A lists some currently treatable congenital heart defects and the palliative and corrective operations commonly employed.

PATHOPHYSIOLOGICAL CONSIDERATIONS

Congenital heart defects have been categorized by a variety of criteria. The most useful classification considers two common pathophysiological consequences: congestive heart failure and systemic arterial hemoglobin unsaturation or cyanosis (see Table 8-3).[2,24,25]

Congestive heart failure occurs in situations where there is *excessive pulmonary blood flow* or *pulmonary venous congestion* caused by inadequate egress of blood from the lungs through

Table 8-3

Pathophysiological Classification of Congenital Heart Disease

I. Congestive Heart Failure
  A. Excessive pulmonary blood flow
    1. Ventricular septal defect
    2. Patent ductus arteriosus
    3. Aorticopulmonary window
    4. Truncus arteriosus
    5. Atrial septal defect
  B. Pulmonary venous congestion or obstruction to forward flow
    1. Hypoplastic left heart syndrome
    2. Coarctation of the aorta
    3. Aortic stenosis or aortic atresia
    4. Mitral stenosis or mitral atresia
    5. Cor triatriatum
    6. Obstructed total anomalous pulmonary venous drainage
    7. Coronary arteriovenous fistula
II. Systemic Arterial Hemoglobin Unsaturation (Cyanosis)
  A. Inadequate pulmonary blood flow
    1. Tetralogy of Fallot
    2. Pulmonary atresia (with or without intact ventricular septum)
    3. Tricuspid atresia
    4. Double-outlet right ventricle with pulmonary stenosis
  B. Intracardiac mixing of pulmonary venous and systemic venous blood*
    1. Atrioventricular canal
    2. Common atrium
    3. Common ventricle
    4. Truncus arteriosus with pulmonary hypertension
  C. Diversion of systemic venous blood back into aorta without passage through the lungs*
    1. Transposition of the great arteries

* Cyanosis and congestive heart failure may coexist.

the left side of the heart. Examples of congenital heart defects causing symptoms of congestive heart failure because of a greater-than-normal pulmonary blood flow include ventricular septal defect, patent ductus arteriosus, aorticopulmonary window, truncus arteriosus, and occasionally even atrial septal defect. All of these defects produce a so-called left-to-right shunt, a situation in which the volume of blood flowing through the lungs is greater than the volume pumped to the systemic circulation. Blood flows from a left heart chamber through an abnormally persisting communication to a right heart chamber because the pulmonary vascular resistance is lower than the systemic vascular resistance.

Congenital heart defects causing congestive heart failure by the mechanism of *pulmonary venous congestion* and *inadequate forward flow of blood* through the left side of the heart include the hypoplastic left heart syndrome, coarctation of the aorta, aortic stenosis, mitral stenosis, cor triatriatum, obstructed forms of total anomalous pulmonary venous drainage, and the anatomic abnormalities producing myocardial ischemia, including coronary arteriovenous fistulae, coronary-arterial-to-right-atrial fistulae, and anomalous origin of a coronary artery from the pulmonary artery.

Physiological considerations of congenital heart disease in the infant must take into account the gradual changes in pulmonary vascular resistance that occur after birth and the alterations in pressures and flows occurring as a consequence of closure of the ductus arteriosus, sinus venosus, and foramen ovale.[26] Intracardiac septal defects and communications between the aorta and pulmonary artery (patent ductus arteriosus or aorticopulmonary window) are usually, *not* recognized at birth. Murmurs are rarely heard; congestive heart failure is not apparent. At this early stage the pulmonary vascular resistance is still elevated to nearly intrauterine levels. Because of the essentially identical pulmonary arterial and aortic pressures, little flow occurs through the anatomic communications described above. As the pulmonary vascular resistance falls progressively over the first few days and weeks of life, the magnitude of the left-to-right shunt increases. Pulmonary blood flow increases, murmurs appear, and symptoms of congestive heart failure become apparent. As long as 18 months to 2 years may be required for pulmonary resistance to fall to normal adult levels. In some circumstances this normal low level of pulmonary resistance may never be reached when pulmonary blood flow remains increased.

A moderate-sized ventricular septal defect or patent ductus arteriosus will usually manifest a murmur and symptoms of congestive heart failure when the child is between 1 and 2 months old. If associated congenital heart defects are present, congestive failure may become a problem earlier and may pose a far greater challenge to treatment. For example, the not uncommon association of coarctation of the aorta, ventricular septal defect, and patent ductus arteriosus usually causes severe congestive heart failure during the first week of life.

In contrast to these severe defects with early presentation of life-threatening symptoms, isolated atrial septal defects are usually recognized only in late infancy or early childhood. A soft murmur may be detected during the first year of life, but little else points to an underlying congenital heart lesion until the child is 2 or 3 years old or even older. Relatively slight differences exist between normal left and right atrial pressures, the defect in the atrial septum simply producing a functional common atrial reservoir. During infancy, both ventricles are quite compliant and capable of accepting atrially presented inflow. Outflow depends only upon the relative resistances of the pulmonary and systemic vascular beds. Thus, in the presence of an atrial septal defect, the increase in pulmonary blood flow is gradual. In contrast to a left-to-right shunt at the ventricular or great vessel level, the left ventricle must pump *no more* than its normal volume of blood in the presence of an atrial septal defect. Symptoms of congestive heart failure are rarely apparent. The increase in pulmonary blood flow caused by an atrial septal defect is usually detected incidentally in a 2 or 3-year-old child found to have an enlarged heart and increased pulmonary vascularity on a chest x-ray taken when pneumonia is suspected or during the evaluation of a soft systolic ejection murmur along the left upper sternal border.

The *signs and symptoms of congestive heart failure in infancy* differ somewhat from those seen in older patients, although the basic pathophysiological changes are similar. Tachypnea, pallor, irritability, poor feeding, and "failure to thrive" are common. Cardiomegaly and increased pulmonary vascularity are usually apparent on chest x-ray. Kerley "B" lines may be seen if pulmonary venous hypertension is present. Sweating during feeding is a manifestation of the stress and catecholamine response produced by eating while attempting to maintain adequate ventilation (see Table 8-4).

Respiratory symptoms may progress in severity from simple tachypnea to flaring of the

Table 8-4

Signs, Symptoms, and Complications of
Congestive Heart Failure in Infants and
Children

Tachypnea	Flaring of alae nasae
Pallor	Grunting
Irritability	Wheezing
Poor feeding patterns	Edema of eyelids
Failure to thrive	Excessive sweating
Retraction of sternum and intercostal spaces	
Recurrent respiratory infections	

alae nasae, grunting, intercostal and suprasternal retractions, sternal and abdominal retractions, wheezing from bronchospasm, rales, and
obviously labored respiration with cyanosis and
circumoral pallor. Ventilatory support may be
required to maintain acceptable arterial blood
gases; inotropic infusions are occasionally
needed to sustain cardiac output, peripheral perfusion, and an adequate urinary output. Rarely
do children with significant congestive heart failure attain normally expected weight gain,
growth, and developmental milestones. Sleep is
restless and intermittent, and anxiety levels are
high in both child and parents. Symptoms of so-
called right-sided failure, including hepatomegaly, periorbital edema, distended neck veins,
peripheral edema, obvious fluid retention, and
"dilutional" hyponatremia, are usually late and
relatively ominous manifestations of congestive
heart failure in infancy. Some improvement can
be expected following treatment with digitalis
preparations and diuretics, but such improvement is often not sufficient. Surgical intervention is required.

The second major pathophysiological consequence caused by some congenital heart defects, *systemic arterial hemoglobin unsaturation*, results from (1) an inadequate volume of
pulmonary blood flow, (2) the intracardiac mixing of systemic venous and pulmonary venous
blood before entry into the aorta, or (3) the
diversion of systemic venous blood directly
back into the aorta without passage through the
lungs. Approximately 30 to 35 percent of children with congenital heart disease will be cyanotic because of one or more of these three
mechanisms.

Inadequate pulmonary blood flow results
when any one of a variety of lesions obstructs

the flow of desaturated systemic venous blood
into the pulmonary vascular bed. The classic
example of such a defect is tetralogy of Fallot
in which the hemodynamic defect is right ventricular outflow tract obstruction (pulmonary
valve stenosis, pulmonary atresia, pulmonary
annular or arterial hypoplasia, or infundibular
stenosis) associated with a ventricular septal defect that allows the unsaturated venous blood to
be shunted from the right ventricle to the left
ventricle and aorta. Since the response of either
ventricle to outflow tract obstruction is the development of myocardial hypertrophy, milder
degrees of pulmonary valve and/or infundibular
stenosis often become more severe with the passage of time, producing the physiological consequences of tetralogy of Fallot in an older child
who may have had only mild pulmonary stenosis, a ventricular septal defect, and a left-to-
right shunt as an infant. Children having such a
combination of lesions may require treatment
with digitalis and diuretics during infancy because of a significantly increased cardiac work
load associated with increased pulmonary blood
flow. They may later become asymptomatic as
the shunt becomes "balanced" and still later
may require total correction of tetralogy of Fallot as progressive infundibular hypertrophy obstructs the right ventricular outflow tract and
causes systemic arterial unsaturation and hypercyanotic episodes.

Other examples of defects causing inadequate pulmonary blood flow include tricuspid
atresia, pulmonary atresia with intact ventricular septum, pulmonary stenosis with a patent
foramen ovale, peripheral pulmonary arterial
stenosis with a patent ductus arteriosus, double-
outlet right ventricle with pulmonary stenosis,
Ebstein's anomaly, and the hypoplastic right
heart syndrome. This mechanism of diminished
pulmonary blood flow resulting from the passage
of blood from a right heart chamber (right
atrium, right ventricle, or pulmonary artery)
through a septal defect (patent foramen ovale,
atrial septal defect, or ventricular septal defect)
or a patent ductus arteriosus is referred to as a
right-to-left shunt. The pulmonary-to-systemic
blood flow ratio (Q_p/Q_s) is *less* than 1:1. This
implies that the pressure in the right heart chamber is higher than or at least as high as the
pressure in the left heart chamber into which the
unsaturated blood is flowing. The *resistance* to
blood flow from the right-sided chamber via its

normal outlet is *greater* than the resistance to flow via the abnormal communication into the left side of the circulation.

Intracardiac mixing of systemic venous and pulmonary venous blood can occur in situations where the total volume of pulmonary blood flow is *normal* or even much *greater than normal.* Examples include complete atrioventricular canal in which there is functionally a two-chambered heart—one large communicating atrium and one large ventricle—and in total anomalous pulmonary venous drainage, common atrium, single ventricle, and truncus arteriosus. In these defects, blood pumped from the heart into the aorta is *not* pure pulmonary venous blood. It is a mixture of varying proportions of well-oxygenated blood from the lungs and desaturated blood that has not passed through the pulmonary circulation. Children with such defects usually manifest symptoms of both cyanosis and congestive heart failure.

The *diversion of systemic venous blood back into the aorta without passage through the lungs* is the mechanism of cyanosis and severe systemic arterial hemoglobin unsaturation active in transposition of the great arteries where the aorta arises from the right ventricle and the pulmonary artery arises from the left ventricle. Complete *separation* of the pulmonary and systemic circulations is incompatible with life, and hence children surviving with transposition of the great arteries must have some form of communication between the right and left heart. At birth, this is usually a patent ductus arteriosus and a patent foramen ovale, the former often but not always remaining patent in response to the hypoxic stimulus. A ventricular septal defect may likewise be present. Of the three possible levels for communication between the pulmonary and systemic circulations in transposition, interatrial communication through a patent foramen ovale is the least likely to produce excessive pulmonary blood flow and congestive heart failure. For this reason the foramen ovale is enlarged at the time of initial emergency cardiac catheterization in the infant with transposition of the great arteries in order to prevent progressive severe systemic hypoxemia, acidosis, cerebral hypoxic injury, and death. This is accomplished by the use of the Rashkind balloon atrioseptostomy catheter[27] which is passed through a systemic vein into the right atrium,

through the foramen ovale, and into the left atrium, where it is inflated with radiopaque contrast material. The balloon is then jerked briskly back into the right atrium while inflated, thus disrupting the interatrial septum and allowing mixing of pulmonary venous and systemic venous blood in the "common atrium" before the mixed venous blood passes to the right ventricle and the body via the transposed aorta. When the balloon septostomy fails to provide adequate mixing, the atrial septum can be surgically excised and the right pulmonary veins directed toward the right atrium (Blalock-Hanlon atrial septectomy).[28]

Congenital heart defects producing (1) inadequate pulmonary blood flow, (2) excessive intracardiac mixing of systemic venous and pulmonary venous blood in infants with normally related great vessels, or (3) inadequate mixing of systemic and pulmonary venous blood in infants with transposed great vessels usually become apparent early in life by the presence of *cyanosis.* This must be distinguished from the common and benign acrocyanosis seen in most normal newborns during the first few days of life. The presence of a potentially lethal "cyanotic defect" may be disguised for several days in infants having a persistent patent ductus arteriosus, or, in the case of transposition of the great arteries, a large patent foramen ovale, ventricular septal defect, or patent ductus arteriosus. Anemia, while making visible cyanosis less apparent, hastens the onset of symptoms of acidosis, cerebral hypoxia, and congestive heart failure because of the associated reduction in oxygen delivery to vital organs. Congestive heart failure is a variable symptom and, as discussed earlier, is related to the magnitude of pulmonary blood flow, myocardial ischemia, and arrhythmias. Respiratory symptoms including tachypnea, grunting, and retractions with labored respiratory effort are common. Seizures suggest cerebral hypoxia, serum electrolyte imbalance, and/or abnormal blood glucose levels. Metabolic acidosis reflects the overall inadequacy of oxygen delivery in the presence of increased respiratory effort. Initial increase in respiratory effort may maintain nearly normal arterial P_{CO_2} levels, but progressive fatigue may lead to respiratory failure and severe combined metabolic and respiratory acidosis (see Table 8-5).

Table 8-5
Signs, Symptoms, and
Complications of Systemic
Arterial Hemoglobin
Unsaturation in Infants and
Children

Cyanosis	Irritability
Clubbing	Cerebral infarction
Polycythemia	Brain abscess
Hemoptysis	Systemic emboli
Squatting	

As early as 4 to 5 months of age, clubbing of the fingertips and toes may become apparent, and polycythemia may progress to the point of producing intravascular thrombosis, cerebrovascular accidents, cerebral infarction, pulmonary infarction, and hemoptysis. Brain abscesses and other focal systemic infections may result from septic emboli. Exercise tolerance is severely limited. Growth and developmental milestones may be delayed. Children with decreased pulmonary blood flow may learn that assuming a "squatting" posture makes them feel better, probably by increasing central blood volume and peripheral vascular resistance with a concomitant transient increase in pulmonary blood flow.

When evaluating a cyanotic newborn, noncardiac causes of hypoxemia must be considered. These include congenital diaphragmatic hernia, tracheoesophageal fistula with aspiration or other forms of pneumonitis, sepsis, upper airway obstruction, hyaline membrane disease, congenital lung cysts, or pneumothorax. The acronym COPS provides a simple mnemonic for use in the evaluation of the cyanotic infant, with C standing for "*c*ardiac disease"; O, for "*o*bstruction of the airway"; P, for "*p*ulmonary *p*arynchymal disease"; and S, for "*s*pace-occupying lesions" (pneumothorax, chylothorax, lung cysts, diaphragmatic hernia, and others). When noncardiac causes of cyanosis have been excluded, the "5 T's and 2 AT's" provide a quick checklist of the cardiac defects most likely to cause cyanosis (see Table 8-6).

Persistence of the fetal circulation (PFC) is a cardiac-related but nonsurgical cause of cyanosis in the newborn.[26] This often-confusing phenomenon, seen relatively frequently in infant victims of neonatal asphyxia, is simply the persistence of a right-to-left shunt through the patent foramen ovale and the patent ductus arter-

Table 8-6
Mnemonics for Differential Diagnosis of the Cyanotic Infant (COPS = Causes of Cyanosis;
5 T's and 2 AT's = Cardiac Causes of Cyanosis)

"C" Cardiac Disease	"O" Obstruction of the Airway	"P" Pulmonary Parenchymal Disease	"S" Space-occupying Lesion
The 5 "T's"	Choanal atresia	Respiratory distress	Diaphragmatic hernia
Tetralogy of Fallot	Pierre-Robin	syndrome	Pneumothorax
Transposition of the	syndrome	Persistence of the	Hemothorax
great vessels	Laryngeal web	fetal circulation	Lung cysts
Tricuspid atresia	Macroglossia	Pneumonia	Chylothorax
Total anomalous	Laryngotracheal	Meconium aspiration	Eventration of
pulmonary venous	malacia	Hyaline membrane	diaphragm
return	Subglottic	disease	
Truncus arteriosus	hemangioma		
The 2 "AT's"			
Aortic atresia			
Pulmonary atresia			

iosus caused by continued elevation of the pulmonary vascular resistance and the pulmonary arterial pressure. This elevated pulmonary vascular resistance may result from the poorly understood stress of hypoxia or immaturity of the pulmonary vasculature. Echocardiography may be helpful in ruling out heart disease, but cardiac catheterization is often necessary to exclude other surgically treatable congenital heart defects in these cyanotic infants. Persistent fetal circulation may respond to positive pressure ventilation, a fall in resistance occurring with further airway recruitment as atelectatic alveoli are expanded. Alkalinization with sodium bicarbonate and direct pulmonary arterial infusion of pulmonary vasodilators such as tolazoline may be of value in the treatment of the PFC syndrome.[29]

Although the above classification is helpful in planning the management of a child with a specific heart defect, there is considerable overlap in the *pathophysiological manifestations of complex defects*. For example, infants with total anomalous pulmonary venous drainage (TAPVD) to the innominate vein, superior vena cava, inferior vena cava, or particularly the portal venous system will often have pulmonary venous obstruction, a greater-than-normal pulmonary blood flow, *and* cyanosis. The only blood reaching the systemic circulation in TAPVD is a mixture of systemic venous (unoxygenated) and pulmonary venous (oxygenated) blood which passes into the left heart through a patent foramen ovale. When the foramen ovale is small or the pulmonary blood flow is very large, signs and symptoms of low systemic cardiac output may be present, including acidosis, hypotension, oliguria, mental obtundation, and profound vasoconstriction.

All defects producing *both* an increase in pulmonary blood flow *and* intracardiac mixing of pulmonary and systemic venous blood, including transposition of the great arteries with septal defects or a patent ductus arteriosus, truncus arteriosus, and complete atrioventricular canal, will cause varying degrees of both cyanosis and congestive heart failure. In cases of anomalous origin of a coronary artery from the pulmonary artery, the complications of myocardial ischemia produced by the "steal" of coronary arterial blood away from the myocardium as a result of the lower resistance of the pulmonary vascular bed may also lead to a sig-

nificant *increase* in pulmonary blood flow. This further complicates the ischemic ventricular arrhythmias, low cardiac output, and mitral regurgitation associated with ischemic papillary muscle dysfunction.

THE ANESTHESIOLOGISTS' RESPONSIBILITIES

Successful management of the child with congenital heart disease demands an efficient and cooperative effort among pediatricians, cardiologists, surgeons, and anesthesiologists. The anesthesiologist encounters unique problems in these critically ill infants and children. A thorough understanding of the pathophysiology of the lesion present, as well as the medical and surgical alternatives for treatment, is invaluable in the anesthetic management of these patients. The "team approach" to the management of cardiovascular disease clearly offers the best chance for patient survival. Superior results are obtained when individuals interested in the problems work together frequently, know and understand each other well, anticipate the requirements for a successful outcome, and follow a preplanned protocol for the conduct of the operation. This protocol should include alternatives for unexpected findings and events. This may, at first glance, seem excessively idealistic. Those who doubt their importance, however, should at least examine their own results in the treatment of the child with congenital heart disease and compare them to the results being obtained today by other well-organized teams. Such a comparison will usually reveal the lack of wisdom in continuing a haphazard and disorganized approach to this critically ill, yet ultimately salvageable group of patients.

A *protocol* for the operative management of patients with congenital heart disease makes the conduct of the procedure easier, more predictable, and far more "teachable." Safety is greatly enhanced, attention being directed to the occasional *extraordinary* events, while *ordinary* events are being managed and potential problems prevented by often simple and repetitious measures. This concept has been proved time and time again by the compulsive use of pilots' checklists in the aviation industry. Although specific lesions and operations dictate the details of anesthetic management, children undergoing elective total correction of complex heart defects on cardiopulmonary bypass, emergency procedures, and palliative operations not requiring the use of the pump oxygenator can be approached using a similar protocol (see Appendix B).

The goals of any anesthetic protocol should include *simplicity, reproducibility,* and *safety*. All individuals who might be involved in the anesthetic management of children with heart disease should be thoroughly instructed in the details of the protocol, including an explanation of the *reasons* for each of the steps and potential problems. Inexperienced personnel must have ample opportunity to implement the protocol under the supervision of skilled cardiovascular anesthesiologists *before* being expected to handle these potentially difficult problems alone. The small size of these infants, the instability of their cardiovascular and respiratory systems, and the relatively large number of monitoring devices and medications required combine to place infant cardiac operations among anesthesiologists' greatest challenges.

The Surgical Environment

The responsibilities of a cardiovascular anesthesiologist begin long before a preoperative encounter with child and family. The physical arrangement of the operating suite, the selection and maintenance of proper monitoring devices, and the assurance of an adequate supply of expendable equipment required in the management of children from infancy to adolescence are among the anesthesiologist's responsibilities. In some programs the anesthesiologist is directly responsible for the training and supervision of perfusionists and for the selection and maintenance of cardiopulmonary bypass equipment and protocols.

The anesthesiologist directing a pediatric cardiovascular surgical program will usually spend more time in the cardiovascular operating suite than any single surgeon, even one whose major effort involves children. A convenient and comfortable physical arrangement will thus be of great concern to him. Critically ill infants may arrive in the operating room in poor condition after a stressful transfer from another hospital or emergency cardiac catheterization under less-than-ideal supportive circumstances. The physical arrangement of the operating room and supplies must be optimal for resuscitation, intubation, ventilation, insertion of intravenous and arterial lines, monitoring, and induction.

It is occasionally necessary for individuals not routinely involved in the administration of anesthesia for elective pediatric cardiac surgery to manage infants and children undergoing urgent operations. Readily available and identifiable supplies and equipment greatly expedite the critical operating room management of such children.

There can be little doubt that the quality of care provided for children with congenital heart disease is improved by having a team of responsible individuals who administer anesthesia and supervise the monitoring of patients undergoing elective or semielective cardiovascular operations. Such a team approach must *not*, however, exclude all other personnel from experiencing and understanding the problems involved. Familiarity with the principles of cardiovascular anesthesia, monitoring techniques, and pharmacology is valuable in the management of any other critically ill child.

In emergency situations, personnel not part of the cardiovascular team may be required to manage difficult cardiac problems. This is particularly true in programs where the pediatric cardiac surgery is conducted in a children's hospital or pediatric unit separate from a large adult unit. Few pediatric cardiac surgical programs exist where the number of children operated upon is sufficient to justify several optimally experienced staff anesthesiologists all sharing "call" for cardiovascular emergencies. In such situations the responsible cardiovascular anesthesiologist must ensure that adequate in-service education and supervised experience are provided to other members of the staff and that emergency "on-call" teams consist of at least one person with appropriate cardiovascular experience.

The establishment of clearly defined protocols for preoperative management, monitoring, induction, and maintenance of anesthesia is helpful in assuring the safe conduct of anesthesia for both elective and urgent operations. Staff members required to administer an occasional anesthetic for a cardiac procedure can use such protocols with full understanding that they represent guidelines agreed upon by the cardiovascular surgical and anesthesia teams.

Preoperative Patient Evaluation

The amount of preoperative information available to the cardiac anesthesiologist is often inversely related to the severity of the illness. Critically hypoxemic newborn infants may be transferred from an obstetric unit or neonatal nursery, evaluated quickly by a cardiologist, catheterized to establish an anatomic diagnosis, operated upon immediately thereafter, and admitted to the intensive care unit for postoperative care—all within a few hours of birth. Mothers are not present; distraught fathers need support but offer little useful information. Emergency teams—in some cases with less than ideal experience—must be assembled. Time is critical in the expeditious management of such infants.

In contrast, older children scheduled for elective cardiac operations are hospitalized 2 days prior to the planned procedure. During these 2 days, consultations are obtained from hematologists, cardiologists, respiratory therapists, and other specialists as indicated. Appropriate laboratory data are accumulated, and the child is observed by the medical and nursing staff for evidence of upper respiratory illness, contagious childhood diseases, diarrhea, febrile episodes, and related contraindications to elective operation. The child's pediatrician is consulted if there has been a need for recent changes in medication or treatment for a noncardiac illness.

For older cooperative children, education and practice in the techniques of postoperative respiratory care and prophylaxis are begun. Parents are oriented to the hospital environment and personnel roles. Parents and child (when of appropriate age) are taken for a visit to the postoperative intensive care unit, and an explanation of the various tubes, respirators, and monitoring devices is provided by a nurse using a familiar "Raggedy Ann" doll.[30] Whenever possible the parents are taken to see another child in the early phases of recovery from a cardiac operation. The shock of seeing for the first time a child with chest tubes, monitors, and mechanically assisted ventilation is always less when that child is *not* one's own! Parents are reassured that they will be kept informed of all major events during and after the operation and are given a realistic but supportive assessment of prognosis.

Mothers are allowed to stay with their children preoperatively and after discharge from the intensive care unit. Reasons for the more limited hourly visitation in the intensive care unit are explained.

Perhaps most important during this preoperative period, an opportunity is provided for the parents to ask questions and express their fears and anxiety to an understanding and knowledgeable listener. In some circumstances, a member of the cardiac parents group—mothers and fathers of children who have undergone cardiac surgery—will visit to offer nonmedical psychological support.

Relatively healthy children undergoing elective cardiac operations for straightforward defects such as patent ductus arteriosus or coarctation of the aorta are hospitalized only 1 day prior to operation, but preoperative management otherwise differs very little.

The anesthesiologist must thoroughly familiarize himself with the patient by reviewing the history, physical examination, cardiac catheterization data, chest x-ray, electrocardiogram, special diagnostic studies, hemoglobin, hematocrit, arterial blood gases, serum electrolytes, blood urea nitrogen (BUN), and creatinine. Blood glucose and serum calcium levels must be determined in neonates.

An adequate understanding of the planned procedure is best obtained by direct conversation with the surgeon or one of his assistants. In dealing with a child with congenital heart disease, one is frequently confronted with the "exception rather than the rule." Plans for unexpected or alternative procedures must be made.

After the chart review and discussion with the surgeon, the patient is visited. When dealing with toddlers and older children, an attempt is made to establish a pleasant rapport between the anesthesiologist and the patient. All aspects of the hospital stay will affect the child psychologically and may indeed have long-term consequences. Children with congenital heart disease have often been exposed to numerous health care professionals, and if their experiences have been relatively atraumatic or even pleasant, they will be approachable and easier to examine than children with less complex problems. The child is told in language appropriate for his age that he is in the hospital in order that the doctors may help to make his heart stronger. In order for this to be done, it will be necessary for him to "take a nap" or be asleep for a short while. The approach should be one of appropriate positive explanation, not denial. This orientation is usually preceded by a longer and more detailed explanation by a nurse or the surgeon as described above. The possibility of postoperative ventilatory support and the tubes required is discussed. Reassurance is given that any discomfort will be minimized, with medications given through intravenous lines, and that he will not have to have many painful injections. At this point, children are often fearful of repeated venipunctures for blood studies, having just experienced this on admission. Reassurance is in order that such blood samples can be obtained painlessly from his indwelling lines.

A more detailed explanation of the anesthetic management may be provided to the parents, in the absence of the child if desired. This discussion should include mention of medications given the night before operation, premedication, transport to the operating room, and expected induction technique. Types and locations of monitoring lines used postoperatively are described. The anticipated duration of the operation and the possibility of postoperative ventilatory support or reexploration for persistent bleeding are explained. Again, the parents are encouraged to ask questions. Good rapport with and parental confidence in the anesthesiologist is always important, especially when the anesthesiologist will be active in the child's postoperative care in the intensive care unit.

During this preoperative visit, a careful assessment of the child's physical abnormalities and his general, cardiovascular, and respiratory status must be made. The upper airway is examined. Loose, missing, capped, or artificial teeth are noted. Any previously unrecognized abnormalities are pointed out to the parents. The precordium and peripheral pulses are palpated, and the lungs and heart are auscultated. Skin lesions that might influence the site of monitoring devices are sought. Allen's test to assess the integrity of the palmar arch is performed bilaterally. The anesthesiology preoperative consultation or data sheet is completed, including notation of all pertinent findings that might influence anesthetic management. Recommendations may be made to the surgical staff for further studies or operative preparation. After determination of the desired anesthetic technique (see subsequent sections of this discussion), orders for the patient's preoperative medications are written and, if necessary, reviewed with the nursing staff.

The anesthesiologist's preoperative evaluation of the child with congenital heart disease may suggest the need for adjunctive measures that often improve overall prognosis. The small infant with torrential pulmonary blood flow from a left-to-right shunt (ventricular septal defect, large patent ductus arteriosus, or truncus arteriosus) may derive considerable benefit from a period of preoperative assisted ventilation using an endotracheal tube and positive end-expiratory pressure or controlled continuous positive pressure ventilation. This is particularly true if atelectasis is present or if pulmonary infection plays a major role in the poor condition of the patient. A course of decongestants, bronchodilators, or antibiotics may be of similar benefit. Vigorous medical management of congestive heart failure with digitalis and diuretics, pharmacologic control of arrhythmias, correction of hypokalemia, or the insertion of a temporary pacing wire may reduce risks associated with inductions. The treatment of anemia with packed red blood cell transfusion or the reduction of hemoglobin concentration in severely polycythemic children by erythrophoresis will often favorably influence the operative outcome. Team cooperation between anesthesiologist, surgeon, and cardiologist is as important during this preoperative phase as it is during the operation itself and the postoperative period.

Premedication

Experience has proved that premedication is not necessary for all children undergoing the usual operations encountered in pediatric surgery. Some children become alarmingly dysphoric with certain premedication regimens. Many children are quite willing to accept an intravenous induction using thiopental and atropine administered through a skillfully introduced small-bore needle rather than experience the painful intramuscular injection of sedative or analgesic medications. In contrast, however, we and others[31-34] feel that the child undergoing a cardiac operation *should* be relatively heavily premedicated using a combination of a sedative or tranquilizer, a narcotic, and an anticholinergic agent—either atropine or scopolamine. Exceptions to this general rule must be made for children in borderline respiratory compensation, for those with low cardiac output states, or for those having significant tachyarrhythmias.

Infants undergoing cardiac operations during the first year of life are premedicated with morphine sulfate (0.2 mg/kg) and scopolamine (0.01 mg/kg) administered intramuscularly 45 minutes prior to arrival in the operating suite.

Children over 1 year of age are premedicated with a sedative or tranquilizer in addition to the above regimen. Pentobarbital or secobarbital (2-3 mg/kg), morphine sulfate (0.2 mg/kg), and atropine sulfate (0.02 mg/kg) *or* scopolamine (0.01 mg/kg) are administered intramuscularly 1 hour prior to induction of anesthesia. If promethazine is administered[33] orally in divided doses the night before operation, the tranquilizer or sedative portion of the premedication regimen is omitted. Diazepam (Valium) (0.1 mg/kg) or Hydroxyzine (Vistaril) (1 mg/kg) can be given in a similar manner at bedtime, with a second similar oral dose given 2 hours prior to administration of the narcotic/anticholinergic premedication.

It is unnecessary and indeed may be harmful to withhold oral feedings from a small infant or polycythemic child for a prolonged period prior to operation. Except in the extremely ill infant, gastric emptying time is sufficiently rapid to allow oral feedings until 3 or 4 hours before induction of anesthesia. If feedings are withheld for a longer period, supplementary intravenous fluids containing dextrose and water should be administered. We prefer routine feedings until 8 hours prior to induction, clear liquids for the next 3 hours as desired, a specific offering of clear liquids at 4 hours before induction, and nothing by mouth during the remaining 4 preoperative hours. Oral tranquilizers, when used, are administered with a small sip of clear liquids.

As indicated previously, certain patients with heart disease may present unusual premedication problems. Children with tetralogy of Fallot who have been experiencing intermittent hypercyanotic episodes ("spells") for which morphine sulfate and oxygen have been administered will require close experienced supervision during the administration of premedication. Hypercyanotic episodes are often precipitated by the trauma, pain, and agitation accompanying

the administration of intramuscular premedications. Orders are written requesting the administration of oxygen by hood or face mask immediately after the premedication is given, and a nurse or physician should be in attendance at all times after premedication. Infants should be placed in the "knee-chest" position after injection. In extreme circumstances, premedication may be omitted altogether or given with the anesthesiologist in attendance.

During the past few years, pharmacologic β-blockade using propranolol has been used to treat and prevent hypercyanotic episodes in labile patients with tetralogy of Fallot.[35,36] This medication has proved lifesaving in terminating the acute infundibular spasm that causes the sudden increase in the magnitude of the right-to-left shunting of blood through the ventricular septal defect. Bradyarrhythmias and asystole, however, have been described during induction in children receiving propranolol.[37] For these reasons, as well as the undesirability of persistent β-blockade at the termination of cardiopulmonary bypass, the risk of discontinuing propranolol must be carefully weighed against the possibility of recurrent life-threatening hypercyanotic episodes in the early perioperative period. Since the half-life of propranolol in the body is approximately 3½ to 6 hours, it should be reasonably safe to discontinue the medication 24 hours prior to surgery if total correction of tetralogy of Fallot is planned. If a palliative procedure (systemic-arterial-to-pulmonary arterial anastomosis) is planned, propranolol need not be discontinued. In fact, the anesthesiologist managing a child with tetralogy of Fallot should be prepared to administer propranolol (0.01 mg/kg) in the event of a hypercyanotic episode that cannot be controlled by more conventional means.[38] These include morphine sulfate, oxygen, volume expansion, and avoidance of hypotension from a fall in systemic vascular resistance as a result of the vasodilating effect of anesthetic medications. The long-term use of propranolol in the management of tetralogy of Fallot has not gained popularity. When the anatomy is favorable, that is, when the pulmonary arteries are of adequate size, early total correction is preferred. In the absence of favorable anatomy, a palliative systemic-arterial-to-pulmonary-arterial anastomosis (Blalock-Taussig or Waterston shunt) is constructed followed by later total correction.

Induction of Anesthesia

PRINCIPLES

Following preoperative evaluation of the patient and of the catheterization data, x-rays, electrocardiograms, and laboratory data, an anesthetic plan must be determined with particular attention being paid to the relationship of the anesthetic agents to the pathophysiology of the cardiac lesion.

Lesions with increased pulmonary blood flow as a result of left-to-right shunting of blood via intracardiac septal defects or large aortico-pulmonary communications cause rapid uptake of inhalation agents from the alveoli, resulting in rapid induction of anesthesia.[31] These same defects lead to a slower induction by the intravenous agents owing to recirculation of blood in the pulmonary vascular bed.

A reciprocal response is seen in patients with diminished pulmonary blood flow (tetralogy of Fallot, tricuspid atresia, or pulmonary atresia). Use of inhalation agents leads to a slow induction; the shorter "vein-to-brain" circulation time via the right-to-left shunt produces rapid induction with intravenous medications. The magnitude of the right-to-left shunt will be accentuated if the systemic blood pressure falls significantly, subjecting the patient to the further risk of severe hypoxemia and relative overdosage with the intravenous agents.

Extreme care must be exercised to avoid systemic hypotension or a fall in systemic vascular resistance in cyanotic patients with diminished pulmonary blood flow. Further reduction in pulmonary blood flow "triggers" the vicious cycle of hypoxemia, acidosis, myocardial depression, bradycardia, pulmonary vasoconstriction, catecholamine release, and in tetralogy of Fallot, progressive infundibular "spastic" obstruction.

The anesthetic management of cyanotic infants with labile circulatory dynamics is extremely hazardous. Noxious stimuli such as venipuncture, intramuscular injections, endotracheal intubation, agitation, or any catecholamine-releasing stimulus—even a cold operating room—may precipitate a hypercyanotic episode. Cautiously administered premedication, ventilatory assistance, prevention or rapid correction of acidosis, and maintenance of adequate central vascular volume and red cell mass are essential. Extreme positive pressure ventilation

and systemic vasodilators[39,40] should be avoided. Prevention or correction of arrhythmias, elimination of absolutely *all* air bubbles from intravenous lines, and the judicious use of intravenous β-blockade with propranolol when indicated are important to the safe conduct of anesthesia in children with cyanotic congenital heart disease. Once the situation has deteriorated to a point requiring inotropic infusions, the vicious cycle is often made worse by the exogenous catecholamines.

Children with transposition of the great arteries will also have a slow delivery to the brain of inhaled anesthetic gases because of the relative separation of the two parallel circulations. Generally speaking, the lower the arterial P_{O_2}, the slower will be the inhalation induction because of the poor intracardiac mixing of pulmonary venous and systemic venous blood. An intravenous induction, however, will be relatively rapid.

PREINDUCTION PROCEDURE

If the child responds as predicted to the premedication, he should arrive in the operating room either asleep or sedated and cooperative. Using the premedication regimen previously outlined, we have found that most children will be asleep and can be moved from the transport stretcher to the operating table with little more response than opening their eyes and looking around. Reassurance, gentleness, and appropriate premedication will help dispel fear caused by separation from parents and the unfamiliar environment. If the child is awake but calm, soothing conversation will allow the necessary monitoring devices to be applied. A smooth induction can be anticipated.

Essential monitoring devices for induction of a child undergoing cardiovascular surgery include (1) a precordial *stethoscope*, (2) a *blood pressure cuff* (usually a Doppler-principle device), and (3) oscillographic monitoring *electrocardiogram* electrodes. The quality of the heart sounds is noted by the anesthesiologist listening with the precordial stethoscope. The volume and quality of the peripheral pulses are assessed by palpation.

With the child on the operating table and the initial monitoring devices applied, induction of anesthesia is carried out in one of several ways, depending upon the lesion present (see previous discussion). The hemodynamic status of the patient is determined from the preoperative evaluation and the child's response to premedication.

INTRAVENOUS INDUCTION
TECHNIQUES

When an induction with thiopental or other intravenous agent is used, children are preoxygenated for 4 minutes prior to the administration of the medication. During this time, it is important for the anesthesiologist to talk reassuringly to the child so that the presence of the mask is not unduly disturbing. If the child refuses to accept the mask applied directly to his face, holding the mask with a high flow of oxygen several inches above his face surrounded by gently cupped hands will accomplish much the same result.

As previously described to the older child at the preoperative visit, intravenous induction is begun after insertion of a large-bore cannula using 1 percent lidocaine injected locally to reduce the discomfort.

For ASA Class II patients—the older child with an ostium secundum atrial septal defect or the asymptomatic child with coarctation of the aorta or a patent ductus arteriosus—sodium thiopental (2-4 mg/kg) is often used, titrating the dose to the point of loss of lid reflex. This can be followed safely by a defasciculating dose of a nondepolarizing muscle relaxant such as pancuronium (0.01 mg/kg) or d-tubocurarine (0.1 mg/kg). Succinylcholine (1-2 mg/kg) is then administered to facilitate intubation. Nitrous oxide with oxygen and either halothane or enflurane in low concentrations are used during the early phases of the anesthetic. We have found this intravenous induction to be safe and effective for reasonably stable patients if conducted smoothly and with frequent monitoring of systemic blood pressure.

Even in Class II patients, an unhurried and controlled induction is necessary; such patients can be easily "overdosed" if the "routine" attributed to the less-than-ideal anesthesiologist is followed—"half the big syringe, all the little syringe, and bag, bag, bag!" This induction technique is deplorable for *any* patient, but children with heart disease *must* be anesthetized very carefully because of the possibility of serious hemodynamic responses to the anesthetic agents.

Intravenous or intramuscular ketamine is used in higher-risk patients in ASA Class III or IV (see below). We rarely, if ever, use sodium thiopental in cyanotic patients. The direct effect of sodium thiopental on the peripheral vasculature is a slight increase in resistance,[41] but an ordinary dose of sodium thiopental causes a fall in cardiac output as a result of direct myocardial depression. The net effect is a decrease in systemic blood pressure, which causes the right-to-left shunt to increase, worsening the hypoxemia. Depending on the degree of right-to-left shunting, the "vein-to-brain" transit time for even a small dose of sodium thiopental may result in central nervous system overdosage.

INTRAVENOUS INDUCTION FOR
CYANOTIC PATIENTS

Ketamine is generally believed to be the drug of choice for induction of anesthesia in cyanotic patients, even those weighing as little as 5 kg. The theoretical disadvantages of ketamine include its sympathomimetic properties, which cause an increase in heart rate and in systemic and pulmonary blood pressures.[42] The possible precipitation of a hypercyanotic episode in patients with tetralogy of Fallot must be considered. If there is a history of hypercyanotic episodes in such patients, propranolol must be readily available for intravenous use in the event that induction of anesthesia precipitates another episode of severe hypoxemia. Intravenous propranolol (0.01 mg/kg) may be employed effectively for a short time in carefully monitored patients with hypercyanotic episodes while preparing for operation, during induction, or during manipulation of the heart.

Ketamine produces a dose-related depression of myocardial function in isolated heart preparations[43, 44] and therefore depends upon an intact sympathetic nervous system to produce an increase in cardiac output and systemic vascular resistance. It has been shown, however, that ketamine can be used safely as an induction agent even in patients being treated with β-blocking drugs including propranolol, as may be the case in children with idiopathic hypertrophic subaortic stenosis (IHSS) or tetralogy of Fallot.[45]

Despite its theoretical disadvantages, we have found ketamine to be safe and effective for induction of cyanotic patients. Ketamine is administered intravenously (2 mg/kg) over 1 minute or intramuscularly (5 mg/kg) into the arterior thigh muscles with a 3/4-inch 25-gauge needle. During 4 years of experience using ketamine as the induction agent for cyanotic patients, many of whom have undergone correction of tetralogy of Fallot, we have not encountered a hypercyanotic episode on induction. The patients must be *properly premedicated*. Inadequate premedication contributes to agitation and fright; excessive premedication will cause hypoventilation and hypercarbia. Both hypercarbia and agitation lead to catecholamine release, which increases the likelihood of a hypercyanotic episode.

MASK INDUCTION FOR THE ACYANOTIC PATIENT

When an inhalation induction is believed to be the method of choice, nitrous oxide and oxygen in a 60:40 ratio is administered for approximately 4 minutes after initial monitoring devices are attached. Low concentrations of halothane or enflurane are then begun, the child being allowed to breathe at his own respiratory rate and depth. Systemic blood pressure, heart sounds, and peripheral pulse amplitude are monitored frequently. After the child has drifted off to sleep, assisted ventilation is begun. The anesthesiologist watches the respiratory pattern, carefully assisting respiratory effort by simply increasing tidal volume with each breath. The concentrations of the gaseous agents are increased slowly to 2 percent halothane or 3 percent enflurane over a period of 5 minutes with assisted ventilation as tolerated by the patient.

Muscle relaxants are administered as outlined above using a defasciculating dose of pancuronium (0.01 mg/kg) or *d*-tubocurarine (0.1 mg/kg). Succinylcholine (1-2 mg/kg) is then given to facilitate intubation, the patient being hyperventilated with 100 percent oxygen just prior to laryngoscopy and intubation. In older children, we usually spray the trachea with a topical anesthetic such as 2 percent lidocaine (2 mg/kg) to decrease coughing stimulated by the endotracheal tube after recovery from succinylcholine paralysis. In the relatively healthy patient (ASA Class II or better), a paralyzing dose of pancuronium (0.08 mg/kg) can be given to facilitate intubation.

Monitoring

GENERAL PRINCIPLES

The purpose of all hemodynamic monitoring techniques is to ensure adequate blood volume, cardiac output, and regional blood flow. Assessment of perfusion is equally important during spontaneous cardiac output and during periods on cardiopulmonary bypass.

In circumstances in which total cardiac output may be less than optimal, monitoring should ensure at least *adequate* perfusion of organs most vulnerable to the noxious effects of ischemia. The brain, is, of course, the organ most sensitive to hypoxic injury. Destructive cellular responses to hypoxia are greatly influenced by temperature. The amount of oxygen required to maintain viability declines exponentially as body temperature is reduced. At 20°C oxygen consumption is reduced to 17 percent of normothermic levels.[46] The importance of this temperature-related phenomenon is clearly demonstrated by the brain's lack of tolerance of more than 4 minutes of total circulatory arrest at 37°C. When body temperature is reduced to 15°C, however, periods of circulatory arrest of 60 minutes are usually tolerated without permanent neurological sequelae.[47-49]

Parameters other than cardiac output and temperature influence oxygen delivery to vital organs. In children with congenital heart disease the level of systemic arterial hemoglobin saturation, total red blood cell mass or hemoglobin concentration, blood viscosity, presence of intravascular thrombosis, and the relative reactivity of the pulmonary and systemic vascular beds all influence adequacy of perfusion.

Basic monitoring devices used during the induction of anesthesia in the child with heart disease include (1) the *electrocardiogram*, (2) an arterial *blood pressure cuff* with a Doppler-principle sphygmomanometer, and (3) the *precordial stethoscope* to assess heart rate, rhythm, and the quality of heart sounds (see "Preinduction").

More accurate and sophisticated monitoring techniques are required for patients undergoing complex operations on the cardiovascular system during which normal autoregulatory mechanisms are altered both intraoperatively and postoperatively.

The monitoring protocol utilized in the

management of a child undergoing a cardiac operation depends upon the preferences of the responsible anesthesiologist. "Adequate monitoring" for a specific patient is the *simplest* system that will allow assessment and maintenance of adequate organ perfusion throughout the induction, operation, and postoperative period. Philosophical differences exist regarding the complexity of monitoring required. Some excellent teams manage large numbers of children with congenital heart disease very successfully using simpler monitoring systems equivalent to the devices used during induction. They rely heavily on "experience, observation, and clinical judgment." Other equally skilled teams, especially those with investigative curiosity, prefer the objectivity of more quantitative monitoring techniques.

Every additional monitoring device or measurement poses a small but definitely increased cost, time requirement, inconvenience, and in most cases, potential monitor-related complications. The anesthetic and surgical team should be convinced that the information provided by each monitoring device justifies the potential disadvantages.

Table 8-7 includes the monitoring techniques and parameters that should be considered for use in patients undergoing operation for treatment of congenital heart defects. Each team should adopt a protocol for monitoring their *routine* patients but should remain open-minded in consideration of additional parameters to be monitored in *specific* patients. As previously discussed, management of congenital heart disease often involves "the exception rather than the rule." Specific monitoring techniques are discussed in more detail in the sections and references that follow.

ELECTROCARDIOGRAM (ECG)

We routinely apply four standard disposable limb-lead electrocardiogram electrodes as well as a V_5 precordial electrode applied directly to the chest and draped out of the operative field using an adhesive-backed waterproof plastic skin towel. This V_5 lead is particularly helpful in recognizing periods of left ventricular ischemia reflected in the ST segments of the recorded electrocardiogram. The electrocardiographic monitor should be equipped with a write-out mode for recording on paper any possible arrhythmia or ST-segment change as it oc-

Table 8-7

Intraoperative Monitoring for the Pediatric Cardiac Surgical Patient

Preinduction
  1. Precordial stethoscope
  2. Electrocardiogram (ECG)
  3. Blood pressure (usually a Doppler-principle device)*
  4. Temperature (cutaneous temperature strip)
  5. Neuromuscular blockade nerve stimulator electrodes
Postinduction, before incision
  1. Esophageal stethoscope
  2. Intra-arterial monitoring catheter†
  3. Central venous pressure catheter
  4. Nasopharyngeal thermistor probe
  5. Rectal thermistor probe
  6. Urinary bladder catheter
  7. Electroencephalogram (EEG)‡
Postrepair, before closure of incision
  1. Atrial pacing wires
  2. Ventricular pacing wires
  3. Right atrial catheter‡
  4. Left atrial catheter‡
  5. Right ventricular–pulmonary arterial catheter‡
  6. Pulmonary arterial thermistor for cardiac output‡

* Applied on contralateral side of previous Blalock-Taussig shunt or on right arm during coarctation repair.
† Inserted on side indicated above.
‡ In selected patients.

curs. Accurate analysis of complex arrhythmias and recognition of ischemia must be made immediately, but retrospective review is also possible if a permanent record has been provided.

A child's resting heart rate is normally more rapid than that of an adult. The definition of undesirable sinus tachycardia must be arbitrarily extended to approximately 140 beats per minute or even faster for the small infant.[50] The ability to increase cardiac rate is one of the vital compensatory mechanisms for maintaining adequate cardiac output.

Arrhythmias contribute considerably toward reduction of cardiac output in both infants and older patients. Prompt recognition and treatment eases the transition to normal cardiac function after cardiopulmonary bypass.

Since many postoperative low cardiac output states are the result of abnormal conduction between the atria and the ventricles, atrial and ventricular pacing wires are routinely attached to the heart after many cardiovascular operations. The atrial pacing wires can be used as bipolar electrocardiographic leads for the electrical amplification of atrial activity and the assessment of supraventricular arrhythmias. Patients with sinus or junctional bradycardia but persistent atrioventricular conduction will benefit greatly from simple atrial pacing. Those patients with complete heart block or abnormal atrioventricular conduction will have a 15 to 25 percent increase in cardiac output when sequential AV pacing is instituted with an appropriate P-R interval.[51]

The ability to accurately and continuously display the heart rate and rhythm is one of the most important means of assessing the various causes of postoperative low cardiac output. The monitoring oscilloscope display should be clearly visible to the anesthesia team, the surgeon, and the perfusionist.

ARTERIAL PRESSURE

The level of systemic arterial pressure measured at any accessible site is determined by blood volume, cardiac output, peripheral resistance, elasticity of the arterial wall, proximal patency of the artery, and characteristics of the recording system. Arterial blood pressure and vital organ perfusion are related through vascular resistance. Satisfactory blood flow and organ perfusion may be present when there is relative hypotension; conversely, vital organ perfusion may be grossly inadequate, while the arterial blood pressure is normal or even elevated. Nonetheless, the accurate recording and display of the direct intra-arterial blood pressure and waveform are important techniques for assessing adequacy of cardiac output.

In the small infant, considerable difficulty may be encountered in obtaining an accurate arterial blood pressure by conventional blood pressure cuff and auscultation of Korotkoff sounds. This problem is accentuated during periods of hypovolemia and hypotension or increased peripheral vasoconstriction. For this reason, we measure intra-arterial blood pressure directly with an indwelling cannula, transducer, and oscillographic display in all operations re-

quiring cardiopulmonary bypass and in nearly all other cardiac operations.

The indwelling arterial cannula is placed in a location convenient to the anesthesiologist to allow frequent arterial blood sampling for measurements of blood gases, hemoglobin, hematocrit, blood glucose, serum electrolytes, activated clotting time, and other hematologic parameters as required.

We usually use the radial artery at the wrist for intraoperative and postoperative monitoring of arterial pressure even in very small infants. It is usually possible to cannulate the radial artery percutaneously using a 1½-inch-long 22-gauge plastic cannula. The percutaneous radial artery puncture is made just proximal to the volar carpal ligament on the palmar aspect of the wrist. Stopcocks are *not* used at the hub connector of the cannula. A T-connector (Abbott Laboratories) with a rubber diaphragm is placed at this point, minimizing the inadvertent injection of air, frequent motion, and arterial trauma produced by turning the stopcock and the risk of bacterial contamination associated with the open areas of the stopcock (see Fig. 8-1). The rubber diaphragm of the T-connector may be punctured quite easily with a small needle, and blood may be obtained after a few drops have been allowed to escape to clear the cannula of flush solution. Little or no negative pressure need be applied to the syringe during sampling. Blood samples not requiring anaerobic collection may be allowed to drip into the collecting tube by the force of arterial pressure alone, thus minimizing thrombogenic trauma to the arterial intima at the point of the cannula tip. This technique may seem unnecessary to those involved primarily in *adult* direct arterial blood pressure monitoring. It is absolutely *essential*, however, in the preservation of long-term function and patency of indwelling arterial cannulae in the tiny infant and child subject to greater-than-normal peripheral vascular resistance and arterial spasm.

The indwelling arterial cannula is connected to a pressure transducer and a constant infusion pump.[52] The cannula is continuously flushed with a solution of normal saline containing 1000 units of sodium heparin and 100 mg of lidocaine per 100 ml at a rate of 1-2 ml per hour. A second T-connector with the rubber diaphragm removed is inserted at the pressure transducer manifold. This arrangement allows continuous

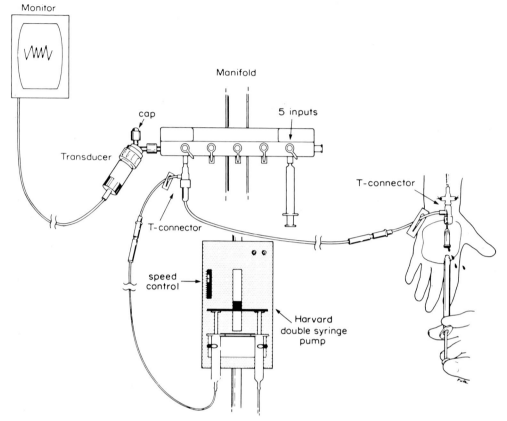

Fig. 8-1. Arterial line set-up for constant infusion of flush solution and continuous readout of pressure tracing (see text).

display of the arterial pressure waveform and simultaneous continuous irrigation of the cannula. The constant infusion pump need *not* be turned off during the brief intervals required for obtaining a blood sample. The "tail" of the T-connector attached to the arterial cannula is simply occluded with the metal clip and the blood sample obtained through the rubber diaphragm with as little negative pressure as possible. Upon completion of sampling the metal clip is released; the slight pressure that has built up within the tubing system during the sampling provides the only flushing required for continuation of waveform recording and maintenance of patency. Application of strong negative pressure in the attempt to aspirate blood from the arterial line will almost always collapse a small artery, damage the intima, induce spasm, and cause permanent thrombosis. Samples should be collected by the force of transmitted arterial pressure alone whenever possible.

The arterial cannula, cannulation site, and T-connector must be conspicuously labeled to avoid inadvertent injection of medications or air into the artery. Loss of hands, arms, and legs has occurred from this error! We use a large piece of red tape to identify the arterial catheter.

Utilizing the techniques described above both in the operating room and in the intensive care unit, we have maintained the functional patency of arterial cannulae in the radial and temporal arteries of newborn infants for as long as 21 days, at which point they were removed electively when no longer needed.

We prefer a constant oscillographic display of *mean* arterial blood pressure both intraoperatively and postoperatively. This is a more stable hemodynamic parameter than either systolic or diastolic arterial blood pressure and is less subject to variation as a function of tubing compliance, arterial elasticity, tiny air bubbles in the pressure-recording system, and the characteristics of the recording system itself. The mean arterial pressure is not significantly influenced by the continuous infusion of the saline-heparin-lidocaine irrigation solution. When more precise phasic pressures are desired for analysis of the waveform or for recording the systolic and diastolic pressures, the metal occluding clamp of the T-connector located near the pressure manifold is occluded, thus excluding the more compliant irrigation tubing, syringe, and pump from the monitoring system. Under these circumstances, a normal-appearing arterial waveform will be displayed. For those preferring continuous display of a normal arterial waveform rather than the sine-wave mean arterial pressure, a Sorenson Intraflo device can be connected permanently to the T-connector in the monitoring manifold or directly to the transducer. The remainder of the infusion system is unchanged, but the Intraflo device eliminates the "damping" caused by the more compliant constant infusion system. We do *not* like to use the Intraflo unit with a pressurized intravenous fluid bag, as is commonly practiced in *adult* arterial line care. Such a system does not allow sufficiently precise control of the volume of fluid administered.

When percutaneous insertion of the cannula cannot be easily accomplished, the artery is exposed and cannulated under direct vision. The use of optical magnification loupes, a surgical headlight, a sitting position for the surgeon, and a small set of microvascular surgical instruments increases the ease and success of direct cannulation of the tiny radial or superficial temporal artery. Insertion of the arterial pressure monitoring catheter is carried out *after* the induction of anesthesia but *before* positioning, prepping, and draping the patient. A careful taping routine for securing the arterial cannula is most important. An arm board is usually not necessary. Adhesive tape properly applied will minimize motion, prevent inadvertent removal of the cannula, and avoid thrombogenic trauma to the arterial intima during blood sampling.

When the radial arteries are thrombosed or when proximal obstruction is present in the brachial arterial system, other arteries must be used for monitoring. The left radial artery should not be used for monitoring during operations for repair of coarctation of the aorta or vascular ring; it may be occluded or sacrificed. When a Blalock-Taussig shunt has been or is being con-structed, the radial artery on the ipsilateral side cannot be used. Alternative sites of arterial monitoring in such circumstances include the superficial temporal arteries bilaterally and the common or superficial femoral arteries. These are usually cannulated by direct surgical exposure, but percutaneous techniques may also be used. The superficial temporal arteries are the preferred alternatives for monitoring during coarctation repair when the right radial artery cannot be used. When an anomalous origin of a subclavian artery has been demonstrated angiographically, an appropriate alternate artery should be used for intraoperative pressure monitoring.

CENTRAL VENOUS PRESSURE

A central venous pressure monitoring catheter is often inserted percutaneously through the brachial vein preoperatively in older children undergoing cardiovascular surgery. This relatively large-bore cannula provides a useful conduit for the injection of irritating medications, including calcium and vasopressors, blood, packed red blood cells, and other volume expanders. It is also useful for assessing the relationship between blood volume and cardiac function.

If this catheter is to be used for the determination of venous pressure in the head and neck during cardiopulmonary bypass, the tip of the catheter must lie near the cephalad end of the superior vena cava. If the catheter tip is passed further down the superior vena cava or into the right atrium, it will be occluded by the tourniquet tightened around the superior vena caval cannula when total cardiopulmonary bypass is instituted.

Percutaneous internal jugular venous catheters are inserted by some teams[53, 54] even in small children. A low incidence of complications is reported by advocates of this technique. Care must again be taken not to insert this cannula too far down into the superior vena cava or right atrium.

We do not feel that the *routine* monitoring of central venous pressure during pediatric cardiac surgery is necessary. This information is useful, however, in certain critically ill infants and in those in whom hypovolemia with subsequent need for central vascular volume expansion during induction is anticipated.

In the presence *or* absence of central venous pressure monitoring, the anesthesiologist must *observe the face and head* carefully during total cardiopulmonary bypass for evidence of obstruction of venous return from the upper portion of the body. If the superior vena caval venous drainage cannula is partially occluded, wedged into the innominate vein or jugular vein, or intermittently kinked by the surgeon, inadequacy of venous return is usually first reflected by loss of volume from the oxygenator reservoir. Shortly thereafter, plethora of the face and head and soft tissue swelling or suffusion of the eyelids, conjunctivae, and neck may be noted. This is a catastrophic event and must be called to the surgeon's attention immediately! Rapid repositioning of the superior caval cannula or correction of other causes for obstruction is essential if the development of significant cerebral edema or lethal intracranial hemorrhage is to be avoided.

Those individuals dealing primarily in the management of adults undergoing cardiovascular surgery may again not be impressed by the need for this constant attention to potential superior vena caval obstruction. In the small child, however, the difference between the size of the venous return cannula and the superior vena cava may be quite small. The relatively frequent occurrence of a persistent left superior vena cava in children with congenital heart defects further accentuates the problem of adequate venous drainage from the head. Changes in position of only a few millimeters in the superior vena caval venous drainage cannula can make the difference between adequate and totally inadequate venous decompression. Movements of the cannula by the surgeon within the operative field may result in sudden changes in the adequacy of venous return. Frequent and repeated observation for facial plethora, petechiae, and conjunctival suffusion is absolutely essential! Even the continuous recording of central venous pressure does *not* obviate the potential complication of superior vena caval obstruction, since position of the monitoring catheter tip may alter the accuracy of the recording. When a central venous pressure catheter is present, however, it is helpful to ask the surgeon to temporarily occlude the superior vena cava or the superior drainage cannula, thus determining the degree to which the central venous pressure catheter can be expected to reveal such obstruction.

Even though the external jugular veins may be prominent in the neck and may tempt per-

cutaneous cannulation, catheters placed through the external venous jugular system are particularly sensitive to changes in position and are extremely difficult and inconvenient to maintain postoperatively in children. We have therefore come to the conclusion that monitoring the venous pressure in the external jugular veins is probably more trouble than it is worth. If catheter passage by the brachial route is unsuccessful, either percutaneously or by cutdown, the intraoperative insertion of right and left atrial lines by the surgeon is easier and more likely to provide accurate hemodynamic data (see below).

Extreme caution must be exercised in the care of central venous catheters—indeed *all* venous lines—in children with *cyanotic* congenital heart disease! Even very small air bubbles in the intravenous tubing and connectors pose a potentially lethal threat to such a child. Air passes directly through a right-to-left anatomic communication into the aorta and on to the coronary arteries or to the *brain*, producing a cerebrovascular accident, seizure, and even permanent neurological deficit. We manage central venous catheters by continuous heparinized flush *exactly* like arterial and left atrial catheters (see Fig. 8-1).

The anesthesiologist managing children with congenital heart defects must develop a keen sense of awareness of air bubbles in the intravenous lines and monitoring devices. The casual attitude toward small air bubbles frequently practiced by those caring for adult cardiovascular patients has absolutely no place in pediatric management. Even in the acyanotic child, an air bubble present in the right heart may find its way through a patent foramen ovale or patent ductus arteriosus during a period of coughing, Valsalva, or positive pressure ventilation with associated elevation in pulmonary arterial and right heart pressures.

The intraoperative and postoperative care of central venous pressure catheters is similar to that previously described for the indwelling arterial cannula and the transthoracic right and left atrial catheters (see below). A continuous flushing system identical to that previously described is used.

TRANSTHORACIC RIGHT AND
LEFT ATRIAL CATHETERS

The direct placement of right atrial and/or left atrial pressure monitoring catheters by the surgeon prior to termination of cardiopulmonary bypass provides useful information during the weaning of the patient from bypass and in the postoperative period.

In the absence of atrioventricular valve stenosis, the mean atrial pressure can be assumed to be an accurate reflection of the end-diastolic pressure in the related ventricle. In accordance with the Frank-Starling relationship, ventricular output is largely a function of ventricular filling pressure or the end-diastolic pressure.[55]

Cardiac output is ordinarily determined by left ventricular performance. The placement of a left atrial catheter will therefore be helpful for determination of the mean left atrial pressure (left ventricular filling pressure). Optimum cardiac output can only be obtained if the left atrial pressure is maintained within the appropriate range determined for the individual patient.

In many congenital cardiac defects the *right* ventricle is more likely to pose a limitation to adequate cardiac output. For example, operation for the total correction of tetralogy of Fallot adds an insulting right ventriculotomy to the previously existing right ventricular outflow tract obstruction and hypertrophic myocardium. In this case, both right atrial *and* left atrial pressure monitoring catheters are desirable. It would not be unusual for the right atrial pressure to remain somewhat higher than the left atrial pressure after repair of such defects or in the presence of pulmonary vascular obstructive disease. Judgment, plus awareness of the pathophysiology of the lesion being treated, must dictate interpretation of the right and left atrial pressures.

In all but the simplest of intracardiac operations, we prefer to monitor both right and left atrial pressures postoperatively. The catheters are passed through the chest wall, secured to the skin, and maintained patent by a flushing system exactly like that previously described for maintenance of indwelling arterial pressure monitoring catheters (Fig. 8-1).

Pressures can be recorded and displayed continuously while the catheters are being used for the infusion of vasopressors, vasodilators, antiarrhythmic medications, or maintenance intravenous fluids. If none of these infusions is required, the catheters should be maintained patent with a constant infusion of approximately 1-2 ml per hour of the previously described irrigation solution. The lidocaine may be omitted

from this infusion if desired, since arterial spasm is not a problem.

When no longer needed, the catheters are simply withdrawn through the chest wall. Bleeding from points of catheter insertion, sepsis, thrombosis, and catheter entrapment have not been significant problems.

Frequent comparison of relative right and left atrial pressures provides useful postoperative information. Simultaneous fall of both right and left atrial pressures suggests either hypovolemia or improvement in myocardial performance. Gradual simultaneous *increases* in both right and left atrial pressures suggest hypervolemia or deterioration in ventricular performance. An abrupt rise in both pressures simultaneously warns of a catastrophic event such as an arrhythmia or ischemic myocardial insult. An abrupt fall in both pressures suggests life-threatening hemorrhage. Of great importance during the early postoperative hours is a disparate *rise* in right atrial pressure with a simultaneous *fall* in left atrial pressure, which suggests either cardiac tamponade or a sudden increase in pulmonary vascular resistance. Elevated right heart filling pressures are particularly suggestive of excessive positive pressure ventilation with associated reduction in pulmonary blood flow in the infant and child.

The selective use of right and left atrial catheters may be particularly useful in patients requiring inotropic support and/or vasodilator infusions. The use of the *left* atrial catheter for the infusion of inotropic medications such as epinephrine allows the desired cardiac effect to be obtained at a lower dose without the undesired pulmonary vasoconstriction associated with the infusion of such medications into right-sided catheters. Conversely, right atrial or direct pulmonary arterial infusion of vasodilator medications such as tolazoline hydrochloride (Priscoline) or sodium nitroprusside (Nipride) may be helpful in the management of the child with elevated pulmonary vascular resistance.

A direct right atrial catheter may be used in conjunction with a small thermistor wire placed in the pulmonary artery for the direct measurement of cardiac output in small infants by the thermodilution principle (see "Cardiac Output" below).

BODY TEMPERATURE

The importance of intraoperative body temperature monitoring for infants and children is well recognized.[56-61] Significant changes in body temperature may occur during anesthesia as a consequence of exposure, reaction to anesthetic agents, extreme vasocontriction or vasodilatation, excessive draping and hot operating room lights, or the infusion of cold intravenous fluids and blood.

Significant uncontrolled hypothermia in the neonate or premature infant will produce metabolic acidosis and myocardial and respiratory depression. Catecholamine release stimulated by hypothermic stress is undesirable in children with cardiac disease.

Hyperthermia is most undesirable in children with cyanotic congenital heart disease and systemic arterial hemoglobin unsaturation. Total body oxygen consumption is directly related to body temperature.[56,62] Increases in oxygen consumption associated with hyperthermia produce metabolic acidosis and myocardial depression. In children subject to hypercyanotic episodes, elevated body temperature may prompt a life-threatening hypoxemic episode (see previous discussion of tetralogy of Fallot).

The use of a servo-controlled overhead warming light or heating mattress is useful in maintaining normal body temperature during induction and exposure associated with insertion of monitoring catheters, prepping, and draping. The ambient temperature of pediatric operating rooms is usually maintained at a level above that used for adult operations. Infants are particularly prone to heat loss because of their large surface-area-to-body-mass ratio.

Cardiovascular surgery poses some unique body temperature monitoring problems. Total body hypothermia—often to extreme degrees—is used to reduce metabolic oxygen requirements of the myocardium, the brain, the kidneys, and other vital organs. The judicious use of both generalized and selective hypothermia minimizes the ischemic insult associated with various surgical manipulations, even during periods of totally interrupted blood flow (see ''Myocardial Preservation'' and ''Profound Hypothermia'' below).

The accuracy of temperature monitors may be difficult to assess because of altered regional blood flow. The temperature being recorded by a probe in one area of the body may not reflect the temperature, perfusion, and protection afforded other vital organs.

We continuously monitor *nasopharyngeal* and/or high *esophageal* temperature and *rectal* temperature using thermistor probes in all patients undergoing cardiovascular operations. The temperature of the *heart* may be measured more accurately by the direct application of a sterile myocardial thermistor, a technique that has been helpful during the use of hypothermia-dependent myocardial preservation techniques. It is also useful in assessing the adequacy of myocardial rewarming during resuscitation, weaning from cardiopulmonary bypass, and when significant differences are apparent between measured nasopharyngeal and rectal temperatures.

Peripheral *skin* temperature is useful in assessing the adequacy of overall perfusion. Reduced cardiac output or inadequate blood volume prompts sympathetic vasoconstriction of the subcutaneous vascular bed. Measured skin temperature falls, an objective confirmation of the cool extremities found in patients with inadequate cardiac output or shock.

Accurately recorded nasopharyngeal temperature probably most closely reflects actual brain temperature.[63] Tympanic membrane thermistors are used in some centers to reflect brain temperature, although damage to the tympanic membrane is possible using these probes even when extreme care is employed on insertion and removal.[64]

Caution is required when cold intrapericardial solutions or ice slush is used as an adjunct to myocardial preservation. In such situations the esophageal temperature will almost always be lower than the temperature in the remainder of the body.

In order to reduce to a minimum the time required to cool or rewarm the body during cardiopulmonary bypass and to minimize the effects of vasoconstriction in various vascular beds, small doses of vasodilator medications (sodium nitroprusside, phentolamine, chlorpromazine, halothane, or enflurane) are useful. We prefer the use of an easily regulated intravenous infusion of sodium nitroprusside for this purpose. An adequate blood volume and a mean arterial perfusion pressure of 40-50 torr should be maintained during vasodilatation for cooling or rewarming. A similar vasodilator regimen may be used to hasten and improve the uniformity of surface-induced hypothermia in infants undergoing operations under conditions of circulatory arrest.

URINARY OUTPUT

The continuous output of a relatively normal quantity of urine is one of the most reliable indicators of adequate hydration, blood volume, cardiac output and perfusion on cardiopulmonary bypass, and absence of inferior vena caval obstruction. All patients undergoing cardiovascular surgery should have a urinary bladder catheter inserted for the accurate timed measurement of urinary output and urine specific gravity or osmolarity. The catheter may be omitted in healthy patients undergoing very short operations such as the ligation of an uncomplicated patent ductus arteriosus.

The newborn's meatus and urethra may be too small to accept an adequate Foley catheter. In such situations we use a small infant feeding tube (8-Fr) inserted just barely beyond the point of first urine drainage. The tube is then sutured to the labial skin in the female child or to the foreskin of the male infant. Further adhesive tape is used to anchor the catheter to the skin, care being taken to avoid penile constriction in the male.

A Foley catheter is used in larger children. Foley catheters smaller than the 10-Fr size should probably not be used, since they drain poorly. When using small Foley catheters, only one-half of the recommended balloon volume should be injected to avoid compression of the catheter lumen.

Catheterization should be performed by someone experienced in the techniques required for small infants. Awareness of previous urologic pathology or instrumentation is important. The external genitalia should be examined for congenital abnormalities before catheterization. Awareness of the significance of hypospadias, meatal stenosis, chordae, posterior urethral valves, and other congenital abnormalities is important.

The catheter should be passed gently into the bladder under sterile conditions and should *not* be secured in position until urine flow is demonstrated. Catheters have often been passed into the vagina rather than the urethra in female children. Foley balloons have been inflated in the prostatic urethra of the male child, and urethral perforations have occurred. When in doubt as to catheter position, a small amount of sterile saline should be injected and quantitatively recovered.

If extreme difficulty is encountered during urinary bladder catheterization, a urologist should be consulted and consideration should be given to cancellation of the operation. The possibility of gram-negative sepsis and subsequent endocarditis following complicated urologic instrumentation is well known.

We prefer the use of intravenous tubing or other small-diameter connections from the catheter to the urine collection bag in infants and small children. The smaller dead space allows more accurate determination of urine volume than one can obtain using the large-volume adult connecting tubing.

Hourly determinations of urine volume are recorded routinely. Determinations of urine output should be made every 15 minutes in patients on cardiopulmonary bypass and during the early unstable period following completion of cardiopulmonary bypass. Adequate urine production is considered to be 1 ml/kg body weight per hour.[32,33,65,66] Complete anuria suggests a malfunction of the catheter or collecting system. In small children the bladder is easily palpated above the pubis. If it is felt to be distended the catheter should be repositioned, or a suprapubic aspiration can be carried out using a small plastic needle.

Inadequate urinary output in the presence of a functioning catheter system suggests low cardiac output, hypovolemia, or inadequate perfusion on cardiopulmonary bypass. If the patient is on complete cardiopulmonary bypass, the position and adequacy of drainage of venous blood through the inferior vena caval cannula should be confirmed by the surgeon and perfusionist. Inferior vena caval obstruction will, of course, lead to elevation of renal vein pressure and cessation of urine output.

During periods of profound hypothermia and/or circulatory arrest, urine output is expected to cease. No treatment is necessary during these periods.

When other treatable causes of oliguria have been excluded, persistent oliguria should be treated by the intravenous administration of furosemide (1 mg/kg) and/or mannitol (0.5 gm/kg). If oliguria continues, it may be treated by the administration of a pharmacologic vasodilator (sodium nitroprusside) and increased doses of furosemide and/or mannitol within reasonable limits. It is very rare for oliguria to persist in the presence of adequate cardiac output or adequate perfusion on cardiopulmonary bypass.

The presence of pink or red urine indicates hemolysis that may be secondary to the excessive use of cardiotomy suction by the surgeon, trauma to red blood cells due to a long period of cardiopulmonary bypass, or a blood transfusion reaction. Hemolysis should be treated by alkalinization using sodium bicarbonate and by administration of crystalloid solutions for hemodilution. If the urine concentration is allowed to increase or if oliguria develops during a period of significant hemolysis, hematin precipitation within the renal tubules and subsequent acute renal failure are likely. Other stigmata of a transfusion reaction should be sought, including "hives" or urticaria. A small amount of hemolysis is not unusual during cardiopulmonary bypass in children.

ARTERIAL BLOOD GASES, ELECTROLYTES, AND HEMOGLOBIN

Blood withdrawn from the arterial pressure monitoring cannula is submitted for analysis of arterial blood gases, potassium, hemoglobin, and hematocrit immediately after insertion of the catheter and as frequently thereafter as desired by the anesthesiologist. No particular interval between blood gas determinations is advocated. The frequency of such analyses must be determined to some extent by the experience of the anesthesiologist and the hemodynamic stability of the patient. It is important to measure arterial blood gases shortly after induction to determine acid-base status and the adequacy of ventilation. While on cardiopulmonary bypass the development of metabolic acidosis suggests inadequate perfusion, just as it suggests low cardiac output in the prebypass and postoperative periods.

If arterial blood gas analysis and other necessary laboratory procedures are not provided in the operating room, the central laboratory must be prepared to report results of such determinations within a maximum of 5 minutes from the time of sampling.

In addition to the serum potassium, serum and ionized calcium levels must be monitored in infants and young children and in all patients undergoing operations on cardiopulmonary bypass. Measurement of ionized rather than total serum calcium is preferred, but the technology for accurate measurement of serum ionized calcium has been subject to a variety of problems.

The appearance of the electrocardiogram (widened QRS complex; prolonged Q-T interval) and an increase in blood pressure or cardiac output in response to a small injection of calcium chloride (5-10 mg/kg) are presumptive evidence of a less-than-optimal ionized calcium level. Ionized calcium plays a vital role in maintenance of electromechanical association within the myocardium.[67] Calcium depletion or chelation by citrate in bank blood can result in severe depression of myocardial contractility and cardiac output.

NEUROMUSCULAR BLOCKADE

Nondepolarizing muscle relaxants are utilized in most cardiovascular operations, unless otherwise contraindicated, either in combination with the potent anesthetic agents (halothane or enflurane) or as an adjunct to the nitrous oxide/oxygen/narcotic technique. Muscle relaxants must be administered in a safe and controlled manner. The choice of pancuronium, d-tubocurarine, or gallamine is made on the basis of the physiology of the lesion present and the expected cardiovascular effects of each of these medications.

For neuromuscular-blockade monitoring, we insert needle electrodes or attach noninvasive cutaneous patch electrodes on the ulnar side of the arm in which the radial arterial catheter has been placed. Muscle-twitch response is measured prior to the administration of any muscle relaxants and is periodically measured throughout the operation; additional muscle relaxant being given when the twitch response returns. Blockade monitoring is important in all cases in which muscle relaxants are used but is especially helpful in those patients for whom postoperative mechanical ventilation is not planned. The nondepolarizing muscle relaxants are reversed at the end of the operation in these patients, the blockade monitor being used as one indicator of the completeness of reversal.

CARDIAC OUTPUT

In the anesthetized patient the previously described parameters of urinary output, arterial blood pressure, left and/or right atrial pressure, arterial blood pH, and the extremity skin temperature provide indirect guidelines as to the adequacy of cardiac output. In the nonanesthetized patient and during the postoperative period, the level of consciousness and the mental status offer additional indirect information. Each of these parameters, however, is significantly influenced by other factors and thus cannot be relied upon as an absolute indicator of the amount of blood being pumped by the heart.

Two techniques—green dye dilution[68] and thermodilution—[69] are in current use for the direct measurement of cardiac output in children in the operating room and postoperatively in the intensive care unit. In the green dye dilution technique, cardiogreen dye is injected through a central venous, right atrial, or pulmonary arterial catheter. The concentration of the dye is measured in blood aspirated continuously through an optical densitometer connected to an indwelling peripheral arterial catheter. Computation of cardiac output may be made manually, applying the Stewart-Hamilton equation to the exponential downslope of the curve and using planimetric methods for measurement of the area beneath the curve. Calculations are now performed automatically by a variety of computerized cardiac output instruments.

The green dye technique is particularly useful for detection of residual intracardiac right-to-left and left-to-right shunts, the former being apparent as an earlier-than-normal appearance time for the green dye, and the latter producing a prolonged, flat recirculation of dye during the inscription of the downslope.

Thermodilution techniques for the measurement of cardiac output have been more widely used in the operating room and the intensive care unit since the development of the flow-directed balloon-tipped Swan-Ganz catheter. This device has been used relatively infrequently in children because of the large size of the catheter. The thermodilution principle, however, is applicable even in very small infants if a thermistor wire is inserted into the pulmonary artery through the anterior wall of the right ventricle during the cardiac operation. A right atrial catheter is inserted through the appendage at the completion of bypass. A small bolus (2-5 ml) of room-temperature or colder dextrose in water solution is then injected through the right atrial cannula. The typical thermodilution curve is recorded from the pulmonary arterial thermistor. Calculations are made immediately by computer. The thermistor and right atrial catheter are left in place and passed through the chest wall for continued use in the intensive care unit. They can be removed safely simply by pulling

them out when no longer required for postoperative monitoring.

The simultaneous measurement of cardiac output, mean arterial blood pressure, mean pulmonary arterial blood pressure, and left and right atrial pressures allow the calculation of both systemic and pulmonary vascular resistances. Knowledge of these values is helpful in the choice of medications needed for the management of low cardiac output in the postoperative period.

ACTIVATED CLOTTING TIME AND COAGULATION FACTORS

Patients operated upon using cardiopulmonary bypass must be systemically heparinized prior to insertion of cardiac and aortic cannulae. The activated clotting time (ACT) is used to monitor the adequacy of heparinization and subsequent reversal with protamine sulfate. A blood sample is obtained from the arterial pressure monitoring cannula while the incision is being made, and the "control" ACT is determined using a Hemochron device.[70] The control ACT is usually in the range of 140 to 160 seconds before heparin is administered. Beef lung sodium heparin (200-300 units/kg or 2-3 mg/kg) is administered through a freely flowing intravenous line as the pericardium is being opened. In reoperations where extensive dissection may be required, the surgeon may request that the heparin be withheld until later in the operation. When surface-induced profound hypothermia is employed in infants, heparin is given during the surface cooling before the incision so that cardiopulmonary bypass can be instituted rapidly if an inadequate cardiac rhythm develops. About 3 minutes after the administration of heparin, another ACT is determined, this one usually exceeding 300 seconds. If the ACT is *less* than 300 seconds, additional heparin is administered, and the institution of cardiopulmonary bypass is delayed until a value exceeding 300 seconds is obtained.

The heparin administered as a component of the pump oxygenator prime adds significantly to the total patient heparin level and hence to the amount of protamine sulfate required for reversal of heparinization at the completion of bypass. This is particularly true in small infants, in whom the ratio of prime volume to patient blood volume is large. The ACT is used to determine the amount of protamine required for reversal, since a variety of factors, including body temperature and duration of bypass, influence the in vivo half-life of heparin. Administration of the appropriate dose of protamine usually restores the ACT to near control levels.[71]

Following completion of cardiopulmonary bypass, reversal of heparin and restoration of the activated clotting time to normal levels, and control of major anatomic bleeding sources, a blood sample is submitted for determination of platelet count, prothrombin time (PT), and partial thromboplastin time (PTT). These values, in addition to the hemoglobin and hematocrit, determine the need for the transfusion of fresh whole blood, fresh frozen plasma, platelets, or packed red blood cells.

ELECTROENCEPHALOGRAM (EEG)

Bifrontal and temporal electroencephalographic electrodes are applied and the signal displayed oscillographically in selected cases during cardiopulmonary bypass. This admittedly crude indication of cerebral activity is useful in those cases in which profound hypothermia is employed. Cerebral activity slows with cooling; at temperatures below 22°C, electroencephalographic activity ceases.[72] With rewarming the EEG pattern returns to preoperative potentials and can be a useful prognostic sign in even the smallest infants.

BLOOD GLUCOSE

Levels of blood glucose are monitored by sampling blood from the arterial monitoring catheter several times during cardiovascular operations. Knowledge of the blood glucose level is particularly important in the very small infant with immature glucose autoregulatory mechanisms and in whom stress, fever, critical illness, or sepsis may provoke life-threatening or neurologically destructive hypoglycemia or significant hyperglycemia. Anesthesia masks many of the usual signs and symptoms of hypoglycemia, including irritability, hypertonicity, listlessness, seizures, and loss of consciousness. Corticosteroids administered to cardiac patients may further complicate glucose metabolism.

Hyperglycemia (blood glucose in excess of 150 mg/100 ml) during cardiopulmonary bypass and in the postoperative period are also potentially harmful.[73] Nonketotic hyperosmolar coma

and polyuria with potassium depletion may be significant problems.

Administration of Intraoperative Fluids

Fluid and electrolyte therapy before, during, and after cardiopulmonary bypass is determined by the patient's age and weight, the type of malformation present, as well as the urinary output determined on an hourly basis. Because of the tendency to absorb fluid during cardiopulmonary bypass, we generally limit the amount of crystalloid administered in the prebypass and bypass periods. Using constant infusion pumps to deliver very accurate amounts of fluid, we are better able to control the net amount of fluid absorbed by the patient in the perioperative period. Using 5 percent dextrose and Ringer's lactate or 5 percent dextrose and 0.25 percent saline, we usually infuse 1ml/kg/hr per I.V. through each of two large-bore plastic cannulae. Although this is a low maintenance dose of I.V. fluids for the small child, who generally requires more fluid than an adult, this dose has been arrived at because of the relatively large amount of crystalloid that is absorbed by the patients during the cardiopulmonary bypass, especially using hemodilution techniques.

If, however, urinary output during the prebypass or early bypass periods is not adequate, an increase in the amount of crystalloid is justified as a challenge to ensure adequate urinary excretion during the operative period. If an increase in crystalloid administration does not result in an increase in urinary output, furosemide is administered (1-2 mg/kg) to stimulate urine output.

Others have suggested the necessity of administering considerably larger amounts of crystalloid fluid during the prebypass and bypass periods in the hope of improving peripheral perfusion during bypass.[33] If the patient is adequately hydrated in the preoperative and immediate perioperative periods, the administration of larger quantities of fluid is considered unnecessary and perhaps detrimental because of the tendency of these small patients to absorb large quantities of fluid from the pump prime in the early phases of the cardiopulmonary bypass.

While no formula is considered absolutely accurate, the major indication of adequate fluid administration and blood volume is adequate urine output, which is generally considered to be ½-1 ml/kg/hr or greater.[32,33,65,66]

In the small infant (less than 5 kg), blood glucose levels must be followed during the surgery to ensure that hypoglycemia or hyperglycemia does not ensue from the administered fluids.[73]

Maintenance of Anesthesia in the Prebypass Period

Once induction of anesthesia is safely accomplished and the patient is intubated, monitoring lines established, and two large-bore plastic intravenous needles inserted, the appropriate level of anesthesia is maintained using nitrous oxide, oxygen, and halothane or enflurane in low concentrations with a nondepolarizing muscle relaxant. Alternatively, a nitrous oxide/oxygen/narcotic muscle relaxant technique is used.

A sump-type pediatric nasogastric tube is inserted, and its position in the stomach is confirmed by injection of air, auscultation, palpation, or aspiration of gastric contents. The nasogastric tube is required to avoid gastric dilatation from swallowed air and anesthetic gases leaking around the usually loosely fitting uncuffed pediatric endotracheal tube. Gastric distention can cause reflex bradycardia and hypotension and can be confused with abdominal distention or liver enlargement from obstructed inferior vena caval flow or high central venous pressure.

A pediatric esophageal stethoscope is positioned behind the heart as the precordial stethoscope is removed for skin preparation. Nasopharyngeal and esophageal temperature probes are inserted.

Arterial blood gases are measured to assess the adequacy of ventilation. Significant metabolic acidosis, if present, is corrected with sodium bicarbonate. If the metabolic acidosis persists, it should be considered an indication of low cardiac output, and an inotropic infusion (dopamine, isoproterenol, or epinephrine) may be required. Excessive positive pressure ventilation is avoided in cyanotic patients with less than normal pulmonary blood flow, since this will further reduce pulmonary blood flow.

The control activated clotting time is measured prior to the administration of heparin, which is given when the pericardium is opened or about 10 minutes prior to cannulation of the heart and aorta. Anticoagulation is considered to be adequate within about 3 minutes after administration of heparin, but we prefer to document an ACT of more than 300 seconds before insertion of cannulae. Bank blood should be available for administration at the time of cannulation in the unexpected event of excessive blood loss from this procedure. It is desirable to institute cardiopulmonary bypass with the patient as nearly normovolemic as possible.

An adequate dose of narcotic is necessary at the beginning of bypass to ensure satisfactory anesthesia and analgesia during bypass when the inhalation agents are withdrawn. Additional doses of narcotic can, of course, be given during bypass, and inhalation agents can be administered through the pump oxygenator.

If the nerve stimulator (blockade monitor) indicates greater than 90 percent neuromuscular blackade prior to bypass, no further muscle relaxants are administered. The initial paralyzing dose has usually fallen to a degree consistent with return of some neuromuscular function, and a small maintenance dose of nondepolarizing muscle relaxant (10-20% of the initial dose) is usually administered at the onset of cardiopulmonary bypass.

CARDIOPULMONARY BYPASS

General Considerations

The use of the pump oxygenator during periods of cardiopulmonary bypass should result in adequate blood flow to vital organs while providing the surgeon with a relatively bloodless intracardiac operative field. The basic components of any cardiopulmonary bypass system include the following apparatus:

1. A *venous cannulae* for collection of blood from the cavae or the right atrium.
2. A *reservoir* to which the venous blood flows by gravity.
3. An *oxygenator* in which blood is equilibrated with oxygen and carbon dioxide.
4. A *heat exchanger* for cooling or warming the blood.
5. A *pump* to return blood to the patient at arterial pressure.
6. A *filter* in the tubing for removal of bubbles and particulate debris.

7. An *arterial cannula* through which the oxygenated blood is returned to the patient's arterial system.

A good cardiopulmonary bypass system for pediatric use must be capable of varying blood flow over a wide range with precise control over small changes in flow. The formed elements of the blood (red blood cells and platelets) must not be unduly damaged by the mechanics of the system. The temperature of the blood must be rapidly variable over a wide range (16°-38°C). The priming volume of the system should be small. Oxygen and carbon dioxide equilibration should be efficient and predictable.

Choice of arterial and venous cannula size is critical in infants and small children. Flow is obstructed when cannulae are either too large or too small (see Tables 8-8 and 8-9 for guidelines).

The technical aspects and theoretical implications of cardiopulmonary bypass are considered elsewhere in this book and will not be discussed in detail here.

We currently use a disposable bubble-type oxygenator with self-contained heat exchanger and a minimally occlusive twin-roller pump for

Table 8-8

Arterial Perfusion
Cannulae Sizes for
Pediatric Cardiac Surgery

Weight of Child	French Size
0–5 kg	10 Fr
5–10 kg	12 Fr
10–22 kg	14 Fr
22–32 kg	16 Fr
32–45 kg	18 Fr
Over 45 kg	20 Fr

all pediatric patients requiring cardiopulmonary bypass. When the anticipated period of cardiopulmonary bypass is less than 30 minutes, perfusion is carried out at nomothermia (35°–37.5°C). For perfusions expected to last from 30 to 60 minutes, temperature is lowered to 30°-33°C (moderate hypothermia) to reduce total body oxygen requirements and allow a lower total blood flow on cardiopulmonary bypass. Damage to formed blood elements is thus reduced. For more complex operations in which bypass time is expected to exceed 60 minutes

Table 8-9

The flow rates listed below are the *maximum* levels that should be counted on when using *two* venous drainage cannulae (Bardic wire-reinforced pediatric lighthouse tipped type) of the size indicated attached to a single venous return line of the size indicated.

Venous Drainage Catheter	Venous Line Sizes		
	1/4 Inch	3/8 Inch	1/2 Inch
16	920 ml/min	1200 ml/min	1200 ml/min
18	1080	1800	1800
20	1280	2300	2300
22	1300	3000	3300
24	1320	3500	4300
26	1650	4100	5300
28	2000	4450	6200
30		4800	7200
32		5100	7200+
34		5200	7200+
36		5300	7200+
38		5300	7200+
40		5300	7200+

and prolonged periods of aortic cross-clamping (total myocardial ischemia) are likely to be required, hypothermic perfusion at temperatures of 22°-28°C is used. When carrying out total correction of complex defects in infants less than 1 year of age, we often use periods of total circulatory arrest of up to 60 minutes at levels of profound hypothermia (16°-20°C), surface cooling with an ice bath being used initially to lower the infants' temperature to 28°-30°C (see "Profound Hypothermia with Circulatory Arrest").

Flow rates required for adequate perfusion are a function of the patient's body surface area, temperature, and the presence of arteriovenous communications, such as the large bronchial arteries often found in children with cyanotic congenital heart disease. Under the usual conditions of moderate hypothermia, we attempt to maintain a perfusion (pump flow) of 2.2-2.6 liters/min/m² of body surface area. Based on body weight, the infant requires a much greater flow per kilogram of body weight than does the adult. For example, a flow of 2.5 liters/min/m² for a 70-kg man would be 4250 ml/min, or about 61 ml/kg/min. A similar flow of 2.5 liters/min/m² for a 3-kg infant would be about 375 ml/min or about 125 ml/kg/min. The use of body surface area rather than body weight as a standard for perfusion "normalizes" these differences between adults and children.

Blood is equilibrated in the oxygenator with a mixture of oxygen and 3 to 5 percent carbon dioxide, attempting to maintain the measured arterial Pco_2 at approximately 34-38 torr when corrected to a temperature of 37°C using a blood gas analyzer.

The composition of the pump-priming volume depends upon the ratio of the priming volume to the patient's blood volume, the anticipated duration of the perfusion, the patient's initial hematocrit reading, the temperature to which the patient will be cooled, and the desired hematocrit value at the conclusion of bypass. Examples of typical pump "primes" are listed in Table 8-10.

Hemodilution is used for all operations, the *degree* of hemodilution being determined by the factors listed above. The disadvantages of hemodilution include (1) a reduction in the total oxygen carrying capacity of the blood, (2) a reduction in the level of platelets and white blood cells, (3) a reduction in the plasma oncotic pressure, and (4) dilution of coagulation factors. The advantages, however, include (1) a reduction in the volume of transfused bank blood with its higher content of microaggregates and hepatitis risk, and (2) the improved flow characteristics at low temperatures of the less viscous dilute prime.[74] The dilute prime prompts a beneficial diuresis, but the response may not be spontaneously sufficient; furosemide or mannitol is used to stimulate urine flow. Fluid must be

Table 8-10
Representative Pump Oxygenator "Primes" for Pediatric Cardiac Surgery

A. Three-kilogram infant with hematocrit value of 40% for operation utilizing deep hypothermia and circulatory arrest:

Packed red blood cells	200 ml
Plasmalyte 148*	500 ml
Mannitol	3 gm
Sodium bicarbonate	15 mEq
Heparin	2000 units

B. Ten-kilogram child with hematocrit value of 65%. Operation planned at 28°C:

Plasmalyte 148*	800 ml
Mannitol	10 gm
Heparin	1000 units

C. Ten-kilogram child with hematocrit value of 30% for operation at 28°C:

Packed red blood cells	250 ml
Plasmalyte 148*	550 ml
Mannitol	10 gm
Sodium bicarbonate	15 mEq
Heparin	2000 units

D. Thirty-kilogram child with hematocrit value of 45% for short operation at near normothermia:

Plasmalyte 149*	1000 ml
Whole blood	200 ml
Sodium bicarbonate	7 mEq
Calcium chloride	250 mg
Mannitol	10 gm

Note: All hematocrits for the above examples are intended to be at approximately 25% during cardiopulmonary bypass.

* Travenol Laboratories' balanced electrolyte solution containing Na, 140 mEq/liter; K, 5 mEq/liter; Mg, 3 mEq/liter; Cl, 98 mEq/liter; acetate, 27 mEq/liter; gluconate, 23 mEq/liter. pH 7.4 and osmolarity 294 mOsm/liter. Antibiotics (Oxacillin 25 mg/kg and cephalosporin 1 gm) are added to the pump prime.

added to the oxygenator during bypass to replace volume lost as urine and into the interstitial space. These problems are usually not significant during short perfusions, but volume loss into the interstitial space may be considerable during long repairs of complex defects. Early postoperative diuresis will be required to mobilize this fluid from the lungs and extracellular space.

For reasons not clearly understood, hypokalemia is common during and after cardiopulmonary bypass. Losses of potassium are greater than can be accounted for in the urine alone. Hypokalemia may be a major factor in the etiology of postoperative ventricular irritability. Potassium is measured frequently during and after bypass, and the level is maintained between 3.5 and 4.5 mEq/liter by the addition of small doses of potassium chloride to the oxygenator during bypass and to the intravenous fluids postoperatively. Metabolic alkalosis tends to accentuate the fall in serum potassium during bypass. For this reason, metabolic acidosis should not be overcorrected.

Blood glucose levels are determined several times during bypass. Serum glucose tends to rise as consumption is lowered during hypothermia and as a response to corticosteroids and sympathetic stimulation during operation and bypass.

The pH of the initial pump prime is adjusted to physiological limits and arterial blood gases and hemoglobin/hematocrit measurements are made after a brief period of equilibration on cardiopulmonary bypass. These measurements are repeated at 20-minute intervals. Metabolic acidosis (base deficit of -5 mEq/liter) is corrected as needed, using sodium bicarbonate. Development of metabolic acidosis during cardiopulmonary bypass always suggests inadequate perfusion, just as metabolic acidosis is a manifestation of low cardiac output in a patient with a spontaneously beating heart. Causes for inadequate perfusion should be sought. (see Table 8-11).

The surgeon *must* obliterate all known large arteriovenous communications, including a patent ductus arteriosus and previously constructed systemic-arterial-to-pulmonary-arterial shunts, simultaneously with the institution of bypass. In most cases, such communications are encircled with a ligature before bypass, the ligature being tied as bypass is begun.

Table 8-11
Causes of Inadequate Perfusion on
Cardiopulmonary Bypass

A. Pump oxygenator malfunction
   1. Inadequate occlusion of tubing by pump rollers
   2. Inaccurate calibration of pump rollers or flowmeter
   3. Thrombosis in pump oxygenator or line filters
   4. Leak in oxygenator, heat exchanger, or tubing
B. Obstruction to arterial inflow
   1. Arterial cannula too small
   2. Improper placement of arterial cannula, i.e., wedged in the innominate artery
   3. Kinked arterial tubing or cannula
   4. Clamp on arterial tubing or cannula
   5. Aortic cross-clamp placed across perfusion cannula
C. Inadequate venous return
   1. Hypovolemia
   2. Venous cannulae too small
   3. Venous cannulae too large, wedged against caval wall
   4. Excessive siphon effect of gravity drainage, collapsing the venae cavae
   5. Inadequate siphon effect; reservoir level too high
   6. Kinked or otherwise obstructed venous cannulae
   7. Caval tourniquets tightened proximal to tip of caval cannulae
   8. Excessive aortic "runoff" via PDA, shunt, or bronchial collateral circulation
   9. Markedly increased peripheral resistance
   10. Markedly decreased peripheral resistance
   11. Intravascular thrombosis

In the presence of a large Waterston shunt (ascending-aorta-to-right-pulmonary-arterial anastomosis) or an aorticopulmonary window, the ascending aorta must be cross-clamped between the perfusion cannula and the shunt shortly after the institution of bypass to avoid flooding of the lungs and systemic hypotension. The shunt is closed surgically by suture, or a patch is placed within the aorta. The clamp can then be removed safely.

Aortic valvular insufficiency, another cause of "aortic runoff" producing hypotension, inadequate systemic perfusion, and cardiac dilatation, must be managed by cross-clamping the aorta shortly after the institution of bypass.

A Potts' shunt (descending aorta-to-left-pulmonary-arterial anastomosis) poses a particularly frustrating problem. The shunt may be occluded with the surgeon's fingertip until a level of profound hypothermia is reached on bypass, at which point the pump flow is reduced to a very low level or even stopped. The left pulmonary artery is opened, and the shunt is obliterated by suture.

Children with prolonged cyanosis may have extremely large bronchial collateral vessels originating from the descending thoracic aorta. These can be demonstrated angiographically and may require surgical obliteration prior to total correction of the underlying defect.[75,76] Multiple small bronchial collateral communications may cause torrential pulmonary arterial blood flow during cardiopulmonary bypass, reducing peripheral blood flow and obscuring the operative field. In such circumstances the perfusate temperature should be reduced to 20°-25°C and the flow rate reduced to one-half or less of the calculated normothermia flow rate.

Institution of Cardiopulmonary Bypass

The responses of individual patients to the institution of cardiopulmonary bypass vary widely. We attempt to initiate total cardiopulmonary bypass gradually, making the transition from the patient's own cardiac output to total maintenance of perfusion by the pump oxygenator over a 3- to 4-minute period. Most operations for correction of congenital heart defects require *total* cardiopulmonary bypass, that is, one cannula in the superior vena cava, another in the inferior vena cava, and tourniquets tightened around each of these cannula to *totally* divert venous blood away from the right atrium and into the pump oxygenator. Each of these tourniquets is tightened separately, adequacy of flow through the two cannulae being examined individually.

Left ventricular ejection gradually disappears from the arterial pressure waveform. Total cardiopulmonary bypass produces a barely pulsatile sine-wave arterial perfusion pressure. The anesthesiologist must observe the head and face carefully for several minutes after the surgeon tightens the superior vena caval tourniquet. The development of plethora or congestion suggests obstruction of the cannula; its position must be rechecked. Development of abdominal distention, hepatomegaly, or a sudden decrease in urine output suggest obstruction of the inferior vena caval venous return.

Ordinarily a period of 4 or 5 minutes is required to establish a "stable" perfusion in a child, that is, full calculated flow with an acceptable mean perfusion pressure. During these initial few minutes, cautious observation rather than pharmacologic intervention is appropriate.

The levels of acceptable arterial perfusion pressure in children vary widely. During relatively short periods on total bypass, a mean arterial pressure of 30-40 torr is acceptable, providing the following other indices of adequate perfusion are present: (1) urine output should continue at normal or above-normal levels, (2) there should be no significant loss of volume from the pump oxygenator reservoir to the patient, (3) metabolic acidosis should be minimal or absent, (4) the difference between P_{O_2} levels measured in the arterial and venous blood should be within normal physiological limits (see Table 8-12).

Arterial blood P_{O_2} levels are normally between 200 and 300 torr on bypass; blood in the venous return lines usually has a P_{O_2} of 40 torr or more. Lower venous P_{O_2} levels suggest that an inadequate volume of blood is being provided to meet the metabolic demands of the body, similar to the wide arteriovenous oxygen differences seen in patients with a low cardiac output. This single parameter cannot be used alone to assess the adequacy of perfusion, however. Very high venous P_{O_2} levels may indicate the presence of significant peripheral vasoconstriction with diminished oxygen consumption in important vascular beds or the presence of arteriovenous communications allowing the blood to return directly to the pump oxygenator without passing through the capillary beds as described earlier. When major arteriovenous communications have been excluded, vasodilator therapy is appropriate to overcome the vasoconstriction resulting in hypertension and a very high venous P_{O_2} level.

Table 8-12
Signs and Symptoms of Possible
Inadequate Perfusion on Bypass

Metabolic acidosis
Respiratory acidosis
Urine output less than 1 ml/kg/hr
Hypotension
Hypertension
Po_2 of venous return blood less than 40 torr
Spontaneous ventilatory effort
Facial plethora
Conjunctival suffusion
Elevation of correctly positioned CVP monitoring catheter
Negative or unreadable CVP from correctly positioned catheter
High pressure in arterial line pump tubing
Vibration of arterial line pump tubing
"Flutter" (vibration) of venous return pump tubing
Wide discrepancy of temperatures measured in the nasopharynx, esophagus, rectum, and skin

Older children and adolescents generally maintain higher perfusion pressures on total cardiopulmonary bypass, ordinarily in the range of 50- 70 torr. Arterial perfusion pressures exceeding these levels at normal calculated flow rates suggest vasoconstriction and may be treated with vasodilator medications such as sodium nitroprusside, phentolamine, halothane, or enflurane. Vasodilator therapy is particularly useful in minimizing the vasoconstrictor effect of core-cooling during procedures carried out under moderate and profound hypothermia. When vasodilators are used, it is often necessary to add volume to the pump oxygenator in order to maintain the same flow rate with the same reservoir level. Tables 8-11 and 8-13 list the major causes of hypoxemia and inadequate perfusion on cardiopulmonary bypass.

Myocardial Preservation

One of the surgeon's most significant problems continues to be the maintenance of normally viable myocardium during the repair of complex congenital heart defects. Most cases of low cardiac output syndrome in the postoperative period can be traced to myocardial injury sustained during the operation.[77]

In the early days of surgical treatment for congenital heart disease, relatively little- attention was paid to what was then an underestimated problem. Most corrective operations were conducted in relatively large children. Flow of coronary arterial blood from the aortic root was rarely or only briefly interrupted. The heart was usually allowed to beat throughout the operation. Occasionally elective electrical ventricular fibrillation was used to minimize the risk of air embolization. Most operations were performed at about 30°- 32°C. Even under these circumstances the incidence of postoperative low cardiac output syndrome was higher than would now be acceptable, in many cases owing to inadequate repair or pulmonary vascular obstructive disease.

During the past decade, emphasis has been placed on earlier total correction of complex congenital heart defects in the infant and small child.[78] More elaborate operations involving conduits with multiple suture lines and the placement of complex intracardiac patches require a longer period on cardiopulmonary bypass. Avoidance of injury to the electrical conduction system and precise placement of such small intracardiac patches and conduits are facilitated by a motionless heart provided only by interruption of coronary arterial blood flow.

The relative disparity between right and left ventricular size and performance in children with congenital heart defects leaves little margin for loss of contractile performance during operation. Extensive systemic-to-pulmonary collateral circulation in children with cyanotic forms of heart disease further complicates the problems of obtaining the bloodless and motionless operative field so desirable for complex intracardiac repairs in small children.

Table 8-13
Causes of Inadequate Oxygenation
on Cardiopulmonary Bypass

Damaged pump oxygenator
Inadequate flow of oxygen from source into oxygenator
Blood flow exceeding limits of oxygenator producing "channeling"
Anemia
Hyperthermia
Thrombosis in oxygenator

Techniques of myocardial preservation requiring the addition of significant tubing and equipment in the operative field are impractical for use in small children; confusion, impaired exposure, and potential injury to the heart and great vessels being introduced by their presence.

The two basic principles of myocardial preservation in common use at present include (1) *hypothermia* and (2) pharmacologically induced asystole (*cardioplegia*). These two approaches are usually combined in one of several techniques, depending upon the nature of the operation to be performed and the surgeons' preferences.[79]

Total body hypothermia is used in all but the briefest operations for congenital heart disease requiring the use of cardiopulmonary bypass. Total body oxygen consumption is reduced under hypothermic circumstances, the total flow required from the heart-lung machine thus being lowered.[80] Myocardial tolerance to periods of aortic cross-clamping is greatly increased even when the temperature is lowered only to 30°C. Total body cooling to lower levels (22°-25°C) is frequently used in operations for congenital heart defects, particularly those in which large bronchial collateral vessels cause flooding of the operative field and hypotension on cardiopulmonary bypass. Under such circumstances the total flow from the heart-lung machine can be reduced to between one-third and one-half the level required at 37°C without harmful oxygen deprivation. Much longer periods of aortic cross-clamping and interrupted coronary arterial blood flow will then be tolerated without significant myocardial injury.

Systemic hypothermia provided by the heart-lung machine and heat exchanger can be supplemented by *topical cooling* of the myocardium.[81] Saline at 4°-5°C is allowed to drip into the pericardial cavity, covering most of the left ventricle and a portion of the right ventricle. The saline is aspirated from the pericardium by a separate sump tube and discarded. When the heart has been opened, this technique can be supplemented by the addition of intracardiac flushing or irrigation with a similar cold solution. This *endomyocardial cooling* is particularly beneficial in the presence of left ventricular and/or right ventricular hypertrophy where simple surface cooling of the heart may not efficiently cool the sensitive endomyocardium.

A great deal of attention to detail is required if this seemingly simple technique of surface cooling is to be relied upon for myocardial preservation. Two atrial cannulae and tourniquets around the superior and inferior venae cavae are required to prevent warmer blood from rewarming the myocardium. Bronchial collateral flow must be relatively low, especially if the heart itself has been opened. An initial large bolus of pericardial saline is required to achieve primary cooling, and direct measurement of myocardial temperature is desirable. When the temperature is actually measured, it is often found to be considerably higher than one might expect from the volume of cold solution being poured into the pericardium.

The use of *cold pharmacologic cardioplegia* for myocardial preservation is probably the single most significant modification in operative technique for congenital heart disease introduced in the past 5 years.[82] It is simple and extremely effective. Although individual surgeons and institutions use personalized modifications, all the common methods involve the intracoronary injection of a cold solution (5°C) containing a cardioplegic agent, the most popular one now being potassium chloride in a concentration of about 25-30 mEq/liter. The solutions are usually made slightly hyperosmolar by the addition of glucose or mannitol or both. Table 8-14 describes the solution that we currently find very effective in this institution. The cold cardioplegic solution is injected through a plastic needle or air-aspiration device inserted into the aortic root proximal to the aortic cross-

Table 8-14
Composition of Cardioplegic
Solution*

NaCl	82.5 mM/liter
KCl	30 mM/liter
CaCl$_2$	1 mM/liter
NaHCO$_3$	27 mM/liter
Dextrose	0.5% (5 gm/liter)
Mannitol	1% (10 gm/liter)

* This is one of many acceptable formulations of a cardioplegic solution and the one presently used in our institution. The cardioplegic agent is potassium. Hyponatremia and hypocalcemia accentuate the effects of hyperkalemia. Dextrose and mannitol contribute to the slight hyperosmolarity of the solution (350–370 mOsm/liter).

clamp. A sufficient volume is injected to induce a completely isoelectric electrocardiogram. Full-thickness myocardial hypothermia and a relaxed asystolic heart are thus induced simultaneously.

When the aortic root has been opened for operations on the aortic valve and/or left ventricular outflow tract, the cardioplegic solution can be injected directly into the coronary arterial ostia. This is particularly important in the presence of aortic valvular insufficiency; a competent aortic valve is required if the fluid injected into the aortic root is to be diverted into the coronary arterial bed. The cold solution may be infused at a slower but continuous rate by gravity drip or a small pump, or additional bolus injections may be given when the ECG demonstrates return of electrical activity.

We presently prefer the very effective combination of systemic core-cooling by the heart-lung machine supplemented by cold hyperkalemic cardioplegia for relatively long open heart operations in children. The mechanics of this system are simple and uncluttered. Excellent exposure of intracardiac structures is provided. Pump flow can be reduced when bronchial collateral blood obscures the operative field. The need for postoperative inotropic support has been greatly reduced by this combination of hypothermia and pharmacologic cardioplegia.

Termination of Cardiopulmonary Bypass

Rewarming is begun in operations utilizing hypothermia at a point when the surgeon believes he will no longer need to cross-clamp the aorta for a prolonged period and when the operation is otherwise relatively close to completion.

Just prior to attempting to wean the patient from cardiopulmonary bypass, calcium chloride (30 mg/kg) is administered into the oxygenator reservoir to further counteract the calcium chelation by citrate in the initial blood prime and to stimulate myocardial contractility. Additional calcium may be required after termination of bypass.

An attempt should not be made to wean the patient from bypass until the body temperature is 34°-37°C and until the ECG looks normal, the ST segments have returned to preoperative position, and the rhythm is stable.

If complete atrioventricular dissociation or heart block is present, an adequate ventricular rate should be obtained by ventricular pacing through wires attached to the heart by the surgeon. Simple atrioventricular dissociation with a normal or only slightly slow ventricular response may be improved or converted to sinus rhythm by the administration of a small dose of atropine (0.015 mg/kg) or isoproterenol (0.1 ug/kg).

Supraventricular bradycardia (junctional, nodal, atrial, or sinus) will usually respond nicely to atrial pacing through wires attached directly to the atrium by the surgeon, maintaining atrial contribution to the stroke volume. Again, atropine or isoproterenol may be useful. The use of a sequential atrioventricular pacemaker connected to both atrial and ventricular pacing wires is useful in the management of patients in atrioventricular dissociation or complete heart block and marginal cardiac output. Restoration of normal atrial and ventricular contraction time relationships may contribute as much as 15 to 20 percent to the stroke volume.[51]

Weaning the patient from cardiopulmonary bypass may be accomplished by simply clamping the venous and arterial lines in a patient with good contractility and normal intravascular volume. The patient's ejection is then immediately apparent in the arterial pressure waveform. We prefer, however, to exercise a bit more caution at this point. In most patients having undergone repair of a complex intracardiac defect, a left atrial pressure monitoring catheter is inserted through the right superior pulmonary vein, the left atrial wall, the foramen ovale, or the left atrial appendage. The pressure in the left atrium is displayed on the monitor, and the patient is transfused from the pump oxygenator until the left atrial pressure is approximately 10 torr (up to 15 torr for suspected poor ventricular function; as low as 5 torr for hearts with nearly normal contractility). The perfusionist then gradually reduces arterial inflow and venous return to the oxygenator over 2 or 3 minutes while maintaining the left atrial pressure within physiological limits as described above.

The patient's inability to maintain a mean arterial pressure of 50 torr with a mean left atrial pressure of 15 torr or less is considered an indication of the need for a supporting inotropic infusion. We prefer dopamine (3-30 μg/kg/min) (see Appendices C&D) as needed if the heart rate is normal or fast or isoproterenol (0.05-0.1

μg/kg/min) if the heart rate is slower than normal or cannot be maintained at a normal rate by *atrial* pacing. During the first year of life, an initial mean arterial pressure of 40 torr would be acceptable. After removal of arterial and venous cannulae from the heart, the arterial pressure often improves, especially in the small infant in whom the aortic perfusion cannula may be a significant source of obstruction.

Fresh blood should be readily available at the time of decannulation so that any unexpected sudden losses or gradual losses due to anticoagulation can be replaced until the heparin has been reversed and all sites of surgical bleeding controlled.

Reversal of Anticoagulation

Protamine sulfate to reverse the heparin anticoagulation is given after removal of cardiac cannulae and control of major surgical bleeding. The activated clotting time is determined, and 1.3 mg/kg of protamine is given for each 100 units of heparin remaining in the patient as calculated from the ACT.[71] Use of the ACT-heparin-protamine graph (see Fig. 8-2) simplifies the determination of the amount of protamine required.

Heparin in the initial pump prime contributes considerably to the total amount of heparin in the circulation, especially in small infants. The activated clotting time may be considerably above predicted levels in these patients. We have found the use of the activated clotting time to be a far better guide to protamine reversal than mathematical formulas relating the protamine dose simply to the amount of heparin given and the time since the last heparin dose.

Protamine can produce significant hypotension if given rapidly as a bolus. We prefer to administer the protamine only after the patient is hemodynamically stable, well vasodilated, and has an adequate central vascular volume as evidenced by the right atrial, left atrial, or central venous pressure. The protamine is then given over a 3- to 5-minute period. Use of the cardiotomy suction returning blood to the pump oxygenator should be terminated as protamine is begun to avoid coagulation of the remaining pump-prime volume.

POSTOPERATIVE CARE

Intraoperative Considerations

It has been stated that "95 percent of postoperative care occurs in the operating room!" There is a great deal of truth in this hyperbole. A skillfully performed operation providing physiological correction or significant palliation of

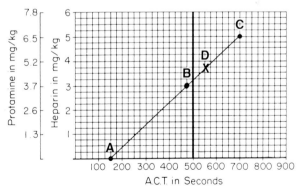

Fig. 8-2. Heparin–Protamine relationship at end of bypass.
The Activated Clotting Time (ACT) is measured before heparin is administered and a point is plotted on the graph.
After heparin is administered, a second point is plotted and the points connected by the line shown.
Point X is at the measured ACT when heparin reversal is desired and corresponds to 3.7 mg/kg units of heparin remaining in the circulation. Protamine dosage is determined by reading the amount needed from the scale on the left.

a congenital heart defect during a properly administered anesthetic usually leaves little more than observation and minimal support for those providing postoperative care.

While the child is in the operating room, all necessary monitoring devices are inserted and carefully secured to avoid inadvertent removal when the child begins to awaken. Assessment of the repair is made by the measurement of intracardiac pressures and Po_2 levels. Atrial and ventricular pacing wires are attached to the heart to allow control of heart rate and diagnosis of arrhythmias. Hemostasis is achieved, minimizing the risk of continued postoperative bleeding and possible cardiac tamponade.

Proper endotracheal intubation, intraoperative tracheal toilet, gastric decompression, judicious fluid administration, and appropriate use of the heart-lung machine minimize the pulmonary complications associated with lesions causing markedly increased pulmonary blood flow or those in which there are many large bronchial collateral vessels.

Compulsive attention to sterile technique on the part of the anesthesia and operative teams reduces the tragic consequences of postoperative sepsis. These patients may have extensive and prolonged mediastinal exposure, abnormally formed intracardiac structures, and implanted prosthetic valves or fabric patches. Sepsis, once established, is difficult or impossible to control.

The personal health of members of the anesthesia staff, surgeons, and nurses is a rarely considered but important factor in the management of children with heart disease. One well-known cardiac surgical pioneer insisted that members of his team be in condition to undergo an *elective* operation *themselves* if they were to participate in any operation! Such attention to detail undoubtedly contributed to the success of cardiovascular surgery prior to the availability of potent antibiotics upon which we now place excessive confidence.

Transfer of the Child from Operating Room to Intensive Care Unit

The two most dangerous periods during any cardiovascular operation are the induction of anesthesia and the transfer from operating room to intensive care unit. In both of these situations the anesthesiologist should remain fully in command, supervising the procedures and monitoring the patients' physiological responses to the rapidly changing environment.

Our patients are transferred from the operating room directly to the intensive care unit while the electrocardiogram and arterial blood pressure are displayed on a portable monitor. The patient is ventilated with 100 percent oxygen during transport. An anesthesiologist is in direct attendance and is responsible for observation and support of the child during the transfer. A member of the surgical team and operating room nursing staff are also in attendance.

Upon arrival in the intensive care unit the anesthesiologist supervises the gradual transfer from portable monitor to permanent monitor and from manual ventilation to the mechanical ventilator, the latter with the assistance of a respiratory therapist. Care is taken to avoid periods during which there is no direct display of a blood pressure, arterial waveform, or electrocardiogram. If such a loss of monitoring should occur, a finger *must* be kept on a palpable peripheral pulse.

A full report of significant problems, laboratory values, fluid administration, pressor requirements, need for pacing, and other pertinent data is given to the intensive care unit nurse by the responsible anesthesiologist. The members of the anesthesia team should leave the intensive care unit only after the patient is fully monitored, ventilation is satisfactory, bleeding seems acceptable, vital signs are maintained in a satisfactory range, medication infusions are properly adjusted, and appropriate nursing and surgical personnel are in attendance and properly informed.

Problems of the Postoperative Period

Postoperative care of a child having undergone a successful cardiovascular operation and smoothly conducted anesthetic involves little more than observation of vital signs, provision of maintenance fluids and electrolytes, and progressive discontinuation of monitoring devices and life-support systems such as the ventilator, endotracheal tube, and thermal regulators.

Postoperative problems, when they do occur, usually relate to (1) inadequate cardiac output, (2) respiratory failure, (3) renal failure, or (4) sepsis. Malnutrition, so often a problem in patients undergoing extensive gastrointestinal surgical procedures or multiple operations for trauma, is rare in the cardiovascular patient. It does occur, however, and is further complicated by the need to restrict fluids in children with significant congestive heart failure. Prolonged failure to thrive preoperatively increases the risks of postoperative malnutrition with poor wound healing and sepsis. Persistent postoperative hypoxemia and/or low cardiac output accentuates the harmful effects of malnutrition in complicating recovery and wound healing.

The most significant postoperative problem is the *low cardiac output syndrome* (LCOS), consisting of *hypotension, oliguria, acidosis, mental obtundation*, and a *low mixed venous oxygen tension*.[83] The two most common causes of postoperative low cardiac output are (1) inadequate intracardiac anatomic and physiological correction and (2) inadequate intraoperative myocardial preservation. Contributing factors include (1) failure to maintain blood volume properly,[84] (2) electrolyte imbalance,[85,86] (3) the occurrence of arrhythmias,[87] and (4) cardiac tamponade.[88,89]

A balance must be maintained between total body tissue oxygen demands and oxygen supply, the latter being determined primarily by the cardiac output. Fever, agitation, seizures, and respiratory effort increase oxygen demand and hence pose additional demands upon the already stressed heart for the delivery of a greater cardiac output.

Tissue oxygen delivery is a function of the amount of blood pumped per minute and the amount of oxygen carried in that blood. The latter, in turn, is determined by the hemoglobin concentration and the oxygen saturation. Persistent intracardiac or intrapulmonary right-to-left- shunts causing hypoxemia obviously lower tissue oxygen delivery and complicate postoperative recovery.

Since adequate delivery of oxygen to the tissues of the body is the goal of maintaining an adequate cardiac output, it is clear from the above facts that factors *increasing* oxygen demand must be minimized, blood hemoglobin levels must be maintained in a normal range, and hypoxemia of pulmonary or intracardiac origin must be avoided whenever possible. Fever is controlled with rectal or oral acetaminophen and, when necessary, surface cooling with a hy-

pothermia mattress. Agitation, fear, and pain are controlled with adequate doses of morphine sulfate. Seizures, if present, are treated immediately with anticonvulsants, and paralysis, with muscle relaxants (with controlled ventilation, of course). The work of breathing is kept to a minimum by controlled ventilation on a volume respirator until there is evidence of completely adequate cardiac output, minimal mediastinal bleeding, and complete neurological integrity.[90]

The following five factors determine cardiac output:[91,92]

1. Heart *rate*
2. Heart *rhythm*
3. Preload (intravascular *volume*)
4. Afterload
   Peripheral vascular resistance (for left ventricle)
   Pulmonary vascular resistance (for right ventricle)
5. Myocardial *contractility*

Each of these five factors must be considered individually and "normalized" in order to assure adequacy of cardiac output.

Heart rate, if slower than optimal for the specific patient, is controlled by atrial pacing when atrioventricular conduction is intact. In the presence of complete heart block, heart rate is controlled by sequential atrioventricular pacing with an appropriate P-R interval or, if a sequential pacer is not available, by simple but less effective ventricular pacing.[51,93] Sinus or junctional bradycardias or both may respond to atropine; atrioventricular dissociation and other slow heart rates may respond to an infusion of isoproterenol.

Tachycardias are more difficult to control.[94] Sinus tachycardia should be viewed as a *symptom* of hypovolemia, pain, fear, agitation, cold, congestive heart failure, or low cardiac output. Treatment of the *cause* usually results in an improvement in the heart rate. Ventricular tachycardia is a true emergency and must be treated immediately by a lidocaine bolus injection followed by a constant infusion. If this is ineffective, electrical cardioversion is required. Serum potassium and calcium levels must be checked and restored to normal if necessary. Supraventricular tachycardias of other than sinus origin may be quite difficult to control. Digitalis is the medication of choice where digitalis intoxication is not a suspected cause of the arrhythmia. Propranalol may be very useful in the management of some supraventricular tachyarrhythmias. Cardiological consultation is advisable in the management of all significant arrhythmias.

Maintenance of an adequate circulating blood volume is important in ensuring optimal cardiac output. Use of the central venous pressure, left atrial pressure, and mean arterial blood pressure in combination usually serves as a satisfactory guide to volume replacement. When cardiac output is measured directly by green dye or thermodilution techniques, the appropriate level of central venous pressure and/or left atrial pressure can be determined at which cardiac output is acceptable (approximately 3 liters/min/m²).

Determination of optimal peripheral vascular resistance and pulmonary vascular resistance is more difficult. An increase in vascular resistance is an expected response to low cardiac output. This is manifest clinically as cool skin, pallor, and blotchy areas of cyanosis (mottling). Severe degrees of vasoconstriction may lead to acidosis. Inappropriate increases in peripheral vascular resistance may result in a higher-than-necessary mean arterial pressure even in the face of low cardiac output. This increase in afterload is detrimental to cardiac performance. Systemic vascular resistance can be determined by the following relationship:

Systemic vascular resistance =

$$\frac{\text{mean aortic pressure} - \text{central venous pressure}}{\text{cardiac output}}$$

Normal systemic vascular resistance is 10–13 units. When the resistance is found to be considerably greater than this value, a trial of vasodilator therapy (nitroglycerin or nitroprusside) should be considered. We use intravenous sodium nitroprusside quite freely in the management of even marginally low cardiac output, often *before* the need for an inotropic infusion. Such therapy seems particularly useful in those patients in whom there is associated elevation of the pulmonary vascular resistance.

Finally, inadequate myocardial contractility may be a cause of low cardiac output. All the other factors described above should be "normalized" if possible before resorting to the augmentation of cardiac output by the administration of inotropic medications such as dopamine, epinephrine, or isoproterenol. Meticulous attention to myocardial preservation during bypass and an adequate anatomic repair should result in little need for postoperative inotropic support. Digitalis is frequently given during the early postoperative period to minimize the likelihood of supraventricular arrhythmias and later congestive heart failure.[95] The importance of ionized calcium in the contractile process is well known.[96] Frequent measurements of calcium and replacement as necessary are important.

When cardiac output remains low after efforts have been made to establish a normal heart rate, rhythm, blood volume, and systemic vascular resistance, a constant infusion of dopamine (3–30 μg/kg/min) should be instituted. If the heart rate is slow, isoproterenol may be used instead. The combination of isoproterenol and dopamine has certain theoretical advantages, but we have found dopamine and nitroprusside in combination to be more useful if inotropic support is indicated.[97] Epinephrine, long a favorite medication for the treatment of postoperative low cardiac output syndrome, is not likely to be effective if dopamine and/or isoproterenol in combination with sodium nitroprusside have failed to generate adequate myocardial contractility and cardiac output.

All inotropic medications should be administered to infants and children by constant pump infusion of a relatively concentrated solution. Dilute solutions result in absorption of excessive fluid. Concentrated infusions given by gravity drip cannot be controlled with sufficient accuracy to prevent wide swings in heart rate and blood pressure or the development of arrhythmias.

The clinical assessment of the adequacy of cardiac output depends upon the detection of acidosis, oliguria, hypotension, and mental obtundation. At best, these are crude and often vague end points. Direct measurement of cardiac output by thermodilution techniques is practical even in the small infant and is highly recommended as a guideline to proper postoperative care.[69]

Cardiac tamponade is one of the most feared complications occurring during the early postoperative hours. Blood accumulating in the mediastinum may cause few if any detectable signs and symptoms until shortly before a fatal fall in cardiac output. The problem of cardiac tamponade in infants and children is even more acute and subtle.[98] In our institution, special precautions are taken in the operating room to minimize the likelihood of tamponade. At least one pleural cavity is opened widely, and a drainage tube is placed into that pleural cavity in addition to the usual two mediastinal drainage tubes. Meticulous attention is paid to control of postoperative bleeding, usually by at least two surgeons working independently. Every effort is made to normalize coagulation parameters. The activated clotting time is restored to normal, and the partial thromboplastin time, prothrombin time, and platelet count are corrected with fresh frozen plasma, platelets, and, if needed, vitamin K.

The signs and symptoms of tamponade include hypotension, low cardiac output, a narrow pulse pressure, pulsus paradoxus (often misleading in patients on ventilators), decreased voltage in the ECG, elevation of right heart pressures (central venous and atrial pressures), and usually a fall in left atrial pressure associated with the rise in right atrial pressure.[95,99,100] Tamponade *must* be high on the list of differential diagnoses when a postoperative cardiac surgical patient is simply "not doing well." The possibility of tamponade must always be considered when the low cardiac output syndrome develops.

The members of our cardiac team have a very low threshold for reexploration of the mediastinum if tamponade is even slightly suspected. We have never regretted mediastinal exploration and have witnessed significant improvement in the clinical condition of a number of patients in whom the classical signs and symptoms of tamponade were not impressive. The surgical team must be prepared to open the lower end of the sternotomy incision (or the entire incision if necessary) in the intensive care unit when life-threatening tamponade develops.

Respiratory failure was once a common postoperative complication following heart surgery in infants and children.[101,102] The development of better volume ventilators and the adaptation of techniques used in the care of infants with hyaline membrane disease have greatly reduced these complications.[90,103–111] We now prefer to maintain almost all patients on controlled volume ventilation for 12 to 18 hours following open heart operations. During this period the patient is kept well sedated and is allowed to awaken gradually as the intermittent mandatory ventilation (IMV) rate is reduced. When cardiac output is adequate, bleeding has stopped, the patient is fully awake, and normal arterial blood gases can be maintained on an F_1O_2 of 0.4 at an IMV rate of 5 per minute, the patient is extubated and placed in a humidified environment (hood or tent) with an F_1O_2 of 0.4. Although anesthesia is administered through an orotracheal tube, we often change to a nasotracheal tube in the operating room at the completion of the operation, especially when prolonged ventilatory support is anticipated. Intensive pulmonary physical therapy is begun in the intensive care unit and continued until discharge from the hospital. Introduction to techniques of chest physiotherapy in the preoperative period makes this better tolerated and more acceptable. Continuous positive airway pressure (CPAP) is occasionally used without intermittent mandatory ventilation (IMV), but this is relatively uncommon. This technique is useful in the treatment or prevention of atelectasis in patients with increased pulmonary blood flow (ventricular septal defect or recently created systemic-to-pulmonary shunt). Excessive CPAP should be *avoided* in children with diminished pulmonary blood flow (tetralogy of Fallot, tricuspid atresia, pulmonary atresia), since it can increase hypoxemia by further reducing pulmonary blood flow.

Renal failure is likewise uncommon following open heart surgery today.[112] Adequate intraoperative perfusion and fluid administration and the use of potent diuretics (furosemide and mannitol) help assure preservation of the kidneys. Moderate hemodilution, limited use of cardiotomy suction with subsequent hemolysis, and the use of moderate hypothermia on bypass probably contribute to the success of renal preservation. We expect to maintain a urine output of *no less than* 1 ml/kg/hr on bypass and during the postoperative period. When less than this level is achieved, causes of low perfusion and/ or low cardiac output are sought. Serum and urine osmolarity are used as a guide to adequacy of hydration. When the cardiac output is proved to be normal and the serum osmolarity is normal or low (after administration of a fluid challenge), oliguria is managed by elimination of potassium from all solutions, careful monitoring of the serum potassium level, and the administration of furosemide (1 mg/kg). Fifty percent glucose and insulin, sodium bicarbonate, and calcium chloride are administered if the potassium is dangerously high. In the event of complete renal shutdown, a situation that we have rarely encountered, preparation must immediately be made for peritoneal dialysis and administration of ion exchange resins.

Data pertinent to postoperative management are recorded on a single four-page flow sheet as a function of time (see Figs. 8-3, 8-4, 8-5, and 8-6). All events, vital signs, observations, laboratory and ventilation data, and input-output data are recorded on a single line corresponding to the time of the data collection. *No other records are maintained.* The entire time course of a patient's progress or problems can thus be reviewed chronologically.

The problems that must be managed during the postoperative course of a child having undergone heart surgery can be categorized and

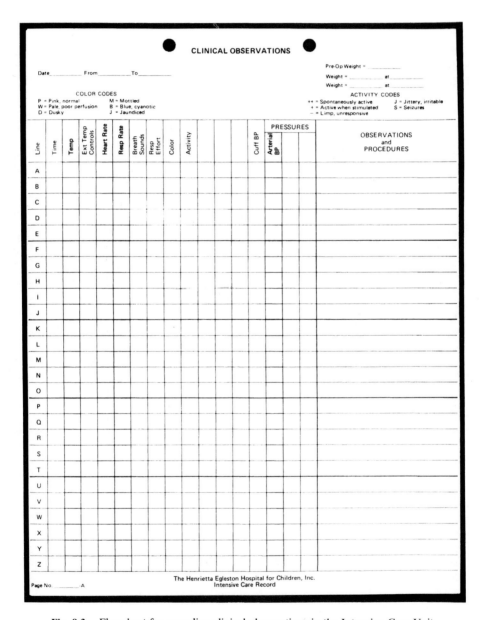

Fig. 8-3. Flowsheet for recording clinical observations in the Intensive Care Unit.

remembered simply by the mnemonic CORKS, where CO refers to "*c*ardiac *o*utput"; R, to "*r*espiratory support"; K, to "*k*idney function"; and S reminds us of "*s*eptic precautions." There are, of course, many other specific and less frequent problems confronting the postoperative care staff, but these are beyond the scope of this discussion.

SPECIAL PROBLEMS IN ANESTHESIA FOR CONGENITAL HEART DISEASE

Profound Hypothermia with Circulatory Arrest

The use of conventional techniques for correction of congenital heart defects using cardiopulmonary bypass and moderate hypothermia

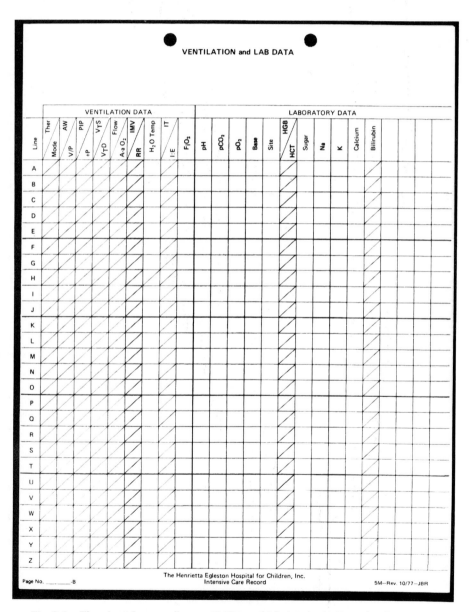

Fig. 8-4. Flowsheet for recording ventilation and lab data in the Intensive Care Unit.

has generally been associated with a higher mortality in infants as compared to older children, while mortality and morbidity have steadily decreased for similar operations in older children and adults. Recent reports have indicated, however, that the risk of intracardiac surgery in infants less than 2 years old has also decreased.[113-122] This improved survival is undoubtedly related, at least in part, to a better understanding of the anatomy and pathophysiology of the defects and to other improvements in surgical and anesthesia techniques,[123, 124] a better understanding of the metabolic alterations that occur,[125-127] and the effectiveness of supportive measures. Incorporation of techniques to induce profound hypothermia (15°- 20°C) has proved useful in the intraoperative management of many patients less than 2 years of age

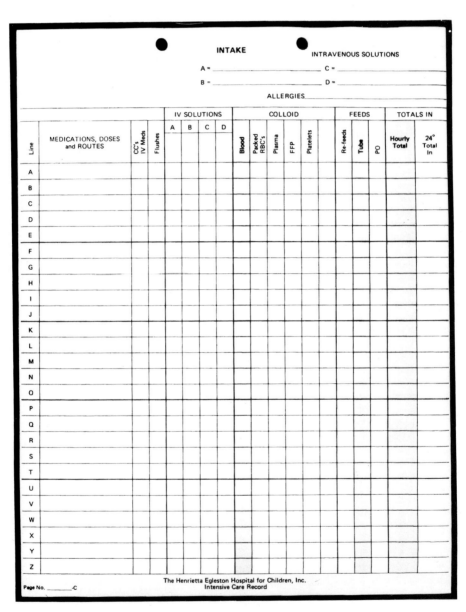

Fig. 8-5.   Flowsheet for recording intake data in the Intensive Care Unit.

undergoing correction of congenital heart defects.

The advantages of profound hypothermia include the following:

1. Excellent surgical exposure is provided when the cannulae are removed from the heart, allowing a relaxed and bloodless field. The cannulae obstruct the surgical field in the very small heart of the infant, in whom surgical repair is often quite complex and difficult.
2. Metabolic demand for oxygen by the heart, brain, and other vital tissues is decreased.
3. The total time on cardiopulmonary bypass is shortened, reducing pulmonary and hematologic complications postoperatively.
4. More uniform cooling of the body is pro-

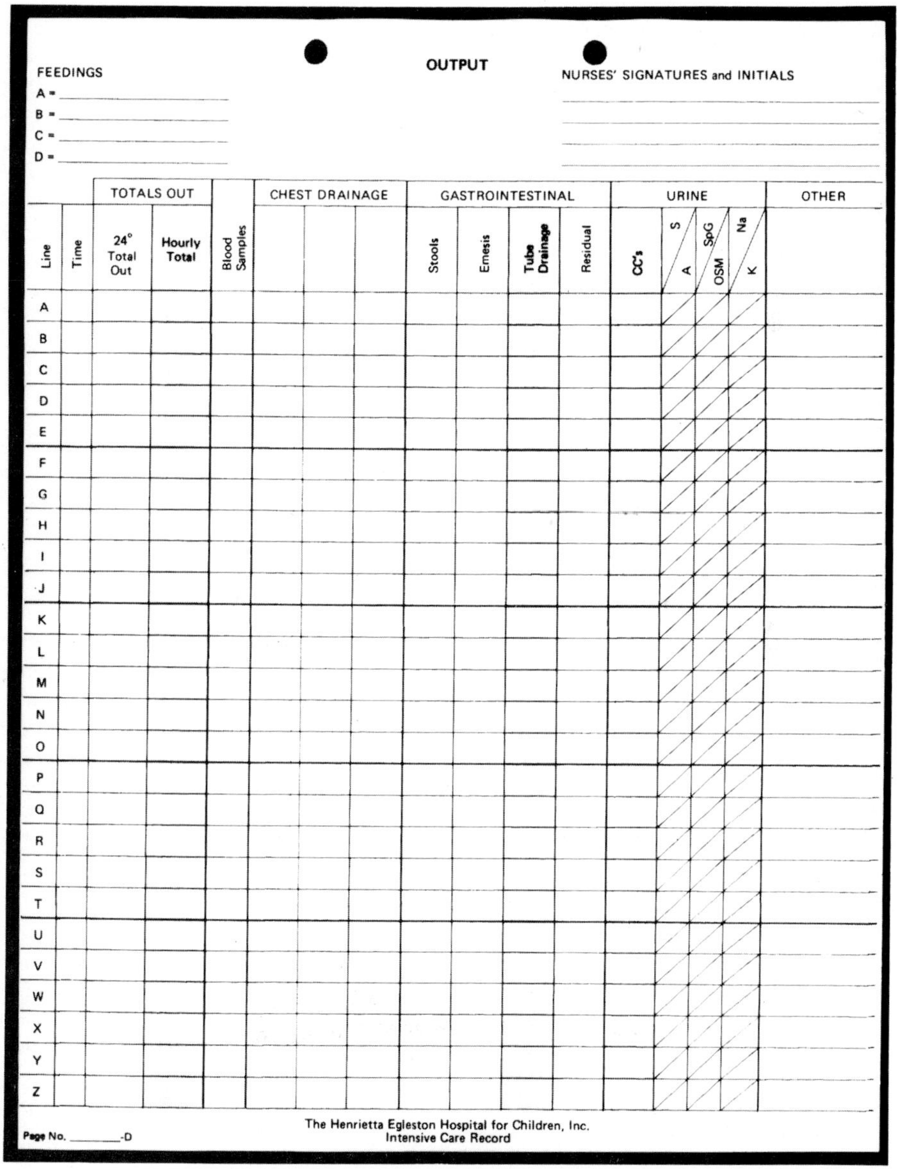
FEEDINGS
A = ______
B = ______
C = ______
D = ______

OUTPUT

NURSES' SIGNATURES and INITIALS

Line	Time	TOTALS OUT: 24° Total Out	Hourly Total	Blood Samples	CHEST DRAINAGE			GASTROINTESTINAL: Stools	Emesis	Tube Drainage	Residual	URINE: CC's	S / A	SpG / OSM	Na / K	OTHER
A																
B																
C																
D																
E																
F																
G																
H																
I																
J																
K																
L																
M																
N																
O																
P																
Q																
R																
S																
T																
U																
V																
W																
X																
Y																
Z																

Page No. ______-D

The Henrietta Egleston Hospital for Children, Inc.
Intensive Care Record

Fig. 8-6. Flowsheet for recording output data in the Intensive Care Unit.

vided, possibly with fewer postoperative metabolic problems.

5. The time required to cool on bypass is reduced.

6. Hypothermia affords excellent myocardial preservation.

The major risks involved in using surface cooling, cardiopulmonary bypass, and subsequent cooling using the pump oxygenator include the following:

1. Prolongation of anesthesia time.
2. Tissue hypoxia (regional and general).
3. Metabolic acidosis.
4. Cerebral dysfunction from changes in cerebral blood flow.
5. Postoperative bleeding due to fibrinolysis.
6. Potential cold injury to the skin and subcutaneous tissues as well as to internal organs such as the kidneys and the liver.

One limitation of the technique of profound hypothermia with circulatory arrest is *time*. We feel relatively safe in utilizing up to 60 minutes of circulatory arrest at 16°-20°C, but no clearly defined limits for neurologically safe circulatory arrest exist.

We employ surface cooling with ice bags or an ice tub plus cooling on cardiopulmonary bypass in many but not all infants requiring open heart surgery who are less than 2 years of age and who weigh less than 10 kg (see Fig. 8-7).

Certain patients require definitive operation in early infancy because of the nature and severity of the defect present. These include infants with critical aortic or pulmonary stenosis, total anomalous pulmonary venous return,[119,124] isolated or combined lesions including ventricular septal defect,[117,119,121,123] tetralogy of Fallot,[128,129] and transposition of the great vessels.[117,119] Some of these may be treated by either a primary or two-stage repair. Because of the improvements already mentioned, a single operation for primary repair may be preferable. The infant with congestive heart failure due to a large ventricular septal defect may be treated in one of two ways. The pulmonary artery may be banded to reduce pulmonary blood flow, with later debanding and closure of the septal defect when the child is older. Alternatively, the ventricular septal defect may be closed primarily in a single operation, thereby avoiding the morbidity and·mortality associated with a second operation and uncertain palliation. Use of profound hypothermia and circulatory arrest allows the surgeon a more accessible operative field and better exposure of the ventricular septal defect and associated conduction tissue areas. It also minimizes the metabolic effects of a prolonged period on cardiopulmonary bypass in an infant already severely stressed from congestive heart failure.

The anesthetic management is discussed elsewhere in the chapter (see above and protocol below) and includes surface cooling to 30°C and core cooling to 16°C using cardiopulmonary bypass. The use of sodium nitroprusside during cooling and rewarming has, in our experience, shortened considerably the time required to reach the desired temperature. Halothane in low concentrations in the inspired gases *may* reduce the likelihood of ventricular fibrillation during the vulnerable period from 26°-30°C, but this has not yet been proved.[130]

Persistent Patency of the Ductus Arteriosus in Premature Infants

Delay in closure of the ductus arteriosus in the premature infant has been well documented.[131–135] Because of improved techniques for maintaining ventilation in premature infants, the survival of these small babies has improved dramatically during the past decade.

Since the vasoconstriction response of the ductus arteriosus to increasing partial pressures of oxygen is proportional to gestational age, it is not surprising that there is a high incidence of persistent patent ductus arteriosus in small preterm infants. Some institutions report that 45 percent of infants having a birth weight of less than 1750 gm show clinical evidence of a patent ductus[131] and in infants weighing less that 1200 gm at birth, the incidence approaches 80 percent.

The clinical manifestations depend upon the magnitude of the left-to-right shunt through the ductus and the ability of the infant to employ mechanisms to cope with the extra volume load. As with other types of left-to-right shunts, the amount of blood entering the pulmonary circulation is determined by the size of the ductus itself and the relationship between pulmonary and systemic vascular resistances. Many premature infants (60 percent)[136] have idiopathic respiratory distress syndrome (RDS); the severity of this condition influences the amount of left-to-right shunting, since pulmonary vascular resistance is increased in relation to systemic vascular resistance.

There are three fairly distinct patterns of clinical presentation in the infants with patent ductus arteriosus.[133]

1. *Patent ductus arteriosus with no lung disease.* These babies show no significant underlying lung disease, and their weight usually exceeds 1500 gm. Systolic murmurs are heard a week or so after birth. As the left-to-right shunt increases, the murmur becomes louder and more prolonged, eventually extending into diastole. If the shunt becomes significantly large, clinical evidence of congestive heart failure (CHF) may appear. There may be an increase in the arterial blood P_{CO_2}. Episodic apnea associated with bradycardia may occur.[137] The chest x-ray may show enlargement of the left atrium and ventricle, but it is common for heart

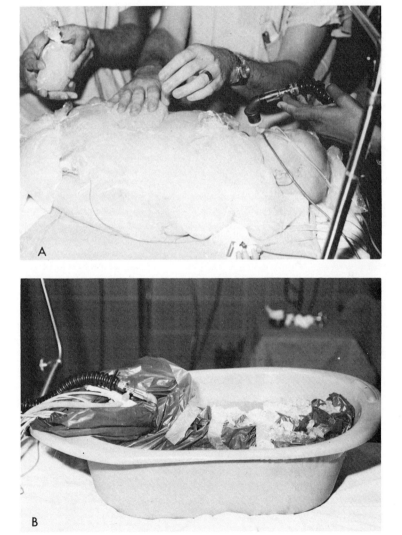

Fig. 8-7. Surface cooling of infant for correction of cardiac defect requiring profound hypothermia and circulatory arrest.

size to remain normal. Pulmonary vascularity is often increased, and cardiac catheterization usually indicates moderate elevation of pulmonary arterial pressure.

The large majority of these infants do not develop severe left ventricular failure, and those who do are generally managed with medical therapy including fluid restriction and maintenance of the hematocrit valve above 45 percent. If untreated surgically, the ductus often closes spontaneously within 2 or 3 months after birth. Rarely, intractable cardiac failure results, and surgical closure is required.

2. *Patent ductus arteriosus in infants recovering from lung disease.* The second most common group of infants may develop left-to-right shunting during recovery from severe or moderately severe RDS. They usually weigh around 1500 gm at birth, and RDS is generally evident within a few hours after birth and begins to improve in 3 to 4 days. As improvement continues, the signs of left-to-right shunting through a patent ductus become evident. It is thought that the ductus has been patent since birth and that pulmonary disease with resultant increase in pulmonary vascular resistance has prevented a significant left-to-right shunt. As pulmonary disease improves, oxygenation increases, and the ductus should begin to constrict. The majority of these infants are quite immature, however, so that good constrictor response to oxygen is not likely. Many are still maintained on ventilators and continuous positive airway pressure, so that careful clinical assessment is required to establish the presence of a shunt through the ductus. Often, murmurs are not audible until the infant is given a brief trial off the ventilator. Since recovery from RDS is often not continuously progressive but is interrupted by periods of exacerbation of the disease and intermittent left-to-right shunting, the murmur may be intermittent for several days. Murmurs may appear and disappear several times within the period of improvement, or there may be only a systolic murmur. As the shunt increases, the murmur extends into diastole and eventually becomes continuous.

The deterioration of the infant recovering from RDS is thought to be an indication of a significant left-to-right shunt through a patent ductus. Other causes of deterioration must be considered and include pneumothorax, sepsis, or infection. Deterioration is often manifest by requirements for an increased inspired oxygen concentration, alterations in ventilator rate and pressure, increased requirements for positive airway pressure ventilation, and an increase in arterial P_{CO_2}. The chest x-ray may show the expected changes resulting from the RDS, and an increase in pulmonary vascularity may be difficult to diagnose. Enlargement of the heart is also difficult to assess but may indicate the presence of a significant left-to-right shunt. The echocardiogram may be helpful in assessing the condition of these babies by showing an increase in the left atrial/aortic ratio if the deterioration is due to an increasing shunt through the ductus and not to worsening of RDS.[138,139]

3. *Patent ductus arteriosus associated with lung disease.* The third group consists of infants who have had severe RDS from birth and have shown little or no improvement in their lung disease. Clinical deterioration may signal the presence of a large left-to-right shunt. Most of these babies weigh less than 1200 gm at birth and require ventilatory assistance using mechanical ventilators and CPAP. Their deterioration is usually manifest by the need for increasing pressures or increasing levels of CPAP to maintain adequate blood gases. In these patients, murmurs are often difficult to hear because the ductus is so large that a murmur is not produced. A change in ventilatory requirements may be due to progression of RDS or to increasing congestive failure from the large shunt.

One of the most important considerations in treating infants with patent ductus arteriosus is the maintenance of adequate hemoglobin and hematocrit values. Reduction of hemoglobin requires increased cardiac output to maintain peripheral oxygenation. With a left-to-right shunt, and with an already compromised myocardium, anemia may further impair cardiac output. Also, since myocardial oxygen delivery is dependent on blood oxygen content, low hemoglobin levels may be associated with myocardial ischemia. Since arterial blood gas sampling is common, the hematocrit reading often falls, and care must be taken to maintain this above 45 volumes percent.[131] Since peripheral tissue oxygen delivery is retarded by fetal hemoglobin, exchange transfusion for replacing fetal hemoglobin with adult hemoglobin may help to facilitate peripheral oxygenation.[140] Most premature infants require repeated blood sampling and transfusion results in essentially exchanging fetal hemoglobin for adult hemoglobin.

Maintenance of electrolyte, glucose, and nutrition (including intravenous and hyperalimentation feedings) is necessary. Fluid administration is generally restricted to low maintenance fluid, since volume overload may result in left ventricular failure. If failure does develop, digitalis and diuretic therapy is effective to varying degrees. If 48 to 72 hours of medical management fails to control congestive heart failure, surgical closure of the patent ductus is probably indicated.[131,137] Ligation is performed rather than division, and surgery can be performed with minimal mortality and morbidity.[136]

Prostaglandin inhibitors such as indomethacin are currently under investigation as an alternative to early surgical intervention, but the effectiveness of this method of treatment is, at present, still undecided.[141-143]

The relationship between presence of a patent ductus and the development of necrotizing enterocolitis in the premature infant has not been clearly defined, but the vascular effects of the large runoff are at least theoretically important.[144,145]

ANESTHESIA

Premature infants tolerate anesthesia for ligation of the patent ductus surprisingly well. Nitrous oxide/air/oxygen, pancuronium, and low concentrations of halothane or small doses of morphine are generally employed.

Protection of the eyes must be ensured by not using high inspired oxygen concentrations during anesthesia and by measuring the Pa_{O_2} during and shortly after surgery to keep the level within the normal range (60-80 torr).[146,147]

Other supportive measures must be meticulously carried out, including maintenance of body temperature, proper administration of fluids, electrolytes, glucose, correction of metabolic acidosis with $NaHCO_3$, as well as careful replacement of blood if the intraoperative loss exceeds 10 percent.

Congenital Heart Disease in the Adult

The problems posed by the adult with congenital heart disease are similar in nature but often more severe than those in children having the same defects. For example, the adult with a cyanotic congenital heart defect almost always has more and larger bronchial collateral vessels and severe polycythemia, which complicate anesthesia induction and perfusion during total repair on cardiopulmonary bypass. The postoperative course of patients with an extensive systemic-to-pulmonary-arterial collateral circulation is also complicated, since the pulmonary blood flow is often excessive following total repair in these patients, and the pulmonary arterial pressure may be higher than normal.[75,76]

Many adult patients with congenital heart disease have had one or more previous palliative operations. Total repair is complicated by the reoperative nature of the surgery, larger blood replacement requirements, lack of veins and arteries for monitoring and intravenous infusion, and the patients' own anxieties prompted by stressful events of previous hospitalizations. Such secondary operations are usually longer and more difficult because previously constructed systemic-to-pulmonary-arterial shunts must be mobilized and closed, pulmonary arterial bands must be removed and the pulmonary artery repaired, or previously inadequate repairs must be radically revised. Closure of a previously constructed Potts' shunt (descending-aortic-to-left-pulmonary-arterial anastomosis) poses a series of problems best solved by the use of circulatory arrest under conditions of profound hypothermia even in the adult.[148] The combination of postoperative fibrosis, pericarditis, and mediastinal or pleural collateral circulation increases blood loss in the heparinized patient. Even the sternotomy incision itself is a far greater risk the second time, and some surgeons prefer to expose the femoral vessels to allow rapid institution of cardiopulmonary bypass in the event of injury to the right ventricle or great vessels.

The adult with coarctation of the aorta is likely to have extensive chest wall collateral circulation and more labile hypertension than the child with an equivalent degree of aortic obstruction. Postoperative blood pressure responses are less predictable and more difficult to control than in the child.[149]

Many adults with long-standing congenital heart defects associated with an increase in pulmonary blood flow or pulmonary venous hypertension (mitral and/or aortic valve disease) will have an increase in pulmonary vascular resistance. Such patients are at greater risk of developing postoperative low cardiac output and pulmonary insufficiency. Prolonged postoperative ventilatory support should be anticipated.

Adults with atrial septal defect and congestive heart failure are particularly susceptible to the development of postoperative supraventricular and occasionally ventricular arrhythmias.[150] Patients with long-standing pressure overload (pulmonary stenosis, aortic stenosis, coarctation of the aorta) have markedly hypertrophic ventricles. The decreased compliance of such hypertrophic ventricles increases the likelihood of postoperative low cardiac output. Subendocardial ischemia is more common in the hypertrophic and hypertensive ventricle and increases the incidence of postoperative ventricular arrhythmias. Intraoperative myocardial preservation is more difficult in the severely hypertrophic ventricle. Patients having long-standing volume overload of the ventricles as a result of valvular regurgitation or a large intracardiac shunt generally manifest at least some degree of low cardiac output in the early postoperative period.[151] The use of inotropic infusions and afterload reduction with vasodilators should be anticipated.

Basic anesthetic principles and techniques for management of the adult and child with congenital heart disease are similar. Anesthetic and surgical challenges exist at the extremes of the spectrum—the tiny infant with a life-threatening defect and the adult with one or more previous palliative operations for a defect present from birth.

Prevention of Infective Endocarditis

The anesthesiologist often encounters patients with rheumatic or congenital heart disease who require anesthesia for noncardiac surgical procedures. It should be remembered that even hemodynamically insignificant defects (e.g., small VSD, minimal pulmonic or aortic stenosis or bicuspid aortic valve, or mild mitral regurgitation from previous rheumatic fever) assume more importance when certain operations are

performed that may result in transitory bacteremia causing bacterial endocarditis or endarteritis.[152] This is one of the most serious complications of heart disease, and preventative measures must be taken to minimize the risk.[153-158]

While anesthesiologists may not be wholly responsible for actually ordering the antibiotic prophylaxis, it behooves them to be aware of the risks involved if prophylaxis is omitted, of the types of operations for which antibiotic coverage is needed, and of the drugs recommended and the dosages.

The Committee on Rheumatic Fever and Bacterial Endocarditis of the Council on Cardiovascular Disease in the Young of the American Heart Association has recently updated its recommendations[159] as to the types of surgery requiring prophylaxis, which patients are at greatest risk, and the drugs most effective in preventing this serious complication in patients with heart disease.

In general, operations that require prophylaxis include the following:

1. Dental procedures likely to result in gingival bleeding. This does not include shedding of decidious teeth.
2. Surgery or instrumentation of the upper or lower respiratory tract, e.g., tonsillectomy, adnoidectomy, bronchoscopy, or any procedure involving disruption of the respiratory mucosa.
3. Genitourinary tract surgery or instrumentation, e.g., cystoscopy, urethral catheterization, prostatic or bladder surgery.
4. Lower gastrointestinal or gallbladder instrumentation with biopsy or surgery.
5. Cardiac surgery.
6. Following cardiac surgery (*exceptions* include patients with *uncomplicated secundum atrial septal defects* closed by direct suturing without a prosthetic patch and those who have had division and ligation of a *patent ductus arteriosus* following a healing period of 6 months after surgery, and patients who have undergone *coronary artery bypass*.)
7. Procedures on any infected or contaminated tissues, e.g., incision and drainage of abscesses.
8. Long-term indwelling vascular catheters.

Patients on long-term rheumatic fever prophylaxis with antibiotics must be given adequate endocarditis prophylaxis for indicated procedures, since the rheumatic fever prevention doses are *inadequate* to prevent endocarditis.

Depending on the type of surgery planned on patients with heart disease and the type of bacteremia that can be expected, the appropriate antibiotic regimen can be chosen. Aqueous penicillin combined with procaine penicillin plus streptomycin, or aqueous penicillin, ampicillin, and streptomycin or gentamycin are the usual drugs employed to prevent endocarditis. These are given 30 minutes to 1 hour prior to surgery and are followed with oral administration of the penicillin portion of the regimen every 6 hours for 8 doses.

In penicillin-sensitive patients, vancomycin or erythromycin, along with or in combination with streptomycin, is administered 30 minutes to 1 hour prior to the procedure and repeated in 12 hours. The dosage of these drugs is adjusted to the age and weight of the patient.

The importance of prophylaxis for the susceptible patient cannot be overemphasized, and the anesthesiologist must make this part of his preoperative evaluation.

HEMODYNAMIC DATA IN CONGENITAL HEART DISEASE

Information obtained during the diagnostic investigation of a child with congenital heart disease is helpful to the anesthesiologist in selecting the proper anesthetic techniques for the surgical procedure. The history, physical examination, electrocardiogram, and chest x-rays are often sufficient to allow a choice of a safe anesthetic and surgical approach. The patient with an uncomplicated patent ductus arteriosus, for example, may not require cardiac catheterization when the history and physical findings clearly indicate a specific diagnosis. In the newborn infant in whom clinical information is often puzzling or at least inconclusive, cardiac catheterization *is* necessary and provides the surgeon and the anesthesiologist with invaluable information.

The anesthesiologist should be particularly familiar with information provided by cardiac catheterization (see Table 8-15).[31,68,160] This includes (1) *anatomic* data and precise diagnoses obtained from the course of catheter passage

Table 8-15
Cardiac Catheterization Data of Interest to the Anesthesiologist

Anatomic data
  Catheter course
  Angiocardiograms
Physiological data
  Pressures in all chambers and vessels
  Oxygen consumption (often estimated in infants and children)[161]
  Oxygen saturation in all chambers and vessels
  Contour of pressure tracings
  Rate of change of left ventricular pressure (dP/dt)
  Indicator dilution curves and magnitude of shunts
  Pharmacologic effects
    Vasodilators (tolazoline, amyl nitrite)
    Oxygen
    Inotropic medications
  Responses to exercise
Derived data and calculations
  Cardiac output (Q_s)
  Pulmonary blood flow (Q_p)
  Pulmonary vascular resistance (PVR or R_p)
  Systemic vascular resistance (SVR or R_s)
  Ratio of pulmonary blood flow to systemic blood flow (Q_p/Q_s)
  Ratio of pulmonary vascular resistance to systemic vascular resistance (R_p/R_s)
  Valve areas
  Ventricular volumes
  Regurgitant volumes
  Ejection fraction or other indices of ventricular function

and angiographic visualization of cardiac chambers and vessels; (2) *physiological* data obtained by measurement of pressures and oxygen saturations in each chamber and vessel; and (3) assessment of *ventricular function* determined by a combination of angiographic and physiological measurements. The rate of change of ventricular pressure as a function of time (dP/dt) and the calculation of the ventricular ejection fraction by comparison of systolic and diastolic frames from cineangiograms are commonly used indices of ventricular function. Derived physiological data include the calculation of (1) cardiac output; (2) systemic vascular resistance (SVR or R_s); (3) pulmonary vascular resistance (PVR or

R_p); (4) the ratio of pulmonary and systemic resistances (R_p/R_s); (5) the direction and magnitude of flow through intracardiac shunts and the ratio of pulmonary blood flow to systemic blood flow (Q_p/Q_s); (6) the magnitude of pressure gradients across stenotic valves and the cross-sectional area of these valves; and (6) the volume of blood being regurgitated backward across incompetent valves.

In our institution, patients are not anesthetized for cardiac catheterization. Heavy sedation is utilized, with local infiltration anesthesia for insertion of catheters.

Pressure gradients in patients with valvular stenosis may suggest the degree of impairment of ventricular function to be anticipated at the termination of bypass. For example, the patient with suprasystemic pressures in the right ventricle may not tolerate even a minor degree of myocardial depression during induction of anesthesia for correction of severe pulmonary valve stenosis. Significant right ventricular failure may ensue with termination of cardiopulmonary bypass in such patients.

As a general rule, anesthetic agents with myocardial depressant properties are avoided for induction of anesthesia in patients with impaired ventricular reserve as seen in severe right or left ventricular outflow obstructive lesions. In those patients with tetralogy of Fallot physiology in whom a decrease in systemic vascular resistance may result in a significant increase in right-to-left shunting and cyanosis, peripheral vasodilators are avoided (halothane or enflurane). It must be remembered, however, that nondepressant drugs such as ketamine may actually *increase* right ventricular outflow obstruction and result in decreased pulmonary blood flow. A hypercyanotic episode may then occur during induction of anesthesia.

All drugs utilized by anesthesiologists have profound cardiovascular effects and must be *titrated* to the desired effect. Both detrimental and desired effects must be considered in each and every patient. Measures must be available to counteract the undesired effects if they occur during induction and maintenance of anesthesia.

CALCULATION OF INTRACARDIAC SHUNT FLOWS

The traditional division of congenital heart defects into cyanotic and acyanotic forms suggests the value of oxygen saturation studies in both the localization and quantification of shunts. The distinction of right-to-left (cyanotic) shunts from left-to-right (acyanotic) shunts can be made on the basis of the peripheral arterial oxygen saturation, assuming the absence of pulmonary disease or hypoxia. Localization of shunts can be determined by detection of abnormal oxygen saturations within the cardiac chambers. For example, in the case of a left-to-right shunt at the ventricular level (VSD), a catheter sampling blood in the right heart would detect an increased oxygen saturation in the right ventricle as a result of the admixture of arterialized blood from the left ventricle. This "arterialization" would persist at all points downstream from the shunt but at no point upstream. Conversely, in a right-to-left shunt, a decrease in oxygen saturation would be detected in the left heart at the site of the "venous admixture" from the right heart and would persist at all points downstream from the shunt, being manifest peripherally as desaturation and, if of sufficient degree, cyanosis.

The amount of oxygen in the blood may be expressed in two different but interconvertible units—percentage of oxygen saturation (percent O_2 Sat) and oxygen content (milliliters of $O_2/100$ ml blood, or O_2 volumes percent). To convert, oxygen content is divided by oxygen capacity:

$$\% \ O_2 \ Saturation = \frac{(O_2 \ content) \ (100)}{(hemoglobin \ in \ grams/100 \ ml) \ (1.34 \ ml \ O_2/gm \ Hgb)}$$

The normal levels of oxygen within the cardiac chambers are shown in Table 8-16. Note that the inferior vena cava (IVC) saturation is greater than the superior vena cava (SVC) saturation as a result of either the excessive oxygen extraction by the brain or the large proportion of the cardiac output of the kidney with its relatively low oxygen extraction or both. The coronary sinus blood has a very low saturation because of the high oxygen extraction by the myocardium. These facts imply the importance of obtaining several right atrial oxygen determinations in order to obtain a true "mixed venous" value. They also indicate the difficulty of evaluating left-to-right shunts at the atrial level, since it is quite difficult to obtain a valid "mixed venous" oxygen saturation value for use in the shunt calculations. The best approximation is

Table 8-16
Normal Oxygen Saturation Values at Rest

Site	$O_2\%$ Saturation	O_2 content
IVC	83% ± 10%	15.6 ml O_2/100 ml blood
SVC	77% ± 10%	14.4
RA	80% ± 6%	15.0
RV	79% ± 4%	14.8
PA	78% ± 5%	14.6
PA wedge, "PC"	79% ± 5%	18.4
LA, LV, aorta peripheral arterial	97.5% ± 2%	18.3

IVC = inferior vena cava; SVC = superior vena cava; RA = right atrium; RV = right ventricle; PA = pulmonary artery; PC = pulmonary capillary; LA = left atrium; LV = left ventricle.

probably a weighted average of the SVC and IVC oxygen saturations. Since IVC flow is greater than SVC flow, a reasonably accurate approximation of the mixed venous oxygen saturation is determined by the following formula:

Mixed venous O_2 Sat =

$$\frac{(\text{IVC } O_2 \text{ saturation} \times 3) + (\text{SVC } O_2 \text{ saturation})}{3}$$

In the absence of intracardiac shunts, the pulmonary arterial blood is most representative of the true "mixed venous" values.

Once the shunt has been localized and the oxygen data obtained, the Fick principle for calculating cardiac output or cardiac index (cardiac output per square meter body surface area) may be applied to estimate the quantity of blood traversing the abnormal opening. The Fick principle is expressed as

Cardiac output =

$$\frac{\text{oxygen consumption}}{\text{Arteriovenous oxygen difference}}$$

If blood is shunted from left heart to right heart, the pulmonary blood flow (Q_p) must be greater than the systemic blood flow (Q_s). If one applied the Fick principle twice, once to the systemic cardiac output and again to the pulmonary cardiac output, the ratio Q_p/Q_s can be obtained as an estimate of the degree of shunting. When ratios alone are desired, it is not necessary to determine the oxygen consumption, since this value cancels out in the calculation (see Table 8-17).

A similar method is used for quantification of a right-to-left shunt, except that the desaturation of the left heart blood makes it impossible to use just any left heart value for oxygenated blood returning from the lungs as was done in the calculation of the left-to-right shunt. Here it becomes necessary to have a value for pulmonary venous blood itself. Since this is difficult to obtain in all catheterizations, one may assume that in the absence of pulmonary disease and pulmonary arteriovenous fistulae the blood will be about 97.5 percent saturated. See Table 8-17 for calculation of a right-to-left shunt.

Table 8-17
Simplified Calculation of Q_p/Q_s with Intracardiac Shunts

I. Calculation of a left-to-right shunt

$$Q_p/Q_s = \frac{\text{arterial } O_2 \text{ sat} - \text{estimated mixed venous } O_2 \text{ sat}}{\text{arterial } O_2 \text{ sat} - \text{pulmonary arterial } O_2 \text{ sat}}$$

II. Calculation of a right-to-left shunt

$$Q_p/Q_s = \frac{\text{arterial } O_2 \text{ sat} - \text{estimated mixed venous } O_2 \text{ sat}}{\text{Real or assumed pulmonary venous } O_2 \text{ sat} - \text{pulmonary arterial } O_2 \text{ sat}}$$

CALCULATION OF VASCULAR RESISTANCE

Vascular resistance may be determined by Poiseuille's relationship:

$$\text{Resistance} = \frac{\text{pressure change}}{\text{flow}}$$

Changes in calculated resistance can be considered significant, however, only when changes in flow have been confined to relatively narrow limits. Hence the calculated change in pulmonary vascular resistance (R_p) after closure of a left-to-right shunt may be grossly misleading as a result of the extreme change in pulmonary blood flow. Also, distinction cannot be made between obliterative disease and vasoconstriction without the use of pharmacologic agents. Pulmonary vascular resistance is influenced by several mechanisms operating upon the pulmonary vascular bed, including reactive vasoconstriction, medial hypertrophy, intimal hyperplasia and proliferation that may progress to obstruction, thromboembolic obstruction of pulmonary vessels, hypoxia, acidosis, and destruction of large area of lung. Effect, not mechanism, is determined by resistance calculations, expressed as

Pulmonary vascular resistance =

$$\frac{(\text{MPAP} - \text{MLAP})}{Q_p}\text{(normal, 0–3 units)}$$

and

Systemic vascular resistance =

$$\frac{(\text{MAoP} - \text{MRAP})}{Q_s}\text{(normal, 10–13 units)}$$

where MPAP = mean pulmonary arterial pressure, MLAP = mean left atrial pressure, MAoP = mean aortic pressure, MRAP = mean right atrial pressure, and Q_p and Q_s represent pulmonary and systemic blood flow, respectively.

APPENDIX A

MORE COMMON TYPES OF OPERABLE HEART DISEASE

Lesion	% Incidence*	Operation
VSD	19–25	Pulmonary artery banding for palliation; Total Correction (CPB)
PDA	12–15	Ligation or ligation and division
CoA	5–8	Patch angioplasty or resection with end-to-end anastomosis.
PS(IVS)	7–8	Pulmonary valvotomy (CPB)
T of F	6–10	Aortico-pulmonary shunt for palliation. Patch closure of VSD, right ventricular outflow reconstruction
AS	5	Aortic valvotomy (CPB)
TGA	4–5	Atrial septectomy for palliation; Mustard's repair (CPB)
ASD(S)	4–10	Suture or patch closure (CPB)
VSD & PS	3–4	Patch closure and pulmonary valvotomy (CPB)
TAPVD	1–2	Anastomosis of collecting vein and enlargement of left atrium (CPB and profound hypothermia)
TA	1–2	Aortico-pulmonary shunt or superior vena cava to pulmonary artery anastomosis for palliation

Abbreviations: VSD (Ventricular septal defect); CPB (Cardiopulmonary bypass); PDA (Patent ductus arteriosus); CoA (Coarctation of the aorta); PS(IVS) Pulmonary stenosis with intact ventricular septum; T of F (Tetralogy of Fallot); AS (Aortic stenosis); TGA (Transposition of the Great Arteries) ASD(S) (atrial septal defect-secundum variety); VSD & PS (Ventricular septal defect and pulmonary stenosis with left-to-right shunt); TAPVD (Total anomalous pulmonary venous drainage); TA (Tricuspid atresia).

* Incidence range data from series from Children's Hospital Medical Center, Boston, and Hospital for Sick Children, Toronto. Nadas, A.S. and Fyler D.C. Pediatric Cardiology (ed 3). Philadelphia, Saunders, 1972, p. 683

APPENDIX B

ANESTHESIA PROTOCOL FOR OPEN HEART OPERATIONS*

Preparation for open heart surgical anesthesia begins with the preoperative visit. Both the child and family are seen the afternoon prior to the scheduled operation. Information pertinent to the conduct of anesthesia is recorded on the Anesthesia Consultation Form, including:

1. Significant *history*
2. Significant *physical findings*
3. Laboratory data
4. Chest x-ray findings
5. Electrocardiographic findings
6. Cardiac catheterization data, including diagnoses and factors contributing to increased risk or influencing anesthetic management
7. Premedication
8. Anesthetic management plan
9. Immediate postoperative management plan

When questions arise as to the specific operation planned or when observations such as fever or abnormal laboratory data suggest that the operation should be deferred, the surgeon or one of his assistants should be consulted. The preoperative medication plan and anesthetic plan should be suited to the requirements of the patient and the specific operation planned. Management should be discussed in appropriate detail with both the child and the parents.

Before arrival of the patient in the operating room the following preparations are made:

1. The standard operating room monitor is turned on and checked for proper function.
2. The standard equipment required for the administration of any general anesthetic is obtained and checked for proper function.
3. *Two* cassette-type constant-infusion pumps are obtained and set up.
4. *One* single-syringe constant-infusion pump with a 50-ml syringe is obtained.
5. Intravenous solutions of 5 percent dextrose

* Henrietta Egleston Hospital for Children, Inc., Atlanta, Georgia.

and 0.25 percent normal saline with burettes are prepared.
6. A heparinized flush solution is prepared (1 unit beef lung sodium heparin per milliliter of normal saline).
7. Two disposable-dome pressure transducers are set up on a five-stopcock manifold and calibrated (see "Protocol for Direct Pressure Monitoring").
8. The standard operating table thermal-regulating mattress is placed and checked for proper function.

The following medications are prepared according to the dilutions required by the age of the patient (see "Protocol for Medication Dilution"):

Atropine sulfate
d-tubocurarine (or pancuronium bromide)
Morphine sulfate
Lidocaine
Succinylcholine
Heparin
Phenylephrine (Neo-Synephrine)
Methylprednisolone (Solu-Medrol)
Oxacillin (or cephalosporin)
Furosemide (Lasix)
Potassium chloride
Calcium chloride
Sodium bicarbonate.

The following medications should be available but need not be diluted or prepared for infusion at this time:

Dopamine hydrochloride (Intropin)
Dextrose 50 percent
Regular Insulin U40
Sodium nitroprusside (Nipride)
Protamine sulfate

After arrival of the patient but *before* the induction of anesthesia, the following monitors are established:

1. Blood pressure cuff (*not* to be placed on side of previous Blalock-Taussig shunt or on side of possible intraoperative occlusion of subclavian artery)
2. Electrocardiogram electrodes
3. Precordial stethoscope

After induction of anesthesia, the following devices are placed:

1. Two peripheral intravenous cannulae (large-

bore plastic) with T-connectors attached to the hubs. One line is infused with solution from the cassette constant-infusion pump; the other line is infused constantly via the single-syringe pump.

2. A central venous catheter (percutaneous or by cutdown if necessary) with attached T-connector.

3. An indwelling plastic arterial cannula, ordinarily in a radial artery that has not or will not be occluded during the operation. The arterial cannula is inserted percutaneously when possible, but cutdown may be required. A T-connector is attached to the hub for sampling, and the line is marked conspicuously with red tape to avoid inadvertent injection of damaging medications. The arterial line is connected to a constant infusion syringe pump via the manifold (see "Protocol for Direct Pressure Monitoring").

4. Esophageal stethoscope.

5. Sump-type nasogastric tube connected to suction.

6. Nasopharyngeal thermistor probe.

7. Rectal thermistor probe.

8. Foley bladder catheter (or infant feeding tube in bladder for infants).

9. Electrocautery ground plate.

As soon as convenient after insertion of the arterial monitoring cannula a blood sample is obtained for measurement of the following:

1. Arterial blood gases
2. Hemoglobin
3. Hematocrit
4. Serum potassium
5. Activated clotting time

Care must be exercised to avoid contamination of the sample with the heparinized flush solution.

All monitoring devices and the endotracheal tube are taped securely and labeled as necessary. All intravenous and arterial lines are maintained by either constant pump infusion at a carefully controlled rate *or* by syringe "heparin lock." No intravenous fluids are allowed to flow by gravity control alone.

All air bubbles in fluid lines must be eliminated! Connectors and injection ports are particularly likely to trap small air bubbles which may later be forced into the patient during an injection. Such bubbles can pass directly to the

cerebral circulation and brain of a cyanotic child!

Methylprednisolone (Solu-Medrol) (30 mg/kg) is administered intravenously at the beginning of open heart operations unless otherwise requested by the surgeon.

Oxacillin (25 mg/kg) (*or cephalosporin,* 25 mg/kg) is administered intravenously at the beginning of open heart operations unless otherwise indicated by the surgeon. Oxacillin (25 mg/kg) (or cephalosporin 25 mg/kg) is diluted in an appropriate amount of fluid and administered continuously throughout the case via the intravenous lines.

Beef lung sodium *heparin* (200 units/kg, or 2 mg/kg) is administered intravenously into a free-flowing intravenous line *when the pericardium is opened* except during reoperations in the mediastinum or when otherwise requested by the surgeon. When possible, the heparin should be given into a central venous line from which blood can be easily aspirated. Otherwise, it must be given into a fully visible intravenous cannula where extravasation would be easily noted. Three minutes following the administration of heparin, another blood sample is withdrawn for measurement of the activated clotting time, which should now exceed 500 seconds. If the ACT is less than 500 seconds, an additional 100 units/kg of heparin is given intravenously. The surgeon is notified 3 minutes after the administration of heparin and is also told when the ACT is in excess of 300 seconds, the latter being considered a "safe" level for insertion of intracardiac cannulae.

Fresh frozen plasma and platelet concentrates (1 unit/5 kg) are requested from the blood bank at the time bypass begins, allowing time for preparation and delivery for administration at the conclusion of bypass.

Arterial blood gases, hemoglobin, hematocrit, potassium, and calcium determinations are made at least every 30 minutes during cardiopulmonary bypass and more often as indicated or requested.

Urine output should be noted every 15 minutes during bypass, and the surgeon should be notified if urine production falls below a rate of 1 ml/kg/hr for any of these 15-minute intervals, that is, 0.25 ml/kg/15 min.

The activated clotting time should be determined immediately after beginning bypass and should be rechecked every 30 minutes thereafter. The ACT should be maintained at a level greater than 500 seconds by the administration of additional heparin according to the ACT nomogram.

During periods of complete cardiopulmonary bypass where ventilation is not required, the lungs should be maintained in a position of slight inflation by approximately 10 cm positive pressure unless otherwise requested.

If pressors are needed to facilitate termination of bypass, they should be administered *only* by a constant infusion pump, and when possible, they should be administered into a central venous catheter. Particular care must be exercised in the injection or infusion of epinephrine, calcium chloride, or 50 percent dextrose; these must *not* be given into a peripheral I.V., since they are highly irritating and can cause tissue necrosis.

After discontinuation of bypass, heparin is reversed with protamine sulfate (1.3 mg/mg of remaining heparin) as determined from the ACT graph.

Fresh frozen plasma (30 ml/kg) and platelet concentrates (1 unit/5 kg) are administered soon after discontinuation of bypass in conjunction with packed red blood cells or whole blood as needed to maintain adequate circulating blood volume as determined by the central venous pressure, left atrial pressure, heart rate, and arterial blood pressure.

While surgical hemostasis has been assured and the incision closed, the portable monitor used for transport of the patient is prepared. ECG and direct arterial blood pressure are monitored during transport to the intensive care unit. One hundred percent oxygen is administered during transport.

The anesthesiologist remains fully in charge during transport to the intensive care unit. Upon arrival the patient is placed on the previously arranged ventilator or, if extubated, is given oxygen by face mask. Transfer is made from the portable monitor to the permanent intensive care unit monitor, care being taken to avoid periods without *some* form of cardiac monitoring (ECG, arterial blood pressure display, finger on a pulse, precordial stethoscope, etc.).

The anesthesiologist reports the following information to the intensive care unit nurse:

1. Type of anesthesia

2. Any problems encountered during anesthesia
3. If narcotics and/or muscle relaxants have been reversed
4. Urine output during the operation
5. Fluids, blood, and blood products administered
6. Any anticipated problems
7. Contents of infusing intravenous fluids, noting especially any pressors, vasodilators, or antiarrhythmic medications
8. Results of recent blood studies in operating room or the fact that specific studies have been obtained and results are pending
9. Results of chest x-ray (if done in operating room)

Appropriate ventilation and stable vital signs should be assured before the anesthesiologist leaves the patient in the intensive care unit.

BRIEF CHECKLIST OF ANESTHESIA PROTOCOL FOR OPEN HEART SURGERY

1. Preoperative Visit
    a. Review record, including cath data, lab data, special studies
    b. Examine patient
    c. Plan
        (1) Premedication
        (2) Anesthetic technique
        (3) Immediate postoperative management (controlled versus spontaneous ventilation, etc.)
    d. Discussion with patient and family
    e. Complete anesthesia consultation form
    f. Preoperative orders
2. Before arrival of patient in operating room:
    a. Check monitor
    b. Check anesthesia machine and supplies
    c. Two cassette-type constant-infusion pumps
    d. One single-syringe constant-infusion pump with 50-ml syringe
    e. One double-syringe constant-infusion pump with 50-ml syringe
    f. Intravenous solutions (5 percent dextrose and 0.25 percent normal saline) with burettes

g. Heparinized flush (1 unit heparin/milliliter normal saline)

h. Two disposable-dome pressure transducers, set up with five-stopcock manifold and properly calibrated. Should be connected to double-syringe constant-infusion pump for heparinized flushing

i. Check temperature-regulating mattress

j. Proper dilutions of appropriate *medications* (see full protocol).

3. After arrival of patient . . .
   a. Blood pressure cuff
   b. Electrocardiogram electrodes
   c. Precordial stethoscope

4. After induction:
   a. Two peripheral I.V.s
   b. CVP catheter
   c. Arterial monitoring catheter
   d. Esophageal stethoscope
   e. Sump-type nasogastric tube to suction
   f. Nasopharyngeal thermistor
   g. Rectal thermistor
   h. Foley bladder catheter
   i. Electrocautery ground plate
   j. Arterial blood sample for:
      (1) Arterial blood gases
      (2) Hemoglobin
      (3) Hematocrit
      (4) Potassium
      (5) Calcium (Ionized and total serum)
      (6) Activated clotting time

k. All devices secured with tape and labeled

l. All air bubbles eliminated from lines

m. All lines to constant infusion pumps or syringes

5. Methylprednisolone (30 mg/kg I.V.)

6. Oxacillin (25 mg/kg I.V.) *or* cephalosporin (25 mg/kg I.V.) (Oxacillin (25 mg/kg) in 50–100 ml fluid to run continuously throughout the case).

7. Heparin (200 units/kg) when pericardium is opened

8. Repeat ACT 3 minutes after heparin. If less than 500 seconds, give 100 units/kg more heparin and repeat ACT

9. Notify surgeon 3 minutes after heparin given *and* when ACT exceeds 300 seconds

10. Order fresh frozen plasma (about 30 ml/kg)

11. Order platelet concentrates (1 unit/5 kg)

12. Repeat ABGs, potassium, calcium, hemoglobin, hematocrit, and ACT every 30 minutes (more often if needed).

13. Maintain urine output at no less than 1 ml/kg/hr (0.25 ml/kg/15 min recording interval)

14. Maintain ACT greater than 500 seconds according to ACT graph

15. CPAP at 10 cm water while on bypass

16. Prepare proper dilutions of pressors or vasodilators if needed

17. Prepared protamine sulfate (1.3 mg/mg of remaining heparin per ACT graph)

18. Blood, packed red blood cells, fresh frozen plasma, and platelets as needed

19. Transport monitor preparation

20. Transport to intensive care unit

21. Information for ICU nurse

APPENDIX C

CARDIOVASCULAR DRUGS

Drug	Preparation	Usual Dose
Epinephrine†	I.V. Drip—8 μg/ml solution Two 1 mg Amps to 250 ml 5% dextrose in H_2O*	0.1 μg/kg/min
Isoproterenol†	I.V. Drip—make 8 μg/ml solution Two 1 mg Amps (1 mg/5 cc)*	0.1 μg/kg/min
Dopamine†	I.V. Drip—make an 800 μg/ml solution. Add one 200 mg Amp to 250 ml 5% dextrose in H_2O*	2–16 μg/kg/min but may reach 50 μg/kg/min
Phenylephrine	100 μg/ml solution. Add one 10 mg Amp (1 ml) to 9 ml of normal saline, discard 9 ml of mixed solution and re-dilute to 10 ml	give 50 μg as bolus and observe effect; repeat as necessary (*rarely necessary*)
Calcium chloride	100 mg/cc	20–30 mg/kg SLOWLY
Calcium gluconate	Available in prepared solution (100 mg/ml)	3–4 mg/kg as bolus
Propranolol	One 1 mg Amp in 10 ml of normal saline (0.1 mg/ml)	Give 0.01 mg/kg as bolus to counteract effect of hypercyanotic spell in tetralogy of Fallot (0.01–0.1 mg/kg/dose) (maximum 1 mg)
Nitroglycerin†	50 μg/ml or 100 μg/ml solution must be prepared by the hospital pharmacy.	0.4 μg/kg/min
Sodium nitroprusside†‡	Dilute 50 mg vial with 2–3 ml of 5% dextrose H_2O and add the resulting solution to 500 ml of 5% dextrose in H_2O. Wrap in foil to protect from light	0.5–8.0 μg/kg/min *Discard after 4 hours*

* This concentration may be doubled, particularly in infants where volume of fluids must be carefully controlled.

† Administration using constant infusion pump (see Vasoactive Drug Dosage regimen below).

‡ Nitroprusside is good for only four hours after preparation and the bottle and tubing are shielded from light with aluminum foil.

Drug	Preparation	Usual Dose
Digoxin	Prepared commercially as 0.25 mg/ml and 0.1 mg/ml vials	Maintenance dose premature 0.007 mg/kg/day newborn 0.011 mg/kg/day 1 wk– 2 yrs 0.015 mg/kg/day 5– 10 yrs 0.011–0.007 mg/kg/day 10– 15 yrs 0.007–0.004 mg/kg/day total digitalizing dose = 3x maintenance dose. For initial total digitalizing dose; give $\frac{1}{2}$ total dose; give $\frac{1}{4}$ total dose after 8 hrs.; and final $\frac{1}{4}$ dose in another 8 hrs.
Lidocaine (Xylocaine)	For bolus. Prepared commercially as 1% and 2%. For I.V. drip, add 500 mg lidocaine to 250 ml of 5% dextrose in H_2O. Now available in 5 ml 2% solution for treatment of arrhythmias.	Bolus: 1–2 mg/kg/I.V. for arrhythmias Drip: 15–30 μg/kg/min should not exceed 5 mg/kg/hour
KCL	10 ml vial—20 mEq.	The Dose of KCL: 1) Determine the extracellular fluid volume by multiplying the body weight × 0.3 (or 0.5 for infants less than one year of age). 2) Determine the K^+ deficit per kg by subtracting the K^+ value from the desired value, e.g., K^+ = 2.5; desired = 4.5 − 2.5 = 2.0 mEq/kg. 3) Multiply the deficit/kg by ECF volume in kgs. to determine total dose of KCL in mEqs. 4) Usually $\frac{1}{2}$ of this dose is given and K^+ value remeasured. 5) Bolus doses should not exceed 1 mEq/min.

APPENDIX D

VASOACTIVE DRUG DOSAGE REGIMEN

Using constant infusion pumps:

Dopamine (Intropin)

ml/Hr.	400 μg/ml	800 μg/ml	1600 μg/ml
1	7.0 μg/min	13.3 μg/min	26.6 μg/min
2	13.0	26.6	53.2
3	20.0	40.0	80.0
4	26.5	53.0	106.0
5	33.0	66.5	133.0
6	40.0	80.0	160.0
7	46.5	93.0	186.0
8	53.0	106.0	212.0
9	60.0	120.0	240.0
10	66.5	133.0	266.0
15	100.0	200.0	400.0
20	133.0	266.0	532.0
30	200.0	400.0	800.0

Standard Dilutions

DOPAMINE (INTROPIN)
100 mg in 250 ml DS$\frac{1}{4}$NS = 400 μg/ml
200 mg in 250 ml DS$\frac{1}{4}$NS = 800 μg/ml
400 mg in 250 ml DS$\frac{1}{4}$NS = 1600 μg/ml
DOSE RANGE 2–16 μg/kg/min

Sodium Nitroprusside (Nipride)

ml/Hr.	200 μg/ml	100 μg/ml
1	3.3 μg/min	1.65 μg/min
2	6.6	3.30
3	9.9	4.95
4	13.2	6.60
5	16.5	8.25
6	19.8	9.90
7	23.1	11.55
8	26.4	13.20
9	29.7	14.85
10	33.0	16.50
15	49.5	24.75
20	66.0	33.00
25	82.5	41.25
30	99.0	49.50
35	115.5	58.00
40	132.0	66.00
45	148.5	74.25
50	165.0	82.50
55	181.5	91.00
60	200.0	100.00
65	214.5	108.00
70	231.0	116.00
75	247.5	124.00
80	264.0	132.00
85	280.5	140.25
90	297.0	149.00
95	313.5	157.00
100	333.0	166.50

To determine dosage being administered per kg per minute, DI-VIDE patient's weight in kilograms into μg/min figure at pump rate being used.

For example: *For Dopamine*
concentration   800 μg/ml
pump rate   8 ml/hour
patients weight   10 kg

$$\frac{106 \ \mu g/min}{10 \ kg} = 10.6 \ \mu g/kg/min$$

Sodium Nitroprusside (Nipride)
50 mg in 500 ml 5%DW = 100 μg/ml
50 mg in 250 ml 5%DW = 200 μg/ml

DOSE	*μg/kg/min*
Average	3
Range	0.5–8
Toxic	10

REFERENCES

1. Nadas A, Fyler D: Pediatric Cardiology (ed 3). Philadelphia, WB Saunders, 1972, p 293
2. Brinsfield D, Plauth W: Clinical recognition and medical management of congenital heart disease. *In* Hurst, JW, Logue RB, Schlant RC, Wenger NK (eds): The Heart. New York, McGraw-Hill, 1978, p 831
3. Mitchell SC, Korones SB, Berendes HW: Congenital heart disease in 56,109 births. Circulation 43:323, 1971
4. Kirklin JW: Advances in Cardiovascular Surgery. New York, Grune & Stratton, 1973
5. Gross RE, Hubbard JP: Surgical ligation of a patent ductus arteriosus. Report of first successful case. JAMA 112: 729, 1939
6. Blalock A, Taussig HB: The surgical treatment of malformations of the heart. JAMA 128:189, 1945
7. Potts WJ, Smith S, Gibson S: Anastomosis of the aorta to a pulmonary artery. Certain types in congenital heart disease. JAMA 132:627, 1946
8. Brock RC: Pulmonary valvotomy for the relief of congenital pulmonary stenosis. Br Med J 1:1121, 1948
9. Gross RE: Coarctation of the aorta. Surgical treatment of one hundred cases. Circulation 1:41, 1950
10. Crafoord C, Nylin G: Congenital coarctation of the aorta and its surgical treatment. J Thorac Surg 14:347, 1945
11. Lillehei CW, et al: Direct vision intracardiac surgery by means of controlled cross circulation or continued arterial reservoir perfusion for correction of ventricular septal defects, atrioventricularis communis, isolated infundibular pulmonic stenosis, and tetralogy of Fallot. *In* Lam CR (ed): Henry Ford Hospital International Symposium on Cardiovascular Surgery. Philadelphia, WB Saunders, 1955
12. Lillehei CW, Cohen M, Warden HE, et al: Direct vision intracardiac surgical correction of the tetralogy of Fallot and pentalogy of Fallot, and pulmonary atresia defects. Ann Surg 142:418, 1955
13. Lewis FJ, Taufic M: Closure of atrial septal defects with aid of hypothermia: experimental accomplishments and report of one successful case. Surgery 33:52, 1953
14. Gibbon JH: Application of a mechanical heart and lung apparatus to cardiac surgery. Minn Med 37:171, 1954
15. Mustard WT: Successful two-stage correction of transposition of great vessels. Surgery 55:469, 1964
16. Bernhard WL, Filler RM: Hyperbaric oxygenation: Current concepts. Am J Surg 115:661, 1968
17. Bernhard WL, Litwin SB, Williams WH, et al: Recent results of cardiovascular surgery in infants in the first year of life. Am J Surg 132:451, 1972
18. Dillard DH, Mohri H, Hessell EA: Correction of total anomalous pulmonary venous drainage in infants utilizing deep hypothermia with total circulatory arrest. Circulation 35 (suppl 1):I—105, 1967
19. Dillard DH, Mohri H, Merendino KA: Correction of heart disease in infancy utilizing deep hypothermia and total circulatory arrest. J Thorac Cardiovasc Surg 61:64, 1971
20. Barratt-Boyes BG, Simpson M, Neutze JM: Intracardiac surgery in neonates and infants using deep hypothermia with surface cooling and limited cardiopulmonary bypass. Circulation 43, (suppl 1):I—25, 1971
21. Hikasa Y, Shirotani H, Satomura K, et al: Open heart surgery in infants with an aid of hypothermic anesthesia. Arch Jap Chir 36:495, 1967
22. Rastelli GC: A new approach to "anatomic" repair of transposition of great arteries. Mayo Clin Proc 44:1, 1969
23. Hallman GL, Cooley DH: Surgical Treatment of Congenital Heart Disease (ed 2). Philadelphia, Lea and Febiger, 1975, p 173
24. Nadas A, Fyler D: Pediatric Cardiology (ed 3). Philadelphia, WB Saunders, 1972, p 684
25. Tyson KTR: Congenital Heart Disease in Infants. Summit, NJ, Ciba-Geigy, 1975
26. Adams FH: Fetal circulation and alterations at birth. *In* Moss AJ, Adams FH, Emmanouilides GC (eds): Heart Disease in Infants, Children and Adolescents (ed 2). Baltimore, Williams & Wilkins, 1977, p 11
27. Rashkind WJ, Miller WW: Creation of an atrial septal defect without thoracotomy: A palliative approach to complete transposition of the great arteries. JAMA 196:173, 1966
28. Blalock A, Hanlon R: The surgical treatment of complete transposition of the aorta and the pulmonary artery. Surg Gynecol Obstet 90:1, 1950
29. Vogel JHK: Pulmonary hypertension. *In* Moss AJ, Adams FH, Emmanouilides GC (eds): Heart Disease in Infants, Children and Adolescents (ed 2). Baltimore, Williams & Wilkins, 1977, p 629
30. Shealy H: Heather Gets Her Heart Fixed. Atlanta, Ga., The Henrietta Egleston Hospital for Children, 1976
31. Moffitt EA, McGoon DC, Ritter DG: The diagnosis and correction of congenital cardiac defects. Anesthesiology 33:144, 1970
32. Laver MB, Bland JHL: Anesthetic management of the pediatric patient during open-heart surgery. Int Anesthesiol Clin 13:3–149, 1975

33. Santoli FM, Pensa PM, Azzolina G: Anesthesia in open-heart surgery for connection of congenital heart diseases in children over one year of age. Int Anesthesiol Clin 14:3–165, 1976

34. Hansen DD: Anesthesia. *In* Sade RM, Cosgrove DM, Castaneda AR (eds): Infant and Child Care in Heart Surgery. Chicago, Year Book Medical Publishers, 1977

35. Ponce FE, et al: Propranolol palliation of tetralogy of Fallot: Experience with long-term drug treatment in pediatric patients. Pediatrics 52:100, 1973

36. Honey M, Chamberlain DA, Howard J: The effect of beta-sympathetic blockade on arterial oxygen saturation in Fallot's tetralogy. Circulation 30:501, 1964

37. Cummings GR: Propranolol in tetralogy of Fallot. Circulation 41:13, 1970.

38. Guntheroth WG, Kawabori I: Tetralogy of Fallot. *In* Moss AJ, Alams FH, Emmanouilides GC (eds): Heart Disease in Infants, Children and Adolescents (ed 2). Baltimore, Williams & Wilkins, 1977, p 287

39. Anderson MN, Kuchiba K: Depression of cardiac output with mechanical ventilation: comparative studies of intermittent positive-negative and assisted ventilation. J Thorac Cardiovasc Surg 54:182, 1967

40. Rudolph AM: Congenital Diseases of the Heart. Chicago, Year Book Medical Publishers, 1974, p 413

41. Price HL: General anesthetics. *In* Goodman LS, Gilman A: The Pharmacological Basis of Therapeutics (ed 5). New York, MacMillan, 1975, p 98

42. Tweed WA, Minuck M, Mymin D: Circulatory responses to ketamine anesthesia. Anesthesiology 37:613, 1972

43. Merin RG: Effects of anesthetics on the heart. Surg Clin North Am 55:759, 1975

44. Schwartz DA, Horwitz LD: Effects of ketamine on left ventricular performance. J Pharmacol Exp Ther 194:410, 1975

45. Traber DL, Wilson RD, Priano LL: The effect of beta-adrenergic blockade on the cardiopulmonary response to ketamine. Anesth Analg 49:604, 1970

46. Rittenhouse EA, Mohri H, Dillard DH, et al: Deep hypothermia in cardiovascular surgery. Ann Thorac Surg, 17:63, 1974

47. Brunberg JA, Reilly EL, Doty DB: Central nervous system consequences in infants of cardiac surgery using deep hypothermia and circulatory arrest. Circulation 50 (suppl 2):II—60, 1974

48. Stevenson JG, et al: Intellectual development of children subjected to prolonged circulatory arrest during hypothermic open heart surgery in infancy. Circulation 50 (suppl 2):II—54, 1974

49. Blackwood MJA, Haka-Ikse K, Steward DJ: Development of children following cardiac surgery under profound hypothermia, abstracted. Presented at 1976 Annual Meeting of American Society of Anesthesiologists, San Francisco, October 1976

50. Nadas AS, Fyler D: Pediatric Cardiology (ed 3). Philadelphia, WB Saunders, 1972, p 191

51. Samet P, Castillo C, Bernstein WH: Hemodynamic sequelae of atrial, ventricular, and sequential atrioventricular pacing in cardiac patients. Am Heart J 72:725, 1966

52. Galvis AG, Donahoo JS, White JJ: An improved technique for prolonged arterial catheterization in infants and children. Crit Care Med 4(3):166, 1976

53. Prince SR, Sullivan RL, Hackel A: Percutaneous catheterization of the internal jugular vein in infants and children. Anesthesiology 44:170, 1976

54. Schartz, AJ, et al: Central venous catheterization in pediatrics (personal communication, in press)

55. Schlant RC: Normal physiology of the cardiovascular system. *In* Hurst JW (ed): The Heart. New York, McGraw-Hill, 1978, p 80

56. Adamsons K, Towell ME: Thermal homeostasis in the fetus and newborn. Anesthesiology 26:531, 1965.

57. Stern L, Lees MA, Ledac J: Environmental temperature, oxygen consumption, and catecholamine excretion in newborn infants. Pediatrics 36:367, 1965

58. Buetow KC, Klein SW: Effect of maintenance of "normal" skin temperature on survival of infants of low birth weight. Pediatrics 34:163, 1964.

59. Gandy GM, Adamsons K, Cunningham N, et al: Thermal environment and acid-base homeostasis in human infants during the first few hours of life. J Clin Invest 43:751, 1964

60. Goudsouzian NG, Morris RH, Ryan JF: The effects of a warming blanket on the maintenance of body temperatures in anesthetized infants and children. Anesthesiology 39:351, 1973

61. Bennett EJ, Patel KP, Grundy EM: Neonatal temperature and surgery. Anesthesiology 46:303, 1977

62. LaFarge CG, Miettinen OS: The estimation of oxygen consumption. Cardiovasc Res 4:23, 1970

63. Gilston A: Anaesthesia for cardiac surgery. Br J Anaesth 43:217, 1971

64. Benzinger M, Benzinger TH: Tympanic membrane temperature. JAMA 209:1207, 1969

65. Sade RM, Cosgrove DM, Castaneda AR: Infant and Child Care in Heart Surgery. Chicago, Year Book Medical Publishers, 1977, p 60

66. Janssen PJ: Anesthesia for corrective open heart surgery of congenital defects beyond infancy. Int Anesth Clin 14:3:205, 1976

67. Drop LJ, Laver MB: Low plasma ionized calcium and response to calcium therapy in critically ill man. Anesthesiology 43:292, 1975

68. Franch RH: Cardiac catheterization. *In* Hurst JW (ed): The Heart. New York, McGraw-Hill, 1978, p 493

69. Alfieri O, Subramanian S: Cardiac output determination in infants and small children after open intra-cardiac operations. Ann Thorac Surg 19:322, 1975

70. Hill JD, Dontigny L, deLeval M, et al: A simple method of heparin management during prolonged extracorporeal circulation. Ann Thorac Surg 17:129, 1974

71. Bull BS, Korpman RA, Huse WM, et al: Heparin therapy during extracorporeal circulation, I. Problems inherent in existing heparin protocols. J Thorac Cardiovasc Surg 69:674, 1975

72. Mohri H, Merendino A: Hypothermia with or without a pump oxygenator. *In* Galetti P, Brecher G (eds): Heart-Lung Bypass. New York, Grune & Stratton, 1962, p 652

73. Mills NL, Beaulet RL, Isom WO, et al: Hyperglycemia during cardiopulmonary bypass. Ann Surg 177:203, 1973

74. Edie RN, Haubert SM, Malm JR: The use of haemodilution and a non-haemic prime for cardiopulmonary bypass. *In* Ionescu MI, Woller GH (eds): Current Technique in Extracorporeal Circulation. London, Butterworths, 1976, p 117

75. McGoon DC and Baird DK: Surgical management of large bronchial collateral arteries with pulmonary stenosis or atresia. Circulation 52:109, 1975

76. De Leval M, Ritter RG, McGoon DC: Anomalous systemic venous connections, surgical considerations. Mayo Clin Proc 50:599, 1975

77. Taber RE, Morales AR, Fine G: Myocardial necrosis and the postoperative low cardiac output syndrome. Ann Thorac Surg 4:12, 1967

78. Kirklin JW (ed): Advances in Cardiovascular Surgery. New York, Grune & Stratton, 1973, pp 85–172

79. Buckberg GD: Left ventricular subendocardial necrosis. Collective review. Ann Thorac Surg 24:379, 1977

80. Enright LP, Staroscik RN, Reis RL: Left ventricular function after occlusion of the ascending aorta. J Thorac Cardiovasc Surg 60:737, 1970

81. Shumway NE, Lower RR: Topical cardiac hypothermia for extended periods of anoxic arrest. Surg Forum 10:563, 1959

82. Hearse DJ, Stewart DA, Braimbridge MV, et al: Cellular protection during myocardial ischemia. Circulation 54:193, 1976

83. Boyd AD, Tremblay RE, Spencer FC, et al: Estimation of cardiac output after intracardiac surgery with cardiopulmonary bypass. Ann Surg 150:613, 1959

84. McClenahan JB: Blood volume studies in cardiac surgery patients. JAMA 195:356, 1966

85. Cohn LH, Angell WW, Shumway NE: Body fluid shifts after cardiopulmonary bypass. I. Effects of congestive heart failure and hemodilution. J Thorac Cardiovasc Surg 62:423, 1971

86. Sade RM, Cosgrove DM, Castaneda AR: Fluid and electrolyte balance. *In* Sade RM, Cosgrove DM, Castaneda AR (eds): Infant and Child Care in Heart Surgery. Chicago, Year Book Medical Publishers, 1977, p 62

87. Roberts NK, Yabek, S: Arrhythmias following atrial and ventricular surgery. *In* Roberts NK, Gelband H (eds): Cardiac Arrhythmias in the Neonate, Infant, and Child. New York, Appleton-Century-Crofts, 1977, p 405

88. Douglas JS, King SB, Hatcher CR, et al: Late cardiac tamponade after open heart surgery: A problem of differential diagnosis. Presented at American College of Cardiology, February 11, 1975

89. Kaplan JA, Bland JW, Dunbar RW: The perioperative management of pericardial tamponade. South Med J 69:4, 1976

90. Pontoppidan H, Geffin B, Lowenstein, E: Acute Respiratory Failure in the Adult. Boston, Little, Brown, 1973, p 57

91. Braunwald E, Ross J Jr, Sonnenblick EH: Mechanisms of Contraction of the Normal and Failing Heart (ed 2). Boston, Little, Brown, 1976, p 92

92. Katz A: Physiology of the Heart. New York, Raven Press, 1977, p 209

93. Castillo C, Lemberg L, Castellanos A, et al: Bifocal (sequential AV) demand pacemaker for SA and AV conduction disturbances. Am J Cardiol 25:87, 1970

94. Gelband H, Myerburg RJ, Bassett AL: Management of cardiac arrhythmias. *In* Roberts NK, Gelband H (eds): Cardiac Arrhythmias in the Neonate, Infant, and Child. New York, Appleton-Century-Crofts, 1977, p 437

95. Logue RB, Robinson PH, Hatcher CR, Kaplan JA: Medical management in cardiac surgery. *In* Hurst JW (ed): The Heart. New York, McGraw-Hill, 1978, p 1777

96. Shine KI: Ionic basis of excitation and of excitation-contraction coupling. *In* Robert NK,

Gelband H (eds): Cardiac Arrhythmias in the Neonate, Infant, and Child. New York, Appleton-Century-Crofts, 1977, p 91

97. Talley RC: A hemodynamic comparison of dopamine and isoproterenol in patients in shock. Circulation 39: 361, 1969

98. Scott RAD, Drew CE: Delayed pericardial effusion with tamponade after cardiac surgery. Br Heart J 35: 1304, 1973

99. Fowler NO: The recognition and management of pericardial disease and its complications. In Hurst JW, Logue RB, Schlant RC, Wenger NK (eds): The Heart. New York, McGraw-Hill, 1978, p 1640

100. Martin JW, Schenk WG: Pericardial tamponade: Newer dynamic concepts. Am Surg 99:782, 1960

101. Bushnell LS: Acute respiratory failure in the surgical patient: physiology and management. In Skillman JJ (ed): Intensive Care. Boston, Little, Brown, 1975, p 203

102. Bendixen HH, Egbert LD, Hedley-Whyte J, et al: Respiratory management in thoracic and cardiac surgery. In Bendixen HH, Egbert LD, Hedley-Whyte J, et al. (eds): Respiratory Care. St. Louis, Mosby, 1965, p 197

103. Sade RM, Cosgrove DM, Castaneda AR: Infant and Child Care in Heart Surgery. Chicago, Year Book Medical Publishers, 1977, p 67

104. Friedberg SA: Tracheostomy and respiratory care. In Goldin, MD (ed): Intensive Care of the Surgical Patient. Chicago, Year Book Medical Publishers, 1971, p 25

105. Shulman M: Postoperative ventilatory management. In Goldin, MD (ed): Intensive Care of the Surgical Patient. Chicago, Year Book Medical Publishers, 1971, p 39

106. Brumley GW: The respiratory distress syndrome of the newborn. In Smith CA (ed): The Critically Ill Child, Diagnosis and Management. Philadelphia, WB Saunders, 1972, p 152

107. Avery ME, Fletcher BD: The Lung and Its Disorders in the Newborn Infant. Philadelphia, WB Saunders, 1974, p 297

108. Bendixen HH, Egbert LD, Hedley-Whyte J, et al: Management of patients undergoing prolonged artificial ventilation. In Bendixen HH, Egbert LD, Hedley-Whyte J, et al (eds): Respiratory Care. St. Louis, Mosby, 1965, p 197

109. Klaus M, Fanaroff A: Respiratory problems. In Klaus M, Fanaroff A (eds): Care of the High-Risk Neonate. Philadelphia, WB Saunders, 1973, p 119

110. Young JA, Crocker D: Principles and Practice of Inhalation Therapy. Chicago, Year Book Medical Publishers, 1970

111. Llewellyn A, Swyer P: Assisted ventilation. In

Klaus M, Fanaroff A (eds): Care of the High-Risk Neonate. Philadelphia, WB Saunders, 1973, p 119

112. Abel RM, Wick J, Beck CH, Jr, et al: Renal dysfunction following open-heart operations. Arch Surg 108:175, 1974

113. Barratt-Boyes BG: The technique of intracardiac repair in infancy using deep hypothermia with circulatory arrest and limited cardiopulmonary bypass. In Inonescu MI, Woller GH (eds): Current Techniques in Extracorporeal Circulation. London, Butterworths, 1976, p 197

114. Barrett-Boyes BG, Subramanian S, Cartmill TB, et al: Profound hypothermia. In Barrett-Boyes BG, Neutze JM, Harris EA (eds): Heart Disease in Infancy, Diagnosis and Surgical Treatment. Edinburgh, Churchill Livingstone, 1973, pp 25–85

115. Mori A, et al: Deep hypothermia combined with cardiopulmonary bypass for cardiac surgery in neonates and infants. J Thorac Cardiovasc Surg 64:422, 1972

116. Barratt-Boyes BG, Simpson M, Neutze JM: Intracardiac surgery in infants and neonates and infants using deep hypothermia with surface cooling and limited cardiopulmonary bypass. Circulation 43 (suppl 1):I—25, 1971

117. Mori A, et al: Operative indication for corrective surgery in cases of complete transposition of the great arteries associated with large ventricular septal defect. J Thorac Cardiovasc Surg 71:750, 1976

118. Subramanian S: Early correction of congenital cardiac defects using profound hypothermia and circulatory arrest. Ann R Coll Surg Engl 54:176, 1974

119. Trusler G, Mustard WT: Palliative and reparative procedures for transposition of the great arteries. Ann Thorac Surg 17:410, 1974

120. Naches WH, et al: Coarctation of the aorta with ventricular septal defect. Circulation 55:189, 1977

121. Blackstone EH, et al: Optimal age and results in repair of large ventricular septal defects. J Thorac Cardiovasc Surg 72:661, 1976

122. Sade RM, Castaneda AR: Recent advances in cardiac surgery in the young infant. Surg Clin North Am 56:451, 1976

123. Steward DJ, Sloan IA, Johnston AE: Anesthetic management of infants undergoing profound hypothermia for surgical correction of congenital heart defects. Anaesth Soc J 21:15, 1974

124. Bland JW, et al: Anesthetic technique using profound hypothermia for correction of congenital heart defects in infants and small children. South Med J 69:831, 1976

125. Johnston AE, et al: Acid-base and electrolyte

changes in infants undergoing profound hypothermia for surgical correction of congenital heart defects. Can Anaesth Soc J 21:23, 1974

126. Ellis RJ, et al: Metabolic alterations with profound hypothermia: Arch Surg 109:659, 1974

127. Harris, EA: Metabolic aspects of profound hypothermia. *In* Barratt-Boyes BG, Neutze JM, Harris EA: Heart Disease in Infancy—Diagnosis and Surgical Treatment. Edinburgh, Churchill Livingston, 1973, p 65

128. Pacifico AD, Bargeron LM, Kirklin JW: Primary total correction of tetralogy of Fallot in children less than four years of age: Circulation 48:1085, 1973

129. Venugopal P, Subramanian S: Intracardiac repair of tetralogy of Fallot in patients under 5 years of age. Ann Thorac Surg 18:228, 1974

130. Volkert WA, Musacchia XJ: Hypothermia induction and survival in hamsters: The role of temperature acclimation and an anesthetic (halothane) Cryobiology 13:361, 1976

131. Heymann MA: The ductus arteriosus. *In* Moss AJ, Adams FH, Emmanouilides GC (eds): Heart Disease in Infants, Children and Adolescents. Baltimore, Williams & Wilkins, 1977, p 168

132. Clarkson PM, Orgill AA: Continuous murmurs in infants of low birth weight. J Pediatr 84:208, 1974

133. Rudolph AM: Congenital Diseases of the Heart. Chicago, Year Book Medical Publishers, 1974, p 176

134. Neal WA, et al: Patent ductus arteriosus complicating respiratory distress syndrome. J Pediatr 86:127, 1975

135. Thibeault DW, et al: Patent ductus arteriosus complicating the respiratory distress syndrome in preterm infants. J Pediatr 86:120, 1975

136. Edmund LH, et al: Surgical closure of the ductus arteriosus in premature infants. Circulation 48:856, 1973

137. Sade RM, Castenada AR: Recent advances in cardiac surgery in the young infant. Surg Clin North Am 56:452, 1976

138. Meyer RA: Echocardiography. *In* Moss AJ, Adams FH, Emmanouilides GC (eds): Heart Disease in Infants, Children and Adolescents. Baltimore, Williams & Wilkins, 1977, p 96

139. Baylen BG, et al: Echocardiographic assessment of severity of patent ductus arteriosus with pulmonary disease. J Pediatr 86:423, 1975

140. Dglivoria-Papadopoulos M, Roncevic NP, Oski FA: Postnatal changes in oxygen transport of term, premature, and sick infants; the role of red cell 2, 3-diphosphoglycerate and adult hemoglobin. Pediatr Res 5:235, 1971

141. Heymann MA, Rudolph AM, Silverman NH: Closure of the ductus arteriosus in premature infants by inhibition of prostaglandin synthesis. N Engl J Med 295:530, 1976

142. Friedman WF, et al: Pharmacologic closure of patent ductus arteriosus in the premature infant. N Engl J Med 295:526, 1976

143. Nadas AS: Patent ductus revisited (Editorial). N Engl J Med 295:563, 1976

144. Davidson M: Neonatal necrotizing enterocolitis. *In* Rudolph AM (ed): Pediatrics. New York, Appleton-Century-Crofts, 1977, p 992

145. Hakanson DO, Oh W: Necrotizing enterocolitis and hyperviscosity in the newborn infant. J Pediatr 90:458, 1977

146. Betts EK, Downes JJ, Schaeffer DB, et al: Retrolental fibroplasia and oxygen administration during general anesthesia. Anesthesiology 47:518, 1977

147. Orzalesi MM, Mendicini M, Bucci G, et al: Arterial oxygen studies in premature newborns with and without mild respiratory disorders. Arch Dis Child 42:174, 1967

148. Kirklin JW, Devloo RA: Hypothermic perfusion and circulatory arrest for surgical correction of tetralogy of Fallot with previously constructed Pott's anastomosis. Dis Chest 39:87, 1961

149. Shumacker HB Jr, King H, Nahrwald DL, et al: Coarctation of the aorta. Curr Prob Surg, February, 1968

150. Tikoff G, Keith TB, Nelson RM: Clinical and hemodynamic observations after surgical closure of large ASDs complicated by heart failure. Am J Cardiol 23:810, 1969

151. Kloster FE, Bristow JD, Griswold HE: Problems in mitral and multiple valve replacement. Prog Cardiovasc Dis 7:504, 1965

152. Dorney ER: Endocarditis. *In* Hurst JW (ed): The Heart. New York, McGraw-Hill, 1978, p 1497

153. Blumenthal S: Infective endocarditis. *In* Moss AJ, Adams FH, Emmanouilides GC (eds): Heart Disease in Infants, Children, and Adolescents. Baltimore, Williams & Wilkins, 1977, p 551

154. Johnson DH, Rosenthal A, Nadas A: A forty-year review of bacterial endocarditis in infancy and childhood. Circulation 51:581, 1975

155. Weinstein L, Schlesinger JJ: Pathoanatomic, pathophysiologic and clinical correlation in endocarditis. N Engl J Med: 291:832, 1122, 1974

156. Durack D: Current practice in prevention of bacterial endocarditis. Br Heart J 37:478, 1975

157. Everett ED, Hirschman JV: Transient bacteremia and endocarditis prophylaxis: A review. Medicine 56:61, 1977

158. Sipes JN, Thompson RL, Hook EW: Prophy-

laxis of infective endocarditis: A re-evaluation. Annu Rev Med 28:371, 1977

159. American Heart Association Committee on Rheumatic Fever and Bacterial Endocarditis: Prevention of endocarditis. Circulation 56:139A, 1977

160. Lees MH: Diseases of the Cardiovascular system. *In* Behrman RE, Neonatology. Diseases of the Fetus and Infant. St. Louis, Mosby, 1973, p 339

161. Nadas AS, Fyler DC: Pediatric Cardiology. Philadelphia, WB Saunders, 1972, p 670

James R. Zaidan, M.D.

9
PACEMAKERS

In the United States today, over 150,000 people have implanted pacemakers. With the projected United States population growth, one can expect 250,000 people to have implanted pacemakers by 1990.[1] It is no wonder that patients with pacemakers are appearing not only for battery replacement but also for surgery unrelated to their pacemaker. For this reason, anesthesiologists must begin learning more about heart block and pacemakers.

ANATOMY OF THE CONDUCTION SYSTEM

The sinoatrial node is found at the junction of the superior vena cava and the right atrium at the lateral aspect. In the sinus node are found two types of cells, P cells and transitional cells.[2,3] The P cells, which are believed to be the initiator of impulse formation, are found in clusters within the node and are joined to each other and to the second cell type, the transitional cell. These transitional cells join to each other and also to cells that form the atrial conduction system. The impulse initiated in the sinus node travels through definite atrial pathways to the atrioventricular node located in the inferior interatrial septum[4,5] (Fig. 9-1). The atrioventricular node also contains P cells and transitional cells, with the latter predominating. These transitional cells have associations with each other and with P cells, internodal pathway cells, and the Purkinje cells of the bundle of His; their importance is obvious since they seem to connect the P cells to the remainder of the heart.[6] Extending from the atrioventricular node is the bundle of His, which divides into the right bundle branch and the left bundle branch. Anatomic studies reveal no further subdivisions in the left bundle branch,[7] but ECG analysis divides the left bundle into an anterior and a posterior division.[8]

The sinus node artery arises from the right coronary artery 55 percent of the time and from the circumflex 45 percent of the time. The atrioventricular node derives its blood supply from the right coronary artery in 90 percent of cases and from the circumflex in the remaining 10 percent.

TYPES OF CONDUCTION BLOCK

Two types of conduction system block are possible: sinoatrial and atrioventricular. In sinoatrial block the block occurs at the sinus node. Since atrial excitation is not initiated, P waves are not found on the ECG. The next beat

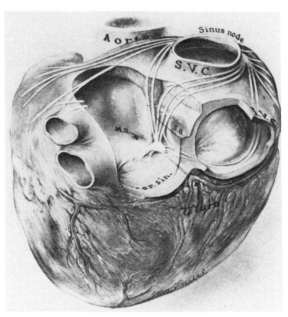

Fig. 9-1. This figure shows definite atrial pathways for impulse conduction. (From James TN: The connecting pathways between the sinus node and AV node and between the right and the left atrium in the human heart. Am Heart J 66:498–508, 1963. Reproduced with permission of publisher and author.)

can be a normal sinus beat, a nodal escape beat, or a ventricular escape beat.

The second type of block is atrioventricular block, which is found in varying degrees of severity. First-degree atrioventricular block is often found in normal hearts but is also associated with coronary artery disease. It is characterized by a P-R interval that is longer than the normal 0.12 to 0.20 seconds. All atrial impulses progress through the atrioventricular node to the Purkinje system.

Second-degree block is associated with the conduction of some, but not all, of the atrial impulses through the atrioventricular node and into the Purkinje system. It is further subdivided into two specific types. Mobitz type I, or Wenckebach block, is characterized by a progressively lengthening P-R interval until an impulse is not conducted and a beat is dropped. This sequence is repetitive. In Mobitz type II second-degree block the regularly occurring - P-R interval prolongation does not occur. The P-R interval is fixed, and the atrial excitation simply is not conducted into the Purkinje system on a regular basis.

Third-degree atrioventricular block, also called complete heart block, occurs when all electrical activity from the atria fails to progress into the Purkinje system. The atrial and ventricular contractions have no relationship with each other, although each can contract regularly. The ventricular rate will be approximately 40 beats per minute. The block can occur in several locations along the conduction system. When the block is in the atrioventricular node, the resulting QRS complex can have a normal appearance if the pacemaker is high in the bundle of His. The block might develop in the bundle of His, at which time the pacemaker will be more distal in the Purkinje system, usually resulting in a widened QRS complex with a slow rate. A complete block can develop even more distally if the right bundle branch and both the anterior superior division and the posterior inferior division of the left bundle branch are blocked. Several ECG changes show blockage of two of the three subdivisions of the bundle of His, indicating that complete blockage might eventually develop.

These ECG changes are as follows:[8–10]

1.   Complete right bundle branch block plus left

axis deviation, which indicates that the right bundle branch and the anterior-superior division of the left bundle branch have been blocked.

2. Complete right bundle branch block plus right axis deviation indicative of blocks in the right bundle branch and in the posterior-inferior division of the left bundle branch.
3. Complete right or left bundle branch block plus first-degree block.
4. Alternating bilateral bundle branch block.
5. Complete left bundle branch block.

The significance of these ECG changes in relation to anesthesia is discussed below.

A common cause of third-degree atrioventricular block is coronary artery disease. Other causes are rheumatic heart disease, congenital block, and cardiomyopathy.[10] The most common causes of complete block in the absence of coronary artery disease are Lev's syndrome[11] secondary to fibrosis and calcification of the cardiac skeleton in the older age groups and Lenegre's disease,[12] a disease of unknown etiology found in younger age groups.

PERMANENT PACEMAKER INDICATIONS

The indications for a permanent pacemaker are given in Table 9-1. Complete heart block is the failure of the electrical activity to progress through the atrioventricular node into the bundle of His. If an impulse is not initiated immediately in the bundle of His or lower in the conduction system, arrest occurs for a brief period, and symptoms such as light-headedness, dizziness, or loss of consciousness, sometimes accompanied by convulsions, occur.[10] About 25 percent of these patients will remain in sinus rhythm between these Stokes-Adams attacks. Despite the sinus rhythm, pacemaker implantation is indicated.

Table 9-1

Indications for a
Permanent Pacemaker

  I. Complete heart block
    A. Acquired
    B. Congenital
 II. Sick sinus syndrome
III. Bradycardia with symptoms

The block can also occur below the atrioventricular node. If the block is trifascicular, then third-degree, or complete heart block exists. The ECG changes associated with eventual development of complete block are listed above. If any of these changes are seen on the ECG and the patient is symptomatic, a pacemaker is indicated.

Congenital block is another indication for a permanent pacemaker. Usually, the heart rate is around 50 per minute, since the impulse arises in the bundle of His, and the QRS complex is narrow with a normal appearance. Only 10 percent of these patients will suffer from syncopal episodes, but they are predisposed to sudden death.[13]

Sick sinus syndrome is the second indication for pacemaker insertion and is characterized by the following:[9]

1. Bradycardia, episodic in nature
2. Episodes of sinus arrest for variable periods not related to drug therapy
3. Atrial fibrillation or atrial flutter alternating with sinus bradycardia
4. Slow return to sinus rhythm after cardioversion

Fast rates are treated with drug therapy, and slow rates are treated with pacing.

Another permanent pacemaker indication is bradycardia, specifically sinus bradycardia, sinoatrial block, and atrial fibrillation or flutter with a very slow ventricular response.[13] If an older patient has a heart rate of 45–50, maintains his pressure, and has no symptoms, then pacemaker insertion probably is not indicated. A slow heart rate with syncope or with ventricular extrasystoles is an indication for pacemaker implantation, however.

TEMPORARY PACEMAKER INDICATIONS

The indications for a temporary pacemaker are listed in Table 9-2. In one study of 276 patients, it was found that 5 percent of patients with an anterior myocardial infarction and 27 percent of patients with a posterior myocardial infarction developed complete heart block.[14] In a review of studies, it was shown that if complete heart block develops during an acute myocardial infarction, then the overall mortality is 58 percent, with a range of 22 to 100 percent.[15]

Table 9-2

Indications for a Temporary
Pacemaker

  I. Heart block associated with acute myo-
     cardial infarction
 II. Conversion of atrial tachyarrhythmias
III. Drug toxicity with slow ventricular rates
 IV. Anesthesia
     A. Emergency surgery
     B. Permanent pacemaker implantation
     C. Bifascicular block-major vascular
        surgery

Of these patients with complete block, 65 to 75
percent have an associated diaphragmatic infarction.[16] During a diaphragmatic infarction,
the pacemaker of the heart is usually high, probably in the bundle of His, resulting in a normal-
appearing QRS complex, with a heart rate high
enough to maintain cardiac output. It has been
shown that if a complete block occurs during
diaphragmatic infarction without other complications, then pacing probably is not necessary.[13]
If other complications such as pulmonary edema
occur along with the block, then, even though
it should be instituted, pacing probably will not
increase survival rate.

An anterior myocardial infarction can involve the ventricular conduction system because it is supplied by the anterior descending
artery. When a complete block appears, it is
sudden in nature and is not always preceded by
second-degree block. Also, the subsequent pacemaker is distal in the Purkinje system and results
in very low heart rates with very wide QRS
complexes. Pacing appears not to increase survival in patients with anterior myocardial infarctions who develop complete block.[13]

As outlined by Furman,[9] temporary pacing
is indicated during an acute myocardial infarction for drug-resistant tachyarrhythmias, for
drug-resistant bradyarrhythmias, for bifascicular block of acute onset, or for Mobitz type II
or complete block during anterior myocardial
infarction. Pacing is not indicated for Wenckebach block or complete block during a diaphragmatic myocardial infarction if the heart rate is
greater than 50 and if ventricular escape beats
do not develop.

It is known that an appropriately timed single atrial electrical stimulus can break episodes

of supraventricular tachycardia caused by a
reentry mechanism.[17] The exact moment at
which this stimulus must be applied to terminate
the tachycardia is variable; therefore, a stimulus
with a frequency of 100 to 1000 stimuli per second is applied for a duration of 50 to 250 msec.
This type of stimulus is not used in the ventricle,
but only in the atrium. Permanent pacemakers
are available for the termination of atrial tachyarrhythmias, but they are rare.

Another possible temporary pacemaker indication is for the treatment of drug toxicity
associated with very slow ventricular rates.

The question of whether to insert a temporary pacemaker specifically for anesthesia is
difficult to answer. If a patient presents for
emergency surgery, cardiac or otherwise, and is
at that time experiencing an acute myocardial
infarction with secondary block or experiencing
digitalis toxicity with very slow ventricular rates,
then a pacemaker probably is indicated. Certainly, a patient in complete block who must
have a permanent pacemaker implanted should
have a temporary transvenous pacemaker before the anesthetic induction.

A question arises concerning pacemaker insertion for patients undergoing surgery if they
have evidence of bifascicular block on the ECG.
Berg and Kotler found that in patients without
a history of syncope, temporary pacemaker insertion is not indicated.[18] Rooney and associates
verify this opinion.[19] If major vascular surgery
is planned, however, and the development of
hypotension, rapid fluid shifts, electrolyte disturbance or acid-base imbalance is a possibility,
then a temporary transvenous pacemaker should
be seriously considered.

TYPES OF PACEMAKERS

The most commonly used pacemakers are
discussed below.[20] To eliminate confusion, the
terms "demand" and "standby" are not used
because they do not indicate the job performed
by the pacemaker.

Asynchronous Pacemakers

Asynchronous pacemakers discharge at a
preset rate that is independent of the inherent
cardiac electrical activity. It can be atrial or
ventricular. If normal sinus rhythm or ventri-

cular systoles reappear, then competition should be expected.[21] Ventricular fibrillation is a potential complication if the pacemaker impulse occurs in the vulnerable period of ventricular repolarization, but ventricular fibrillation appears to be uncommon unless electrolyte imbalance or myocardial ischemia occur.[22] The asynchronous ventricular pacemaker is useful in the presence of complete block that is continuous in nature, so that competition with sinus rhythm does not occur. Atrial asynchronous pacemakers are useless if atrioventricular block is present but are used during bradycardia with normal atrioventricular conduction.

Synchronous Pacemakers

There are three types of synchronous pacemakers: ventricular triggered, ventricular inhibited, and atrial. *Ventricular-triggered* pacemakers sense the QRS complex and then discharge into the absolute refractory period, therefore not triggering another contraction. If normal electrical activity does not occur, the pacer will fire at a preset rate to trigger the contraction. This type of pacer has a refractory period of 0.4 seconds, so that if a premature beat occurs, the pacemaker will not fire in the vulnerable period of the premature beat.[22]

The *ventricular-inhibited* pacemaker is suppressed by the normal electrical activity of the heart. A normal QRS complex prevents a pacing spike from occurring. In addition, it is possible that both P waves and T waves can suppress this type of pacer. Ventricular-triggered and ventricular-inhibited pacemakers are useful in

the patient with complete block who occasionally returns to sinus rhythm. When sinus rhythm is present, these pacemakers do not compete. They can be converted to ventricular asynchronous by application of a magnet.

The *atrial* pacemaker functions in the following way. Through a double electrode system the P wave is sensed, and then, after a prolonged refractory period that can be set, the ventricle is stimulated to contract. If a rapid atrial rate occurs, a rapid ventricular rate is prevented by the long refractory period. The highest ventricular rate allowed is about 140. When the P wave is not sensed, the pacemaker converts to the ventricular asynchronous mode.

Sequential Pacemakers

In sequential pacing, the atria are stimulated to contract first; then, after an adjustable refractory period corresponding to the P-R interval, the ventricle is stimulated to contract (Fig. 9-2). Similar to this and more sophisticated is the atrial sequential ventricular-inhibited pacer. During a normal sinus conduction in this system, the pacemaker will be in a standby mode. If the P wave is not sensed, the atrium is stimulated to contract. Following this event, the electrical activity might be conducted normally. If so, the pacemaker remains in the standby mode during ventricular contraction. If the P wave is not conducted normally, the ventricle is stimulated to contract. This type of pacemaker is converted to a ventricular asynchronous mode by application of a magnet.

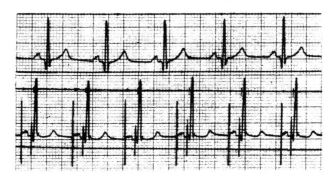

Fig. 9-2. Top tracing shows normal sinus rhythm with a P-R interval of 0.15 seconds. Bottom tracing shows AV sequential pacing in the same patient at a more rapid rate but with the same P-R interval.

BENEFITS OF PACING

To understand the benefits of pacing, one must understand the pathophysiology of complete heart block.[23] Cardiac output depends on preload (the volume of blood in the ventricle at the end of diastole), afterload (the resistance against which the ventricle must move the preload), contractility, and heart rate. Atrial contraction may contribute 15 to 25 percent of the preload to the ventricle; therefore, if the atrial and ventricular contractions are not properly timed, preload decreases, causing a secondary decrease in stroke volume. When stroke volume decreases and heart rate does not increase substantially, cardiac output decreases. Asynchronously contracting atria and ventricles are found in complete heart block. Occasionally, the atrial contraction will accidently occur at the appropriate time in the cardiac cycle and increase the preload, but this situation is the exception (Fig. 9-3).

As heart rate decreases, the stroke volume can increase to maintain a relatively normal cardiac output if the ventricle is normal; but a limit to this compensating mechanism exists, and as the heart rate approaches 40 per minute, cardiac output decreases. This decrease in cardiac output in turn causes several changes to occur. As flow decreases, the arteriovenous oxygen difference increases. During the period of decreased flow, the coronary arteries do not fill appropriately, and the O_2 supply to the myocardium cannot meet the O_2 demand. The myocardial contractility decreases, and pulmonary artery and wedge pressures increase, resulting in pulmonary edema with a further reduction in arterial oxygenation. Renal and cerebral circulations are compromised as well, resulting in decreased urine output and fluid retention, plus CNS symptoms such as light-headedness, dizziness, or even coma.

The answer to the problem is pacing. The pacing can be atrial if atrioventricular block is absent and the ECG shows bradycardia. If atrioventricular block is present, then ventricular or sequential pacing is indicated.

As outlined by Segel and Samet, cardiac output is maintained once the heart rate approaches normal values.[23] A further increase in heart rate above 90 beats per minute will result in a progressive decrease in stroke volume so

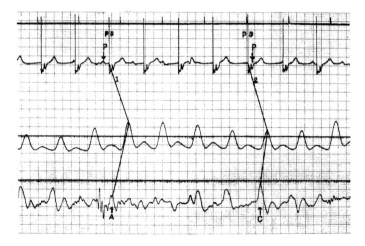

Fig. 9-3. *Line 1:* P-R interval is normal (accidentally). Following line 1, notice that the systolic pressure is the highest point and that the height of the a wave is negligible compared to the mean CVP. *Line 2:* The P wave is in the ventricular complex. With loss of normal timing of atrial contraction, the systolic pressure is the lowest point above the mean and cannon waves appearing on the CVP. P = P wave; A = a wave; C = cannon waves; PS = pacing spike. Notice that the P wave is moving through the ventricular complex. The ventricle is being paced asynchronously. This tracing is also an example of asynchronous pacing. (Frazier, Wesley, personal communication reproduced with permission)

that cardiac output is fairly constant. If metabolic requirements increase, then the stroke volume also increases to meet these metabolic demands. Therefore, atrial pacing during bradycardia will increase the cardiac output, but further increases in the heart rate above normal values probably will not result in a greater increase in cardiac output.

Hartzler et al. have shown in a series of 10 patients that atrial pacing increased cardiac output 26 percent over the cardiac output during ventricular pacing, and atrioventricular sequential pacing increased cardiac output 34 percent over the cardiac output during ventricular pacing.[24] It is interesting that in 8 patients with normally occurring atrioventricular conduction, sequential pacing and shortening of the P-R interval resulted in a cardiac output that was 18 percent higher than with atrial pacing and 50 percent higher than with ventricular pacing. The P-R interval in this study ranged from 50 to 250 msec.

Yoshida et al. have shown that coronary artery blood flow increases and coronary artery resistance decreases during atrial pacing not only in patients without coronary artery disease but also in patients with coronary artery disease paced up to the angina threshold.[25] The paced patients with coronary artery disease who developed angina had only a negligible increase in flow and no decrease in resistance.

ANESTHETIC CONSIDERATIONS

It is important to understand that in regard to anesthesia, the presence of the pacemaker usually is not the problem. The problem is the presence of some disease process that necessitates the pacemaker, most commonly coronary artery disease. Other commonly associated diseases are diabetes mellitus and hypertension,[9] but, of course, any other disease process may exist.

Evaluating the Pacemaker

It is helpful to know the following information about the pacemaker. Is it synchronous or asynchronous? When was it implanted, and what was the rate at that time? It is known that mercury-zinc pacemakers have a life span of 18 to 36 months, and one must be suspicious of a

pacemaker of this age.[26] Lithium-powered pacemakers, in contrast, have never been changed because of power failure. In a study by Luceri et al., it was shown that pacemaker patients could be divided into four groups according to threshold changes.[27]

1. Forty-three percent of patients will have a 0.7 percent increase in pacemaker threshold per year.
2. Seventeen percent will have a 5 percent decrease in threshold.
3. Twenty-one percent will have a variable threshold that, on the average, increases about 1.9 percent annually.
4. Nineteen percent of patients will have a 14 percent increase in pacemaker threshold annually.

One can see then that 80 percent of patients will have essentially stable thresholds, while 20 percent will have a very large increase in pacemaker threshold annually. It is this last group that is potentially difficult to manage during anesthesia because of possible anesthetic drug effects on the pacemaker threshold.

Rate of discharge is the most important indicator of power source dysfunction. The rate can become either rapid, with rates up to 300,[28] or slow, with rates below physiological levels.[26] Simon has suggested that the rate of the pacemaker should be within 2 beats per minute from the initial rate and that a 10 percent rate reduction is a sign of power failure.[10] History is important in determining the ability of the pacemaker to capture the ventricle. Symptoms of dizziness, light-headedness, and fainting will return if the pacer no longer stimulates the ventricle. Palpitations might show that inadequate sensing and competitive rhythms exist in the previously normally functioning synchronous pacemaker.[29]

To evaluate the ability of the ventricular-triggered or ventricular-inhibited pacemaker to capture the ventricle, one must slow the intrinsic heart rate to a rate below that of the pacemaker. This is done with carotid massage, or, if this is contraindicated, by a Valsalva maneuver. If the rate does not slow enough for the pacemaker to take over the ventricle, a magnet can be applied over the pacemaker to convert it to the asynchronous mode, and captured beats can be observed by watching the ECG and palpating the pulse. A pacing spike in the vulnerable period should not cause ventricular fibrillation in the absence of myocardial ischemia or electrolyte imbalance. To cause ventricular fibrillation a stimulus of about 30 milliamperes is needed, but the pacing spike is only a fraction of this stimulus.[21] If a question concerning the pacemaker function exists, then pacemaker pulse width and waveform can be evaluated by special testing.

Drug–Pacemaker Interactions

An area of great concern to the anesthesiologist is the ability of drugs to change the facility with which the pacemaker can stimulate the ventricle to contract. If it becomes more difficult for the pacemaker to stimulate the myocardium, then the pacemaker threshold is increased. If it becomes less difficult for the pacemaker to initiate a contraction, then the pacemaker threshold is decreased.

Potassium. From the Nernst equation

$$emf = -62 \log \frac{K_I(\text{inside the cell})}{K_O(\text{outside the cell})}$$

one can calculate the normal resting membrane potential (RMP) to be -90 if $K_I = 150$ and $K_O = 5$. If the potassium concentration outside the cell becomes larger, then resting membrane potential becomes less negative. As the RMP approaches the cell's threshold potential, it becomes easier for the pacemaker to stimulate the ventricle. In other words, the pacemaker threshold is decreased. Clinically, when can this occur? If a patient is total body depleted of potassium from chronic diuretic therapy, the K_I/K_O ratio might be maintained even though the absolute values are decreased. When potassium is given acutely and the potassium outside the cell increases, the ratio decreases, and the ventricle can be stimulated to fibrillation by the pacemaker stimulus acting on the highly excitable myocardium. With time, however, some of the potassium outside the cells enters the cells, and the ratio is restored, as is the resting membrane potential. The likelihood for ventricular fibrillation then decreases. One can see, therefore, that potassium replacement therapy should be accomplished slowly over a period of several hours if possible so that the serum potassium does not increase abruptly. One method of fa-

cilitating potassium entrance into the cells is to administer glucose and insulin.

Steroids. Mineralocorticoids have been shown to increase the threshold by 25 percent, while glucocorticoids are known to decrease the pacemaker threshold by 25 percent.[21,30] Hydrocortisone has a combined action of a glucocorticoid and a mineralocorticoid but has no significant effect on the pacemaker threshold.

Sympathomimetics. In general, sympathomimetic drugs cause an increase in membrane excitability and therefore decrease the pacemaker threshold. This effect is blocked by propranolol. In higher doses, these drugs increase the pacemaker threshold.[22,30]

Antiarrhythmics. Quinidine, procainamide, and lidocaine have no effect on the pacemaker threshold at therapeutic levels.[30]

Succinylcholine. Because of the possibility of arrest, intermittent doses of succinylcholine might be contraindicated; however, this technique has been used successfully.[31] Redd et al. have also reported that isometric contractions of muscle groups near the implanted pacemaker generator may inhibit the otherwise normally functioning pacemaker.[32] Only the unipolar pacemakers were affected. This response might be important during succinylcholine fasciculations in pectoralis or abdominal muscles. Defasciculation with a nondepolarizing relaxant prior to the administration of succinylcholine is suggested.

Halothane and enflurane. Atlee has shown that atrioventricular conduction is slowed in response to halothane, especially between the atria and the bundle of His, but also from the bundle of His to the Purkinje system at higher MAC levels.[33] Enflurane prolongs the conduction through the atrioventricular node.[34] There are no studies to show the effects of these inhalational anesthetics on the pacemaker threshold. At present, these agents are not contraindicated in the pacemaker patient and have been used safely.

Thiopental. Thiopental (Pentothal) causes hyperpolarization of the membrane, which in turn could cause an increase in the pacemaker threshold. This problem is not obvious clinically, however, and thiopental has been used with good success.

Ketamine. To date, there are no studies to show the effect of ketamine on the pacemaker threshold. This drug has been used successfully in low doses to provide analgesia for pacemaker insertion.

Anesthetic Management

The immediate preoperative evaluation should include at least the following:

1. History and physical: Look for unrelated disease processes. Watch also for signs of congestive failure in the patient with coronary disease. Ask about return of prepacemaker symptoms or palpitations.
2. Determine allergies.
3. Evaluate the airway.
4. List the medications. Expect to see antiarrhythmics, antihypertensives, anticoagulants, diuretics, digoxin, and β-blocking drugs.
5. Evaluate the laboratory data. Check specifically the electrolytes for potassium balance, the ECG for correct pacing, and the chest x-ray for pacing wire placement and integrity.
6. Determine the functioning of the pacemaker as outlined above.
7. Have the magnet supplied with the synchronous pacers sent to the operating room with the patient. If it is to be placed in the operative field, the magnet can be gas sterilized. Movement of the magnet over the pacemaker can turn off the pacemaker; therefore, once the magnet is in place, do not move it except to completely remove it from the pacemaker site.

Intraoperative Management

Inhalational anesthesia, balanced technique, and neuroleptanesthesia have all been used successfully in the patient with a pacemaker; therefore, the choice of an anesthetic agent can be made in relation to other diseases and not necessarily to the pacemaker. Personal preference enters into the decision also. Presently, there are no studies to indicate the effect of anesthetic agents on the pacemaker threshold. Consider spinals if the patient is not on anticoagulants, or blocks for surgery on the extremities. Several reasonable methods for general anesthesia are suggested below:

1. Induction with incremental doses of thiopental and maintenance with an inhalational anesthetic
2. Neuroleptanesthesia technique
3. Narcotic-relaxant technique

At Emory Hospital, a thiopental induction with enflurane maintenance is being used with excellent success. Succinylcholine (1 mg/kg) after defasciculation with a competitive blocker is a reasonable technique for intubation.

Intraoperative Monitoring

1. ECG—The ECG must be monitored to follow the possibility of developing acute myocardial ischemia or pacemaker failure during anesthesia. The T wave can be followed to help in the management of potassium balance. Consider using not only the standard limb leads but also a V_5 lead, where most ischemic changes are found during anesthesia.
2. Fluids—Consider a Foley catheter and a central venous pressure line to help in the fluid management of these patients.
3. Electrolytes—Serum potassium must be kept within the normal range so that acute changes in pacemaker thresholds do not occur. Serial determinations of serum electrolytes are easily accomplished in the operating room.
4. Arterial blood gases—These should be determined frequently to be sure that the patient is well oxygenated, well ventilated, and has normal acid–base status. The presence of acidosis, either from metabolic or from respiratory causes, will result in a corresponding increase in extracellular potassium and a decrease in intracellular potassium. As the K_I/K_O ratio falls, the resting membrane potential becomes less negative, implying a more irritable myocardium with the possibility of ventricular fibrillation. The opposite occurs when alkalosis is present.

As the K_I/K_O ratio increases, the resting membrane potential becomes more negative, therefore making it more difficult for the pacemaker to stimulate the myocardium to contract—an increased pacemaker threshold. Myocardial hypoxia secondary to decreased perfusion from coronary artery disease causes localized metabolic acidosis within the myocardium with the associated changes mentioned above.

5. Temperature—Temperature monitoring is advisable because a cold patient increases the oxygen consumption. It is possible that a patient with coronary artery disease who becomes cold will not be able to supply adequate oxygen to the myocardium to meet the demand. Ischemia develops, as does irritability and the possibility of fibrillation if the pacemaker impulse falls on the vulnerable period of the T wave.

6. Electrocautery—Bipolar indicates that two electrodes are placed directly on the myocardium, while unipolar indicates one electrode on the myocardium and the second electrode distant from the heart. With continuous use of the electrocautery, synchronous unipolar pacemakers will convert to the asynchronous mode and continue pacing. Intermittent use of the electrocautery, however, will cause this type of pacemaker to become inhibited. It was recently reported that a ventricular demand pacemaker was inhibited by the use of a cutting current but not with the use of a coagulation current during a transurethral resection of the prostate.[35] Asynchronous pacemakers should be unaffected. Despite sophisticated monitoring, the best monitor available to determine if inhibition is taking place is a hand on a pulse. The surgeon must be reminded constantly of this problem. Simon suggests that the return plate for the electrocautery be placed far away from the pacemaker and that the use of the electrocautery be limited to 1-second bursts every 10 seconds.[10] One method of preventing inhibition is to apply the magnet to the pacemaker so that it is converted to the asynchronous mode.

Intraoperative Failure of Pacemaker Capturing

If the pacemaker suddenly stops capturing the stimulated chamber during the anesthetic, the following possible causes should be considered:

1. Drug effects—Evaluate what drugs have been given and determine the possible effects of those drugs on the pacemaker threshold. Consider reducing the inspired concentration of the inhalational anesthetics and increasing the F_IO_2.

2. Acid–base balance—Arterial blood gases are necessary to ensure normal pH balance. Adjust the pH appropriately by adequate ventilation and bicarbonate administration.

3. Potassium balance—If the change in potassium is related to the pH change, adjust the pH first and reevaluate the serum potassium in a few minutes. With hyperkalemia in the presence of the normal pH, consider glucose (25 gm) plus insulin (10 units regular I.V. push). Hypokalemia is treated with the slow administration of KCl at approximately 10 mEq over 1 hour given through a central I.V., provided that renal function is adequate.

4. Generator failure—If the pacemaker has been properly evaluated preoperatively, the chances are that generator failure will not occur. If this remote possibility does occur, then proceed with a replacement. If a question exists concerning generator failure versus anesthetic drug effects, wake the patient as quickly as possible and reevaluate the pacemaker.

5. Broken lead—This can be determined by a chest x-ray and should be replaced (Fig. 9-4). Carefully watch a lead that is close to the surgical field, as that lead might be damaged.

6. Displaced lead—If the pacemaker begins capturing intermittently and has a varying amplitude on the pacing spike, consider the possibility of a displaced lead. Also, if the pacing is intermittent and the diaphragm is being stimulated, the myocardium may have been perforated.

7. If pacing stops during anesthesia and cannot be corrected quickly by one of the above measures, consider an isoproterenol infusion starting at 1–3 μg/min. This infusion can be mixed conveniently by adding 1 mg of isoproterenol to 250 ml of 5 percent dextrose in water. Isoproterenol decreases pacemaker threshold in lower dosages and also

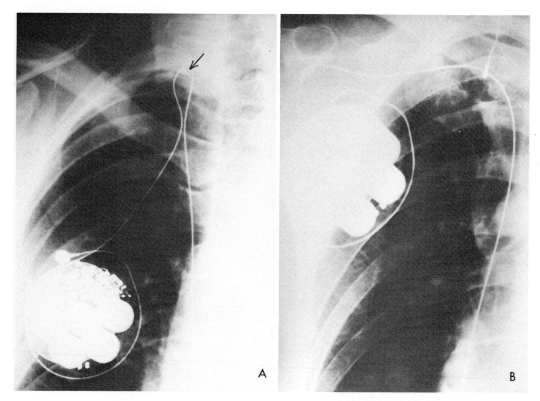

Fig. 9-4. (A) The arrow points out the break in the pacemaker lead wire. (B) Same patient after lead and pacemaker replacement. (From Mansour, K: Complications of cardiac pacemakers. Am Surg 43:132, 1977. Reproduced with permission of publisher and author.)

provides a positive chronotropic and inotropic action on the ventricle.

Postoperative Period

Continue the intraoperative monitoring until the patient is awake and stable. A 12-lead ECG with a rhythm strip should be considered immediately following surgery to ensure continued pacing.

Anesthesia for Pacemaker Insertion

The same precautions should be taken for anesthesia for pacemaker insertion as for any anesthetic. If a transvenous pacemaker is to be placed into the right ventricular endocardium, then local anesthesia is useful. When bipolar lead placement to the epicardium is planned through the transthoracic approach, general anesthesia is necessary, and once again various anesthetics are useful. At Emory, the transxiphoid approach is commonly used and can be accomplished with either general or local anesthesia.[36]

A transvenous temporary pacemaker is necessary if a complete block or severe bradycardia is present before induction of anesthesia. When the patient is in sinus rhythm at the time of induction, a temporary pacer probably is not necessary. The sudden development of a complete block after induction is treated with isoproterenol. For convenience, consider using an infusion pump.

The external temporary transvenous pacemaker gives a direct connection from external electrical sources to the endocardium. If this pacemaker is placed on an electrical device with a faulty ground, then ventricular fibrillation is a definite possibility. A rubber glove or gauze around the metal container will guard against

Table 9-3

Complications of Epicardial Implantation in 100 Consecutive Patients

Complications	Number
Pericarditis	3
Pneumonia, atelectasis, or both	3
Pleural effusion	1
Hemorrhage	1
Threshold increased	5
Erosion of skin	0
Infection (battery)	4
Deaths (due to acute myocardial infarction)	2
Total	19
Average stay in hospital	10 days

Source. Reprinted from Mansour K et al: Cardiac pacemakers: comparing epicardial and pervenous pacing. Geriatrics 28:151, 1973, with permission of author and publisher.

Table 9-4

Complications of Pervenous Implantation in 100 Consecutive Patients

Complications		Number
Displacement of catheter		14
Early (in 1 week or less)	10	
Late (in 1 month to 2 years)	4	
Erosion of skin		6
Infection (battery)		5
Inability to pace		7
Would not pace	4	
Failed to sense	2	
Inconsistent	1	
Threshold increased		2
Myocardial perforation		2
Ventricular fibrillation		1
Postoperative hemorrhage in neck		1
Deaths		2
Failed to capture	1	
Stimulation of diaphragm		5
Endocarditis		2
Total		47

Source. Reprinted from Mansour K et al: Cardiac pacemakers: Comparing epicardial and pervenous pacing. Geriatrics 28:151, 1973, with permission of author and publisher.

the introduction of an unwanted current into the myocardium. In the operating room, place the pacemaker by the patient's shoulder and keep all electrical devices away from this area.

After the leads have been placed and the implanted pacemaker properly positioned, the temporary pacemaker should be turned off. Keep a finger on the pulse, and if the pulse does not continue at the rate of the new pacemaker within 1 or 2 seconds, restart the temporary pacemaker.

During the process of lead insertion, ventricular arrhythmias can occur and can be treated with lidocaine (1 mg/kg I.V. push) and, if necessary, with a lidocaine infusion at 1–3 mg/min.

Mansour has reported the complications with 100 consecutive epicardial pacemakers and with 100 consecutive endocardial pacemakers. His results are outlined in Tables 9-3 and 9-4.[37]

There were no anesthesia-related deaths during his studies.

Massive bleeding necessitating cardiopulmonary bypass during epicardial lead placement has been reported.[38] Endocardial leads have been reported to cause right atrial thrombi with secondary pulmonary emboli and failure to pace,[39,40] and adhesive endocarditis.[41] Despite these rare complications, both endocardial and epicardial pacemaker electrodes are extremely safe in experienced hands.

APPENDIX

CLINICAL USE OF PACEMAKERS

The following figures show a representative sample of external pacemakers that one might encounter in clinical practice.

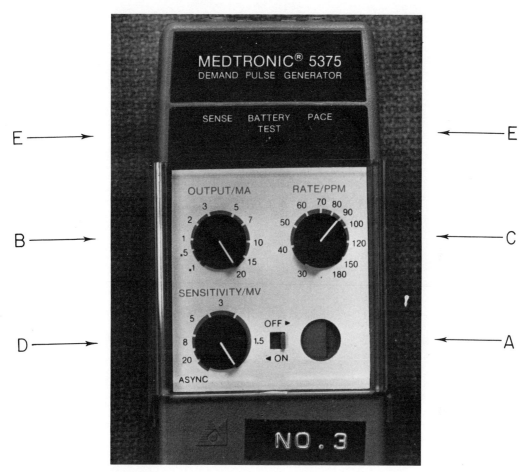

Fig. 9-5. Medtronic 5375.

A. On-off—To turn off the pacer, push down the button in the opening to the right of the switch, then move the switch to the right.
B. Output/MA—This control is the current in milliamps that the pacer can supply to the myocardium and varies between 0.1 and 20 ma.
C. Rate/PPM—This controls the number of impulses per minute.
D. Sensitivity/MV—This pacer is ventricular inhibited. The sensitivity in millivolts indicates the ease with which the pacer will be inhibited by the QRS proceeding through the conduction system. The higher the number on the sensitivity, the more difficult it is to inhibit this pacer. At a sensitivity of 20 mv it is approaching the asynchronous mode in which it is never inhibited. As an example, a sensitivity setting of 5 mv would be inhibited by a QRS of 6 mv but not by a QRS of 4 mv. If the QRS of 4 mv caused a contraction, competition with the external pacemaker would be expected.
E. Sense-Pace indicators—While pacing, the pacing light should appear and while sensing, the sensing light should appear.

The above nomenclature is used in Figures 9-6 and 9-7.

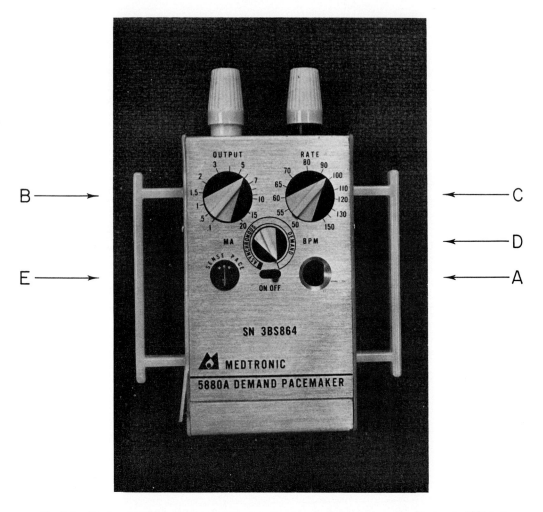

Fig. 9-6. Medtronic 5880A. This pacemaker has the same basic controls as the Medtronic 5375 just described and can be used as an asynchronous or ventricular inhibited pacemaker.

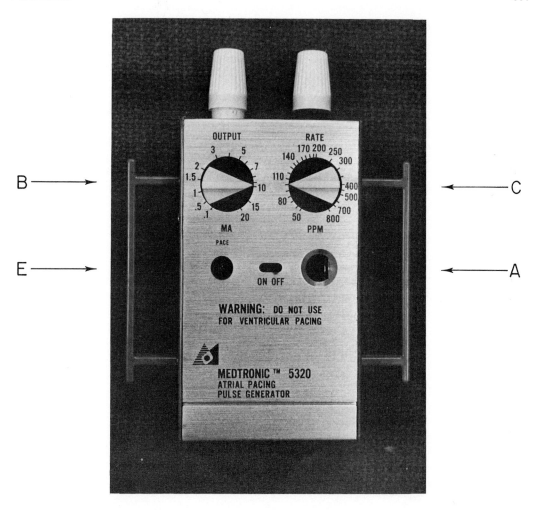

Fig. 9-7.   Medtronic 5320 Atrial Pacemaker. Since this pacemaker has no sensitivity control it functions in an asynchronous mode. The rate control allows up to 800 beats per minute and is used to convert supraventricular tachycardias to sinus rhythm. An atrial wire must be in place. Slowly increase the rate control to a point at which the atrial tachycardia is converted to NSR then turn off the pacer. Notice the warning that this pacer should not be used for ventricular pacing.

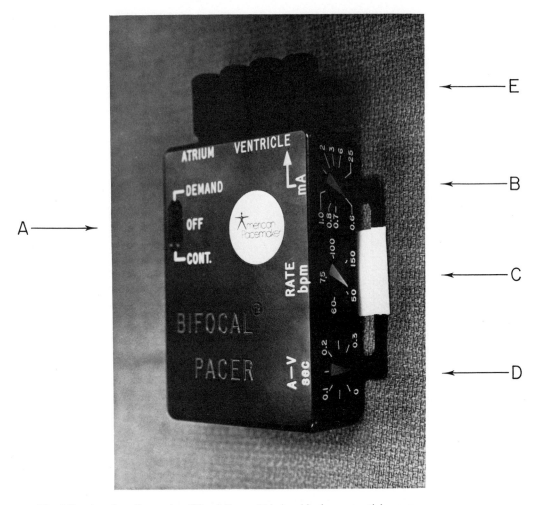

Fig. 9-8. American Pacemaker Bifocal Pacer. This is a bipolar sequential pacer.

A. On-off switch—"Demand" indicates a ventricular inhibited mode and "Cont." indicates the asynchronous mode. There is no sensitivity control.

B. MA—This controls the output of the pacer as previously described.

C. Rate-bpm—This is the heart rate control.

D. A-V-Sec—This control is unique to the sequential pacer. It indicates the time in seconds between the atrial impulse and ventricular impulse, or the PR interval. If it is in the "demand" or ventricular inhibited mode, then, after the atrium is stimulated synchronously, the pacer senses the QRS. If it is in the "cont." mode then the pacer does not sense the QRS, but simply fires into the ventricle at a continous rate.

E. Connections for myocardial leads—Notice that there are two sets, one for the atrial wires and one for the ventricular wires.

This pacemaker is used after cardiac surgery for sequential pacing and probably will not be used in other areas of anesthesia because both atrial and ventricular wires are necessary and because it is a bipolar pacer.

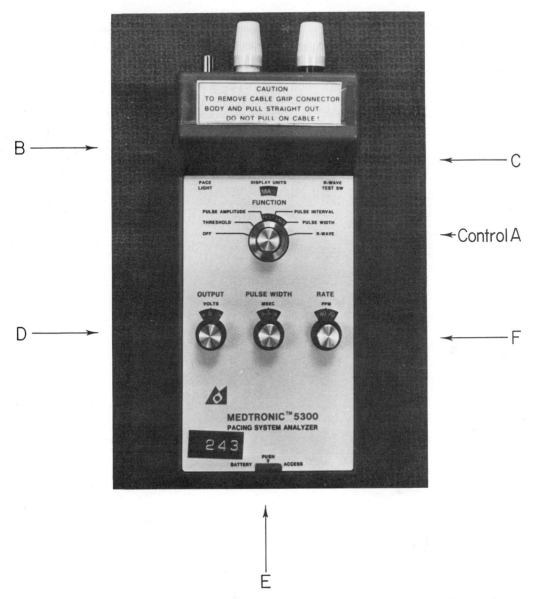

Fig. 9-9. Medtronic 5300 Pacing System Analyzer. This system analyzes the pacing wires, not the pacemaker itself, and is used just after the electrodes have been applied to the myocardium to measure the threshold and the sensitivity of the electrodes. Instructions for use:

1. With control A in the off position adjust the output to 6–7 volts, the pulse width to 0.5 msec, and the rate control to a rate approximately 10% above the resting heart rate, or if the patient is in complete block, to a physiological level.
2. Assure that the cable is connected negative to negative and positive to positive.
3. Turn control A to "Threshold." The analyzer is now acting as an asynchronous pacemaker. A digital readout will appear in the screen. This number is the number of ma necessary to capture the ventricle. Begin decreasing the voltage with the output control until the ventricle is no longer paced, then increase the voltage until pacing begins. This is the minimum number of volts necessary to pace the ventricle. Now read the number of ma in the digital readout. This is the

(*continued*)

minimum number of ma necessary to pace the ventricle. Divide voltage by ma to obtain the resistance. This is the resistance to the passage of the current from the electrode into the myocardium. A high resistance indicates that the electrode should be in a different position.

4. Now turn control A to "R-wave." The analyzer will continue to function as an asynchronous pacer. Push the button marked R-wave Test located to the right of the digital readout. When this control is pushed, the analyzer no longer paces, but begins sensing the QRS complexes proceeding through the ventricle. The number of millivolts in the QRS is found in the digital readout. Record the highest number as the QRS. A high number of mv indicates that the electrode can pick up the QRS voltage appropriately. Remember that while the button is depressed the patient is not being paced. After the electrodes are analyzed, the pacemaker is connected to the electrodes and implanted.

Controls:

A. On–off and threshold—R-wave selection
B. Digital readout
C. R-wave test button
D. Output in mv
E. Pulse width in msec
F. Rate in beats per minute

Fig. 9-10. Medtronic 5837 R-Wave Coupled. This pacer is a research instrument but is occasionally found in the cardiac anesthesia setting. A detailed description of the functional possibilities of this model is beyond the scope of this text. Instead, some of the more common uses will be presented.

1. Simple Ventricular Pacing
   a. Connect the patient cable to output 2 (13)
   b. Set stimulation output 1 (17) to 0 and stimulation output 2 (18) to the desired milliamps
   c. Set Refractory Period–Rate control (14) to desired rate by reading the bottom scale
   d. Set output switch (11) to "separate"
   e. Set function switch (1) to "paired"
   f. Readjust stimulation output 2 (18) to a level just above the threshold.
2. Sequential Pacing
   a. Connect atrial cable to output 1 (12)
   b. Set stimulation output 1 (17) and stimulation output 2 (18) to the desired milliamps
   c. Set Refractory Period–Rate control (14) to the desired rate by reading the bottom scale. Then set the desired P-R interval by adjusting the Delay interval (3)
   d. Set output switch (11) to "common"
   e. Set function switch (1) to "paired"
   f. Set sensitivity switch (2) to 10
   g. Readjust both stimulation outputs (17) and (18) to the appropriate level

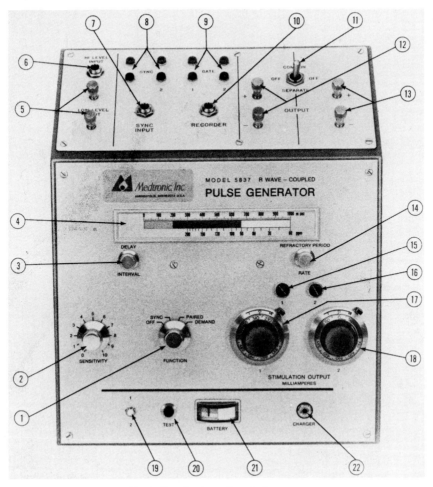

Fig. 9-10. See legend on facing page.

REFERENCES

1. Furman S: Controversies in cardiac pacing. *In* Corday E (ed): Controversies in Cardiology. Philadelphia, FA Davis, 1977, p 313
2. James T, Sherf L: Ultrastructure of the myocardium. *In* Hurst JW (ed): The Heart. New York, McGraw-Hill, 1978, pp 57–70
3. Massing G, James T: Anatomy and Pathology of the Conduction System. *In* Samet P (ed): Cardiac Pacing. New York, Grune & Stratton, 1973, pp 18–19
4. James T: The connecting pathways between the sinus node and AV node and between the right and the left atrium in the human heart. Am Heart J 66:498, 1963
5. Sano T, Yamagishi S: Spread of excitation from the sinus node. Circ Res 16:423, 1965
6. James T: Anatomy of the Conduction System of the Heart. *In* Hurst JW (ed): The Heart. New York, McGraw-Hill, 1978, pp 47–57
7. Demoulin J, Kulbertus, H: Histopathological examination of concept of left hemiblock. Br Heart J 34:807, 1972
8. Rosenbaum M: The hemiblocks: Diagnostic criteria and clinical significance. Mod Concepts Cardiovasc Dis 38:141, 1970
9. Furman S: Cardiac pacing and pacemakers 1. Indications for pacing bradyarrhythmias. Am Heart J 93:523, 1977
10. Simon A: Perioperative management of the pacemaker patient. Anesthesiology 46:127, 1977
11. Lev M: Anatomic basis for atrioventricular block. Am J Med 37:742, 1964
12. Lenegre J: Etiology and pathology of bundle branch block in relation to complete heart block. Prog Cardiovasc Dis 6:409, 1964
13. Lown B, Kosowsky B: Artificial cardiac pacemakers. N Engl J Med 283:971, 1970
14. Norris RM: Heart block in posterior and anterior myocardial infarction. Br Heart J 31:352, 1969
15. Friedberg CK, Cohen H, Donaso E: Advanced heart block as a complication of acute myocardial infarction. Prog Cardiovasc Dis 10:466, 1968
16. Julian DG, Lassers BW, Godman MJ: Pacing for heart block in acute myocardial infarction. Ann NY Acad Sci 167:911, 1969
17. Spurrell RAJ, Sowton E: Pacing techniques in the management of supraventricular tachycardia. J Electrocardiol 8:287, 1975
18. Berg G, Kotler M: The significance of bilateral bundle branch block in the preoperative patient. Chest 59:62, 1971
19. Rooney S, Goldiner P, Muss E: Relationship of right bundle branch block and marked left axis deviation to complete heart block during general anesthesia. Anesthesiology 44:64, 1976
20. Dorney E: The use of pacemakers in the treatment of cardiac arrhythmias. *In* Hurst JW (ed): The Heart. New York, McGraw-Hill, 1978, pp 698–705
21. Lown B, Kosowsky B: Artificial cardiac pacemakers, part I. N Engl J Med 283:907, 1970
22. Dorney E: Home evaluation of permanently implanted pacemakers. South Med J 64:784, 1971
23. Segel N, Samet P: Physiological Aspects of Pacing. *In* Samet P (ed): Cardiac Pacing. New York, Grune & Stratton, 1973, pp 74–113
24. Hartzler G, Maloney J, Curtis J, et al: Hemodynamic benefits of AV sequential pacing after cardiac surgery. Am J Cardiol 40:232, 1977
25. Yoshida S, Ganz W, Donaso R, et al: Coronary hemodynamics during successive elevation of heart rate by pacing in subjects with angina pectoris. Circulation 44:1062, 1971
26. Furman S: Cardiac pacing and pacemakers. The pacemaker follow-up clinic. Am Heart J 94:795, 1977
27. Luceri R, Furman S, Hurzelen P, et al: Threshold behavior of electrodes in long-term ventricular pacing. Am J Cardiol 40:184, 1977
28. Nassallah A, Hall RJ, Garcia E, et al: Runaway pacemaker in seven patients: A persisting problem. J Thorac Cardiovasc Surg 69:365, 1975
29. Furman S: Cardiac pacing and pacemakers: VI. Analysis of pacemaker malfunction. Am Heart J 94:378, 1977
30. Preston JA, Judge RD: Alteration of pacemaker threshold by drug and physiological factors. Ann NY Acad Sci 167:686, 1969
31. Scott DL: Cardiac pacemakers as an anesthetic problem. Anaesthesia 25:87, 1970
32. Redd R, McAnulty J, Phillips S, et al: Demand pacemaker inhibition by isometric skeletal muscle contraction. Circulation 49, 50 (suppl III); 957, 1974
33. Atlee J, Rusy B: Halothane depression of AV conduction studied by electrograms of the bundle of His in dogs. Anesthesiology 36:112, 1972
34. Atlee J, Rusy B: Atrioventricular conduction times and atrioventricular nodal conductivity during enflurane anesthesia in dogs. Anesthesiology 47:498, 1977
35. Batra YK, Bali IM: Effect of coagulating and cutting current on a demand pacemaker during transurethral resection of the prostate. A case report. Can Anaesth Soc J 25:65, 1978
36. Mansour K, Fleming W, Hatcher C: Initial experience with a sutureless, screw-in electrode for cardiac pacing. Ann Thorac Surg 16:127, 1973
37. Mansour K, Dorney E, Tyras D, et al: Cardiac pacemakers: Comparing epicardial and pervenous pacing. Geriatrics 28:151, 1973
38. Sutton J, Smith C: A near-fatal complication of

sutureless electrode placement. JAMA 238:2717, 1977

39. Landon A, Runge P, Balsam R, et al: Large right atrial thrombi surrounding permanent transvenous pacemakers. Circulation 40:661, 1969

40. Reynolds J, Anslinger D, Yore R, et al: Trans-venous cardiac pacemaker, mural thrombosis, and pulmonary embolism. Am Heart J 78:688, 1969

41. Friedberg D, D'Cunha G: Adhesions of pacing catheter to tricuspid valve: Adhesive endocarditis. Thorax 24:498, 1969

Ronald W. Dunbar, M.D.

10
Thoracic Aneurysms

Aneurysms of the thoracic aorta have been recognized as a potentially lethal disease for centuries. The first available description of a dissecting aneurysm of the thoracic aorta was given in 1761; in 1862, Laennec coined the term "dissecting aneurysm" to mean a tear of the intima of the aorta allowing blood to enter and permeate between the walls of the vessel and hence produce a false lumen extending for various distances. As early as these were described, there was no treatment available for several decades.[1,2]

It was not until after World War II that attempts were made to treat aneurysms of the thoracic aorta surgically. It was in the mid-1950s, however, before successful treatment of dissecting aneurysms of the thoracic aorta were reported. Mortality rates varied considerably from institution to institution, but, in general, there was a high mortality, particularly in those cases involving the ascending aorta. The survival rates were considerably improved in patients who had surgery on the descending aorta. The reason for these better results as compared to dissections of the ascending aorta was that a major portion of the operations on the descending aorta was performed after the acute dissection. Generally, the mortality for all cases of dissecting aneurysms of the thoracic aorta varied from a low of 5 to 6 percent for patients

having elective delayed resection of their dissecting aneurysms to as high as 15 to 45 percent for those having surgery during the acute dissection of the aneurysm (see Appendix).

ETIOLOGY AND PATHOGENESIS

Many causes have been postulated to explain the occurrence of a dissecting aneurysm. A high preponderance of patients are hypertensive (>80 percent), and many of these patients also have associated arteriosclerosis. Another cause is the cystic medial necrosis associated with Marfan's syndrome. This cystic medial necrosis has also been seen in patients with coarctation of the aorta. Still another cause frequently encountered is trauma, such as occurs from automobile accidents or from dissection during aortic cannulation for extracorporeal circulation and during femoral artery cannulation for extracorporeal circulation.

It is generally believed that degeneration of the media of the aorta is the primary mechanism causing acute dissection. This entity, associated with concomitant hypertension and arteriosclerosis, generally leads to the pathogenesis of dissecting aneurysms of the aorta and the descending aorta distal to the left subclavian artery.

CLASSIFICATION

In 1965, DeBakey and his associates proposed the most accepted classification for dissecting aneurysms of the thoracic aorta.[3] Type I dissection begins in the ascending aorta and extends for varying distances past the aortic arch and below the diaphragm. Type II dissection also starts in the ascending aorta, but ends proximal to the left subclavian artery. Type III aortic dissection generally starts just distal to the left subclavian artery, extends for varying distances, and may even include the iliac arteries. Type I aortic dissection is by far the most common dissecting aneurysm of the aorta, occurring in approximately 70 percent of all cases of aneurysms of the thoracic aorta. A very high initial mortality (38 percent), however, with many cases unable to get to surgery, makes this type seem rare to most anesthesiologists. Type II aortic dissection is frequently seen in patients with Marfan's syndrome. Type III dissections of the aorta occur in approximately 20 percent of aortic dissections. Because these are generally managed conservatively and have elective resection, however, they are quite commonly seen by anesthesiologists.

In addition, approximately half of the patients with type I aortic dissection also have involvement of the aortic valve. This results in aortic valve replacement or resuspension in approximately half the patients with this lesion.

SURGICAL TECHNIQUE AND COURSE OF THERAPY

Many series have been published describing the management of type I and type II dissections of the thoracic aorta.[3-5] Surgical therapy is currently the method of choice for type I and type II dissections. The best results show a survival rate of over 90 percent, with a general average mortality of 10 to 15 percent in the larger centers. Medical management of acute dissections of the type I or type II variety has a much greater early and late mortality.[6] Therefore, current opinion in dissections of the ascending aorta is to perform surgery immediately. This results in the best statistics for long-term survival. Surgery is performed using cardiopulmonary bypass with cannulation of either the right atrium (preferably) or the femoral vein. If at all possible, the femoral artery is cannulated for retrograde perfusion to avoid having to use the already damaged aorta. The operative procedure generally consists of replacing the ascending aorta with a Dacron prosthesis if the lesion is limited to the ascending aorta. When the dissection extends into the transverse aortic arch or further, the technique includes approximation of the walls of the true and false lumen. This results in reestablishing the true lumen when pressure is restored. In addition, resuspension or replacement of the aortic valve is performed if necessary.

Patients with acute dissections originating in the descending aorta (type III) are generally not considered surgical emergencies.[1,6] An exception to this is if there is a rupture of the aorta or worsening of the patient's condition. It is thought that initially the aorta is fragile and holds sutures poorly. This makes an emergency resection technically quite difficult, particularly if the dissection extends far down the aorta. Generally, these patients are treated by vasodilators to produce controlled hypotension, allowing them to survive the acute phase of the dissection. Long-term results from many investigators have confirmed that this is the method of choice for type III dissections. Once the patient has stabilized, elective resection of the chronic type III dissection results in a much greater long-term survival.

ANESTHETIC MANAGEMENT OF TYPES I AND II

Anesthetic management of types I and II aortic dissections is generally performed on an urgent or semiemergency basis. These patients are acutely ill and are an anesthetic challenge. Frequently, because of their lesion, cardiac catheterization and outlining the extent of the disease is technically difficult. Venous or, preferably, retrograde arterial angiography must be done, however, to confirm the diagnosis of a type I or II dissecting thoracic aneurysm.

These patients should all be monitored with direct arterial pressure in the left radial artery and a central venous or pulmonary artery catheter. Because of the difficulty in ascertaining the presence or absence of left ventricular failure in these patients, it is our general preference to monitor these patients with a pulmonary artery (Swan-Ganz) catheter. This is inserted through the right internal or external jugular vein and advanced through the right ventricle into the pulmonary artery and hence into the wedge position. With a thermistor on the tip, the Swan-Ganz catheter makes it possible not only to follow the pulmonary capillary wedge pressure, which reflects the filling pressure of the left ventricle, but also to perform serial cardiac outputs to monitor the patient's hemodynamic status both intraoperatively and postoperatively.

Needless to say, at least two very large cannulae are necessary for intravenous infusions. A temperature probe is inserted to monitor the intraoperative temperature fluctuations, and in addition, a Foley catheter is inserted, and diuretics such as mannitol (0.5–1.0 mg/kg) and/or furosemide (20–80 mg) are used to assure adequate urine output. In addition, a precordial electrocardiographic lead (V_5) is also monitored to determine any evidence of left heart ischemia.

Our anesthetic technique consists of morphine sulfate (0.5–1.0 mg/kg) supplemented with diazepam (0.25–0.5 mg/kg) and nitrous oxide and oxygen. Inhalational agents such as enflurane or halothane are used as needed to supplement the anesthetic while observing cardiac function. Intubation is accomplished with the use of pancuronium bromide (0.1 mg/kg), and respiration is controlled to maintain a normal metabolic state and oxygenation. Vasodilators such as nitroglycerin or nitroprusside are infrequently used, as hypertension is generally not a complication of these acute surgical emergencies. If there is an elevation of pressure, however, vasodilators are used to maintain a mean pressure of approximately 70–80 torr.

The femoral artery is exposed and cannulated prior to the median sternotomy. If at all possible, after the median sternotomy, the right atrium is cannulated and extracorporeal bypass instituted. Temperature is lowered to 28°–30° C. The aorta is cross-clamped to allow surgical repair of the lesion. Myocardial preservation is accomplished with systemic cooling, as well as with hypothermic, hyperkalemic cardioplegic solutions, or, rarely, with perfusion of the coronary arteries. Following surgical repair of the dissection, aortic valve suspension or replacement, and coronary reimplantation, the patient is removed from cardiopulmonary bypass. Constant monitoring of urine output to see that reapproximation of the aortic walls did not compromise renal blood flow and monitoring of the

carotid as well as the radial pulses determine adequate reconstruction of the true lumen. Serial cardiac outputs are routinely performed, and pulmonary capillary wedge pressure is altered to provide optimal left ventricular performance. At this point, vasodilators such as nitroprusside are frequently used to maintain mean arterial pressure at approximately 70–80 torr in an effort not to stress the suture lines. This is subsequently continued into the postoperative period if necessary.

The patient is usually left intubated with controlled ventilation over the next 12 to 24 hours. At that time, appropriate studies are performed to determine the feasibility of extubation.

TYPE III DISSECTIONS OF THE AORTA

Type III dissection of the aorta, beginning distal to the left subclavian artery and extending various distances down the aorta, is generally managed conservatively if possible.[1,6] Conservative management generally consists of monitoring the arterial pressure and pulmonary capillary wedge pressure. Vasodilators such as trimethaphan or nitroprusside, plus propranolol to decrease dP/dt, are used to maintain a mean arterial pressure of 70–80 torr. Urinary output is also constantly monitored, and appropriate osmotic or other diuretics are administered to maintain adequate urine volume.

Surgical management of type III dissection of the aorta presents some rather unique anesthetic situations, depending upon the surgical technique.

General guidelines

1. Surgical incision consisting of a left thoracotomy with or without an extension below the diaphragm
2. Pressure measurements above and below the area of cross-clamping
3. Establishment and maintenance of urinary output
4. Frequent blood gas determinations to evaluate adequacy of ventilation
5. Heparinization as needed, depending upon the surgical technique
6. Vasodilators and/or vasopressors as necessary to maintain adequate perfusion above and below the area of cross-clamping of the aorta.

Prior to the induction of anesthesia for a type III dissecting aortic aneurysm, it is necessary to communicate with the surgeon about the technique and method of perfusion that will be used below the aortic cross-clamp during the operative procedure.[7,8] Generally, the most common methods of perfusion with heparinization are either femoral vein–femoral artery partial cardiopulmonary bypass or partial left heart bypass (left atrium to femoral artery), using pump outputs of 35 ml/kg.[9] Recently, techniques not requiring heparinization have been developed. One method is the femoral venoarterial bypass without an oxygenator which does not require systemic heparinization.[10] Instead, a set of nonthrombogenic tubing and cannulae is used. Another common method is the use of the tridodecylmethylammonium chloride (TDMAC) heparin-coated shunt as a temporary bypass during the operative procedure on the aorta and great vessels.[11-13] This has been used very satisfactorily by Gott and associates to provide temporary perfusion of the distal aorta, thereby avoiding the need for systemic heparinization. The proximal end of the shunt is generally inserted into the subclavian artery or into the ascending aorta, or even occasionally into the apex of the left ventricle. The distal end of the shunt is then inserted distal to the aneurysm. Frequently, the femoral artery is exposed, and the distal shunt is inserted into it. A 9-mm × 90-cm shunt is generally preferred, but occasionally a 7-mm × 66-cm shunt has been used successfully. This provides nonpulsatile flow, with the added problem of kinking of the shunt.[14] All of these techniques have been developed in an effort to provide adequate perfusion to the organs distal to the aortic cross-clamp, especially the kidneys and spinal cord, since renal failure and paraplegia have been major complications in the past (Fig. 10-1).

SUMMARY OF GENERAL PRINCIPLES OF ANESTHETIC MANAGEMENT

1. A Carlen's tube or other endobronchial tube is used to allow ventilation of the right lung and to allow collapse of the left lung for adequate exposure.[15,16]
2. Blood gas monitoring every 10 to 15 minutes is necessary, particularly with the use of the Carlen's tube.
3. Monitoring of the arterial pressure from the *right* radial artery as well as distal to the dissection is mandatory to ascertain perfusion proximal to the aortic aneurysm as well as distal perfusion pressures.
4. Accurate and constant monitoring of the urinary output is necessary.

In addition to the specific recommendations outlined above, we routinely monitor either the central venous pressure or the pulmonary capillary wedge pressure or both. The latter is monitored if there is any indication of left ventricular failure. We feel there is a definite advantage in monitoring the pulmonary capillary wedge pressure in that we can ascertain the strain on the left ventricle as reflected by an elevation in the wedge pressure upon cross-clamping of the aorta.[17] In addition, it allows serial determinations of cardiac output in the preoperative, intraoperative, and postoperative course. As mentioned, the right radial artery is cannulated with a 20-gauge Teflon catheter, and the femoral artery opposite to that being cannulated for perfusion is cannulated with an 18- or 20-gauge Teflon catheter for continual monitoring of the distal perfusion pressures. Temperature monitoring is also essential, as are frequent blood gas determinations to assure adequacy of oxygenation as well as an adequate metabolic state.

The anesthetic management of these patients generally consists of morphine sulphate (0.5–1 mg/kg), diazepam (0.25–0.5 mg/kg), nitrous oxide and oxygen. Occasionally, depending upon pulmonary capillary wedge pressure, cardiac output, and general status of the patient, an inhalation agent may be used. The patient is paralyzed with pancuronium bromide and intubated with a Carlen's or Robertshaw tube to isolate the right lung. Every effort is made with osmotic diuretics as well as furosemide to establish and maintain adequate urine output preoperatively as well as intraoperatively.

If partial (femoral-femoral or left atrium-femoral) cardiopulmonary bypass is used, it is necessary to heparinize the patient, and the oxygenator will maintain adequate oxygenation of the perfusate of the lower part distal to the dissection. If the unheparinized femoral venoarterial bypass is used without an oxygenator, it is also necessary to monitor oxygenation and acid–base status of the distal part of the body. If a TDMAC heparin-coated polyvinyl chloride

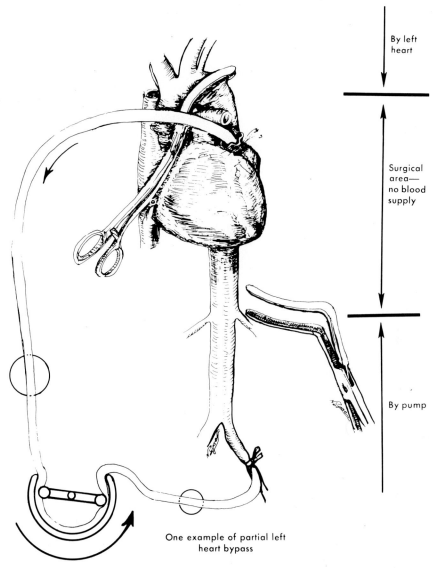

By left
heart

Surgical
area—
no blood
supply

By pump

One example of partial left
heart bypass

Fig. 10-1. Partial left heart bypass is demonstrated. Blood is taken from the left atrium, oxygenated, and pumped back into the femoral artery. One-half the calculated cardiac output is taken through the bypass circuit and the other half of the cardiac output is ejected by the heart. (Reprinted with permission of the author and publisher from Nosé, Manual on Artificial Organs. Vol. II. The Oxygenator. C. V. Mosby, St. Louis, 1973.)

shunt is used, the pressures above and below the shunt must be monitored at all times. Vasopressors and/or vasodilators may be used to assure adequate perfusion of the areas above and below the aortic dissection and the aortic cross-clamp. It is generally accepted that arterial systolic pressure of the upper part of the body should be kept at about 150 torr. The lower part of the body, either with a shunt or partial bypass, will have a lowered perfusion pressure. The mean arterial pressure distal to the aneurysm should be maintained in the general range of 50–70 torr. These precautions result in improved surgical results as well as in fewer postoperative complications such as acute tubular necrosis and neurological deficits.

If adequate oxygenation cannot be maintained with the use of the Carlen's catheter ventilating only the right lung, it may be necessary to intermittently inflate the left lung with 100 percent oxygen. This can be accomplished through a separate circuit and sometimes will continue to allow intermittent deflation of the left lung to facilitate the surgical procedure. Another useful technique is to put 5–10 cm H_2O of positive end-expiratory pressure (PEEP) on the right lung circuit. This has been shown to improve oxygenation during thoracotomy.[18]

SUMMARY

The anesthetic and surgical considerations of the various types of aortic dissections have been discussed. Types I and II are generally surgical emergencies requiring total cardiopulmonary bypass and constant monitoring. Type III dissection of the aorta is generally managed conservatively, with repair done on a more elective basis. The most important concept in anesthetic management is to ensure adequate perfusion of all the vital body organs via careful monitoring.

APPENDIX

Acute Aortic Dissection
(Emory University 1965–
1974, 106 consecutive cases)

Ascending aorta involvement	70
Limited to descending aorta	36

Source. From Douglas JS Jr: Acute aortic dissection: One hundred and six consecutive cases. Circulation 52 (suppl II): 2-10, 1975.

Clinical Course of Ascending
Aortic Dissection

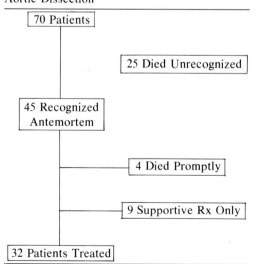

Treatment of Ascending Aortic Dissection

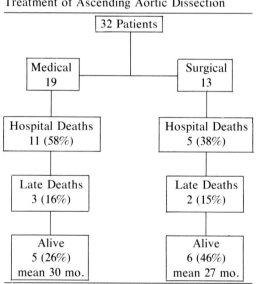

Descending Aortic Dissection

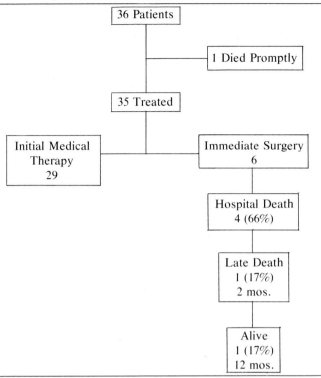

Descending Aortic Dissection

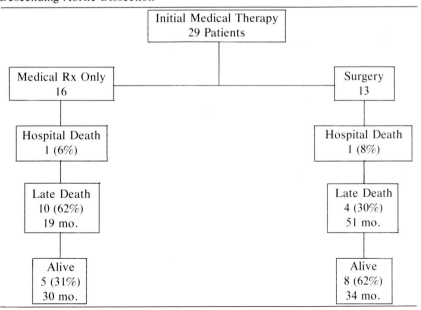

REFERENCES

1. Anagnostopoulos CE, Prabhakar MJS, Kittle CF: Aortic dissections and dissecting aneurysms. Am J Cardiol 30:263–273, 1972

2. D'Allaines C, Blondeau P, Piwnica A, et al: Surgery for aortic dissection: 53 operated cases with 32 in the acute phase. J Cardiovasc Surg 18:261–266, 1977

3. DeBakey ME, Hewley WS, Cooley DA, et al: Surgical management of dissecting aneurysms of the aorta. J Thorac Cardiovasc Surg 49:130–149, 1965

4. Ruben JC: Dissecting aneurysms of the ascending aorta. J Cardiovasc Surg 18:267–272, 1977

5. Singh MP, Bentall HH: Complete replacement of the ascending aorta and the aortic valve for the treatment of aortic aneurysm. J Thorac Cardiovasc Surg 63:218–225, 1972

6. McFarland J, Willerson JT, Dinsmore RE, et al: The medical treatment of dissecting aortic aneurysms. N Engl J Med 286:115–119, 1972

7. Pasternak BM, Boyd DP, Ellis FH: Spinal cord injury after procedures on the aorta. Surg Gynecol Obstet 135:29–34, 1972

8. Crawford ES, Rubio PA: Reappraisal of adjuncts to avoid ischemia in the treatment of aneurysms of descending thoracic aorta. J Thorac Cardiovasc Surg 66:693–704, 1973

9. Neville WE, Cox WD, Leininger B, et al: Resection of the descending thoracic aorta with femoral vein to femoral artery oxygenation and pertusion. J Thorac Cardiovasc Surg 56:39–42, 1968

10. May IA, Ecker RR, Iverson LIG: Heparinless femoral venoarterial bypass without an oxygenator for surgery on the descending thoracic aorta. J Thorac Cardiovasc Surg 73:387–392, 1977

11. Donahoo JS, Brawley RK, Gott VL: The heparin-coated shunt for thoracic aortic and great vessel procedures: A ten-year experience. Ann Thorac Surg 23:507–513, 1977

12. Wolfe WG, Kleinman LH, Wechsler AS, et al: Heparin-coated shunts for lesions of the descending thoracic aorta. Arch Surg 112:1481–1487, 1977

13. Connors JP, Ferguson TB, Roper CL, et al: The use of the TDMAC-heparin shunt in replacement of the descending thoracic aorta. Ann Surg 181:735–741, 1975

14. Kopman EA, Ferguson TB: Intraoperative monitoring of femoral artery pressure during replacement of aneurysm of descending thoracic aorta. Anesth Analg 56:603–605, 1977

15. Das BB, Fenstermacher JM, Keats AS: Endobronchial anesthesia for resection of aneurysms of the descending aorta. Anesthesiology 32:152–155, 1970

16. Sabawala PB, Strong MJ, Keats AS: Surgery of the aorta and its branches. Anesthesiology 33:229–259, 1970

17. Carroll RM, Laravaso RB, Schauble JF: Left ventricular function during aortic surgery. Arch Surg 111:740–743, 1976

18. Brown DR, Kafer ER, Roberson VO, et al: Improved oxygenation during thoracotomy with selective PEEP to the dependent lung. Anesth Analg 56:26–31, 1977

Joel A. Kaplan, M.D.
Ronald W. Dunbar, M.D.

11

Anesthesia for Noncardiac Surgery in Patients with Cardiac Disease

Patients with cardiac disease frequently must be anesthetized for noncardiac surgery. These patients may be just as sick or sometimes sicker than patients undergoing cardiac surgery. Numerous complications involving the cardiovascular system may occur during surgery, anesthesia, or the postoperative period. The incidence of and risks associated with such complications are determined by the type and severity of the cardiovascular disease, the surgical procedure, and the expertise of the operative team. The following discussion highlights the unique features associated with each category of heart disease that influence the anesthetic management of patients undergoing noncardiac surgery.

CORONARY ARTERY DISEASE

Ischemic heart disease is the most common and most serious health problem in the United States.[1] From a statistical standpoint, it is very likely that many patients over the age of 40 undergoing anesthesia have some element of coronary artery disease. In only the more seriously ill patients is this manifest as angina pectoris, which generally signifies disease of two or more of the coronary arteries. There is a spectrum of patients with coronary atherosclerotic

heart disease who undergo surgery. The first are patients with *potential* coronary artery disease who are over 45 years of age and are either obese, hypertensive, smokers, or have a family history of coronary artery disease. Second are the patients with *probable* coronary artery disease. They have other vascular lesions such as carotid insufficiency or abdominal aortic aneurysms but demonstrate no signs or symptoms of coronary insufficiency. Third are patients with *known* coronary atherosclerotic heart disease, that is, those with angina pectoris or previous myocardial infarction. This latter group may be subdivided into patients with good left ventricular function who have only angina pectoris or patients with poor left ventricular function who have angina and signs and symptoms of congestive heart failure.

During a recent 12-month period at Emory University Hospital, 8238 adult patients underwent noncardiac surgery.[3] Ten percent (873 patients) had a diagnosis of known coronary artery disease based on the presence of either angina pectoris, ischemic electrocardiographic changes, or prior myocardial infarctions. Seventy-five of those 873 patients (8.6 percent) had had a prior myocardial revascularization operation. We can expect to see more patients who have had coronary artery surgery, since 70,000 of these operations are being performed annually in the

United States. These patients are coming to surgery mainly for urologic procedures, pacemakers, or superficial chest wall procedures required secondary to the coronary artery surgery. Theoretically, these patients should be better surgical risks than they were prior to coronary revascularization.

In the past, the patient with coronary artery disease has presented a major problem to the anesthesiologist and surgeon.[4–6] Previous results have shown a high incidence of infarction during the perioperative period. Tarhan studied 32,877 patients undergoing general anesthesia for noncardiac surgery at the Mayo Clinic between 1967 and 1968.[7] Patients without a previous myocardial infarction (32,455) had only a 0.13 percent incidence of a myocardial infarction within the first postoperative week. In 422 patients who had had a prior myocardial infarction, there was a 6.6 percent incidence of reinfarction in the first postoperative week. The incidence of reinfarction was 37 percent in those operated on within 3 months, and 16 percent when the operation was performed within 3 to 6 months of the prior infarction. The incidence was approximately 4 to 5 percent when the previous infarction occurred more than 6 months before surgery. The largest percentage of infarctions, 33 percent, occurred on the third postoperative day, while only 18 percent occurred on the first postoperative day. The mortality was 54 percent, with 80 percent of the deaths occurring within 48 hours. Reinfarction was more frequent in surgery in the thorax or the upper part of the abdomen and was independent of the type of anesthesia.

Steen and Tarhan repeated the study between 1974 and 1975, since new anesthetic agents and monitoring techniques were introduced after the first study in 1968.[8] They studied the records of 587 patients who had documented evidence of prior myocardial infarctions. None of these patients had undergone prior coronary artery revascularization. The results were very similar to the first study. There was a 27 percent reinfarction rate in patients operated upon within 3 months of the acute myocardial infarction and an 11 percent rate in patients operated upon within 3 to 6 months of the old infarction. The reinfarction rate was 4.1 percent when surgery was performed more than 6 months after the prior infarction. Mortality with a reinfarction was still very high, at 69 percent.

In our recent study of 873 patients with significant coronary artery disease, there were 72 perioperative complications. These included acute myocardial infarctions in 10 patients, progressive ischemia in 18 patients, significant arrhythmias in 35 patients, congestive heart failure in 8 patients, and 1 patient with a stroke. Five of the 10 patients with acute myocardial infarctions died, as did 2 of the 35 patients with severe arrhythmias. Two patients had intraoperative cardiac arrests associated with their disease process, and 1 died. Of the 10 patients sustaining acute myocardial infarctions, 7 developed intraoperative hypotension and 5 had rate-pressure products greater than 15,000. No relationship was apparent between complications and the type of anesthesia or surgery.

Therefore, the following appear to be major factors in determining the incidence of reinfarction:[9]

1. The time interval since the myocardial infarction. From Tarhan's study, it appears that 6 months is a safe period to wait after a myocardial infarction for elective surgery.
2. The type of infarction. The risk appears to be much greater with a transmural infarction than with a subendocardial infarction.
3. Complications after the myocardial infarction, such as congestive heart failure and arrhythmias.
4. The type of surgery. Diagnostic procedures with general anesthesia hold very low risk as compared to major surgical procedures.
5. Location of the surgery. Thoracic and upper abdominal procedures have higher complication rates than peripheral procedures.
6. The length of surgery. Reinfarction rates increased from 1.9 percent for 0- to 1-hour procedures to 15.6 percent for procedures lasting over 5 hours.
7. Wide swings in vital signs. Hypotension, defined as a 30 percent lowering of the systolic blood pressure, increased the reinfarction rate from 3.2 to 15.2 percent.

Two factors may improve on past results:

1. The skill of the anesthesiologist in dealing with patients with acute cardiovascular disease. Modern monitoring equipment, such as the Swan-Ganz catheter, allows the anesthesiologist to evaluate the functions of the heart during surgery much more precisely.

2. The use of the intra-aortic balloon pump, which may be placed before induction of anesthesia in patients with acute myocardial infarction brought for emergency surgery. A few of these patients have survived emergency surgery within days of acute myocardial infarction utilizing this technique.[10]

The current mortality of a myocardial infarction incident to anesthesia and surgery is more than three times greater than that occurring unrelated to operations and treated in the coronary care unit. These figures are incongruous in view of the reasonably small risk of coronary artery bypass surgery performed in patients with severe disease, and even occasionally in the presence of a recent myocardial infarction. The application of the same type of care given the coronary patient in the coronary care unit or postcardiac surgical intensive care unit would undoubtedly reduce the mortality of myocardial infarction incident to surgery. Thus, constant monitoring of the heart rhythm, control of arrhythmias, early detection and treatment of left-sided heart failure, and careful monitoring of the filling pressures of the heart clinically (S_3,rales) or by the Swan-Ganz catheter would surely reduce the distressing mortality.

Many of the patients have concurrent peripheral vascular disease involving the aorta or carotid, iliac, femoral, or renal arteries. In addition, these patients frequently are hypertensive, obese, diabetic, and have chronic obstructive pulmonary disease. All of these factors, plus drug interactions, make the anesthetic management of these patients with coronary artery disease very challenging. In many ways, these cases are just as difficult to manage as cardiac surgical procedures.

The major problem in cerebral vascular disease is prevention of cerebral vascular accidents. Patients should be questioned regarding symptoms of cerebral ischemia, transient ischemic attacks, and cerebral vascular accidents; and the carotid arteries should be examined for the presence of bruits. If a bruit is found, it may be advantageous to perform a carotid arteriogram and, if necessary, to fix the carotid artery obstruction *prior to* the other anticipated elective surgery. This has proved to be the best policy in patients with bruits scheduled for coronary artery surgery and may well apply to the noncardiac surgical patient.[11] It is essential to avoid hypotension and wide swings in arterial oxygen and carbon dioxide tensions during surgery in patients with known cerebral vascular disease, since these factors regulate the cerebral blood flow. Hypotension and arrhythmias should be aggressively treated. The blood pressure should be maintained at the upper limits of normal for the patient, and the arterial carbon dioxide tension should be reduced to 30–35 torr.

Patients with pulmonary disease have an increased anesthetic risk and are subject to postoperative complications. Hypoxia, hypercarbia, and atelectasis are common in the postoperative period. These are especailly dangerous in association with coronary artery disease. Those patients with chronic bronchitis due to smoking have increased pulmonary secretions and bronchospasm and are particularly prone to develop atelectasis and pneumonia. These patients should stop smoking for several days to weeks preoperatively. All cardiac patients with signs and symptoms of significant pulmonary disease should have preoperative pulmonary function tests and arterial blood gases. Signs of increased risk include the following:[9]

1. Maximum voluntary ventilation or maximum breathing capacity less than 50 percent of predicted
2. Forced expiratory volume in 1 second less than .50
3. Maximum mid-expiratory flow less than 0.6 liters/sec
4. Maximum expiratory flow less than 100 liters/min
5. Vital capacity less than 1 liter
6. Severe hypoxia with arterial oxygen tensions less than 55 torr
7. Elevations of arterial carbon dioxide tensions
8. Failure to improve after bronchodilators

Preoperative therapy of the cardiac patient with chronic obstructive pulmonary disease may be needed and may involve postponing surgery until the patient is in optimal shape for the procedure. Expectorants, bronchodilators, chest physical therapy, and intermittent positive pressure breathing may be used to improve the vital capacity, clear secretions, and correct bronchospasm.

Recent studies have demonstrated that pulmonary function is altered after an acute myocardial infarction.[12-13] The derangement of pulmonary function is related to the severity of hemodynamic dysfunction. Abnormalities of pulmonary function occur even in patients without clinical or radiological evidence of congestive heart failure. A small increase in lung water produces hypoxemia as a result of ventilation-perfusion mismatch and increased shunting. There is also evidence for dysfunction of small airways for up to 4 weeks after infarction with the mean values for closing volume exceeding 125 percent of predicted values.

For a discussion of the preoperative evaluation and management of hypertension, renal and hepatic disease, diabetes and coagulopathies, see Chapters 5 and 7.

VALVULAR HEART DISEASE

Patients with valvular heart disease can pose serious problems for the anesthesiologist. Aortic valve disease of a mild or moderate degree is usually well tolerated by the patient. Severe aortic valve disease leads to the symptom complex of congestive heart failure, angina pectoris, and syncope. These patients are at increased risk when awake as well as during anesthesia and frequently die of ventricular fibrillation. Patients with mitral valve disease have an increased risk of developing congestive heart failure and pulmonary edema during and after surgery. Care must be taken to avoid overloading with blood and intravenous fluids in order to avoid this complication. Supraventricular tachyarrhythmias are poorly tolerated by patients with mitral stenosis. Patients with valvular heart disease should receive prophylactic antibiotics before all surgical procedures. For further detail about valvular heart disease, see Chapter 6.

CONGENITAL HEART DISEASE

Patients with congenital heart disease with left-to-right shunts (e.g. atrial septal defects) usually tolerate anesthesia quite well. These patients are at increased risk if they develop pulmonary hypertension secondary to their increased blood flow and start to reverse their shunt (Eisenmenger's syndrome). Actually, all shunts are bidirectional at times, and bubbles must be carefully avoided in all intravenous in-

fusions. Patients with cyanotic congenital heart disease, such as tetrology of Fallot, have right-to-left shunts and are a greater anesthetic risk. Their hypoxemia is obvious and must not be made worse. Decreasing the left ventricular afterload with vasodilators or producing myocardial depression with halothane or enflurane can be detrimental. The right-to-left shunt can increase and hypoxemia worsen. A peripheral vasoconstrictor is occasionally needed to increase peripheral vascular resistance and to decrease the right-to-left shunt in order to increase the arterial oxygen tension. Ketamine is a very effective drug for children with right-to-left shunts and has been used in noncardiac procedures by our group with great success. For further detail about congenital heart disease, see Chapter 8.

CONGESTIVE HEART FAILURE AND ARRHYTHMIAS

Compensated congestive heart failure may produce a moderate increase in risk. The cardiac reserve should be estimated by determining whether the patient is able to carry on normal activities without symptoms of congestive heart failure. If the patient develops dyspnea on walking one block or has paroxysmal nocturnal dyspnea, the operative risks may be increased. If he can climb several flights of steps without symptoms, his cardiac reserve is adequate and his operative risk should not be increased. It is useful to classify the patient's functional status according to the criteria of the New York Heart Association (see Chapter 7).

Systolic (forward) failure is present when ventricular ejection is subnormal or when an adequate supply of blood is not delivered to the periphery. Diastolic (backward) failure is present when the pulmonary venous pressure cannot be maintained at normal levels. This is seen when the left ventricular chamber becomes stiff (noncompliant). Failure may also result from overload of the heart. The overload can be either by volume (acute intravascular volume expansion) or by pressure (aortic stenosis or essential hypertension).

Congestive heart failure is defined as the inability of the heart to deliver a blood supply adequate for the metabolic demands of the body.[14] Thus, in congestive heart failure (cardiac output ≠ peripheral demands) treatment is directed at improving the cardiac output and/or decreasing the peripheral demands to meet a reduced cardiac output. The digitalis glycosides are the standard therapy to augment cardiac output. Recently, vasodilators have been added to reduce preload and afterload and thus reduce peripheral demands.

Digitalization should be accomplished several days prior to surgery so that a maintenance dose of digitalis free of toxicity can be established. Digitalis is indicated in the following situations:[9,15]

1. Where there is a history of recent congestive heart failure
2. When there is evidence of myocardial failure, such as a ventricular gallop rhythm, pulses alternans, rales, neck vein distention, or interstitial edema on x-ray
3. In some patients with nocturnal angina
4. In patients with atrial fibrillation or flutter
5. In patients with frequent atrial or nodal tachycardia

We believe that patients with the above indications will benefit by preoperative digitalization. We do not feel, however, that patients should be prophylactically digitalized just because they are over 60 years of age, undergoing thoracic surgical procedures, or have coronary artery disease. When atrial fibrillation is present, the ventricular rate should be in the range of 80 at rest and no greater than 100 with mild activity. In cases in which digitalization has been previously carried out, the patient's status should be reviewed to determine whether additional drug is needed, or whether the dose should be temporarily omitted or reduced because of evidence of toxicity.

Premature ventricular beats are commonly related to anxiety and require no therapy. If there are frequent premature ventricular beats, however, lidocaine may be given as a bolus dose of 1.5 mg/kg and then as an infusion of 1–4 mg/min. Premature ventricular contractions should be treated if they are frequent (more than 5 per minute), multifocal, have the R-on-T phenomenon, or if short runs of ventricular tachycardia are present. Procainamide or quinidine sulfate may be added to the preoperative drug regimen to control these arrhythmias.

The significance of right or left bundle branch block depends on the type and extent of heart disease. Bundle branch block per se does not increase surgical risk. Studies on patients under the age of 40 years have demonstrated that bundle branch blocks may frequently be present with no other obvious evidence of cardiac disease.[16] Of those patients with complete right bundle branch block, 97 percent had no evidence of cardiac disease, and of those with complete left bundle branch block, 89 percent had no obvious cardiac disease. The presence of right bundle branch block and left anterior or posterior hemiblock with or without a prolonged P-R interval may increase the risk of the development of complete heart block. Prophylactic pacing may be indicated if there is a history of dizziness or syncope. When complete heart block is present, a pacemaker is necessary for the safe conduct of surgery and anesthesia.

PREOPERATIVE MEASURES

It is necessary for the anesthesiologist to adequately evaluate all patients prior to surgery. The American Society of Anesthesiologists Physical Status Scoring System is routinely used to evaluate patients. This is an excellent predictor of noncardiac perioperative complications, but not necessarily of cardiac problems. Recently, Goldman has proposed the use of a new multifactoral index of cardiac risks in noncardiac surgical procedures.[17] The Cardiac Risk Index is calculated using the scale shown in Table 11-1.

Four risk categories are defined by this system. In the progression from Class 1 to Class 4, Goldman found a statistically significant stepwise increase in the proportion of patients who had life-threatening complications. Over one-half the cardiac deaths were found in Class 4 patients. The ASA Physical Status Classification could not match the Cardiac Risk Index Score's ability to isolate the high-risk cardiac patient.

In our recent study of patients with coronary artery disease, we compared the Cardiac Risk Index with the Physical Status Scoring systems.[3] In 510 of 873 patients who were classified Physical Status 3 or 4, there was no significant relationship demonstrated between perioperative complications and physical status. In contrast, the incidence of life-threatening complications correlated closely with Cardiac Risk Index. The Cardiac Risk Index was low in most

Table 11-1

Cardiac Risk Index Score

Factors	Points
1. History: Age > 70	5
MI < 6 months	10
2. Physical exam: S_3 or JVD	11
3. ECG: Any rhythm other than sinus	7
>5 PVCs/min	7
4. General information: $Po_2 < 60$	
$Pco_2 > 50$	
$K^+ < 3$	
BUN > 50	3
Creat > 3	
Bedridden	
5. Operation: Emergency	4
Intrathoracic	
Intra-abdominal	3
Aortic surgery	
Total	50

CLASS 1: 0–5 points
     2: 6–12 points
     3: 13–25 points
     4: 26 points or more

Source. Goldman L, Caldera DL, Nussbaum SR, et al: Multifactorial index of cardiac risk in non-cardiac surgical procedures. N Engl J Med 297:845–850, 1977

patients after coronary artery revascularization, while the Physical Status Score was high. Most of these patients had a very benign operative course. We believe this new index is a useful tool in helping to evaluate pateints with cardiac disease.

Preoperative drug therapy should, as a general rule, be continued up until the time of surgery. The only exception to this are the MAO inhibitors, which should be stopped 1 to 2 weeks before elective surgery.

All antihypertensive therapy should be continued at full dose right until the time of surgery.[18] Terazi has shown that hypertensive patients not taking antihypertensive drugs have a decreased plasma volume.[19] This may be accentuated in those patients on chronic diuretic therapy and adds to the risk of surgery and anesthesia. The blood pressure should be recorded with the patient lying and then standing in order to detect postural hypotension. When such hypotension is detected, it may be corrected by administration of crystalloid or colloid solution prior to surgery.

The dangers of general anesthesia for patients taking antihypertensives was first reported in 1955.[20] This was based on a few individual case reports and the theoretical dangers of catecholamine depletion in the face of reserpine therapy. Since that time, a number of studies have shown the following:[21]

1. That the hypertensive patient, even in the absence of treatment, frequently has marked fluctuations of blood pressure during general anesthesia.
2. That the patient maintained on his therapy until surgery has the lowest incidence of both hypotension and hypertension.

There is no evidence that discontinuing drug therapy 1 to 2 weeks preoperatively decreases the likelihood of hypotension or other complications during anesthesia. Preoperative use of antihypertensive agents such as alpha-methyldopa or guanethidine may affect the anesthetic course, but the discontinuation of an effective therapeutic regimen may result in more serious sequelae. If a pressor drug is required during surgery, one with a direct action is preferable in reduced dosage. Most anesthesiologists today consider the drug-treated hypertensive patient as a relatively good risk candidate for anesthesia. The most unstable situation is the withdrawal of an antihypertensive medication, such as clonidine, in which a rapid rebound hypertensive response may occur about the time the patient is to undergo anesthesia and surgery. It is also important to reinstate drug therapy immediately after surgery so that the patient does not become hypertensive in the postoperative period.

Hypertensive patients frequently become more hypertensive during surgery and in the immediate postoperative period. Their marked elevations of blood pressure must be controlled acutely in order to prevent myocardial or cerebral damage. Intraoperatively, sodium nitroprusside, trimethaphan, nitroglycerin, or phentolamine may have to be used. Postoperatively, the intravenous infusions may be continued or therapy changed to intermittent bolus doses of diazoxide or other standard antihypertensive medications. If used, diazoxide should be given in reduced doses (150 mg) in the immediate postoperative period, since it may cause profound hypotension.

Propranolol is an important drug in the medical management of patients with angina pectoris, hypertension, cardiac arrhythmias, thyrotoxicosis, pheochromocytoma, and obstructive cardiomyopathies. An increasing number of patients can be expected to present for surgical anesthesia while taking this β-adrenergic blocking agent. Patients taking propranolol are in an analogous situation to patients taking antihypertensive medication. If they require the drug for the control of their disease, they should be continued on it until the time of operation. We reviewed the cases of 73 patients taking propranolol who were anesthetized for noncardiac operations in order to determine whether there were any intraoperative or postoperative complications.[22] Of these 73 patients, 72 percent took propranolol to within 24 hours of the operation, and 84 percent took it to within 48 hours. The mean dosage of propranolol was 77 mg/day (range 10–320 mg/day). Anesthetic techniques and agents included enflurane, halothane, nitrous oxide/narcotic/relaxant, and spinal anesthesia. There were only three episodes of hypotension, all of which responded to a decreased depth of general anesthesia, intravenous fluid administration, and in 1 patient, a small dose of a vasopressor. There were no intraoperative or postoperative deaths in these patients undergoing all types of noncardiac surgery. It was concluded that propranolol should be continued up until the time of surgery if it is required for adequate medical control of the patient's disease.

Digitalis preparations also should be continued until the time of surgery. Digitalis intoxication must be ruled out, however, in all patients about to undergo surgery. It is especially important to check the serum potassium level in patients taking both digitalis and diuretic preparations. Toxicity may be evidenced by symptoms, but more often is indicated by frequent premature ventricular contractions, atrioventricular block, or other arrhythmias. Serum levels of digoxin may be useful when there is a question of digitalis toxicity.

Many patients with cardiac disease should have a preoperative cardiology consultation. The purpose of this is to have the cardiologist decide if the patient is in the best possible medical condition for surgery, not to tell the anesthesiologist how to give anesthesia. The resting ECG should be reviewed by the cardiologist.

The problem of identification of the patient with asymptomatic coronary disease is difficult, since even in the presence of a history of angina pectoris the ECG is normal in more than half of the patients. Furthermore, a documented history of prior myocardial infarction is more reliable than electrocardiographic demonstration of such an event. Most subendocardial infarcts produce no electrocardiographic changes, and even when such are present, they generally subside within weeks. In one study of 175 patients with myocardial infarctions with only ST-T-wave changes, the ECG returned to normal within one year in 54 percent, while 5.6 percent with Q-wave abnormalities returned to normal.[23]

Premedication should be carefully selected in patients with cardiac disease. A "verbal premedication" can go a long way to reduce the patient's anxiety and decrease the need for depressant drugs. Minor tranquilizers can be added to further reduce anxiety and produce amnesia. We have found diazepam (5–10 mg P.O.) or lorazepam (1–4 mg P.O.) to be very effective. Morphine may be added to potentiate the sedation. In older patients (over 65 years), we avoid barbiturates and scopolamine, since they may produce agitation, severe depression, hypoventilation, and hypotension. Nitrates are used in the preoperative period in all patients with coronary artery disease. These may be given sublingually or preferably in the form of nitroglycerin ointment 2 percent (1–2 inches of Nitrol ointment) for long-lasting effect. This has an onset in 45 minutes and lasts for 4 hours.[24]

MONITORING

Part of the increased safety and improvement in the management of all patients has resulted from the use of sophisticated modern monitoring techniques. In order to adequately evaluate what is occurring with these patients, it is necessary to monitor them in accordance with the extent of their cardiac disease. Obviously, there are complications of any type of monitoring, but these are minor compared to the cardiac complications patients may develop if they are inadequately monitored. With the information gained from careful preoperative assessment, the necessity of adequate intraoperative and postoperative monitoring can be determined. Most patients with significant cardiac disease having upper abdominal, chest, major vascular, or any other major surgery involving potentially large blood loss or a long duration should be monitored essentially the same way as the patient undergoing open heart surgery. Many patients for coronary artery revascularization are relatively young, have no concomitant disease other than restricted blood flow in one of their coronary arteries, and have normal pulmonary status, and yet they are monitored extensively, both intraoperatively and postoperatively. If we consider the very low mortality of less than 1 percent in these patients and that the operations generally last only 2 to 3 hours, it makes one wonder why the more seriously ill patient with concomitant disease undergoing noncardiac surgery is not entitled to the same type of monitoring! The appropriate monitoring should fit the patient and his cardiac condition, not the surgical procedure.

In many instances, patients with significant cardiac disease should have a percutaneous radial artery catheter placed prior to induction of anesthesia. This is used to monitor blood pressure continually during the operative procedure and to allow frequent arterial blood gases to be obtained. In patients with good left ventricular function, a central venous pressure catheter may be placed in the right internal jugular vein, and in these patients the pressure is found to correlate quite well with left ventricular filling pressures. In patients with poor left ventricular function, a thermal dilution Swan-Ganz catheter is placed via the jugular vein and positioned in the pulmonary artery. (See Table 3-1 in Chapter 3 for specific indications for the Swan-Ganz catheter in noncardiac surgery.) In these patients, it is important to be able to watch the pulmonary artery and pulmonary wedge pressures as well as the central venous pressure. Thermal dilution cardiac output measurements are made at frequent intervals to monitor the status of the cardiovascular system. Using these monitoring techniques in patients with poor left ventricular function, it is possible to use the Starling curve to follow their cardiovascular function in response to therapeutic interventions. Therapy can be directed at either the preload, afterload, or myocardial contractility.[25-27] The use of the Starling curve is especially indicated in patients requiring either vasodilators, inotropic infusions, or the intra-aortic balloon.

The electrocardiogram is monitored in all patients with cardiac disease. The standard six leads (I, II, III, AVR, AVL, and AVF) are monitored. In the past, the most commonly used lead in the operating room was lead II. This was monitored because it was very helpful in differentiating supraventricular from ventricular arrhythmias. This is a poor lead to monitor ischemic changes of the anterior and lateral walls of the myocardium, however. Recently, the precordial V_5 lead has been monitored at our institution in all patients with coronary artery disease undergoing both cardiac and noncardiac surgery. We have seen many patients develop severe ischemic changes in the V_5 lead with minimal or no changes in lead II.[28] When the patients develop significant ST-segment depression in lead V_5, it is usually caused by changes in the rate-pressure product, and appropriate therapeutic interventions are then taken in order to reduce either the blood pressure or the heart rate (see Chapter 7).

It must be remembered that there may be a normal heart rate and rhythm when there is virtually no cardiac output and cardiac arrest is impending. In this situation, there is a dissociation between the electrical activity of the heart and its mechanical pumping. This emphasizes the need for careful monitoring of both heart tones and blood pressure along with the electrocardiograph.

The arterial line allows the frequent measurement of arterial blood gases during surgery and has been a major advance. Arterial oxygenation can be measured accurately, and a falling PO_2 used to warn of inadequate inspired oxygen, ventilation perfusion mismatches, increasing shunting, or decreasing cardiac output. The adequacy of ventilation during anesthesia can be very difficult to judge, but measurements of the arterial carbon dioxide tension allow easy correction of respiratory acidosis or alkalosis. Metabolic acidosis is common during surgery, and accurate treatment with sodium bicarbonate can be undertaken with frequent determinations of the pH and base excess.

ANESTHETIC TECHNIQUES

Although no ideal anesthetic agent or technique exists, certain general principles can be applied in the selection of agents and techniques.[29] Local anesthetic techniques produce minimal cardiovascular changes if the dosage is low so that vasomotor effects are limited. In large doses these drugs may be absorbed into the general circulation and produce significant cardiovascular effects, including reduction of myocardial contractility and vasomotor tone. When excessive amounts of local anesthetics are absorbed, they may produce cerebral excitement and convulsions and cardiovascular depression. A small subcutaneous dose of a local anesthetic such as lidocaine (50–100 mg) should produce little cardiovascular effect, whereas large doses, such as 500 mg of lidocaine, may have substantial systemic effects.

Many patients with cardiac disease can have surgery with local anesthesia if it is supplemented with some degree of sedation (the so-called local-standby case). These patients should have anesthesia personnel in attendance at all times, be carefully monitored with an ECG and frequent blood pressure and heart rate checks, receive supplemental oxygen and appropriate verbal stimulation to keep respirations adequate, and receive adequate local anesthesia and sedation to keep them comfortable.

Because of the propensity to hypotension due to vasodilatation, high spinal anesthesia should be used with caution in patients with significant coronary artery disease, pulmonary hypertension, or marginal blood volume. Caudal, lumbar epidural, or low spinal anesthesia may be useful in perineal or lower extremity surgery in patients with cardiac disease. Epinephrine should not be added to local anesthetics in patients with coronary artery disease, since its β-adrenergic effects will increase oxygen demand and decrease oxygen supply.

All general anesthetic agents (1) reduce myocardial contractility, (2) impair ventilation, and (3) affect the autonomic nervous system in either its sympathetic or parasympathetic branches. Since a patient's tolerance to drugs can be determined only by trial, rapid reversibility is a highly desirable property of an anesthetic agent selected for patients with impaired cardiovascular reserve. In this regard, inhalation agents have a marked advantage over intravenous agents because the former can be removed by ventilation. On the other hand, intravenous agents provide a much smoother induction, which may be important in certain apprehensive patients.

A general anesthesic plan for patients with severely limited myocardial reserve and in whom muscle relaxation is required for the surgical procedure can be safely based on a nitrous oxide/muscle relaxant/narcotic technique. In recent years, morphine has become the most commonly used anesthetic agent for patients with decreased left ventricular function. Administered slowly (5 mg/min), hypotension is seldom a problem, and morphine causes no myocardial depression. Since morphine by itself does not guarantee amnesia, it is frequently combined with diazepam and/or scopolamine. Nitrous oxide is added for further amnesia and analgesia. Nitrous oxide causes some myocardial depression and increases pulmonary artery pressure. Fentanyl may be substituted for morphine in shorter operative procedures. It has similar hemodynamic effects to morphine, except for causing less venodilatation.

Patients who have coronary artery disease and a history suggestive of good left ventricular function frequently become hypertensive if anesthetized with a light anesthetic technique based on morphine. They require an anesthetic that depresses their myocardium, such as halothane or enflurane. Halothane has minimal effects on total peripheral resistance, while enflurane decreases peripheral resistance. These agents are administered by the inhalation route and thus have the advantage of ready reversibility. Halothane may cause arrhythmias, since it sensitizes the myocardium to both exogenous and endogenous catecholamines, while enflurane, being an ether drug, tends to stablize the myocardium, and thus arrhythmias are less common.

Endotracheal intubation is a time of marked cardiovascular stress and one of the more dangerous periods during an operative procedure for any cardiac patient. It is frequently associated with hypertension, tachycardia, and various arrhythmias. Adequate anesthesia should be obtained prior to laryngoscopy and intubation. The use of a laryngotracheal anesthetic with lidocaine or intravenous lidocaine may depress airway and cardiovascular reflexes during the intubation. It is not commonly realized that the time of extubation may be equally stressful to the heart.

Muscle relaxants are frequently used during many operative procedures. All of these drugs have significant cardiovascular effects and must be selected with the patient's underlying cardiac disease in mind. For example, succinylcholine may produce bradycardia and arrhythmias; curare may produce hypotension, which would be detrimental in patients with stenotic valvular lesions; pancuronium may cause a rapid increase in the heart rate, which would be detrimental in patients with mitral stenosis and atrial fibrillation or in patients with coronary artery disease; and gallamine may cause an undesirable tachycardia. Dimethyl tubocurarine may be an advantageous drug to use in patients with cardiac disease. Zaidan has demonstrated that there are minimal cardiovascular effects associated with this muscle relaxant.[30] It produces less ganglionic blockade and hypotension than curare and less tachycardia than pancuronium. It may be the drug of choice in patients with coronary artery disease as well as those with mitral stenosis and atrial fibrillation. All the nondepolarizing muscle relaxants frequently require reversal with neostigmine and atropine. This reversal should be done slowly, since it may produce severe cardiovascular derangements with the occurrence of either tachycardia or bradycardia.

POSTOPERATIVE CARE OF THE CARDIAC PATIENT

The following immediate problems are faced in the postoperative period by the cardiac patient:

1. Respiratory depression as a result of the continued action of anesthetic agents and muscle relaxants.
2. Hypovolemia or hypervolemia.
3. Hypotension resulting from myocardial depression, hypovolemia, myocardial ischemia, or heart failure.
4. Hypertension resulting from pain, anxiety, hypervolemia, or heart failure.
5. Tachycardia resulting from pain, agitation, shivering, or hypovolemia.
6. Hypothermia with shivering and markedly increased oxygen demands (up to 800 percent). Benzinger has shown that lowering the skin temperature to 33°C, 32°C, and 31°C increases oxygen consumption by 500 percent, 600 percent, and 800 percent, respectively.[31]

In the postoperative period the patient should be monitored just as extensively as he was intraoperatively. This monitoring should include measurements of blood pressure, heart rate, filling pressures, urine output, chest x-ray, daily electrocardiograms, daily enzyme measurements and any other indicated parameters. Blood gases should be checked frequently postoperatively in patients with cardiac disease to detect hypoxia and/or hypercarbia. In the immediate postoperative period these patients are at marked increased risk secondary to their pain, marginal ventilation, and increase in catecholamine production. Oxygen therapy should be maintained in all patients with cardiac disease for at least the first day, and probably through the second or third postoperative day. Hypoxia and ventilation-perfusion mismatch are common even on the third postoperative day.[32] This is when most patients with coronary artery disease had their reinfarctions in Tarhan's studies.[7]

Many of these patients undergoing noncardiac surgery should go to an intensive care unit postoperatively. This, however, is frequently not done. Patients with cardiac disease are not made better by their noncardiac surgery. They are, in fact, stressed to an extreme degree by their surgery! This is different from the cardiac surgical patient, such as the coronary bypass patient, who has had his cardiac lesion corrected by the surgery. Therefore, the chance of postoperative complications is probably higher in patients with cardiac disease undergoing noncardiac surgery than it is after cardiac surgery. Unfortunately, the routine in many hospitals is that patients with cardiac disease undergoing noncardiac surgery, such as upper abdominal surgery, go to the recovery room postoperatively and then back to the floor instead of to an intensive care unit. This is one area where marked improvement could be made in the future, thereby lowering the perioperative morbidity and mortality associated with surgery in patients with cardiovascular disease.

PERIOPERATIVE COMPLICATIONS

Cardiac Arrests

In the past, cardiac arrests associated with anesthesia occurred once in every 3000 anesthetics. It occurred once in every 1000 elderly or poor-risk patients, and once in 5000 healthy, good-risk patients.[33] It was even more common in infants less than 1 year of age, developing in 1 out of 700 operations.[34] With the dramatic improvements in preoperative preparation of patients, anesthetic management, intraoperative management and monitoring, and postoperative care, intraoperative cardiac arrests are now a rare event. Today, in fact, intraoperative deaths are quite rare, and are usually related to the patient's underlying disease state.

Acute Myocardial Infarction

As emphasized earlier, the incidence of postoperative myocardial infarction is small in patients without previous symptoms of coronary artery disease but does occur in 5 to 6 percent of patients with a history of preoperative atherosclerotic heart disease.[7] Electrocardiographic monitoring should be continued for several days in the postoperative period in patients with symptomatic coronary artery disease. Myocardial ischemia and cardiac arrhythmias may be recognized with greater facility using a continuous oscilloscopic display. It must be remembered that pain is a symptom in less than half of the cases of postoperative myocardial infarction and that the manifestations are notoriously atypical. In one series, half of the postoperative infarctions would have been missed without routine postoperative electrocardiograms.[35] An ECG should be made routinely in the postoperative period in all patients with a prior history of angina or myocardial infarction and is indicated when any of the following situations are present:

1. Unexplained hypotension during or after surgery
2. Development of signs and symptoms of congestive heart failure
3. Development of an arrhythmia
4. Complaints of chest, back, arm, or shoulder pain
5. Unexplained syncope

Serial tracings may be needed if the initial tracing is minimally abnormal and there is suspicion of a myocardial infarction. Serum enzymes such as the CPK-MB should be obtained for three postoperative days.

Pulmonary Edema

Acute pulmonary edema is not uncommon in the recovery or postoperative phases of an operation. This may be due to the large amounts of crystalloid and colloid fluids administered during anesthesia to patients who are vasodilated and receiving positive pressure ventilation. Cooperman found that most of the cases of pulmonary edema occurred in the first 30 minutes after discontinuing the anesthetic.[36] He found there were 6 changes occurring at the end of an anesthetic to produce this:

1. Cessation of positive pressure respiration
2. Increased cardiac output
3. Increase $Paco_2$
4. Decreased Pao_2
5. Airway obstruction
6. Hypertension

These changes are poorly tolerated in patients with cardiovascular disease. Patients who develop pulmonary edema should be treated by placing them in the semi-Fowler's position; administering oxygen, possibly with positive pressure ventilation; giving rapid-acting intravenous diuretics such as furosemide (Lasix); administering opiates, especially morphine in small doses; giving digitalis in undigitalized patients; and using vasodilators such as nitroprusside or nitroglycerin in hypertensive patients. It may even be necessary to perform a rapid phlebotomy of 300–500 ml of blood to obtain prompt improvement in the patient's condition.

Pulmonary Embolism

Thrombophlebitis of the calf veins may be detected in 30 to 40 percent of patients after general abdominal or hip surgery. Fortunately, only a small percentage of these thrombi dislodge and embolize to the central circulation. The frequency of pulmonary embolism may be decreased by early ambulation after surgery. Mini-dose heparin and dextran may also be used in an effort to decrease the incidence of pulmonary embolism. The use of elastic stockings and frequent movement of the lower extremities while the patients are in bed is quite important.

The clinical findings of a pulmonary embolism are frequently quite subtle, and the diagnosis is of necessity imprecise and based on clinical suspicion in many instances. The following symptoms may indicate a pulmonary embolism:[9]

1. Chest pain
2. Unexplained dyspnea
3. Syncope
4. Unexplained bronchospasm
5. Palpitations
6. Arrhythmias
7. Unexplained anxiety
8. Fever

Blood gases frequently show severe hypoxemia and, in some instances, a decrease in the carbon dioxide tension. Massive pulmonary embolism may be associated with dyspnea, cyanosis, chest pain, shock, and acute cor pulmonale.

Chest x-ray may show an increased radiolucency of an area of a lung, blunting of a costophrenic angle, pleural effusion, dilatation of one of the pulmonary arteries, platelike atelectasis, or wedge-shaped densities. A lung scan commonly will show diagnostic changes when the chest film is relatively normal. The electrocardiogram may be perfectly normal during a pulmonary embolism. In some cases there will be inverted T waves in leads V_1 through V_4, a right bundle branch block, right axis deviation, right ventricular hypertrophy, and tall P waves in leads II, III, and AVF.

SUMMARY

Patients with cardiac disease undergoing noncardiac surgery should be evaluated preoperatively and managed intraoperatively and postoperatively in a similar manner to patients having cardiac surgery. The delicate balance between myocardial oxygen supply and demand must be maintained at all times in patients with coronary artery or valvular heart disease. Sophisticated modern equipment, techniques, and drugs should be as readily available to these patients as to the cardiac surgical patient, including precordial ECG monitoring, pulmonary artery catheterization, vasodilator and inotropic therapy, and even the intra-aortic balloon if indicated.

In order to be able to care for these sick patients adequately and completely, the anesthesiologist and his assistants should be experienced in modern *cardiac anesthesia* skills. The anesthesiologist must be able to insert the monitoring devices (e.g., Swan-Ganz catheter), interpret the data (e.g., Starling curve), interpret the ECG (e.g., ischemia, complex arrhythmias), utilize the new pharmacotherapy (e.g., vasodilators in heart failure), and understand the patient's basic pathophysiology. The anesthesiologist who cannot do all of these probably should not be anesthetizing cardiac patients even for noncardiac surgery.

REFERENCES

1. Hillis CD, Braunwald E: Myocardial ischemia. N Engl J Med 296:971–977, 1034–1041, 1093–1096, 1977
2. Kaplan JA: Anesthesia for patients with coronary artery disease. Surg Rounds 1:46–52, 1978
3. Kaplan JA, Hug CC: Anesthesia for non-cardiac surgery in patients with coronary artery disease. Abstract presented at the Association of University Anesthetists, 1978
4. Knapp RB, Topkins MJ, Artusio JF: The cerebrovascular accident and coronary occlusion in anesthesia. JAMA 182:332–334, 1962
5. Arkins R, Smessaert AA, Hicks, RG: Mortality and morbidity in surgical patients with coronary artery disease. JAMA 190:485–488, 1964
6. Mauney FM, Ebert PA, Sabiston DC: Postoperative myocardial infarction: A study of predisposing factors, diagnosis and mortality in a high risk group of surgical patients. Ann Surg 172:497–502, 1970
7. Tarhan S. Moffitt EA, Taylor WF, et al: Myocardial infarction after general anesthesia. JAMA 20:1451–1454, 1972
8. Steen PA, Tinker JH, Tarhan S: Myocardial reinfarction after anesthesia and surgery. JAMA 239:2566–2570, 1978.
9. Logue RB, Kaplan JA: Surgery in patients with heart disease: Medical management in non-cardiac surgery. In Hurst JW (ed): The Heart (ed 4). New York, McGraw-Hill, 1978, pp 1762–1777
10. Miller MG, Hall SV: Intraaortic balloon counterpulsation in a high risk cardiac patient undergoing emergency gastrectomy. Anesthesiology 42:103–105, 1975
11. Mehigan JT, Buch WS, Pipkin RD, et al: A planned approach to coexistent cerebrovascular

disease in coronary artery bypass candidates. Arch Surg 112:1403–1409, 1977

12. Hales CA, Kazemi H: Pulmonary function after uncomplicated myocardial infarction. Chest 72:350–358, 1977

13. Hales CA, Kazemi H: Small airways function in myocardial infarction. N Engl J Med 290:761–765, 1974

14. Wagner S, Cohn K: Heart failure: A proposed definition and classification. Arch Intern Med 137:675–678, 1977

15. Lemberg L: Digitalis in congestive heart failure: Fact or fancy. Arch Intern Med 138:451–452, 1978

16. Rotman M, Treblasser JH: A clinical follow-up study of right and left bundle branch block. Circulation 51:477–484, 1975

17. Goldman L, Caldera DL, Nussbaum SR, et al: Multifactorial index of cardiac risk in non-cardiac surgical procedures. N. Engl J Med 297:845–850, 1977

18. Prys-Roberts C, Meloche R, Foex P: Studies of anesthesia in relation to hypertension. I. Cardiovascular responses of treated and untreated patients. Br J Anaesth 43:122–136, 1971

19. Terazi RC, Frolich E, Dustin HP: Plasma volume in man with essential hypertension. N Engl J Med 278:762–765, 1968

20. Foster MW, Gayle RF: Dangers in combining reserpine and electroconvulsive therapy. JAMA 159:1520–1522, 1955

21. Ominsky AJ, Wollman H: Hazards of general anesthesia in the reserpinized patient. Anesthesiology 30:443–446, 1969

22. Kaplan JA, Dunbar RW: Propranolol and surgical anesthesia. Anesth Analg 55:1–5, 1976

23. Burns-Cox GJ: Return to normal of electrocardiogram after myocardial infarction. Lancet 1:1194–1197, 1967

24. Parker JO, Augustine RJ, Burton JR, et al: Effect of nitroglycerin ointment on the clinical and he-

modynamic response to exercise. Am J Cardiol 38:162–166, 1976

25. Forrester JS, Swan HJC: Acute myocardial infarction: A physiological basis of therapy. Crit Care Med 2:283–293, 1974

26. Crexells C, Chatterjee K. Forrester JS, et al: Optimal level of filling pressure in the left side of the heart in acute myocardial infarction. N Engl J Med 289:1263–1266, 1973

27. Forrester JS, Diamond G, Chatterjee K, et al: Medical therapy of acute myocardial infarction by application of hemodynamic subsets. N Engl J Med 295:1356–1362, 1404–1413, 1976

28. Kaplan JA, King SB: The precordial electrocardiographic lead (V_5) in patients with coronary artery disease. Anesthesiology 45:570–574, 1976

29. Kaplan JA, Steinhaus JE: The heart and anesthesia. In Hurst JW, Logue RB (eds): The Heart (ed 4). New York, McGraw-Hill, 1978, pp 1758–1762

30. Zaidan J, Philbin DM, Antonio R, et al: Hemodynamic effects of metocurine in patients with coronary artery disease receiving propranolol. Anesth Analg 56:255–259, 1977

31. Benzinger TH: Heat regulation: Homeostasis of central temperature in man. Physiol Rev 49:671–759, 1969

32. Siler JN, Rosenberg H, Kaplan JA, et al: Hypoxemia after upper abdominal surgery. Ann Surg 179:149–155, 1974

33. Stephenson HE, Reid LL, Hinton JW: Some common denominators in 1200 cases of cardiac arrest. Ann Surg 137:731–744, 1953

34. Rackow H, Salanitre E, Green LT: Frequency of cardiac arrest with anesthesia in infants and children. Pediatrics 28:697–704, 1961

35. Driscoll A. Hobika JH, Etstein BE, et al: Postoperative myocardial infarction. N Engl J Med 264:633–639, 1961

36. Cooperman LH, Price HL: Pulmonary edema in the operative and postoperative period: A review of 40 cases. Ann Surg 172:883–891, 1970

PART III

Support of the Circulation

Donald C. Finlayson, M.D.
Joel A. Kaplan, M.D.

12
Cardiopulmonary Bypass

The conduct of cardiopulmonary bypass (CPB) is a complex and sophisticated process. Nevertheless it is, today, relatively safe, efficient, and commonplace. Its historic roots go back to LeGallois, who, in 1812, first suggested the idea of tissue perfusion, and to Von Frey and Gruber, who, in 1858, built the first heart-lung machine.[1,2] The physiology of organ system perfusion was intensively studied for many years by workers such as Alexis Carrel, but the numerous suggestions for a surgical approach to many of the cardiovascular disorders were to no avail.[3] It was not until 1951, with the development of heparin, protamine, the sophisticated plastics, and modern electronics, together with the knowledge gained from the basic science laboratories and heart catheterization, that all of these were drawn together to permit the first use of cardiopulmonary bypass for open heart surgery in man.[4-6]

To examine this process, we will discuss the equipment, the prime, the physiological events accompanying its use, and the conduct of bypass from the standpoint of perfusion and the patient.

EQUIPMENT

The equipment basically consists of the following apparatus:

Pump
Tubing and other circuit components: connectors, filters, heat exchangers, reservoirs
Oxygenator
Sensors: transducers and monitors that permit assessment and control of the process

Pump

The pump of the oxygenator circuit should have the capacity to provide the equivalent of a basal cardiac output under the circumstances of perfusion, working against a moderate pressure gradient. It should be easily calibrated and controlled and operable manually or by a self-contained power source if necessary. It should provide flow with minimal development of turbulence and shear forces and minimal risk to the integrity of the blood.

Many pumps have been used for perfusion.

If one were to start with a desire to imitate nature, then a pulsatile flow apparatus giving reasonably physiological pulse contours would seem to be desirable. Indeed, just such a pump was designed by Hooker in 1911.[7] However, the small size of the arterial inflow connectors in the conventional heart-lung machine in relation to the larger size of the aorta to which it is connected would tend to dampen these physiological contours and render them less physiological. In addition, it is well known that nonpulsatile flow is present and reasonably well tolerated with severe coarctation of the aorta. As a consequence, pulsatile flow, although considered essential for long-term isolated organ perfusion, has not been thought to be essential for routine cardiopulmonary bypass.[8,9] Developmental efforts in this area therefore led to a variety of continuous-flow nonpulsatile pumps and the eventual adoption of the double-roller type in most common use today (Fig. 12-1).

This apparatus has rollers at either end of an arm pierced in the center by the power drive shaft. The rollers are driven in a circular course, half of whose traverse is through a shaped, semicircular channel containing the blood-filled pump tubing. The tubing is firmly attached at each end of the channel to prevent "creeping" or forward displacement by the rollers, which by compression of the tubing drive the contents forward. Also, they may be adjusted to produce

significant negative pressure to aspirate blood from the surgical field and the heart chambers, returning it to the oxygenator.

These pumps are rugged, dependable, and convenient. Their clinical performance has been such that there has been, until recently, little interest in other varieties, either pulsatile or nonpulsatile. A recent exception has been the nonpulsatile centripetal noncompressing pump reported by Olsen and associates.[10]

Another exception has been the continuation of counterpulsation during bypass to give pulsatile perfusion in those patients in whom the balloon was present preoperatively. Operation of the balloon pump can be continued after the heart has been arrested by the use of a triggering device. This may be (1) a built-in or an added-on pacemaker component of the balloon pump itself; (2) an ECG simulator, with its signal output connected to the IABP; or (3) a separate pacemaker, if the IABP circuit does not have a capacity to reject the very short pacemaker spikes. This can be done by putting the pacemaker signal adjacent to or through the leads of the balloon ECG cable. Another approach has been the pulsatile assist device proposed by Bregman.[11] It is a compressible conduit placed in the arterial line just proximal to the inflow cannula. It contains a one-way valve system inside a rigid chamber and is subject to intermittent square-wave pneumatic compression.

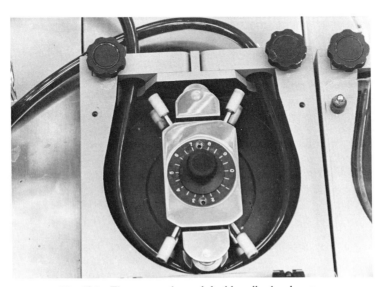

Fig. 12.1   The commonly used double-roller head pump.

This has the effect of giving a pulsatile flow in the aorta downstream from the aortic cannula. This has a disadvantage of exaggerating what is often a very severe degree of cannula-to-aorta pressure gradient and in applying acute acceleration forces to the stream of blood going through the cannula during periods of peak applied pressure. These forces are accompanied by high degrees of shear, turbulence, and jet forces, possibly with cavitation and microbubble formation during the period of peak flow and acceleration.[12–20] Their potential hazard in relation to expected benefits is not yet clear. On a short-term basis the benefits would appear mainly to apply to the kidney and be capable of reducing renin–angiotensin activity and aldosterone secretion. Longer-term, pulsatile flow would appear to be clearly superior for the preservation of organ function.[3] It is therefore possible that the efforts to use bypass procedures

for longer periods of time in the management of such conditions as acute respiratory failure will lead to the further examination of these problems.

With the conventional use of a bubble or disc oxygenator, there is usually one pump for arterial inflow, one for venting or emptying of the heart, and one or two for aspiration of free blood from the surgical field (Figs. 12-2, 12-3). The venous blood will be returned to most oxygenator systems by gravity. Some of the membrane oxygenators, however, e.g., Travenol (Modulung), will require a further pump to maintain the transit of venous blood through the oxygenator to the arterial side. Accessory pumps will also be required (usually two in number) if separate perfusion of the coronary arteries is to be carried out in an attempt to preserve myocardial tissue during such procedures as aortic valve replacement. These will take arterialized

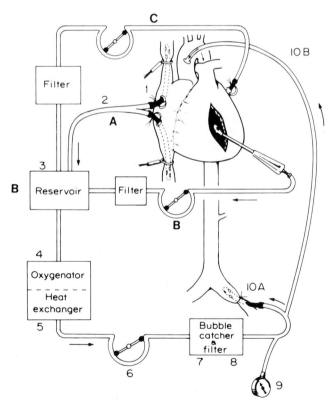

Fig. 12-2. A commonly used cardiopulmonary bypass circuit is demonstrated. The blood may be returned either to femoral artery or the ascending aorta. (Modified and reproduced from Nose Y: The Oxygenator, St. Louis, CV Mosby, 1973, with permission of the author and publisher.)

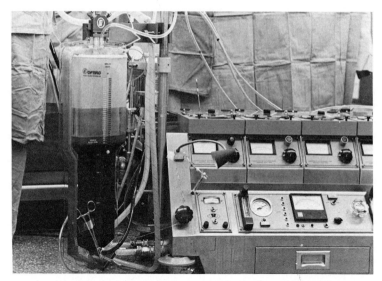

Fig. 12-3. Actual cardiopulmonary bypass circuit is shown. The system consists of an optiflo I bubble oxygenator, and 4 Cinco modular roller pumps.

blood from the heart-lung machine into a reservoir and through each pump head independently into the coronary artery perfusion cannulae.

The amount of trauma to blood cells from apparatus of this sort is relatively small. The application of positive pressure to the cells being driven forward is generally low and well tolerated, especially when the pump head is minimally or just incompletely occlusive. The negative pressures used during suction are significant, however, and may be on the order of several hundred millimeters. Forces of this magnitude are less well tolerated. It must be noted that much of the damage to red cells during bypass is associated with the frothing, violent turbulence, acceleration, and shear forces of negative pressures generated by the suction apparatus and is associated only to a lesser degree with the action of the pumps producing forward flow, or even with the gas interface system to be found in the oxygenator itself.[21-23] Tissue lysosomes and blood left in the pericardial or pleural cavities for prolonged periods also contribute to the cell damage. In addition, there may be enough trauma to the plastic tubing so as to displace small particles of plastic.[24] Most of it will be picked up by the arterial filtering system. All this would seem to indicate that the ordinary roller pump and oxygenator may be

used for some time with minimal risk to red blood cells. The risk–hemolysis will depend for the most part upon the amount and duration of the suction used during a procedure[25] (Fig. 12-4).

Tubing and Other Circuit Components

Other components of the extracorporeal circuit are the tubing, interlinking connectors, filters, and heat exchanger. Although each has its specific effects, they should, in general, be considered in relation to their thromboresistance and effects on flow.

The tubing should have the following characteristics:

1. Be clear, nonwettable, and have a low surface tension
2. Be chemically inert and thromboresistant
3. Have a smooth internal finish and low resistance to flow
4. Tolerate the use of a roller pump without change in shape, undue disruption, or particle release into the perfusate
5. Have minimal priming volumes

The present pump tubing, Tygon S-50-HL or B-44-3, has fair thromboresistance and can be used for relatively long periods of time with minimal risk to the integrity of the formed elements and proteins of the blood. Thromboresistance has been thought to be conferred mainly by materials with nonwettable surfaces; however, there is still a great deal of dispute in regard to the characteristics needed for thromboresistance.[26] Indeed, many of the more recent materials have been developed, at least in part, by trial and error.

An attempt to categorize these materials has been made by Gott.[27] They are described as falling into three basic categories:

1. Those made of inert materials
2. Those possessing an electronegative surface charge
3. Those containing surface-bound heparin or heparinoids

These newer materials have appeared in such equipment as the intra-aortic balloon and might reasonably be expected to appear in other cardiopulmonary bypass components in the near future.[28,29]

Resistance to flow and priming volumes will govern the diameter of tubing used. Smaller tubes can be used in children; that is, when lower blood flows are required and when smaller priming volumes should be used. These are illustrated in Table 12-1.

The structural integrity of pump tubing is threatened to some degree by the continuous use of a roller pump, and some fragmentation of the inner surface can occur. The embolization of plastic particles downstream has been reported by Hubbard.[24]

Filtration in the CPB circuit would appear to be necessary.[30] Very high levels of particles have been demonstrated by such techniques as Doppler counting and by filtration studies.[19,31-36] The particles are principally red cell debris and aggregates of platelets and leukocytes. There have also been repeated histological demonstrations of air, fat, silicone, and lint fragments in all tissue beds. Many of these will come from the surgical field. As a consequence, the use of a filter on the cardiotomy and suction systems might be expected to, and in fact does, remove the majority of the particles. The use of a filter

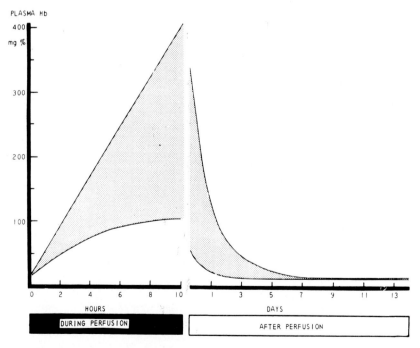

Fig. 12-4. The elevation of plasma hemoglobin during and after cardiopulmonary perfusion is shown. (Reproduced from Galetti PM: Heart-Lung Bypass: Principles and Techniques of Extracorporeal Circulation, New York, Grune & Stratton, 1962, with permission of author and publisher.)

Table 12-1

Patient Weight (kg)	Acceptable Arterial Line Diameters (inches)	Priming Volumes (ml/ft)
Up to 25 kg	¼	9.65
25–40 kg	³/₈	21.71
Above 40	½*	38.61

* Venous tubing in larger children and adults is customarily ½″ in diameter

Note: The customary adult circuit, including a Pall filter in the arterial line, will contain approximately 300 ml on each side—600 ml in total.

on the arterial side will arrest most of the remainder. Small air bubbles, globules of fat, and silicone antifoam material may still pass. With recently improved design, however, the new arterial line filters serve as traps capable of removing most of these latter as well. The Ultipor barrier arterial filter (Pall Corp.) is commonly used. It has a 645-cm² filter area, a pore size of 25–40 μm, and can be used at low resistances with high flows without the development of increased resistance as a result of obstruction by debris.

The Swank Dacron wool filter has a pore size of 80–100 μm, but because it works in part by adsorption of particles on to the fibers of the filter, it functions as though the pore size were much smaller. This results in significant buildup of filtered material which increases flow resistance under some circumstances especially if used at high flows. This phenomenon is most marked at the beginning of bypass or during bypass with episodes of hypotension. This type of filter is most commonly used on the venous cardiotomy system, but a version with a larger filtering surface has been developed for the arterial side of the pumping circuit. Micropore filtration of this sort is also used for the bank blood added to either the perfusion system or directly to the patient.

The development of better materials for manufacture of the heart-lung machine components and more adequate filtration have resulted in less hematologic disturbances and have been associated with a continuing reduction in the risk of disturbance in all organ functions. This has been particularly apparent in regard to brain and lungs but must have been of benefit to every organ system.

The heat exchanger is an essential component of each bypass circuit. The Brown-Harrison and Sarns models have been used for many years, are made of stainless steel and are thus reusable, but they increase the priming volume and may present problems related to their cleaning, e.g., pyrogenic reactions or logistic difficulties (Fig. 12-5). They have sufficient resistance to flow to necessitate their placement on the arterial side and thus, with rewarming, pose the risk of bubble generation owing to the reduction of gas solubility in the blood being rewarmed. For bubble oxygenators, these considerations have led to the inclusion of the heat exchanger in one of the oxygenator chambers. This has had the dual value of simplifying and reducing the internal volume of the circuit, and, as a consequence, reducing its priming volume. The risk of bubble formation is still present however—hence the continued necessity for a distal bubble trap.

The heat exchanger is just that—an energy-exchanging system whose function may be described in terms of its heat transfer coefficient

$$\text{Heat transfer coefficient} = \frac{\text{blood temperature change: inlet - outlet}}{\text{inlet temperature difference: blood - water}}$$

To enhance efficiency, the flows of blood and water are usually arranged in a countercurrent fashion. The temperature control and source of the water are the ordinary hot and cold water system, which can be augmented by active water cooling if necessary.

Figure 12-6 presents the mean warming times of two extracorporeal bubble oxygenators' integral heat exchangers. One set of curves rep-

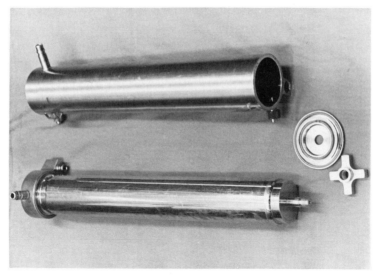

Fig. 12-5.   The Sarns heat-exchanger is shown disassembled for sterilization.

resents a more effective caloric heat-exchange device, the Bentley Laboratories Inc., BOS 10; and the other curves represent the Cobe Laboratories Inc., Optiflo I.[37]

Two matched groups of 10 male coronary bypass patients were exposed to identical extracorporeal circuits except for the blood oxygenator and integral heat exchanger. Patient body surface area, weight, age, and cardiac index during warming were similar in each group. The temperature gradient between water into the heat exchanger and venous blood into the oxygenator was maintained at 10°C or less, and the water-in temperature was not allowed to exceed 42°C.

The esophageal temperature leads the rectal temperature after the initiation of warming. The warming curves are not linear with time. As the temperature gradient between venous blood-in and water-in decreases, the heat flow to the patient decreases, hence warming curves show an exponential rise. The BOS 10 delivers more kilocalories per minute at the same temperature gradient, blood flow, and heat exchanger water flow; therefore, the BOS 10 group reached 37° more rapidly with a similar total number of kilocalories being delivered to the patient in both groups.

Physiological response to rapid warming of a patient on total CPB must be monitored carefully with the use of greater capacity heat-ex-change devices. Patients warmed more rapidly in this protocol had substantially lower peripheral vascular resistance at the termination of bypass and the immediate postbypass period. In the patients warmed at a slower rate, the total body oxygen consumption was, on the average, 40 percent greater at the same temperatures during the warming period suggesting a more uniform temperature distribution. Rapid warming of a hypothermic patient may not be indicated if oxygen consumption during warming is to be maximized, thus avoiding a late oxygen debt and large carbon dioxide production at the end of warming.

The connectors linking the components of the system and the patient should be designed and finished so as to maintain smooth laminar rather than turbulent flow, without significant development of eddy currents, or cavitation caused by abrupt interior contour changes due to such things as stenoses, or ridges at tubing junctions. One problem of this type is seen in the arterial connections. Aortic arch cannulae usually have a smoothly curved right-angle bend leading to a narrowed segment that is inserted into the aorta. Those for the femoral artery taper internally and have a double curve, which permits them, with their tubing, to lie flat on the outside of the leg. High pressures may be required to deliver the pump output through such stenoses.[38] The relationship between pumping

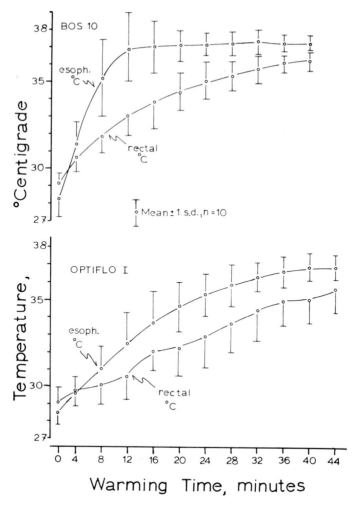

Fig. 12-6. Warming times of two extracorporeal oxygenators internal heat exchangers are shown. See text for details.

pressures and flow volumes with some of the commonly used aortic cannulae is illustrated in Figure 12-7. There is also marked flow acceleration of the stream of red cells through the narrowed segment, with their exit in the case of the aorta, into a vessel of markedly larger diameter with the consequent development of shear forces, convection and eddy currents, and a marked fall in pressure. This has the potential for microbubble generation and red cell and platelet disruption and may be one of the factors leading to the destabilization of blood.[19]

In addition, aortic cannulation may lead to dissection, brought about either mechanically or by the stream of blood in the presence of atherosclerotic lesions. The stream of blood itself may, with improper placement, direct the flow largely at the ostium of the innominate artery, leading to very high pressures and flows in the distribution of that side of the cerebral circulation and low pressures in the rest of the arterial tree, or the stream of blood may be so placed as to lead to hypoperfusion in that side of the cerebral circulation.[39] When the femoral artery is used, the flow is exiting into a vessel of small size leading to a larger one and whose lumen may be further compromised by atherosclerotic disease. This may preclude adequate pump output and may also lead to arterial dissection.

Oxygenator

Blood may be made to take up oxygen and eliminate carbon dioxide in several ways. The basic types of apparatus for this purpose may be categorized in terms of their interface with blood:

1. With gas interface
   a. Disc
   b. Vertical screen
   c. Bubble
2. Without gas interface
   a. Membrane
      (1) Solid
      (2) Microporous
         (a) Sheet-membrane
         (b) Expanded-membrane
   b. Fluid–Fluid-using fluorocarbon liquid

Except for the experimental fluid-fluid oxygenators, the others, at least in rudimentary or crude form, were developed at the outset of open heart surgery and further refined with the passage of time. The disc and vertical screen oxygenators have proved somewhat cumbersome to clean, prepare, and re-sterilize. As cardiovascular surgical services have become busier, reusable equipment has been gradually, but progressively, displaced by the more convenient disposable units. In the main, these latter were initially bubble oxygenators, but with increasing sophistication in design and production, the membrane types have become more economical, more efficient, and less traumatic to blood. Currently available bubble oxygenators are shown in Figures 12-8, 12-9 and 12-10 and listed in Table 12-2.

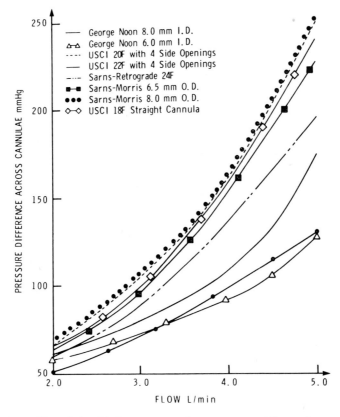

Fig. 12-7. The relationship between pumping pressures and flow volumes with some commonly used aortic cannulae is demonstrated (Reproduced from Hwang NHC: Hydraulic studies of aortic cannulation return nozzles. Trans Am Soc Artif Intern Organs 21:234, 1975 with permission of author and publisher).

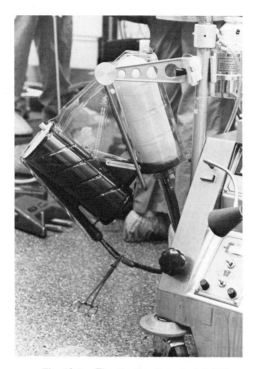

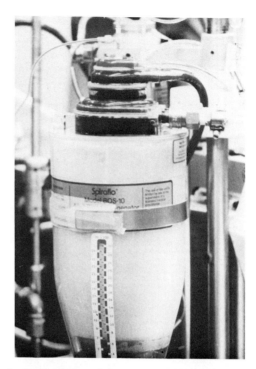

Fig. 12-8. The Bentley-Temptrol Q-200 oxygenator is shown in (A) and the new Bentley Bos-10 in (B).

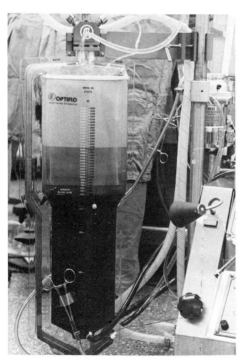

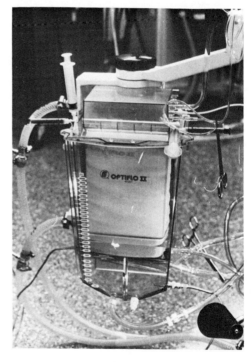

Fig. 12-9. The Galen-Cobe Optiflo I oxygenator is demonstrated in (A) and the new Optiflo II in (B).

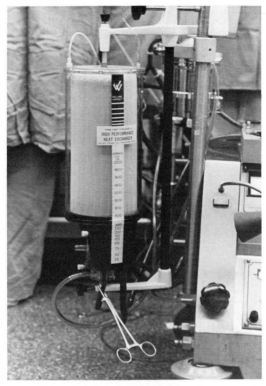

Fig. 12-10. The Harvey oxygenator is demonstrated.

Table 12-2
Critical Volumes for a Variety of Bubble Oxygenators

Manufacturer	Priming Volume (ml)	Oxygenator Column Dynamic Hold-up Volume at Gas:Blood Q 1:1
William Harvey Research		
H 1000	700	200
H 800	450	150
H 400	400	100
Cobe Laboratories		
Optiflo I	800	300
Optiflo II	750	350
Bentley		
Bos 10	650	175
Q 200 A	900	350
Q 110	800	300
Q 130	550	250
Shiley Laboratories		
S 100	700	200

In the bubble oxygenator, the ventilating gases, O_2 and CO_2, are passed through multiple perforations in a diffusing plate, giving rise to bubbles 2–7 mm in diameter which exit into the venous blood at the bottom of what is usually a columnar reservoir.[17,40,41] This produces frothing and turbulence which assists in driving the now partly arterialized blood forward into a debubbling section. The perforations in the diffusing plate and the consequent bubble size are carefully controlled to give bubbles that are not too small, the larger being more readily removed,[42] and not too large, that is, reasonably effective in terms of gas transfer.[40,41] The relationship between bubble size, their numbers produced by 1 ml of gas, and their surface area is illustrated in Figure 12-11.

The balance of gas exchange, ranging from 25 to 65 percent, may occur in the debubbling section. Therefore, care must be taken to ensure that it is not allowed to become too full. This reduces the area available for gas exchange, rendering it less efficient. This is most likely to occur to a significant degree in a larger patient or in those in congestive failure, that is, with larger blood volumes; and may be worsened by the administration of α-adrenergic vasopressors. These drugs can cause marked constriction of venous capacitance vessels in the patient, with the consequent displacement of blood from the patient's circulation into the heart-lung machine.

Oxygenation in the bubbler is not membrane-limited as in the normal lung or membrane oxygenator, but depends upon the gas-blood surface contact area, the thickness of the blood film, the mean red blood cell transit time, and

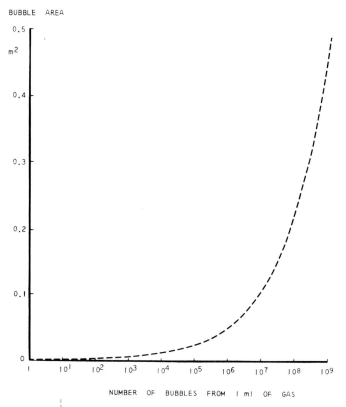

Fig. 12-11. The relationship between bubble size, their number produced by 1 ml of gas and their surface area are illustrated. (Reproduced from Galletti PM: Heart-Lung Bypass: Principles and Techniques of Extracorporeal Circulation. New York, Grune & Stratton, 1962, with permission of author and publisher.)

the partial pressure of oxygen used.[43–45] The gas-blood interfacial surface contact area is usually in the range of 15 m[2].[46] It is governed by the total gas flow and bubble size, since any single amount of gas broken up into a greater number of bubbles will have a greater surface area. The thickness of the blood film will, from a functional standpoint, depend upon the degree of turbulence, and therefore mixing, engendered by the ventilating gasses and apparatus design. The smallest of bubbles will have a much larger surface area and be much more efficient, but they are more stable and thus more difficult to remove.[42] As a compromise, larger bubbles are used. This approach results in an effectively thicker film. Since the time required for oxygenation is a function of the square of the film thickness, and the process is therefore less efficient, a red cell mean transit time of 1 to 2 seconds, longer than that of the normal lung (.1 to 0.75 seconds), is also used. The result for most bubblers in current use is a flow of gas through the oxygenator column that must be at least equal to the flow of blood to maintain both reasonable flow and gas exchange. Because of its increased solubility, this exchange is much more efficient with respect to CO_2 elimination than O_2 uptake. This is true for most bubble oxygenators. In fact, with O_2 flows sufficient to produce acceptable arterial O_2 tensions, in almost all bubble oxygenators, the addition of carbon dioxide is required to avoid hypocarbia and maintain normal arterial tensions.

Initially in many centers, fixed O_2-CO_2 mixtures were used. It soon became apparent, however, that this was an unsatisfactory approach to the problem. Carbon dioxide solubility varies inversely and CO_2 output varies directly with the temperature. As a consequence, with rapid cooling, more carbon dioxide will be needed for addition to the mixture to maintain a normal P_aCO_2; with rewarming, less CO_2 will be needed. Optimal control thus demands separate flowmeters for both O_2 and CO_2. The importance of precision in the control of the P_aCO_2 lies, for the most part, in its effects on the metabolic state, the autonomic nervous system, catecholamine secretion, and thus on organ system blood flow and function. Using the central nervous system as an example, it has been known for many years that low levels of P_aCO_2 are capable of producing significant reductions in cerebral blood flow and tissue oxygen tensions.

Further, the oxyhemoglobin dissociation curve may be markedly shifted under the circumstances of bypass, and double leftward shifts, such as those produced by alkalosis and hypothermia, are not at all uncommon (Fig. 12-12). It can be seen from inspection of the oxyhemoglobin dissociation curve that at a pH of 7.60 and a temperature of 28°, the shift would have reduced the available oxygen to extremely low levels, thus making very little available for respiratory activity in tissue. This might be expressed in a number of ways: as an increase in oxygen affinity or as a reduction in the P_{50}. In any case, one must realize that hypothermia and alkalosis are a double hazard to be avoided at all costs.

For most adult oxygenators, 6 liters/min of flow output can be maintained with adequate oxygenation. However this flow requirement may be exceeded if the lean body mass is particularly large or if the peripheral demand, in the face of hemodilution and reduced oxygen delivery, is so great as to produce marked venous desaturation. Under these circumstances the venous oxygen content may be so low that, even with longer oxygenator transit time, it may not be possible to add significant amounts of oxygen to raise the tension to normal levels. The result will be an oxygen debt marked initially by ven-

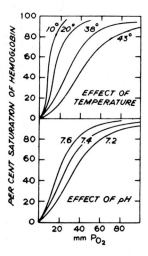

Fig. 12-12. The hemoglobin dissociation curves are shown at normal pH and with the effects of temperature and pH. Alkalosis and hypothermia produce a double leftward shift of the curve. (Reproduced from Comroe JH: Physiology of Respiration, Chicago, Yearbook Medical Publishers, 1965, with permission of author and publisher.)

ous desaturation and shortly thereafter by lowered arterial oxygen tensions. Impairment of oxygen exchange may also be brought about by overfilling of the debubbling section in which, for many oxygenators, much of the total gas exchange may be taking place.

The bubble oxygenator conducts venous blood by gravity to the bottom of the oxygenator column through which is passed a stream of fine bubbles. The bubbles and a certain minimal total gas flow are necessary to carry the blood up the column and to produce sufficient turbulence so as to increase the gas-bubble contact in the form of froth in which a significant part of the gas exchange may take place.

The oxygenator must therefore contain a section in which the exhaled gases can be vented and the bubbles removed. The exhalation port on most devices is a simple duct, usually in the debubbling section, from which the exhaust gases can be directed into a scavenging system if inhalational agents have been used.

Debubbling is effected by a combination of settling and defoaming. The blood is allowed to settle through a smooth flow pathway to the reservoir area at the most dependent part of the oxygenator. As the bubbles are brought into this section, they are broken up by contact with surfaces treated with a surface-tension-reducing agent, most commonly, Dow Corning Medical Antifoam-A. The treated surface is usually in the form of a sponge, a mesh, or a woven material with a relatively large area for surface contact. With gas exchange completed, the blood descends to the reservoir area often containing the heat exchanger and then exits to the arterial pumping system.

One of the measures used to improve the efficiency of oxygenators has been the use of high partial pressures of oxygen. The partial pressure in the oxygenator atmosphere can be estimated by the expression

$$P_{pump} O_2 = (1 \text{ atm} - P_ICO_2 - P_IH_2O) \approx > 650 \text{ mm}$$

The resulting hyperoxia has been the subject of a number of investigations, most of which have concluded that the risk was insignificant, at least for short-term use. As a consequence, oxygenators are ventilated with 100 percent oxygen. In an early study, however, Hyman suggested that high oxygen tensions might be toxic to cytochrome-oxidase and other enzyme systems.[47] Another study by Ashmore and his associates noted that the leukopenia seen with cardiopulmonary bypass could be largely prevented by ventilation of the oxygenator with air rather than oxygen.[31] An increased risk of hemolysis with increased serum hemoglobin levels has also been shown to be associated with high oxygen tensions.[20,48,49] These studies lend support to the need for methods of precise blood gas control, such as in-line O_2 electrodes, which would permit the maintenance of more physiological arterial O_2 tensions (150 torr or less).

Another method of achieving this objective might be the addition of the inert gases, either nitrogen or nitrous oxide, to the oxygenator gas mixture. This has generally been avoided because it was feared that there might be a risk of more stable, less easily eliminated bubbles using an insoluble gas in a patient whose body stores were largely saturated with this gas.[50] The risk is obviously greater in bubble rather than membrane oxygenators. Also, it was feared that there might be lack of fine control of the final oxygen tension levels with the consequent risk of hypoxia. However, the arterial filtering systems currently in common use would appear to reduce the risk of the former and the newer in-line polarographic and chromatographic oxygen analyzers would appear to permit a sufficient degree of control of oxygen tension.

Volatile anesthetic agents may also be added to the ventilating gas mixture of the oxygenator. This is usually done by the insertion into the gas line of a flow- and temperature-compensated anesthetic vaporizer. When this is done, although little information is available in this area, several things must be kept in mind. The oxygenator is somewhat inefficient, and this might be reflected in some degree of inhibition of drug-to-blood transfer. Anesthetic transport and behavior might be altered by the changes in blood-gas partition coefficient brought about by hemodilution and hypothermia.[51] With hypothermia, the coefficient may rise as much as 40 or 50 percent. This rise is prevented by hemodilution. The final value at normothermia in these circumstances is below normal. At a constant inspired gas concentration, investigators have noted an increased rate of rise of tissue anesthetic tensions in vessel-rich tissues. Finally, it must be remembered that an insufficient amount of the agent may have been vaporized. Accuracy in terms of volume percent output of many such vaporizers falls off very markedly with gas flows below 4 liters/min. Even if accurate in terms of concentration, at lower gas flows the absolute amount of the agent being vaporized in milliliters may also be inadequate (Fig. 12-13).

Current membrane oxygenators and their priming volumes are shown in Table 12-3. The membrane oxygenator does not have a true blood gas interface; instead, blood passes between layers of membrane on the other side of which is the gas phase. The membrane is arranged in flat, stacked or coiled sheets, or in a tubular array. The idea that membrane surfaces could be used medically for gas exchange during cardiopulmonary bypass might obviously be expected to follow the contemplation of nature. Gas transfer across dialysis membranes was noted in the early artificial kidney by Kolff.[52] Indeed, animal lungs were used in some of the original investigations of membrane surfaces.[53] With the rapid advance of technology in this area, however, the membranes have become more efficient, more reliable, and less expensive.[54,55]

The membranes are basically of two types: (1) solid or (2) microporous (Fig. 12-14). Although the search for membrane materials has encompassed many types of materials, the solid types are mainly varying forms of silicone rubber. They depend in part for their function on the gas-transfer characteristics of this material

and the technology permitting its manufacture in sheets thin enough to be effective, since diffusion is to some extent a function of membrane thickness; and strong enough to maintain its integrity. It is a matter of good fortune that silicone rubber, one of the first materials to be investigated in relation to its diffusing capacity for oxygen and carbon dioxide, proved to be one of the most satisfactory materials.

The microporous types are (1) simple, that is, formed in plain thin sheets, or (2) expanded, slightly thicker and more matted formulation. The microporous materials are mainly polypropylene, Teflon, and polyacrylamide. They contain a multitude of small pores 0.1–5.0 μm in size, which, in the initial contact with blood, induce a mild degree of protein denaturation and platelet agglutination. This appears to combine with the protein lying immediately above it to give a relatively fixed and nonmoving layer that is essentially cell-free, in effect becoming part of the membrane-bending nature to the purpose of art and, in the process, giving rise to a very efficient system.[33,46] A system that, from a functional point of view, behaves as though no blood-gas interface were present; instead the barrier acts like a true membrane. The protein layer, once formed, "cures" or stabilizes the membrane, reducing its subsequent reactivity with respect to blood. The protein-membrane surface tension effectively isolates the blood and

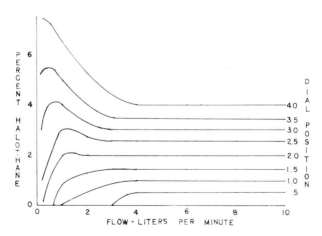

Fig. 12-13. The performance of the Fluotec Mark II vaporizer is demonstrated at different flow rates. (Reproduced from Dorsch JA: Understanding Anesthesia Equipment. Baltimore, Williams & Wilkins, 1975, with permission of author and publishers.)

Table 12-3
Priming Volumes of Available Membrane
Oxygenators

Manufacturer	Type	Priming Volume (ml)
Travenol		
TMO Membrane	Microporous	200
Advanced Sci-Med		
Kolobow Membrane (2.5 m²)	Solid	200
Edwards Laboratories		
Lande-Edwards Membrane	Solid	400

gas phases, preventing their mixing. Mixing "pulmonary edema" can develop if the system is primed with a crystalloid or protein-free solution and then allowed to stand for a protracted period or if the perfusion pressure exceeds the membrane surface tension. The Travenol microporous lung can tolerate pressures in the blood phase of 125 torr at flows in the range of 6 liters/min. However, function of this membrane is compromised with time. Its gas exchange capacity deteriorates significantly after 5 hours.[46] These changes are not seen with the solid membranes.

Gas exchange through a membrane device is limited by characteristics of the membrane,[54-56] and the degree of convection and mixing in the film of blood on its other side. The silicone membranes have $CO_2:O_2$ transfer capacities of 5:1 or 6:1 rather than the lower ratios characteristic of other materials and thus more closely resemble the situation in the lung. As the gas-transfer characteristics of the membrane have improved, another obstacle has become apparent. The boundary layer, the thin layer of plasma immediately adjacent to the membrane, moves slowly enough in relation to the movement of the remainder of the film of blood to act as a significant impediment to gas exchange—more to O_2 than CO_2, because of oxygen's lower solubility. Recent changes in design have been directed at the production of a variety of irregularities in the blood film pathways that would

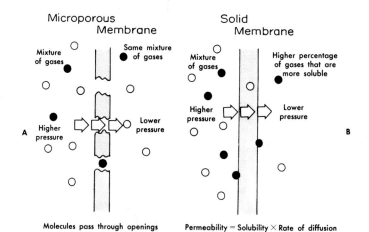

Fig. 12-14. The two basic types of membrane-oxygenators are demonstrated. On the left, the microporous membrane and on the right the solid membrane. (Reproduced from Nose Y: The Oxygenator, St. Louis, CV Mosby, 1973, with permission of author and publisher.)

induce convection and mixing sufficient to reduce the effective thickness of the boundary layer or to thin the layer by external compression of the membrane ("shim pressure" mechanism in the Travenol lung).

These changes are a necessary compensation for the fact that it has not proved possible to produce membranes or capillary tubes with a film thickness comparable to those found in human capillaries. The boundary layer is not a significant impediment to CO_2 exchange, but it is for oxygen. As a result, despite the higher gas-to-blood partial pressure differences for oxygen in the apparatus, the higher solubility of CO_2 results, in many membranes, in an effective gas permeability ratio for $CO_2 : O_2$ of 20:1, which is analogous to that of the lung.

After it initially reacts with and becomes coated by the blood proteins, a membrane oxygenator should be, and in fact is, less disruptive to blood than is a bubble oxygenator. For use in routine perfusions, the membrane lung appears to produce some changes that may be of immediate benefit to the patient in terms of lessened morbidity—principally, less risk of bleeding.[57] Again, however, it must be emphasized

that for short-term use, the greatest contribution to the disruption of the integrity of blood probably comes from the suction system common to both oxygenators. Whether due entirely to this or not, it has proved difficult to demonstrate a substantial benefit from a membrane rather than a bubble oxygenator for these short-term perfusions.

The blood flow requirements for patients during CPB that any type of oxygenator should be able to satisfy may be described in terms of milliliters per kilogram of body weight or milliliters per square meter of body surface area. One such example is shown in Figure 12-15.

In one of the earlier specifications for heart-lung machines, the suggested flow capacity was 3.1 liters/min/m² or 60–85 ml/kg of body weight per minute. In evaluating any single level of pump "cardiac" output, it must be born in mind that the oxygen delivery equation

$$O_2 \text{ Delivery} = Q \times (CaO_2 \times Hgb \times 1.34) + (P_aO_2 \times 0.003)$$

indicates that delivery is a function of cardiac output and oxygen-carrying capacity and that

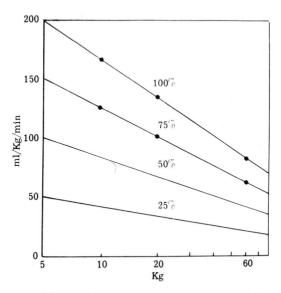

Fig. 12-15. Blood flow requirements for patients on cardiopulmonary bypass are demonstrated. They are described in terms of milliliters per kilogram of body weight per minute. Flow rates are shown that will produce between 25 and 100 percent of normal cardiac outputs. (Reproduced from Peirce EC: Extracorporeal circulation for open-heart surgery. Springfield, Ill., 1969, Charles C. Thomas, with permission of author and publisher).

there is a certain basal requirement of oxygen that must be satisfied. A more satisfactory way of describing the process, in fact, might be in terms of the amount of oxygenated hemoglobin pumped per minute. With dilution of carrying capacity, the output must be increased or the total demand reduced (e.g., by hypothermia) in order to match supply with demand. It must be assumed that, at normothermia, total tissue oxygen delivery may be insufficient, even with increased peripheral oxygen extraction. Standard flow rates on CPB are:

Adults: 2.2–2.5 liters/min/m², or 50–80 ml/kg/min

Children: 2.2–2.6 liters/min/m²;
           Reduce flow by 7 percent for each degree celsius decrease in body temperature (Fig. 12-18).

PHYSIOLOGY OF CARDIOPULMOMARY BYPASS

Prime of the Heart-Lung Machine

Many solutions have been used to prime the oxygenator. These have ranged from all-blood primes to the use of a variety of solutions such as 5 percent dextrose and water, alone or in combination with saline, balanced electrolyte solutions, albumin, dextran, polyvinylpyrrolidone (PVP), hydroxyethyl starch, the buffers $NaHCO_3$ and THAM, and mannitol.[58-63] In addition, at least on an experimental basis, the antiplatelet drugs dipyrridamole, sulfinpyrazone, and aspirin have been used.[64-67]

The usual prime for adult patients at Emory University Hospital is as follows:

Balanced salt solution Plasmalyte 148-Baxter	1000 ml
Dextran 40	500 ml
Mannitol 15 percent	300 ml
Total volume	= 1800 ml
Osmolarity	= 320 mOsm
pH	= 7.32 − 7.35

The priming volumes vary with the size of the oxygenator used and the tubing volume; most oxygenators for use in adult patients have priming volumes of 1500–2000 ml. Those used for children are scaled down, and a number of sizes may be used, with priming volumes as small as 140 ml. The extra volumes required for the priming of the tubing, external heat exchangers, or coronary perfusion apparatus must be added to the volume for the oxygenator. Typical priming volumes for a variety of apparatus in current use are given in Tables 12-2 and 12-3.

The *basic principle* governing the management of the connection of a patient to the cardiopulmonary bypass circuit is to do so in a fashion requiring minimal metabolic adaptation on the part of the patient. In terms of ideal prime composition, this of necessity means primes as close in composition to that of extracellular fluid as possible. For most purposes, this has been interpreted to mean the use of a balanced salt solution with or without supplemental Ca^{++} and Mg^{++}. Calcium has been omitted by many groups in the hope of reducing oxygen demand in the myocardium and the oxygen debt associated with ischemia. The addition of oncotically active material is not considered universally necessary and, for short-term use, appears to make little difference in terms of lung function specifically or clinical results in general.[68,69] It seems clear, however, that the use of a prime with a reduced oncotic pressure is associated with the need to administer significantly larger amounts of fluid to the patient than would have been the case had the oncotic pressure been maintained at a normal level. For longer procedures, especially when hemodilution of serum proteins has been great enough to produce a significant oncotic reduction, the risk of disruption of fluid exchange at the capillary level in all the organ systems may be a real one. The risk of disturbances of capillary exchange with the associated need to infuse large amounts of fluid into the patient must be balanced against the risk of reactions to the compounds used to bring about the oncotic effect and tempered with the knowledge that their use, under most circumstances, does not appear to be of special benefit. The maintenance of oncotic activity might well be considered to be of value in patients in whom congestive heart failure or renal insufficiency might already be present or anticipated postoperatively, that is, in patients who might be unable to handle significant changes in body compartment size. It must also be borne in mind that primes that are grossly abnormal from a metabolic standpoint have been used with success by many groups. The resulting disturbances appear reasonably well tolerated if accompanied by good surgical and perioperative management.

In the early days of open heart surgery, heart-lung machines were primed entirely with blood. The poor results and difficulties with all-blood primes soon became apparent.[58,70] Prime mixtures resulting in varying degrees of hemo-dilution have since been the rule.[71]

In general, blood should be added to the oxygenator if the patient is markedly anemic or if the volume of the heart-lung machine circuit is large in relation to that of the blood volume of the patient. A good rule of thumb in this regard is that the blood volume of the bypass circuit should not be greater than 30 to 40 percent of that of the patient. In other words, the resultant dilution should not reduce the hema-tocrit value to levels below the range of 20 to 25 percent. Although the hemoglobin dependence of oxygen delivery must be borne in mind, ad-equate delivery of oxygen to tissue can usually be assured even with hemodilution, with the reduction of oxygen demand by 6 or 7 percent per degree celsius brought about by moderate hypothermia (Fig. 12-18). This being the case, hemodilution would appear to have few risks and many benefits.

Despite the increase in plasma viscosity produced by hypothermia, the total viscosity is reduced by the dilution of blood cells and pro-teins. Dilution of the normal patient to hema-tocrit values of 20 to 25 percent is usually ac-companied by a fall in the mean pressure, generally, in the range of 40 percent. Examina-tion of one such group of patients showed that the systemic vascular resistance, corrected for the change in viscosity, did not change signifi-cantly after bypass had been established and that the change in pressure was due to the vis-cosity change alone.[62]

The Effects of Hemodilution

With hemodilution, serum protein concen-tration also falls. Unless there is some substitute for its oncotic pressure in the prime, it can be seen from the consideration of the Starling equa-tion that the transcapillary shift of water to tis-sue will be increased in all organ systems.[72]

$$Q_f = K_f (P_{cap} - P_{int}) \, \partial \, (\pi cap - \pi int)$$

An exception to this may be the lung which, after the start of bypass, is largely isolated by virtue of the use of total CPB, since the bron-chial blood flow is usually such a small part of the cardiac output (1 to 2 percent). This risk in the lungs might be increased in circumstances in which the systemic bronchial artery blood flow was increased (i.e., in some of the congen-ital heart conditions), or with increases in pul-monary artery pressure resulting from circum-stances in which blood gained access to the pulmonary vasculature either in larger amounts than normal, or with progress prevented by mal-functioning venting systems. A Swan-Ganz catheter would be useful in the detection of these problems.[68] Detection would then hope-fully be followed by correction of the circum-stances that led to their development. Excess tissue shifts of fluid will be made evident by the need to continually add fluids to the CPB circuit in order to maintain the same blood level in the oxygenator, that is, to replace the same volume taken up by the patient. This need to add fluid can be minimized by the addition of osmotically active materials to the circuit. Most commonly, these have been albumin, plasma protein frac-tion, plasma, dextran, or mannitol. Other com-pounds, such as hydroxyethyl starch and PVP, have also been used for this purpose. All appear capable of minimizing water transfer to tissues, again expressed as the need to add less crystal-loid solution to the heart-lung machine during bypass. Nevertheless, it is not clearly apparent that they have a significantly beneficial effect in the postoperative period and their use is not without risk.

The changes in body composition associ-ated with the use of hemodilution are very dif-ficult to separate from those of bypass, and in-deed from operation itself.[73-76] Interpretation is made even more difficult by differences in oxy-genator prime and patient management and by the presence or absence of congestive heart fail-ure (CHF) and of its change consequent to op-eration. Several facts about these patients must be kept in mind, however. The cardiac patient with CHF will present with some degree of ex-pansion of the extracellular fluid (ECF) com-partment including the blood volume, with an elevated red blood cell mass, and with impaired handling of the Na^+ and water in this expanded volume. The patient not in failure will be normal in all of these areas and may even be hypovolemic.

With operation, there will be moderate expansion of the ECF compartment in all patients. This increase might be expected to be related to the duration of bypass and to the oncotic pressure of the prime. Part or all of this ECF increase might be nonfunctional and represent a third space. The size of the functional part of this compartment—at least as reflected by the size of its blood volume moiety—may be expanded, normal, or reduced, and the response of the volume regulatory mechanisms may be equally variable. It must be assumed, however, that, as with any other operation, increased levels of glucocorticoids and mineralocorticoids will be seen postoperatively. Despite isotonic expansion of the blood and total ECF at the end of bypass and the maintenance of adequate urinary output, the net effect of the development of a third space and the activation of these mechanisms is to produce moderate degrees of sodium and water retention.

These changes, primarily involving aldosterone, also tend to significantly increase the perioperative rate of potassium loss and may contribute to low serum K^+ values.[77,78] These losses may range from levels of 29 mEq, reported in one group, to over 100 mEq.[74] Other factors that may contribute to this situation are the use of diuretics, hyperventilation, and ECF expansion with fluids isotonic with respect to sodium at a time in which sodium-retaining mechanisms are active. This latter mechanism might be expected to lead to increased rates of intrarenal Na^+-for-K^+ exchange and thus increased K^+ loss. Careful monitoring of the serum and urine K^+ levels is indicated where losses are suspected of being large (e.g., in the patient receiving steroid and diuretic therapy). Monitoring of the P_aCO_2 should permit the avoidance of significant hyperventilation. This monitoring should be accompanied by a program of adequate potassium replacement.

Body compositional changes entailing reductions in Ca^{++}, Mg^{++}, $PO_4^=$, and zinc may also be seen accompanying hemodilution.[79-83] Their significance in the clinical setting is difficult to assess. In the absence of Ca^{++} and Mg^{++} in the prime, total values will decrease with hemodilution, paralleling the decrease in serum proteins; the ionized portions will also fall but to a lesser extent, reflecting the reduced level of protein binding. The addition of citrated bank blood will produce a further marked reduction in ionized Ca^{++}; however, elevated levels of ionized Ca^{++} may have a deleterious effect on myocardial and smooth muscle energy and function. Hypocalcemia, although commonly present, is usually not significant during bypass; nevertheless on occasion administration of Ca^{++} may be a useful adjunct in the management of the hypotension often seen at the start of perfusion.

The role of magnesium is not clear. In the clinical setting, reductions in the total magnesium, and presumably the ionized faction, occur with hemodilution. Intracellular magnesium declines in the anoxic heart. Diuretics may cause magnesium deficiency. Magnesium deficiency may make the heart prone to the development of arrhythmias, especially those associated with the use of digitalis, and its use as an adjunct to therapy may be helpful.

As is evident from consideration of the oxygen delivery equation

$$O_2 \text{ delivery} = Q \times (C_aO_2 \times \text{hemoglobin} \times 1.34) + (P_aO_2 \times 0.003)$$

red blood cell dilution and hematocrit reduction lower oxygen-carrying and delivery capacity, unless cardiac output (Q) is raised to a degree corresponding to the degree of hemoglobin dilution. If, for example, the hemoglobin level is reduced by 50 percent, cardiac output must double. However, cardiac outputs of this magnitude are rarely used during CPB; they are usually kept within the normal range. Therefore, while normothermic, oxygen delivery will be abnormally low. This may be partially compensated for by increased oxygen extraction. In addition, the metabolic acidosis resulting from the O_2 debt will lead to a reduction in red cell oxygen affinity. However, reduction in oxygen demand by hypothermia is the mainstay of the methods used in the attempts to deal with this problem.

Hypothermia

Hypothermia was originally induced by surface cooling, a tedious process that cools the vital organs less effectively than fat and muscle.[42,84] Internal cooling, using the heat exchanger system of the heart-lung machine, is much more effective, since, using this mode, the best perfused organs are exposed to the greatest temperature change, both cooling and rewarming more readily than fat and muscle. Quantitation of the reduction in oxygen demand is very difficult.[85] The cooling–rewarming process is not a steady state. It is nonuniform in terms of its temperature distribution from one organ system to the other in the body; it differs in timing for each patient; the patients differ from one another in terms of body composition; and supplemental surface heating and cooling is often used. Temperatures are measured in the rectum and esophagus in most patients. Nasopharyngeal and skin temperatures are also often followed. Because of the differences in time course, organ blood flow, and resulting organ temperatures, core or "average" temperatures can only be estimated. Formulas for their estimation are, of necessity, inaccurate. Direct measurement of total body oxygen consumption is the only way to assess the precise amount of change and to determine an average body temperature. One study of oxygen consumption and temperatures at a variety of body sites found that the nasopharyngeal temperature most closely followed the changes in oxygen consumption during cooling and rewarming (Figs. 12-16 and 12-17).[86]

The fall in oxygen consumption with reduction in temperature is not a linear process. Oxygen consumption will be reduced to 50 percent at 30°C, to 25 percent at 25°C, to 15 percent at 20°C, and to 10 percent at 15°C (Fig. 12-18).

With normothermic hemodilution, however, oxygen-carrying capacity will be abnormally low. Therefore, after rewarming, under circumstances in which oxygen transport might be critical, (e.g., low cardiac output state), the avoidance of alkalosis and decreases in the hemoglobin concentration may be essential. Respiratory alkalosis should be avoided because of its undesirable leftward shift in the oxyhemoglobin dissociation curve and the consequent increase in affinity of hemoglobin for oxygen.[87] Since oxygen affinity may be increased as a result of the addition of bank blood at this time, further measures that might exacerbate the problem, such as respiratory alkalosis, should be avoided. The hemoglobin concentration may be raised by the infusion of packed cells. Ordinary whole blood and autologous blood can also be used, since their hemoglobin level will undoubtedly be higher than that of the patient at this time. In addition, if blood is to be used from the oxygenator, various methods of removal of plasma are possible in order to give the patient the equivalent of packed cell suspensions. If circumstances permit, the simplest way to remove the excess fluid volume from the administered hemodiluted oxygenator blood is simply by the use of diuretics. In any case, attempts must be made to raise the O_2 transport capacity of the patient to the range required for normal

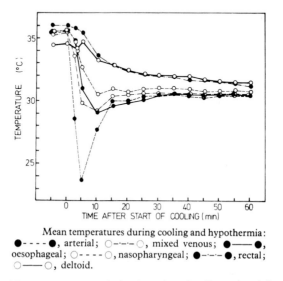

Mean temperatures during cooling and hypothermia: ●- - - -●, arterial; ○–·–·–○, mixed venous; ●———●, oesophageal; ○- - - -○, nasopharyngeal; ●–·–·–●, rectal; ○———○, deltoid.

Fig. 12-16. Mean temperatures during hypothermia. (Reproduced from Davies FM: Thermobalance during cardiopulmonary bypass with moderate hypothermia in man. Br J Anaesth 49:1127, 1977, with permission of author and publisher.)

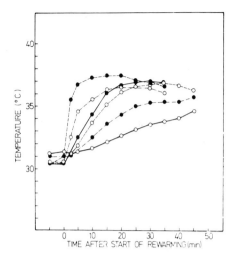

Fig. 12-17. Mean temperatures during rewarming from hypothermia. (Reproduced from Davies FM: Thermobalance during cardiopulmonary bypass with moderate hypothermia in man. Br J Anaesth 49:1127, 1977, with permission of author and publisher).

leftward shift in the oxyhemoglobin dissociation curve. By constriction of the body's capacitance vessels, hypothermia also leads to complex changes in the size and distribution of the blood volume. The blood volume is, in general, reduced in a nonuniform fashion that is undoubtedly related to the temperature and the reduced oxygen demand of each particular organ system. This relative hypovolemia may be significant early in the postoperative period when, with rapid rewarming, equally rapid volume repletion might prove necessary.

Rewarming in the postoperative period may also be accompanied by vigorous shivering. The increase in total body oxygen consumption that may result was found by one group of investigators to be between 135 and 486 percent of normal.[88] This is significant in that it must be matched by corresponding increases in cardiac output in order to maintain oxygen delivery at the normal rate. In the presence of significant hemodilution, the increased peripheral oxygen extraction may result in marked venous desaturation. This may be a significant contribution to systemic arterial hypoxemia. Another such factor might be the increased cardiac output, which might lead to a shortened pulmonary red blood cell mean transit time.[89] The combination of marked red cell desaturation with a shortened oxygen contact time in the lung could easily lead to marked reductions in arterial oxygen tension.

homeostasis and to do so as soon as possible.

Hypothermia, in addition to reducing oxygen consumption, may have other effects. Like hemodilution, it enhances the stability of blood and serum lipids, and reduces the risk of subsequent hematologic disruption after bypass. In addition, as noted in the preceding sections, it alters red cell respiratory function, producing a

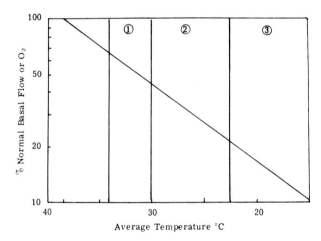

Fig. 12-18. The relationship between oxygen consumption and body temperature is demonstrated. (Reproduced from Peirce EC: Extracorporeal circulation for open-heart surgery. Springfield, Ill., 1969, Charles C. Thomas, with permission of author and publisher).

Profound Hypothermia

Profound hypothermia, that is, a reduction in temperature to the range of 18 to 20°C, was one of the approaches first suggested in the early attempts to operate on the heart. Its potential benefits are based on the marked reductions in total oxygen consumption that result from this degree of temperature reduction (Fig. 12-18) and upon the possibility of stopping the circulation entirely. This combination of circumstances permits the removal of the tubing and cannulae from a surgical field that is motionless and bloodless. As a consequence, the technique has been used principally for the correction of complex congenital disorders in infants.[90] At a "core" temperature of 15°–20°C, it has been suggested that the circulation may be halted for 90 minutes. The early attempts to use this technique were accompanied by what was considered at that time a prohibitively high incidence of complications, most of which affected the central nervous system. With further progress in our understanding of the pathophysiology of cardiopulmonary bypass, most particularly with regard to system filtering, hemodilution, and monitoring, the techniques have again experienced more widespread use and have contributed to what have been considered acceptable results with a reasonable degree of risk.

Specific Hematologic Effects

The interaction between patient blood and the foreign surfaces of the heart-lung machine involve the proteins and the formed elements of the blood in a complex series of processes that are only partly blocked by the use of heparin.[23,91–100] Both the adult-size membrane and the bubble oxygenators may have internal surfaces giving rise to 10–12 m² of contact area. In addition, in the bubble oxygenator, there may be an almost equal amount of gas-blood interfacial contact. These two foreign surfaces, the plastic and the gas interface, give rise to protein denaturation and the adhesion and agglutination of platelets. The proteins adhere to the plastic. The denatured protein layer then attracts platelets, which also become adherent. These reactions with the plastic cause a loss of coagulation proteins and platelets but are largely self-limiting. Once the plastic becomes coated, further extension of the process is largely halted.

In contrast, the reactions at the air-blood interface, which also alter the coagulation proteins and consume platelets, continue as long as the oxygenator is in use. It is this circumstance that largely underlies the superiority of the membrane oxygenator. Again, however, it must be emphasized that in short-term use, a major factor in the hematologic disruption probably stems from the cardiotomy suction common to both types of oxygenators.

The red cell changes may range from simple shortening of survival time to absolute destruction.[13–16,22] The most important factors would appear to be the violent turbulence, negative pressures, foaming, and shear forces generated by the use of the suction. Another would be the high oxygen tensions found in the system. The other factors producing damage are the foreign surfaces, the blood-gas interface, and the mechanical trauma produced by the pumps in the sytem. The arterial pumps are kept incompletely occlusive and therefore produce little in the way of trauma. With the suction excluded from the circuit, the currently available oxygenators can be used for many hours with little in the way of damage to red cells. The risk of damage with membrane oxygenators is even less, but neither is greatly traumatic in the absence of extensive use of the suction. With incomplete damage, shortened red cell survival time is seen. This is usually manifested as a fall in hematocrit in the absence of bleeding in the early postoperative period. A reticulocyte response occurs about the same time and, given adequate iron stores, will rapidly correct the problem. If iron stores are not adequate, supplemental iron may be given. Greater degrees of damage and cellular disruption lead to the production of red cell ghosts that must be removed from the circulation. In the absence of the lungs from the CPB circuit, and with the possibility of reduced perfusion of the liver, those particles that do gain access to the circulation will have their greatest potential impact on the brain (the organ best perfused with the lungs and heart excluded). The avoidance of this risk has been a high-priority goal that appears in large measure to have been reached by the use of the filters incorporated in the circuit of the present-day extracorporeal circuit.

Destruction of red cells will also release free hemoglobin into the circulation.[101,102] Initially this hemoglobin will be protein-bound, largely to haptoglobin, and will subsequently be removed by the reticuloendothelial system. As the binding sites become occupied, more hemoglobin will remain free in the circulation. Above a threshold in the range of 100 mg/100 ml, it will be excreted by the kidney, usually with little difficulty. However, with low rates of renal tubular flow and aciduria, significant amounts of hemoglobin may be converted into acid hematin crystals, with the consequent risk of tubular damage. Although there remains some controversy in regard to this area, this possibility would support the maintenance of higher rates of output of alkaline urine during and after bypass in the presence of hemoglobinuria.

At the beginning of cardiopulmonary bypass, white blood cell levels fall to a degree in excess of that expected solely from hemodilution. In addition, opsonification and phagocytic activity appear to be reduced in the remaining cells.[103–105] The same factors, for example, the foreign surfaces and the gas-blood interface, undoubtedly operate to bring this about. There is some suggestion that the increased PaO_2 under which most of these systems operate may also be a factor.

Platelet counts also fall with exposure to the foreign environment of the heart-lung machine.[64–67] This would appear to be caused mainly by aggregation, adhesion, and the release reaction induced by the foreign surfaces and the blood-gas interface. This process is still present but appears to have been reduced by the newer plastics and the use of membrane oxygenators. Platelet changes are not significantly inhibited by heparin and indeed may, in some respects, even be facilitated by its presence.[98–100] Especially in higher concentrations, the presence of heparin may lead to the release reaction and primary agglutination in platelet-rich mixtures. This is an ADP-release reaction that can be inhibited by aspirin, dipyrridamole, sulfinpyrazone, and other drugs and may be partly reversible.[97]

The development of nonreversible aggregation and adhesion may be potentiated by the insults to platelet integrity in the presence of heparin. Such insults might also include red cell ghosts, damaged white cells, and damage to the cellular elements of the reticuloendothelial system. Studies using Cr^{51}-tagged platelets have shown their disappearance into various tissue capillary beds with some degree of subsequent reappearance after bypass, suggesting that the damage leading to their initial disappearance was not entirely irreversible. Changes in platelet charactertistics may also occur with bypass. The most viable and active platelets may well react and disappear with the initial insult of going on bypass. Those remaining might then be assumed to be functionally less capable. However, platelet damage is not usually clinically significant. Counts fall with all types of perfusion apparatus—more with bubble than with membrane oxygenators but rarely with either below the levels clinically required for hemostasis. Furthermore, platelet infusions widely used by some groups have not been shown to be effective in influencing the amount of bleeding in the immediate perioperative period in unselected cases. However, when more specific indications for their use are present (i.e., preexisting platelet abnormalities resulting from drugs or disease) then, just as in any other patient, they should be used.

The increasing volume of cardiac surgery, especially coronary artery bypass procedures, has placed a large demand on our blood banks for more blood and blood products. The use of fresh autologous blood has previously been suggested as a means of decreasing the need for banked blood products.[106,107] Reducing homologous blood transfusions should also decrease the incidence of serum hepatitis and transfusion reactions.

Multiple coagulation abnormalities have been reported following cardiopulmonary bypass. These have been thought to be secondary to trauma to the platelets and clotting factors induced by the extracorporeal circuit and to the effects of simple dilution of those factors. Withdrawal of fresh autologous blood prior to cardiopulmonary bypass and subsequent reinfusion after bypass has also been recommended as a method to prevent coagulation abnormalities during cardiac surgery.

A variety of methods have been employed at different institutions to obtain and administer fresh autologous blood after bypass. The techniques have included withdrawal of blood prior to cardiopulmonary bypass from peripheral or central veins, from peripheral arteries, or from the extracorporeal tubing on the arterial or venous side of the circuit. The blood has been stored in either acid-citrate-dextrose (ACD), citrate-phosphate-dextrose (CPD), or heparinized solutions at room temperature and reinfused after cardiopulmonary bypass either directly into the heart or into a peripheral vein.

A recent study was undertaken at Emory University Hospital to reevaluate three methods of autologous blood transfusion.[107] Before bypass, 13 to 15 percent of the patient's estimated blood volume was removed and stored with either CPD or heparin at room temperature and returned via a peripheral vein after bypass. All patients had significant abnormalities in their PTT, PT, and platelet counts after bypass. Heparinized autologous blood removed from the vena cava cannula [Pump (HEP)] was the only technique that significantly improved the PTT and platelet count (Fig. 12-19). Total blood bank requirements were significantly less for the autologous blood groups than for controls. There was a saving of 18 percent in banked blood requirements. Fresh frozen plasma and platelets were not found to be routinely needed during cardiac surgery.

Our data support the majority of previous studies showing that autologous blood transfusion does reduce banked blood requirements during cardiac surgery. The autologous blood

groups received 500 ml less banked blood products than the other two groups. This represented an 18 percent saving of banked blood, which is similar to Hallowell's figure of 25 percent and Cohn's figure of 20 percent.[108,109] Coagulation parameters were also improved by reinfusion of heparinized autologous blood which was drawn off the vena cava by gravity and stored at room temperature during bypass. This was the only autologous technique that led to significant improvement in the platelet count and PTT. This method of removing autologous blood also took the least time (2 to 10 minutes) and caused the least inconvenience to the surgical team. There were minimal hemodynamic changes during the blood withdrawal as a result of the previous blood volume expansion with 500 ml of plasma protein fraction and 1000 ml of 5 percent dextrose in Ringer's lactate.

Autologous blood drawn off the radial artery [Rad (CPD)] or internal jugular vein [Jugular (CPD)] did not have all the advantages of the heparinized technique. The coagulation parameters were not significantly improved, probably because of the clots seen in some of the CPD bags which used up some of the clotting factors in the autologous blood. In the 10 patients in these 2 groups who had clots in the bags, the mean rise in platelet count after reinfusion was only 7900 per cubic millimeter. In addition, these techniques required the loss of either continuous arterial blood pressure or central venous pressure monitoring during the period of withdrawal (15 to 45 minutes). These techniques were also very time-consuming for the anesthesia personnel often threatening to distract them from their other duties.

The group receiving fresh frozen plasma and platelets had the best clotting studies but the largest utilization of banked blood products. In a survey of 380 hospitals doing cardiac surgery in 1973, Roche and Stengle found that 13 percent administered fresh frozen plasma routinely (average volume of 630 ml) and 9 percent administered platelets routinely (average volume of 120 ml).[110] Another 15 percent used fresh frozen plasma, and 30 percent used platelets when indicated. The small difference in the clotting studies between this group (FFP and PLTs) and those of the pump (HEP) group does not justify the routine use of fresh frozen plasma and platelets in cardiac surgery. Further arguments against the routine use of fresh frozen

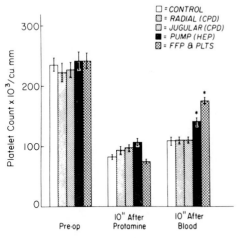

Fig. 12-19. Platelet counts are shown at the three periods of coagulation studies. Ten minutes after protamine the platelet counts are significantly decreased in all five groups. Only groups 4 [pump (HEP)] and 5 [FFP and PLTs] show significant improvement after blood products. FFP = Fresh Frozen Plasma and PLTs = Platelets. (Reproduced from Kaplan JA: Autologous blood transfusion during cardiac surgery. J Thorac Cardiovasc Surg 74:4, 1977, with permission of author and publisher).

plasma and platelets are that: (1) postoperative chest drainage and blood bank requirements were not reduced in the FFP and PLTs, (2) blood bank inconvenience and cost are high, (3) the possibility of transfusion reactions exists, and (4) serum hepatitis can be passed by these blood products.

Serum hepatitis is still a major problem after cardiac surgery. In 1972, the National Transfusion Hepatitis Study found that 2.3 cases of symptomatic hepatitis occurred postoperatively for each 100 patients undergoing cardiac surgery with cardiopulmonary bypass.[111] The use of autologous blood in our study decreased blood bank requirements by 18 percent, and therefore the serum hepatitis risk was also decreased.

CONDUCT OF CARDIOPULMONARY BYPASS

Connection of the Patient to the Circuit

The most common cardiopulmonary bypass circuit is illustrated in Figures 12-2 and 12-3. The surgical procedures for cannulation are shown in Table 12-4.

The arterial inflow connection is usually made by insertion of a cannula into the ascending aorta. This site offers significant advantages over more distal ones such as the femoral artery. Larger cannulae and forward flow with larger volumes are both possible. Retrograde displacement of atheromatous material more proximally in the circulation, for example, to vascular beds of the central nervous system, can be avoided. Potential risks do not appear greater—but benefits do. The arterial connection is completed first in order to establish a route for rapid transfusion should injury to the heart and brisk hemorrhage occur with the remaining part of the dissection for venous cannulation and vent placement. In the event of such a problem, partial bypass and cardiac support can be secured using the suction and venting systems of the pump as the venous return to the oxygenator and then returning oxygenated blood through the arterial line to the patient.

Venous drainage to the oxygenator is customarily taken from separate cannulae placed in the superior and inferior venae cavae. As an alternative method, a single cannula can be used. This type varies somewhat in design but basically functions by taking blood from both cavae together or usually as the streams of blood come together in the right atrium. The single cannula has the advantage that it may be placed through a single opening in the atrium, but it has

Table 12-4

Prebypass Surgical Procedures

---

1. Pericardium open and secured.
2. Tape superior vena cava (SVC) (optional)
3. Tape inferior vena cava (IVC) (optional)
4. Tape aorta (optional)
5. Heparin administered (3 mg/kg via CVP)
6. Assistant surgeons preparing tubing for bypass as above being completed
7. C-Clamp on aorta—observe systemic pressure and carotid pulses
8. Appropriate incision in aorta, two purse-strings used
9. Cannulation of ascending aorta and check on proper position of tip
10. Connection of aortic cannula to arterial limb of pump *after all air removed*
11. SVC cannula via atrial appendage after purse-string
12. IVC cannula via atrial wall after purse-string
13. Pressure on lungs to fill cannulae
14. Venous connections to pump completed
15. Check arterial line pressure
16. Prepare right superior pulmonary vein vent site (optional prior to bypass)

---

the disadvantage that its function is not quite as predictable in providing uniform drainage, without significant resistance to either the inferior or superior vena caval streams of blood. Its position is critical, since small changes may produce low-grade degrees of obstruction in the drainage of the superior or inferior vena cava. These obstructions to venous outflow usually produce only modest elevations in venous back pressure. With the usual dilution of oncotic activity brought about by the use of hemodilution primes, however, even modest increases in back pressure may be associated with the development of tissue edema. The single cannula represents one less incision into the myocardium and a saving of time, but despite meticulous attention in placement, it may give rise to potentially serious problems, particularly in respect to the head. Venous return in most circuits proceeds by gravity to the heart-lung machine, although in some membrane oxygenators, active venous pumping is required. After the venous cannulae are in position, encircling tapes may be placed around the cavae near their tips or around the pulmonary artery to ensure that all the caval drainage is returned to the collecting system of the oxygenator and does not gain access to the lungs.

Upon completion of these connections, the apparatus is ready for use. Initially, some of the venous drainage may pass through the cardiac chambers to the lungs. This situation is described as "partial bypass." To secure "total bypass," the encircling tapes placed around the cavae or the pulmonary artery are tightened so as to direct all caval blood to the oxygenator.

Under these circumstances, relatively little blood gains access to the heart or lungs. However, even without encircling tapes, access will still be minimal in the nonbeating heart. Therefore, in the event that tapes are deliberately not used or cannot readily be placed, as is sometimes the case when the patient has had a previous cardiac procedure, operation with total bypass is still possible.

With total bypass, there is still some return by way of the bronchial and thebesian veins to be considered. The volumes reaching the left ventricle may be particularly large when the bronchial circulation is larger than normal, as is often the case in congenital heart lesions such as tetralogy of Fallot. It may also be very large when competency of the aortic valve is not maintained as a result of either position of the heart or disease of the valve itself. To avoid overdistention of the heart, measures must be taken to ensure that it is kept empty. After arterial and venous cannulation, most particularly in closed heart procedures (e.g., aortocoronary bypass), the heart is customarily kept empty or vented by a cannula inserted into the left ventricle most commonly by way of the right superior pulmonary vein and left atrium. If this area is not accessible, use of the apex of the left ventricle may be necessary.

Going on Bypass

Items similar to those listed in Table 12-5 should be checked by the anesthesiologist prior to instituting cardiopulmonary bypass. When all

Table 12-5
Prebypass Anesthesia Checklist

1. Has heparin been given? ACT value >400 seconds?
2. Has cannulation been successfully completed?
3. Is the prime satisfactory for the patient?
4. What is the calculated pump flow?
5. Are all monitors working and accurate?
6. Is the level of anesthesia adequate?
7. Have pupil size and EEG pattern been checked?
8. Should more muscle relaxant be administered?
9. Has autologous blood been removed?
10. Has prebypass fluid administration and urine output been recorded?
11. Is phenylephrine (100 μg/ml) and a vasodilator prepared?

Table 12-6
Initiating Bypass

1. Ensure all clamps removed
2. Give command to begin bypass
3. Check line pressure and aorta
4. Check mean and venous pressures
5. Determine adequacy of venous return and cannulae position—begin cooling with pump to 28°C
6. Insert sump (vent) through left ventricular tip or superior pulmonary vein
7. Full bypass by securing caval tapes—ventilation by anesthesia stops
8. 5–10 cm H_2O pressure maintained on lungs
9. Ensure all aspects of perfusion are satisfactory—pressures, etc.
10. Cold Ringer's on heart if being used
11. If aorta is cross-clamped, cardioplegic solution injected into aortic root.
12. Cardiotomy

of these factors are checked, the surgeons will initiate bypass (Table 12-6).

The arterial connection should be tested after insertion by pumping a small amount of oxygenator contents toward the patient and observing the aorta for evidences of dissection and for the direction of blood flow while simultaneously checking the arterial line pressure for any evidence of obstruction. The clamps are then removed from the venous cannulae, and the arterial pump is started, gradually increasing its output over a few minutes to full rates of flow. Moderate continuous positive airway pressure (Valsalva) should be applied at the time of vent placement to ensure that air does not enter the ventricle. Air in the blood will demonstrate axial streaming and on leaving the ventricle, will thus go preferentially to the head. After placement of the vent and with the use of hypothermia, ventricular fibrillation may develop spontaneously or can readily be induced, usually by applying a cold saline solution to the surface of the heart.

With the heart empty and arrested and the venous return directed to the oxygenator, that is, with total bypass, there is no need to continue the ventilation of the patient's lungs. Continued ventilation would only be necessary under circumstances in which the systemic bronchial circulation might be expected or known to be very large, for example, in some of the cyanotic patients with shunts. Many approaches have been used in an attempt to protect the lungs during bypass, from simple disconnection of the circuit, leaving them open to air, to continued ventilation with a variety of gases.[112] None appear to have conferred any particular advantage. Advantage would appear to lie in the maintenance of at least minimal bronchial and possibly pulmonary parenchymal blood flow. It is our practice to maintain a moderate degree of lung expansion with oxygen during bypass using 5–10 cm of PEEP.

Monitoring During Bypass

Monitoring should be even more extensive during CPB than in the prebypass period. The following factors are observed during bypass.

CLINICAL OBSERVATIONS

1. Capillary refill—should remain brisk.
2. Pupillary size—should remain small and equal.
3. Level of anesthesia—the patient should not respond to verbal stimuli. Anesthetic depth may be increased by hypothermia.
4. Diaphragmatic motion—usually means light anesthesia or increased Pa_{CO_2}.
5. Electroencephalogram (EEG)—used in all patients in whom cerebral problems may occur, for example, elderly patients or those with calcific valvular heart disease. Usually have an alpha rhythm (8–13 cps) at nor-

mothermia and a theta rhythm (4–7 cps) at hypothermia to 28°C. Poor perfusion with hypoxia, hypotension, or venous engorgement causes a flattening of the EEG and very slow delta waves (0.5–3 cps). Emboli may cause a wave-and-spike seizure pattern.

6. Electrocardiogram (ECG)—depending on the operative procedure and technique, the ECG pattern will vary.

    a. RSR—Maintained in cases done at normothermia on a beating heart, for example, atrial septal defect. It is important to watch for the development of ischemia or conduction disturbances.

    b. Ventricular fibrillation—occurs in hearts maintained at hypothermia with coronary perfusion or external hypothermia (ice saline bath).

    c. Asystole—maintained by cardioplegic solutions during most operations today. Reduces oxygen consumption to a minimum. It is important to watch for the return of ventricular fibrillation (increased oxygen demand) so more cardioplegic solution can be used. Upon reperfusion of the coronary circulation, many types of conduction defects can be seen.

7. Temperature—measured in the esophagus or nasopharynx as well as in the rectum.

HEMODYNAMIC MONITORING

1. Mean arterial pressure—usually maintained between 60 and 100 torr. MAP = CO × TPR; since CO is fixed, the MAP varies directly with the TPR and is altered by administering drugs that increase or decrease TPR.

2. Central venous pressure—should be measured in the *superior* vena cava *above* the venous return line in order to be able to diagnose obstruction to venous return from the head. Persistent elevated venous pressures can lead to cerebral edema. The CVP should be zero or very low on bypass, since venous return to the pump should be by unobstructed gravity flow.

3. Pulmonary artery, pulmonary capillary wedge, or left atrial pressure—should all be low or zero on bypass. If these become elevated, it means the left ventricle is becoming distended as a result of inadequate venting.

4. Cardiac output—pump flow is maintained at 2.2–2.5 liters/min/m² during the bypass. It may be varied by ±20 percent, depending on body temperature and blood gases.

5. Total peripheral resistance (TPR)

$$TPR = \frac{MAP - CVP}{CO} \times 80$$

This should be maintained in the normal range when corrected for viscosity for the best perfusion and reflected, as well, by blood gases and urine output.[62]

$$TPR_{corrected} = \frac{3.5 \times TPR}{\eta}$$

η = blood viscosity; normal value = 3.5

6. Urine output—should be maintained above 1 ml/kg/hr by adequate perfusion. Severe hemolysis with hemoglobinuria should be treated by increasing urine output further with diuretic agents and alkalization of the urine.

BLOOD STUDIES

1. Arterial blood gases—should be obtained 5 minutes after going on bypass, 5 minutes before coming off bypass, and every 15 to 30 minutes while on bypass. The Pa_{O_2}, Pa_{CO_2}, and pH should be fully temperature-corrected to the patient's body temperature. The Pa_{O_2} should be maintained in the 100–150 torr range; Pa_{CO_2}, 35–45 torr; and pH, 7.35–7.45. The frequency of blood gases can be reduced if in-line arterial P_{O_2} and/or P_{CO_2} electrodes are used in the pump circuitry.

2. Venous P_{O_2}—should be obtained from the venous tubing at the oxygenator with each arterial blood gas sample and temperature-corrected. Normal range of values is 40–45 torr. Low values mean increased extraction and may imply poor perfusion. High values are evidence of arteriovenous shunting.

3. Hematocrit—measured with each blood gas and maintained between 20 and 30 percent on bypass.

4. Electrolytes—Na+, K+, and Ca++ measured by flow through electrodes with each blood gas. Potassium may be low as a result of hemodilution, urine output, and fluid shifts and may require supplementation while on

bypass to maintain it over 4.5 mEq/liter. With the use of hyperkalemic cardioplegic solutions, the K^+ is frequently high on bypass and may require therapy to lower the myocardial K^+ level at the end of bypass. The normal value for ionized Ca^{++} is 1.9–2.2 mEq/liter. With hemodilution, the ionized Ca^{++} frequently falls to about 1.5 mEq/liter. Banked blood further reduces it. The ionized Ca^{++} is brought back to normal at the end of bypass by administering 1–2 gm of $CaCl_2$ or other calcium-containing solutions (Table 12-7).

5. Activated clotting time (ACT)—measured at 30-minute intervals after heparin administration. It should be maintained above 400 to 450 seconds; below 300 seconds, fibrin strands and clots may be seen in the blood.

6. Blood sugar—measured in all diabetic patients at one-half–hourly intervals. It is also measured when therapy with glucose-insulin-potassium (GIK) is used.

A brief period of hypotension out of proportion to the reduction of viscosity is often seen with the institution of bypass.[62,113] Several factors may be involved. Vasoactive materials may be released as a consequence of the initial reaction of the serum proteins, blood cells, and platelets with the foreign surfaces of the heart-lung machine.[114] In addition, with blood-free primes, the initial perfusion material will be low in viscosity and almost devoid of oxygen. This will result in a significant oxygen debt, leading to vasodilatation and venous desaturation.[115] This, in turn, may be potentially of a degree great enough to prevent complete arterialization in the oxygenator. This particular problem should disappear within a few minutes, especially if hypothermia is used and the oxygen demand thereby reduced.

The use of vasopressors under these circumstances is common, but their effectiveness

is somewhat difficult to assess in what often seems to be a problem of only limited duration. From the standpoint of therapy, there are two general objectives: (1) the repayment of any oxygen debt, and (2) raising the systemic vascular resistance and thus the mean arterial pressure. The former will usually require moderate hypothermia and an initial rate of pump flow above that predicted from the customary nomograms (Fig. 12-15), until the patient is moderately cool. The nomograms of Galletti are based on flows with normal oxygen-carrying capacity. When the capacity is halved by hemodilution, the demand must also be halved by hypothermia (or the flows doubled). The nomograms must be considered in relation to the amount of oxygenated hemoglobin delivered per minute. The hypotension associated with this mechanism is accompanied by marked venous desaturation. A lowered mixed venous Po_2 will be seen, and successful therapy will be accompanied by its improvement. When considering the administration of vasopressors to raise the mean arterial pressure, it must be remembered that there is no universal agreement in regard to the blood pressure that should be maintained during bypass when there is adequate maintenance of flow.[116] Does an adequate pump output mean adequate blood flow to all vital organs no matter what the pressure? Some have answered yes, others, no; most have chosen a middle course. In the patient with diffuse atherosclerotic disease, there may well be many areas in which lowered pressures may be associated with poor perfusion. This appears to be true for the brain. Stockard noted impairment of cerebral function after bypass in a group of patients in whom the product of the total mean aortic pressure below 50 torr, multiplied by the number of minutes at this pressure, was greater than 100 torr-min.[117] In other studies of the flow distal to significant stenoses in the coronary arterial tree, significant reductions in flow and function were seen when the perfusions were carried out at 50 torr rather than at 100 torr pressures.[118] Maintenance of arterial pressure above these limits would therefore seem advisable, especially for the patient most particularly at risk, that is, the patient with diffuse atherosclerotic disease. With specific reference to the patient with cerebral vascular disease, the risk would appear to be especially high, and hypotension and other than moderate hemodilution should be avoided. Maintenance

Table 12-7
Calcium Solutions

Salt	Weight	Ca^{++}
Calcium chloride 10%	1 gm	13.6 mEq*
Calcium gluconate 10%	1 gm	4.6 mEq
Calcium gluceptate 23%	1.1 gm	4.5 mEq

* 1 mEq = 20 mg.

of hemoglobin levels above certain limits might also be advisable in order to assure the delivery of O_2 to areas distal to stenoses in the arterial tree, especially during normothermia.[119]

It is fortunate that the blood pressure almost invariably returns to a stable level soon after the start of bypass. Little change thereafter would be the rule in most cases. With the fixed cardiac output of the arterial pump, the resulting pressure will vary with changes in autonomic nervous system activity, thereby affecting peripheral resistance.

The mean arterial blood pressure should remain between 60 and 100 torr. Pressures below this after the first 5 to 10 minutes of bypass and accompanied by inadequate pump flow and hematocrit values are treated as noted above by increasing bypass flows temporarily above the predicted norms, by the reduction of body temperature, and by the use of small amounts of primarily α-adrenergic vasopressors. In adults, phenylephrine is used in aliquots of 100 μg, or methoxamine is used in 5-mg increments. When the situation is found to be associated with hematocrit levels below 20 percent, blood is added to the prime to bring about an increase in the hematocrit reading. This measure would be of little value and unnecessary during hypothermia. The pressure rise that usually accompanies its use may result mainly from its effect on viscosity. The pressure, in fact, frequently rises when other colloids are added to the pump, for example, albumin. The increase in oxygen-carrying capacity, however, may be useful at temperatures above 30°C and during active rewarming; and it may be necessary to deliver oxygen past stenotic areas in the vascular tree. A confirmation of adequacy of flow may be sought in examination of urine output, which should be greater than 1 ml/kg/hr; mixed venous P_{O_2}, above 35 torr; and acid–base status, which should remain within normal limits. In addition, it may prove useful to examine the patient's head for evidence of adequate capillary refill and for pupillary size and responsiveness.

Significant pressure rises, that is, above 100 torr in the presence of predicted flows and hematocrit values, results from increased peripheral vascular resistance and signifies increased levels of autonomic nervous system activity, usually the result of inadequate anesthesia. The problem can be managed in a number of ways, *none of which should include reduction of pump*

flows. As noted earlier, an anesthetic vaporizer can be included in the circuit and utilized if a bubble or membrane oxygenator is in use, but evaluation of its use with the membrane lung is not yet available. Varying intravenous combinations of scopolamine, diazepam, and narcotics may be used as supplements. One may also add vasodilator drugs, such as nitroglycerin or sodium nitroprusside, and α-blockers, such as phentolamine, phenoxybenzamine, or chlorpromazine.[120–122] The inhibition of α-adrenergic vasoconstriction during bypass may be of some benefit. In patients with hypertension on bypass (MAP > 100 torr), oliguria, acidosis, and a low P_vO_2 frequently coexist. This situation can frequently be corrected by maintaining pump flow and administering 1 mg of chlorpromazine, phentolamine, or a vasodilator.

Increases in the central venous, pulmonary artery, or pulmonary capillary wedge pressure should direct immediate attention to the mechanisms for the diversion of venous blood to the oxygenator, especially those decompressing the ventricle, that is, the venous cannulae and the vent. Such increases usually signify some degree of obstruction. With hemodilution, there will be alteration of the Starling forces, and the potential for increased transmembranous movement of water at lower-than-normal hydrostatic pressures. Any degree of obstruction at the venous return sites carries with it the risk of the development of edema; obstruction to superior vena cava output affecting the brain; left ventricular obstruction affecting the lungs and ventricle. The pressures reflected by these catheters should normally be at or below zero during bypass. Pressure changes denoting obstruction are usually accompanied by some loss of venous return to the oxygenator, the need for supplemental fluid addition to the prime, and the loss of fluid outside the vascular compartment, presumably resulting in edema. Attempts to correct the problem should be made immediately.

The normal mixed venous P_{O_2} has a value between 40 and 45 torr.[123] Its level during bypass is a reflection of the adequacy of oxygen delivery to tissues; reductions signify increased oxygen extraction. Levels below 35 torr should be considered to represent inadequate oxygen delivery and are usually associated with the development of increasing levels of metabolic acidosis. When low mixed venous P_{O_2} levels are seen, frequent assessment of acid–base status should be carried out. Corrective measures should be directed at improving the adequacy of perfusion. Adequacy of hemoglobin delivery per minute by the pump should first be assured and then inquiry made for other factors that may be involved. The other factors are most commonly vasoconstriction reducing tissue perfusion, which usually can be overcome by adequate anesthesia and, if necessary, vasodilator drugs; and changes in the oxygen affinity of red cells brought about by concomitant hypothermia, alkalosis, and the use of banked blood. These latter changes can usually be improved by adjustment of the Pa_{CO_2}. As noted earlier, the combination of alkalosis and hypothermia should be avoided.

Urine output greater than 1 ml/kg/hr is usually seen during bypass despite the alteration in renal hemodynamics brought about by nonpulsatile flow. If the levels are below this and are not improved by the general measures taken to assure circulatory adequacy, diuretics should be given to assure reasonable rates of flow. Drugs such as furosemide, ethacrynic acid or osmotic diuretics such as mannitol may be used. The maintenance of adequate renal function during bypass is essential and may contribute to the avoidance of renal failure. Renal failure under these circumstances carries with it a very grave risk to the patient.[124]

In administering mannitol, it must be remembered that it is isotonic at approximately the 5 percent level and can usually be excreted by adults at approximately 1 gm/min. Dosage rates in excess of this may expand the blood volume. This should produce no great problem to the patient on bypass. However, hypervolemia resulting from its injudicious use may present a significant hazard afterward. Every milliliter of 20 percent mannitol must be diluted to isosmolar levels and thus represents a 4-ml blood volume expansion.

The appearance of hemoglobin in the urine should elicit measures directed at the alkalization of the urine and increases in its rates of flow. Alkalization may be affected by bicarbonate or the organic buffer, THAM.[125]

The hematocrit should be monitored continuously during the procedure. Unexplained decreases signify unrecognized blood loss. A search should be made for the site from which the blood is being lost and the problem corrected. This may be unnoticed bleeding at a surgical site (e.g., the leg) or unrecognized escape of blood from the surgical field into an open pleural cavity. In any case, recognition should be accompanied by a search for and treatment of the cause.

Myocardial Preservation

The protection of the myocardium during CPB depends upon the extent to which it is possible to control surgical trauma and the effects of ischemia. The trauma can be reduced by meticulous attention to the way the heart is handled and by keeping to a minimum surgical intervention involving the ventricles. The risk of ischemia can be approached in several ways: by satisfying oxygen demand by maintenance of coronary perfusion or by reduction in the oxygen demand.[126,127]

Coronary perfusion through a separate heat exchanger, although inconvenient and less popular in recent years, is effective and can be carried out via the aortic root or into the coronary arteries directly if the aortic root is opened.[128,129] The perfusate is usually taken from the oxygenator to the patient by way of a separate reservoir and pump system but may, on occasion, be taken directly from the arterial line by way of a T-connector. This latter method is not recommended; it may ensure a certain level of pressure but not of measured flow. For this, a separate pumping system is needed. Among the factors that have reduced the popularity of this technique which uses the oxygenator contents are the questionable adequacy of perfusion of the subendocardial layer of the heart, surgical difficulty resulting from the intrusion of the cannulae into the operative field, the risk of injury to the coronary arteries, and adequacy of perfusion via the aortic root in the presence of any degree of aortic insufficiency. As a consequence, the technique is now largely restricted to the continuous infusion by gravity flow or active pumping of cold cardioplegic solutions into the aortic root during periods of crossclamping.

There are circumstances when cross-clamping of the intact aorta is unavoidable and myocardial ischemia otherwise inevitable. This, for example, is often the case during mitral valve procedures in order to control the regurgitant flow through the aortic valve brought about by disease of the valve or impairment of its integrity by changes in the position of the heart. Ischemia at normal temperatures is poorly tolerated. Even after relatively brief periods such as 15 or 20 minutes, it is followed by varying degrees of diffuse cellular damage and subsequent fibrosis and impairment of function. Oxygen consumption is a function of chamber size, wall thickness, and the rate and pressure range in which the heart is working. Although when empty oxygen demand may have fallen as much as 75 percent, the empty beating heart still has a significant metabolic requirement. This demand does not change significantly after the induction of ventricular fibrillation but can be reduced by the use of hypothermia and cardioplegia. Reduction in myocardial temperature and oxygen consumption may be induced by the use, singly or in combination, of systemic hypothermia, by the local application of cold irrigant solutions to the external surface and chambers of the heart, or by the intermittent or continuous infusion of cold solutions, usually via the aortic root into the coronary arterial tree.[128,129] With this approach it is possible to produce myocardial temperatures ranging between 14 and 16°C. With reductions in temperatures of this order, final oxygen consumption will, understandably, be very low.

Oxygen consumption may be further reduced by the production of flaccid cardioplegia. Cardioplegia, with its provision of a relaxed heart, allows optimal conditions for surgery. Examination of the methods for its production began in the early days of heart surgery. Melrose reported the use of a 25 percent solution of potassium citrate in 1955.[130] The use of this solution produced considerable myocardial damage, and interest in this approach to the reduction of metabolic demand languished. It was rekindled by studies which suggested that the damage from the original solution might have been due to its high potassium concentration; over 200 mEq/liter with a tonicity greater than 400 mOsm/liter.[131–136] Subsequent investigations have suggested that a number of features might contribute to the benefits to be seen with the use of cardioplegia. Lysosomal and cell membrane stabilization may be facilitated by the concomitant administration of steroids or their inclusion in the perfusing solution and by the inclusion of small amounts of calcium and procaine.[133,137,138] Slight alkalosis would also appear to be of benefit. For this purpose, several groups have used either THAM or bicarbonate to raise the pH to levels between 7.4 and 7.8. Energy substrate support may be conferred by the inclusion of glucose and insulin.[139] Similarly, a slight increase in osmolality appears to be useful in minimizing intracellular water accumulation. Most workers have added sorbitol, mannitol, or glucose to the electrolytes to produce a concentration of 300–370 mOsm/liter.[140] Although there may be some hazard with higher levels of tonicity, Kirsch has used a solution of 463 mOsm/liter.[131] The cardioplegia itself is brought about by the addition of 10–30 mEq/liter of potassium. Magnesium also may be used for cardioplegia and in Kirsch's solution is present as magnesium aspartate in a concentration of 160 mEq/liter. Some of the cardioplegia solutions in current use are shown in Table 12-8.

The place of each of these manipulations is not yet clear. They all seem of some value singly, however, and appear additive in combination.[133] The use of solutions absolutely devoid of essential cation would seem unwise until the situation is clarified.[134] Despite the questions that still remain in this area, it has become apparent that the measures to produce myocardial hypothermia and flaccid cardioplegia have been shown to be of value and should be used continuously or with a frequency sufficient to maintain the heart cold, flaccid, and without ECG evidence of electrical activity.

Heparin

The first experimental studies of perfusion apparatus used blood that was defibrinogenated. More recent studies have also been done using the same approach.[141,142] Nevertheless, heparin must still be considered a fundamental necessity in the conduct of CPB. It was discovered by McClean in 1916, investigated over the next several decades, and introduced into clinical practice in the 1940s.[143,144] It is a mucopolysaccharide, the strongest organic acid found in the body, and most commonly prepared from bovine lung and porcine or bovine intestinal mucosa.[100] Heparin in the presence of its cofactor leads to the almost instantaneous production of a thrombin-antithrombin complex deactivating the thrombin. The heparin-antithrombin cofactor complex appears also to inactivate factor X_a. Most of the series of linked proteolytic reactions that make up the coagulatin cascade

Table 12-8
Myocardial Preservation Solutions

	Emory	Bretschneider[132]	Kirsch[131]	Jynge[134]	Buckberg[133]	Roe[136]	Tyers[135]
Na⁺ (mEq/liter)	108.1	12.0	0	91.6	140.0	27.0	138.0
Ca⁺⁺ (mEq/liter)	0	0	0	1.2	5.6	0	1.0
K⁺ (mEq/liter)	27.9	10.0	0	14.8	30.0	20.0	25.0
Mg⁺⁺ (mEq/liter)	0	2.0	160	17.4	0	3.0	3.0
Membrane stabilization	0	Procaine 200 mg/100 ml	Procaine 300 mg/100 ml	Procaine 27 mg/100 ml Calcium	Calcium	0	Calcium
Final pH	7.68 (NaHCO₃)	5.5–7.0 (no buffer)	5.8–7.0 (no buffer)	7.4 (NaHCO₃)	7.7 (THAM)	7.6 (THAM)	7.8 (KHCO₃)
Osmotic activity	Mannitol	Mannitol	Sorbitol	None	Glucose	Glucose	None
Osmolarity (mOsm/liter)	278–370	320	463	300	370	347	275
Energy substrate	Glucose	0	0	0	Glucose Insulin	Glucose	0
Temperature (°C)	4	4	4	4	12	4	15

would, in fact, appear to be inhibited by this same mechanism (factors IX_a, X_a, XI_a, and XII_a).

Heparin is protein-bound and thus distributed in the plasma volume.[145,146] It has a biological half-life of approximately 100 minutes in normothermic man, a time that is increased with increasing dosage and decreasing temperature (Fig. 12-20). Details of its elimination are as yet unclear but appear to depend upon a first-order process involving biodegradation in the reticuloendothelial system.

The anticoagulant response to any administered dose is variable and depends upon such factors as body temperature, age, and body composition, most particularly the lean body mass. Heparin has been used conventionally in doses of 3 mg or 300 units/kg of body weight, assuming an initial serum concentration of at least 2–4 units/ml of whole blood. Various regimens have been used empirically for subsequent doses. Most of these have been based on the assumption of a biological half-life of 100 to 150 minutes. In addition to the above factors, however, this latter figure varies with the amount of hypothermia and the average body temperature.[147] As a consequence there is, not surprisingly, a marked individual variation in both initial effect and half-life. Therefore, it would seem indicated to assess precisely the initial effect and rate of decline, that is, the half-life, in each patient. Many tests have been suggested for this purpose, for example, the PTT, heparin assays, and heparin-protamine titrations.

One such method that can be easily and conveniently used by personnel with little laboratory training in an operating room setting is the celite activated clotting time (ACT) test first described by Hattersley.[148] A baseline value is determined prior to the administration of heparin, and the test repeated just after giving heparin and at 30-minute intervals thereafter. With the dose of heparin in milligrams per kilogram on the vertical axis and the ACT in seconds on the horizontal axis, a dose–response curve can be constructed (Fig. 12-21). Bull et al. have advocated that the heparin be given initially in a dose of 2 mg/kg, an ACT determined, and the line extrapolated to give a value of 480 seconds.[149,150] They suggested using the line drawn from this point through the original value to calculate the remaining dose of heparin required. The rate of decline of the ACT can be used to estimate, by further extrapolation, the need for subsequent doses. These are administered to maintain values of at least twice control and not less than 350 seconds. Above these levels the processes of coagulation should be adequately opposed and the risk of disseminated intravascular coagulation minimal.

Recently, Cohen has described a modified thrombin time test as a specific heparin assay.[147] Also, a sophisticated protamine titration machine has become available for intraoperative use. These techniques are much more cumbersome than the ACT. They have the advantage, however, of being specific for only the heparin activity, while the ACT is a nonspecific coagulation assay. Nevertheless, we have found a very good correlation between the ACT and the thrombin time (Fig. 12-22).

The use of protamine as a heparin antagonist was first suggested in 1937.[151] Protamine in vivo binds almost milligram-for-milligram with heparin. In the absence of heparin, it has an anticoagulant activity of its own, most probably a result of its capacity to activate the coagulation mechanism and produce a consumption coagulopathy.[152] Part of this involves its effect on platelets. It leads to the release reaction with aggregation and adhesion that is not necessarily reversible, in contradistinction to the reversible changes brought about by heparin. There are

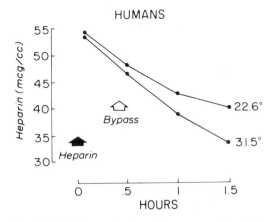

Fig. 12-20. The graph shows the average rate of heparin loss at different temperatures during cardiopulmonary bypass in patients. (Reproduced from Wright JS: Heparin Levels during and after Hypothermic Perfusion. J Cardiovasc Surg 5:244, 1964, with permission of author and publisher).

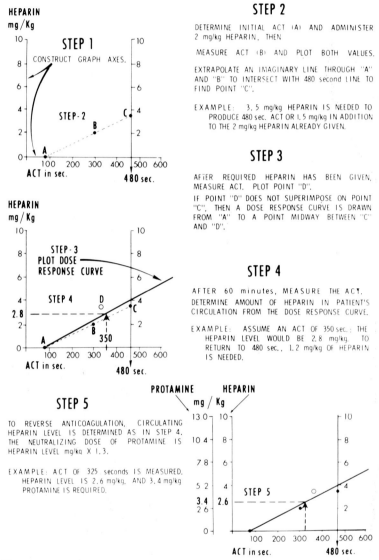

Fig. 12-21. The procedure for and construction of the ACT dose-response curve is shown. (Reproduced from Bull BS et al: Heparin therapy during extracorporeal circulation. J Thorac Cardiovasc Surg 69:78, 1975, with permission of author and publisher).

many questions as yet unanswered concerning the precise physiological effects of protamine administration in the absence of heparin; however, the drug is known to activate coagulation, agglutinate platelets, and increase resistance across capillary beds.[153] In recent studies, much of the pulmonary vasoconstriction seen with protamine was blocked by acetylsalicyclic acid (ASA) administration despite ASA's failure to

block platelet agglutination, which suggests a strong contribution by released humoral compounds (perhaps prostaglandin) in this phenomenon.[114] The humoral and the mechanical effects of the release reaction, platelet aggregation, rouleaux formation, and stasis might be expected to lead to increases in peripheral resistance across capillary beds, as has been demonstrated to be the case in the lung and in the liver. This process could lead to increases in capillary blood volume and corresponding reduction in the blood volume in the venous side of the circulation. The result of this process might be a potentially significant, albeit temporary, reduction of venous return. Direct myocardial depressant effects of the protamine are open to question, and the precise etiologic mechanisms for its hypotensive effects are not entirely clear. The deleterious effects are seen, however, if the rate of administration is too rapid or if a significant excess is given. It would therefore appear more logical to administer the drug on the basis of measured residual heparin activity. The empiric administration of heparin has been associated with degrees of anticoagulation at both ends of the spectrum, both too little and too much. The empiric administration of protamine might logically be expected to be equally unsatisfactory. A variety of dosage schedules have been used, without apparent risk for many years. Nevertheless, common sense would suggest a measurement of heparin activity and the use of protamine on the basis of the measured results. The ACT test, as noted, can be used to estimate the biological half-life of heparin and therefore

the amount remaining. It can then serve as a guide to the further administration of any needed heparin and its reversal by protamine.

Theory suggests that heparin neutralization should proceed on an equal milligram basis; however, this has not been the case in clinical practice. Many dosage regimens have been used, in part because accurate estimations of the amount of heparin remaining was difficult if not impossible in the absence of testing and in part because use of moderate excesses of protamine could apparently be given with relative safety. In addition, although it has not been confirmed, the mode of administration may affect the amount required for heparin reversal. Injection of protamine in a bolus leading to a local blood concentration significantly in excess of the amount of heparin present may result in binding of protamine at sites other than those involving heparin. The protamine present in excess of heparin may lead to the deleterious effects noted above. After dosage selection, in our hands, in an amount equal to the amount of heparin remaining, the protamine administration should begin and the drug should be injected *slowly* with due regard for the mixing time of

Correlation of Heparin Units with Activated Coagulation Time

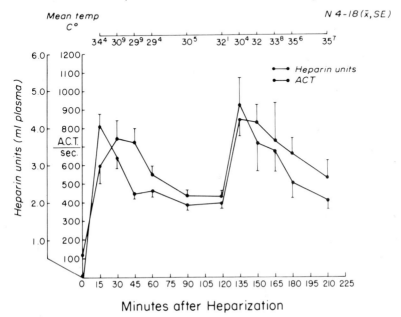

Fig. 12-22.   The correlation between the thrombin time, heparin units, and the activated coagulation time is shown to be excellent. Data taken from 18 patients on cardiopulmonary bypass.

any indicator in the circulation. Uniform mixing in the circulation at the end of bypass should be assumed to be longer than the normal 7- to 10-minute period. It should be injected at a rate slow enough so that its blood level should not greatly exceed that of the heparin at its site of injection. Pharmacokinetic studies to describe this process are not available. Nevertheless, the injection of the calculated amount of the drug over 15 to 30 minutes (the projected mixing time for an indicator in the circulation under these circumstances) is generally well tolerated, in spite of its capacity to produce circulatory disturbances and disturbances in coagulation. After a period of 15 to 30 minutes, the ACT can be repeated and a subsequent dose of protamine given as indicated.

COMING OFF BYPASS

Near the end of the surgical repair, the patient is rewarmed to normal temperature as measured by the nasopharyngeal and rectal probes. If the heart does not spontaneously defibrillate, it is electrically defibrillated with 10–60 w/sec applied internally across the ventricles. During this period of the procedure, the anesthesiologist should be checking many factors (Table 12-9). All of these factors should be corrected and all preparations made before attempting to discontinue bypass. The surgeon carefully removes all air from the cardiac chambers and

coronary grafts and vents the aortic root. A gradual weaning process from the extracorporeal circuit is then begun. This may take 5 minutes or several hours, depending on the patient's status.

1. Oxygenation and ventilation: The lungs are ventilated and are checked to be sure that both sides move equally. The compliance of the lungs is evaluated, and then the ventilator is attached to the anesthesia circuit.
2. Blood gases and electrolytes are corrected to normal: The pH is brought slightly above 7.40 by fully correcting any base deficit with $NaHCO_3$. This is done because cardiac function is improved by mild alkalosis, and the catecholamines (especially epinephrine) are most effective at 7.40–7.45 pH.
3. Cardiac rhythm is restored: if the heart remains in ventricular fibrillation, increasing voltage is used up to 60 w/sec. Blood gases, electrolytes, and temperature are rechecked, and xylocaine is administered (1–2 mg/kg). Rarely, it may be necessary to give incremental doses of propranolol (0.5–1.0 mg) or KCl 0.5 to 2.0 mEq to treat recurrent ventricular tachycardia and fibrillation.

If supraventricular tachyarrhythmias are present, they may be treated with cardioversion, rapid atrial pacing, digoxin

Table 12-9
Checklist for Coming off Bypass

1. Are the blood gases satisfactory?
2. Is the hematocrit value above 20 percent?
3. Is the K^+ above 4.0 mEq/liter?
4. Is the body temperature above 35°C?
5. Has $CaCl_2$ been given to correct the Ca^{++} to normal?
6. Is the depth of anesthesia adequate?
7. Has the vaporizer on the pump been shut off?
8. What is the ACT?
9. Is protamine available? Dose?
10. Is adequate blood available?
11. Have the monitors been recalibrated?
12. What is the ECG pattern?
13. Is a pacemaker available?
14. Are inotropes and/or vasodilators prepared?
15. Is the intra-aortic balloon pump likely to be needed?

(0.25–0.5 mg), ouabain (0.1–0.2 mg), or propranolol.

Potassium cardioplegia frequently leads to various forms of heart block (2°, 3°, or LBBB) at the end of bypass. These usually correct themselves when coronary blood flow is reestablished. In some patients, however, the hyperkalemia requires treatment with $CaCl_2$, $NaHCO_3$, GIK, or pacing.

Various pacemaker modalities may be employed. Ventricular pacing leads to the worst cardiac output, since the atrial contribution is lost; atrial pacing is good if it will be conducted across the AV node. AV sequential pacing is the best modality, since it allows variation of the P-R interval to obtain the best conduction time and cardiac output (Figs. 12-23 and 12-24). A heart rate of 90 beats per minute frequently gives the best cardiac output.

4. Administer $CaCl_2$ (1–2 gm in pump): This is given when the heart starts to contract in an effort to raise the Ca^{++} level, increase myocardial contractility, and reverse potassium cardioplegia. In the presence of digitalis, calcium should be given at a rate consistent with the size of the vascular compartment into which it is being injected. In the adult, 10–20 mEq/kg of calcium chloride may be given at the end of bypass in a relatively short period with minimal risk. The risk lies in the development of arrhythmias in the digitalized patient. It should therefore be given cautiously and with close observation of the ECG in the digitalized patient after bypass. It must be borne in mind that the benefits from its administration will be temporary and that 50 percent of it must be expected to have left the vascular compartment in 30 to 60 minutes, and 65 percent within 2 hours. Obvious benefit from injection of each aliquot and the apparent need for repeated injections should suggest the need for supplemental digitalis.

5. Remove left ventricular vent and place a left atrial line (if desired): The heart should have volume in it when the vent is removed, and positive pressure should be maintained on the lungs to avoid air entrapment in the atrium. The left atrial pres-

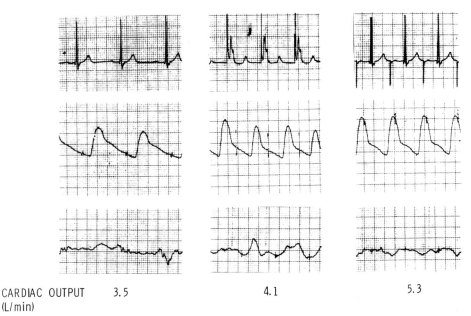

CARDIAC OUTPUT   3.5   4.1   5.3
(L/min)

Fig. 12-23. The hemodynamic effects of atrial and ventricular pacing are demonstrated. The left-hand panel is the patient in normal sinus rhythm with a cardiac output of 3.5 liters/min. The middle panel shows ventricular pacing, and the right-hand panel shows atrial pacing which markedly increases the cardiac output. The third tracing down is the CVP.

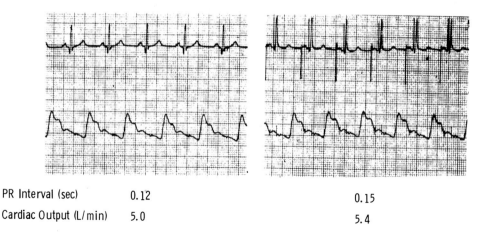

| PR Interval (sec) | 0.12 | 0.15 |
| Cardiac Output (L/min) | 5.0 | 5.4 |

Fig. 12-24. The value of AV sequential pacing is demonstrated, even in a patient with sinus rhythm. By optimizing the P-R interval the cardiac output is further increased.

sure or the pulmonary wedge pressure is observed while discontinuing bypass. In patients with good left ventricular function, the CVP may be used carefully while observing for signs of left ventricular failure (e.g., S_3, rales).

6. Reduce pump flow gradually to half the calculated flow and observe the degree of ventricular function and blood ejection.

7. Use the Starling curve: As the pump flow is gradually reduced, the heart is filled to a left atrial pressure (LAP) of 12–18 torr but not above this. Each increment of volume should lead to an increase in the LAP and the blood pressure (BP) (see Chapter 3). Then, if the BP and arterial upstroke are adequate, the perfusion is discontinued. All pressures are checked and recorded and the cardiac output measured.

8. Inotropic therapy: This is used if bypass cannot be discontinued or if the cardiac output is very low. If the heart rate is rapid, more $CaCl_2$ or ouabain may be used. If the intrinsic rate is slow, isoproterenol (1–10 μg/min) may be infused (especially if β-blocked). Usually either dopamine (5–20 μg/kg/min) or epinephrine (2–10 μg/min) is used. Epinephrine is preferred initially and then is frequently switched to dopamine for long-term therapy. Dopamine has produced many supraventricular tachyarrhythmias and is therefore often not initially our drug of choice. After discontinuing the bypass, the hemodynamics are checked and further therapy utilized as needed.

9. Vasodilator therapy: This is added if the cardiac output is low and afterload (mean arterial pressure or total peripheral resistance) is high or if preload is elevated with a decreased or normal blood pressure. If the problem is increased afterload, nitroprusside is utilized, while if increased preload is the problem, nitroglycerin is used. The addition of the vasodilator frequently corrects the hemodynamic abnormality and may even allow discontinuation of the inotropic drug. Our results in surgery with vasodilators have been similar to the many beneficial reports of the use of vasodilators in patients with low-output syndromes after acute myocardial infarctions. Nitroprusside is especially useful for decreasing afterload in patients who had severe mitral regurgitation and in whom a mitral valve replacement has been performed. In many patients the combination of an inotrope and a vasodilator will correct the abnormal hemodynamic situation. In these cases, the IABP is not needed. We prefer either "Dopride"—dopamine (5–20 μg/kg/min) plus nitroprusside (0.5–1 μg/kg/min); or "Epipride"—epinephrine (2–10 μg/min) plus nitroprusside (0.5–1 μg/kg/min). Nitroglycerin is used instead of nitroprusside when the left atrial pressure is very high or when ischemia/infarction is present. The dosage of nitroglycerin is 25–100 μg/min.

Figure 12-25 is an algorithm of the steps taken to discontinue cardiopulmonary bypass. It is a general plan and may

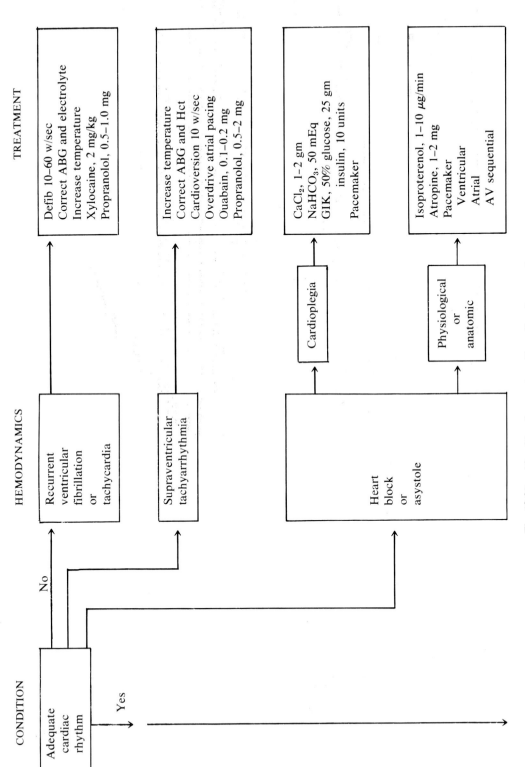

Fig. 12-25. Algorithm for coming off cardiopulmonary bypass.

CONDITION

HEMODYNAMICS

TREATMENT

Adequate cardiac rhythm

Yes

No

Recurrent ventricular fibrillation or tachycardia

Defib 10–60 w/sec
Correct ABG and electrolyte
Increase temperature
Xylocaine, 2 mg/kg
Propranolol, 0.5–1.0 mg

Supraventricular tachyarrhythmia

Increase temperature
Correct ABG and Hct
Cardioversion 10 w/sec
Overdrive atrial pacing
Ouabain, 0.1–0.2 mg
Propranolol, 0.5–2 mg

Heart block or asystole

Cardioplegia

CaCl$_2$, 1–2 gm
NaHCO$_3$, 50 mEq
GIK, 50% glucose, 25 gm insulin, 10 units
Pacemaker

Physiological or anatomic

Isoproterenol, 1–10 μg/min
Atropine, 1–2 mg
Pacemaker
  Ventricular
  Atrial
  AV sequential

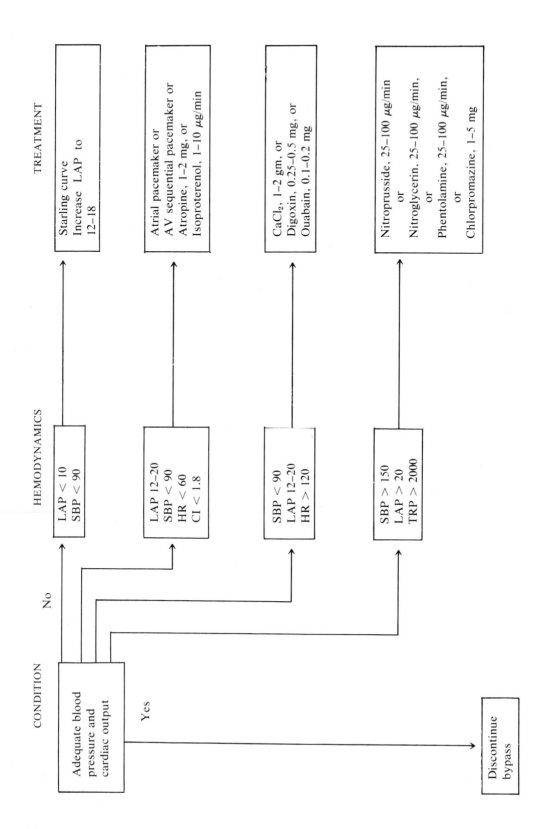

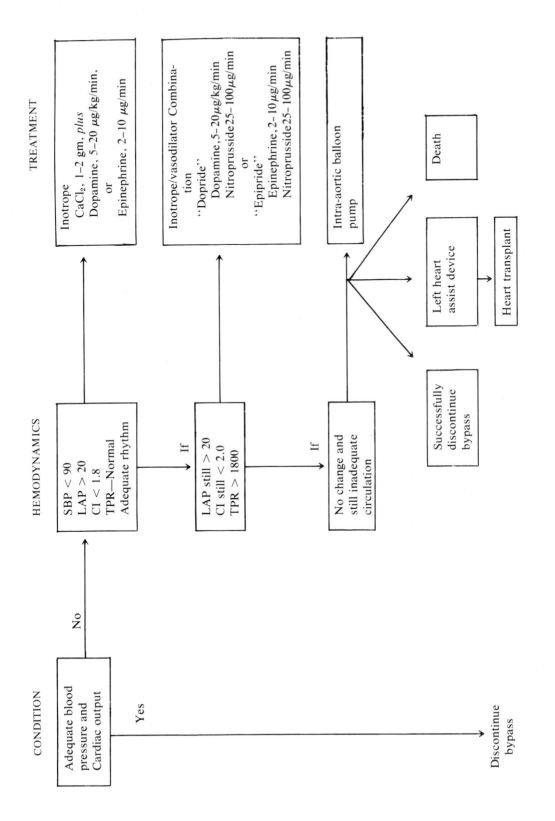

not be applicable to all patients. In some cases, there may be other variables, such as differences between the LAP and LVEDP or PCWP, artificial valves altering gradients between chambers, inability to

measure all desired variables, and combinations of hemodynamic situations.

10. In some patients the above pharmacologic approach fails and then the intra-aortic balloon is required.

REFERENCES

1. LeGallois J-JC: Expériences sur le principe de la vie. Paris, D'Hautel, 1812

2. Von Frey M, Gruber M: Untersuckungen uber den stoffwechsel isolierter organe. Ein respirations—apparat für isolierte organe, Virchow. Arch Physiol 9:519, 1885

3. Carrel A, Lindbergh CH: The culture of whole organs. Science 81:621, 1935

4. Comroe JH, Dripps RD: Ben Franklin and open heart surgery. Circ Res 35:661, 1964

5. Dennis C: Pump oxygenator to supplant the heart and lung for brief periods. Surgery 29:697, 1951

6. Gibbon JH, Jr: Artificial maintenance of circulation during experimental occlusion of pulmonary artery. Arch Surg 34:1105, 1937

7. Hooker DR: A study of the isolated kidney—the influence of pulse pressure upon renal function. Am J Physiol 27:27, 1910

8. Boucher JK, Rudy LW, Edmunds LH: Organ blood flow during pulsatile cardiopulmonary bypass. J Appl Physiol 36:86, 1974

9. Dunn J, Kirsch MN, Harness J, et al: Hemodynamic, metabolic, and hematologic effects of pulsatile cardiopulmonary bypass. J. Thorac Cardiovasc Surg 68:138, 1974

10. Olsen DA, Kletschka HD, Rafferty EH, et al: Design considerations for a non-pulsatile blood pump. JAMA 227:735, 1974

11. Bregman D: Mechanical support of the failing heart. Curr Prob Surg 13:12, 1976

12. Shea MA, Indeglia RA, Dorman FD, et al: The biologic response to pumping blood. Trans Am Soc Artif Intern Organs 13:116, 1967

13. Hendry EB: Erythrocyte fragility: Vertebrates. In Dittmer DS (ed): Blood and Other Body Fluids. Washington DC, Fed Am Soc Exp Biol, 1961

14. Sutera SP, Croce PA, Mehrjardi M: Hemolysis and subhemolytic alterations of human red blood cells induced by turbulent shear flow. Trans Am Soc Artif Intern Organs 18:335, 1972

15. Velker JA, McIntyre LV, Lynch EC: Alteration of erythrocyte deformability due to shear stress as assessed by micropore filters. Trans Am Soc Artif Intern Organs 23:732, 1977

16. Mortensen JD: Evaluation of tests for blood damage produced by oxygenators. Trans Am Soc Artif Intern Organs 23:747, 1977

17. Harrison D, Leung LS: Bubble formation at an orifice in a fluidized blood. Nature (London) 190:433, 1961

18. Goldsmith HL: The effects of flow and fluid mechanical stress on red cells and platelets. Trans Am Soc Artif Intern Organs 20:21, 1974

19. Bass RM, Longmore DB: Cerebral damage during open heart surgery. Nature 222:30, 1969

20. Andersen MN, Kuchiba K: Blood trauma produced by pump oxygenators. J. Thorac Cardiovasc Surg 57:238, 1969

21. Cheesman DF, Davies VT: Physiochemical and biological effects of proteins at interfaces. Adv Protein Chem 9:439, 1954

22. Galletti PM: Blood interfacial phenomena: An overview. Fed Proc 30 (5):1491, 1971

23. Conference on mechanical surface and gas layer effects on moving blood. Fed Proc 30:1485, 1971

24. Hubbard LC, Kletschka HD, Olsen DA, et al: Spallation using roller pumps and its clinical implications. J Extracorp Tech (in press)

25. Okies JE, Goodnight SH, Litchford B, et al: Effects of infusion of cardiotomy suction blood during extracorporeal circulation for coronary bypass surgery. J Thorac Cardiovasc Surg 74:440, 1977

26. Salzman EW: Non-thrombogenic surfaces: Critical review. Blood 38:509, 1971

27. Gott EV, Furose A: Antithrombogenic surfaces: Classification and in vivo evaluation. Fed Proc 30:1674, 1971

28. Leininger RI, Crowley JP, Falb RD, et al: Three years experience in vivo and in vitro with surfaces and devices treated by the heparin complex method. Trans Am Soc Artif Intern Organs 18:156, 1972

29. Bloom JR, Snyder MT, Peterson R, et al: Platelet life span and gas exchange during perfusion with spiral coil membrane lung coated with ethyl cellulose perfluorobutyrate. Trans Am Soc Artif Intern Organs 22:119, 1976

30. Mason KG, Hall LE, Lamoy RE, et al: Evaluation of blood filters: Dynamics of platelets and platelet aggregates. Surgery 77:235, 1975

31. Ashmore PG, Svitek V, Ambrose P: The inci-

dence and effects of particulate aggregation and microembolism in pump oxygenator systems. J Thorac Cardiovasc Surg 55:691, 1968

32. Clark RE, Margraf HW, Beauchamp RA: Fat and solid filtration in clinical perfusions. Surgery 77:216, 1975

33. Dimmick JE, Bove KE, McAdams AJ, et al: Fiber embolization—a hazard of cardiac surgery and catheterization. N Engl J Med 292:685: 1975

34. Dutton RC, Edmunds LH: Measurement of emboli in extracorporeal perfusion systems. J Thorac Cardiovasc Surg 65:523, 1973

35. Reed CC, Romagnoli A, Taylor DE, et al: Particulate matter in bubble oxygenators. J Thorac Cardiovasc Surg 68:971, 1974

36. Valentin N, Vilhelmson R: Blood and tissue silicone in extracorporeal circulation. J Thorac Cardiovasc Surg 17:20, 1976

37. Riley J, Young M: Personal communication

38. Hwang NHC, Borik, Noon GP, et al: Hydraulic studies of aortic cannulation return nozzles. Trans Am Soc Artif Intern Organs 21:237, 1975

39. Krons HG, Mansfield PB, Sauvage LR: Carotid artery hypoperfusion during open heart surgery. J Thorac Cardiovasc Surg 66:118, 1973

40. Hammond GL, Borley WW: Bubble mechanics in oxygen transfer. J Thorac Cardiovasc Surg 71:422, 1976

41. Galletti PM, Brecher GA: Heart-Lung Bypass. New York, Grune & Stratton, 1962

42. Selman MW, McAlpine WA, Ratan RS: The effectiveness of various heart-lung machines in the elimination of microbubbles from the circulation. J Thorac Cardiovasc Surg 53:613, 1967

43. Dorsen WJ, Larsen KG, Elgas RJ, et al: Oxygen transfer of blood: Data and theory. Trans Am Soc Artif Intern Organs 17:309, 1971

44. Galletti PM, Richardson PD, Snider MT, et al: A standardized method for defining the overall gas transfer performance of artificial lungs. Trans Am Soc Artif Intern Organs 18:359, 1972

45. Draft proposal: Standard for blood-gas exchangers. Trans Am Soc Artif Intern Organs 22:734, 1976

46. Bartlett RH, Fong SW, Woldanski C, et al: Hematologic response to prolonged extracorporeal circulation (ECC) with microporous membrane devices. Trans Am Soc Artif Intern Organs 21:250, 1975

47. Hyman ES: A method of introducing blood into a reservoir. Trans Am Soc Artif Intern Organs 5:238, 1959

48. Chartrand C, Langevin L, Forest F, et al: Hyperoxemia in extracorporeal circulation. Can J Surg 18:84, 1975

49. Vervloet AFC, Edwards MJ, Edwards ML, et al: Minimal apparent blood damage in Lande-Edwards membrane oxygenators at physiologic gas tensions. J Thorac Cardiovasc Surg 60:774, 1970

50. Hlastala MP, Van Liew H, Ashmore, et al: Absorption of in vivo inert gas bubbles. Respir Physiol 24:147, 1975

51. Feingold A: Crystalloid hemodilution, hypothermia and halothane blood solubility during cardiopulmonary bypass. Anesth Analg 56:622, 1977

52. Kolff WJ, Berk HTJ: Artificial kidney: Dialyzer with great area. Acta Med Scand 117:121, 1944

53. Mustard WT: Clinical and experimental experience with homologous and heterologous lung perfusions. Trans Am Soc Artif Intern Organs 1:94, 1955

54. Davids SG, Engell HC: Physiological and Clinical Aspects of Oxygenator Design. Amsterdam, Elsevier, 1976

55. Kronenthal C: Polymers in Medicine and Surgery. New York, Plenum Press, 1975

56. Bartlett RH, Drinker PA, Galletti PM: Mechanical Devices for Cardiopulmonary Assistance. Adv Cardiol, Basel, Karger, 1971

57. Heimbecker RO: Progress in extracorporeal circulation. J Thorac Cardiovasc Surg 70:157, 1977

58. Neptune WB, Bongas JA, Panico FG: Open heart surgery without the need for donor blood priming in the pump oxygenator. N Engl J Med 263:111, 1960

59. Miyauchi Y, Inoue T, Paton BC: Comparative study of priming fluids for two hour hemodilution perfusion. J Thorac Cardiovasc Surg 52:413, 1966

60. Messmer K, Schmid-Schonbein H: Hemodilution: Theoretical basis and clinical application. Adv Cardiol, Basel, Karger, 1972

61. Verska JJ, Ludington LG, Brewer LA: A comparative study of cardiopulmonary bypass with non-blood and blood primes. Ann Thorac Surg 18:72, 1974

62. Gordon RJ, Ravin M, Daicoff GR, et al: Effects of hemodilution on hypotension during cardiopulmonary bypass. Anesth Analg 54:482, 1975

63. Lee WH, Rubin JW, Huggins MP: Clinical evaluation of priming solutions for pump-oxygenator perfusion. Ann Thorac Surg 19:537, 1975

64. Mielke CH, deLeval M, Hill JD, et al: Drug influence on platelet loss during extracorporeal circulation. J Thorac Cardiovasc Surg 66:845, 1973

65. Birek A, Duffin J, Glynn MFX, et al: The effect of sulfinpyrazone on platelet and pulmonary responses to onset of membrane oxygenator perfusion. Trans Am Soc Artif Intern Organs 22:94, 1976

66. Addonizio VP, Macarek EJ, Niewiarowski S, et al: Preservation of platelets during extracor-

poreal circulation with prostaglandin E. Trans Am Soc Artif Intern Organs 23:639, 1977

67. Nuutinen LS, Pihlajaniemi R, Saarela E, et al: The effect of dipyridamole on the thrombocyte count and bleeding tendency in open heart surgery. J Thorac Cardiovasc Surg 74:295, 1977

68. Byrick RJ, Kay JC, Noble WH: Extravascular lung-water accumulation in patients following coronary artery surgery. Can Anaesth Soc J 24:332, 1977

69. Barash P, Ramireddy O: Osmotic profiles during open heart surgery: The effect of a colloid prime. Abstract presented at ASA, 1977

70. Gadboys HL, Slonim R, Litwak RS: The homologous blood syndrome: Preliminary observations of its relationship to clinical cardiopulmonary bypass. Ann Surg 156:797, 1962

71. Kamat V, Baker CB, Wilson JK, et al: Openheart surgery in Jehovah's Witnesses: Experiences in a Canadian hospital. Ann Thorac Surg 23: 367, 1977

72. Staub NC: Pulmonary edema. Physiol Rev 54:678, 1974

73. Cleeland J, Pluth JR, Tauxe WN, et al: Blood volume and body fluid compartment changes after closed and open intracardiac surgery. J Thorac Cardiovasc Surg 52:698, 1966

74. Dieter RA, Neville WE, Pifarre R: Serum electrolyte changes after cardiopulmonary bypass with Ringer's lactate solution used for hemodilution. J Thorac Cardiovasc Surg 59:168, 1970

75. Beattie HW, Evans G, Garnett ES, et al: Sustained hypovolemia and extracellular fluid volume expansion following cardiopulmonary bypass. Surgery 71:891, 1972

76. Utley JR, Todd EP, Wachtel CC, et al: Effect of hypothermia, hemodilution, and pump oxygenation on organ water content and blood flow. Surg Forum 27:217, 1976

77. Harris EA, Seelye ER, Barratt-Boyes BG: Respiratory and metabolic changes during cardiopulmonary bypass in man. Br J Anaesth 42:912, 1970

78. Hocking MA, Bain WH: Effect of amiloride on metabolic alkalosis after cardiopulmonary bypass surgery. Br Heart J 36:597, 1974

79. Abrahams N, Johnston AE, Taylor J, et al: A comparison of the effects of two haemodiluents on monovalent and divalent cations in children undergoing cardiopulmonary bypass and open heart surgery. Can Anaesth Soc J 20:153, 1973

80. Calverley RK, Jenkins LC, Griffiths J: A clinical study of serum magnesium concentrations during anaesthesia and cardiopulmonary bypass. Can Anaesth Soc J 20:499, 1973

81. Schaer H: Effects on ionized calcium of a correction of acidosis with alkalinizing agents. Br J Anaesth 48:327, 1976

82. Fuchs C, Brasche M, Spieckermann PG, et al: Divalent ions and myocardial function during cardiopulmonary bypass (CPB): Changes of total calcium, ionized calcium, and magnesium in plasma. J Thorac Cardiovasc Surg 16:476, 1975

83. Chipperfield B, Chipperfield JR: Magnesium and the heart. Am Heart J 93:679, 1977

84. Pierce EC: Extracorporeal Circulation for Open Heart Surgery. Springfield Ill, Charles C Thomas, 1969

85. Fisher A, Foex P, Emerson PM, et al: Oxygen availability during hypothermic cardiopulmonary bypass. Crit Care Med 5:154, 1977

86. Davis FM, Parimelazhagan KW, Harris EA: Thermal balance during cardiopulmonary bypass with moderate hypothermia in man. Br J Anaesth 49:1127, 1977

87. Shappel SD, Lenfant CJM: Adaptive, genetic and iatrogenic alterations of the oxyhemoglobin-dissociation curve. Anesthesiology 37:127, 1972

88. Bay J, Nunn JF, Prys-Roberts C: Factors influencing arterial PO_2 during recovery from anesthesia. Br J Anaesth 40:398, 1968

89. Kelman GR, Nunn JF, Prys-Roberts C: The influence of cardiac output on arterial oxygenation: A theoretical study. Br J Anaesth 39:450, 1957

90. Steward DJ, Sloan IA, Johnston AE: Anesthetic management of infants undergoing profound hypothermia for surgical correction of congenital heart defects. Can Anaesth Soc J 21:15, 1974

91. Szymanski IO, Dean HM, Valeri CR, et al: Measurement of erythrocyte survival during open heart surgery. Trans Am Soc Artif Intern Organs 16:168, 1970

92. Hochmuth RM, Mohandas N, Spaetha EE, et al: Surface adhesion, deformation and detachment at low shear of red cells and white cells. Trans Am Soc Artif Intern Organs 18:325, 1972

93. Kvarstein B, Cappelen C, Osterud A: Blood platelets and leukocytes during cardiopulmonary bypass. Scand J Thorac Cardiovasc Surg 8:142, 1974

94. Brown CH, Lemuth RF, Hellums JD, et al: Response of human platelets to shear stress. Trans Am Soc Artif Intern Organs 21:35, 1975

95. deLeval MR, Hill JD, Mielke CH, et al: Blood platelets and extracorporeal circulation: Kinetic studies on dogs on cardiopulmonary bypass. J Thorac Cardiovasc Surg 69:144, 1975

96. Tamari Y, Aledort L, Puzkin E, et al: Functional changes in platelets during extracorporeal circulation. Ann Thorac Surg 19:639, 1975

97. Wandall HH, Sivertsen U: The puzzle of blood platelets in extracorporeal circulation. Scand J Thorac Cardiovasc Surg 9:140, 1975

98. O'Brien JR: Heparin and platelets. J Curr Ther Res 18:79, 1975

99. Barrer MJ, Ellison N: Platelet function. Anesthesiology 46:202, 1977

100. Gans H, Castaneda AR: Problems in hemostasis during open heart surgery: VII. Changes in fibrinogen concentration during and after cardiopulmonary bypass with particular reference to the effects of heparin neutralization on fibrinogen. Ann Surg 165:551, 1967

101. Sears DA: Disposal of plasma hemoglobin in normal man and patients with intravascular hemolysis. J Clin Invest 49:5, 1970

102. Litwin MS, Walter CW, Jackson N: Experimental production of acute renal tubular necrosis. (III) acid hematin, the etiologic pigment. Ann Surg 152:1016, 1960

103. Silva J, Hoeksema H, Fekety TR: Transient defects in phagocytic functions during cardiopulmonary bypass. J Thorac Cardiovasc Surg 67:175, 1974

104. Scovill WA, Saba TM, Kaplan JE, et al: Disturbances in circulating obsonic activity in man after operative and blunt trauma. J Surg Res 22:709, 1977

105. Alexander JW, McClellan MA, Ogle CK, et al: Consumptive opsoninopathy: Possible pathogenesis in lethal and opertugenic infections. Ann Surg 184:672, 1976

106. Sherman MM, Dobnik DB, Dennis RC, et al: Autologous blood transfusion during cardiopulmonary bypass. Chest 70:592, 1976

107. Kaplan JA, Cannarella C, Jones EL: Autologous blood transfusion during cardiac surgery. J Thorac Cardiovasc Surg 74:4, 1977

108. Hallowell P, Bland JHL, Buckley MJ, et al: Transfusion of fresh autologous blood in open-heart surgery. J Thorac Cardiovasc Surg 64:941, 1972

109. Cohn LH, Fosberg AM, Anderson WP, et al: The effects of phlebotomy, hemodilution and autologous transfusion on systemic oxygenation and whole blood utilization in open-heart surgery. Chest 68:283:1975

110. Roche JK, Stengle JN: Open-heart surgery and the demand for blood. JAMA 225:1516, 1973

111. National Transfusion Hepatitis Study: Risk of post-transfusion hepatitis in the United States: A prospective comparative study. JAMA 220:692, 1972

112. Pennock JL, Pierce WS, Waldhausen JA: Management of the lungs during cardiopulmonary bypass. Surg Gynecol Obstet 145:917, 1977

113. Fowler NO, Holmes JC: Blood viscosity and cardiac output in acute experimental anemia. J Appl Physiol 39:453, 1975

114. Radegran K, McAslan C: Circulatory and ventilatory effects of induced platelet aggregation and their inhibition by acetylsalicylic acid. Acta Anaesthesiol Scand 16:76, 1972

115. Jacobsen E, Jessen C, Sivertsen U: Continuous measurement of arterial Po_2, Pco_2 and pH during autotransplantation of canine hearts. Acta Anaesthesiol Scand 19:265, 1975

116. Garman JK: Survey: Association of cardiac anesthesiologists. Personal communication, 1976

117. Stockard JJ, Bickford RG, Schauble JF: Pressure dependent cerebral ischemia during cardiopulmonary bypass. J Neurol 23:521, 1973

118. Engelman RM, Spencer FC, Boyd AD, et al: The significance of cornonary arterial stenosis during cardiopulmonary bypass. J Thorac Cardiovasc Surg 70:869, 1975

119. Hagel S, Heimisch W, Meisner H, et al: The effect of hemodilution on regional myocardial function in the presence of coronary stenosis. J Basic Res Cardiol 72:344, 1977

120. Evans PJD, Reuygrock P, Seelye ER, et al: Does sodium nitroprusside improve tissue oxygenation during cardiopulmonary bypass? Br J Anaesth 49:799, 1977

121. Mandelbaum I, Silbert N, Berry J: Phenoxybenzamine (Dibenzylene) and renal blood flow during extracorporeal circulation. J Thorac Cardiovasc Surg 8:73, 1967

122. Burack B, Marcs D, Miyamoto A, et al: Response of Class IV patients to alpha blockade prior to open heart surgery. Am Heart J 84:456, 1972

123. Stanley TH, Isern-Amaral, J: Periodic analysis of mixed venous oxygen tension to monitor the adequacy of perfusion during and after cardiopulmonary bypass. Can Anaesth Soc J 21:454, 1974

124. Abel RM, Buckley MJ, Austen WG, et al: Etiology, incidence, and prognosis of renal failure following cardiac operations. J Thorac Cardiovasc Surg 71:23, 1976

125. Schaer H: Effects of acidosis with alkalinizing agents. Br J Anaesth 48:327, 1976

126. O'Connor F, Castilono-Olivaries JL, Romero G, et al: Anoxic cardiac arrest: Its effect on myocardial metabolism. J Cardiovasc Surg 16:493, 1975

127. Bentall H: Protection of the myocardium during surgery. J Cardiovasc Surg 16:228, 1975

128. Bercot M, Deloche A, Piwnica A, et al: Selective cardiac hypothermia versus coronary perfusion. J Cardiovasc Surg 16:232, 1975

129. Brainbridge MV, Chayen J, Bitensky L, et al: Cold cardioplegia or continuous coronary perfusion. J Thorac Cardiovasc Surg 74:900, 1977

130. Melrose DG, Dreyer B, Bentall AJ, et al: Elective cardiac arrest. Lancet 2:21, 1955

131. Kirsch U, Rodewald G, Kalmar P: Induced

ischemic arrest: Clinical experience with cardioplegia in open heart surgery. J Thorac Cardiovasc Surg 63:121, 1972

132. Bretschneider HJ, Hubner G, Knoll D, et al: Myocardial resistance and tolerance to ischemia: Physiological and biochemical basis. J Cardiovasc Surg 16:241, 1975

133. Follette D, Fey K, Mulder D, etal: Prolonged safe aortic clamping by combining stabilization, multidose cardioplegia, appropriate pH, re-perfusion. J Thorac Cardiovasc Surg 74:682, 1977

134. Jynge P, Hearse DJ, Brainbridge MV: Myocardial protection during ischemic cardiac arrest. J Thorac Cardiovasc Surg 73:848, 1977

135. Tyers GFO, Manley NJ, Williams EH, et al: Preliminary clinical experience with isotonic hypothermic potassium-induced arrest. J Thorac Cardiovasc Surg 74:674, 1977

136. Roe BB, Hutchinson JC, Fishman MH, et al: Myocardial protection with cold, ischemic potassium-induced cardioplegia. J Thorac Cardiovasc Surg 73:366, 1977

137. Krause BL, Hassan MA, McMillan AB, et al: Protective effect of methyl-prednisolone on ischemic myocardium assessed by ventricular function. Thorax 32:185, 1977

138. Venas JF, Fewel JT, Grover FL, et al: Effects of methylprednisolone on coronary blood flow and myocardial metabolism during cardiopulmonary bypass. J Surg 81:646, 1977

139. Hewlitt RL, Lolley DM, Adroumey GA, et al: Protective effect of glycogen and glucose on the anoxic arrested heart. J Surg 75:1, 1974

140. Vlahakes GJ, Powell WJ: Effect of hyperosmotic mannitol on myocardial oxygen consumption. J Appl Physiol 233:444, 1977

141. Bergline, Hannson AJ, Teger-Nilsson AC, et al: Proceedings: Anti-coagulation during six hours of extracorporeal perfusion. Comparison between heparinization and defibrinogination. Anesthetist 34:578, 1975

142. White JJ, Bell W, Matthews P, et al: Arvin anticoagulation for prolonged extracorporeal membrane oxygenation. Anesthetist 25:526, 1976

143. McLean J: The discovery of heparin. Circulation 19:75, 1959

144. Best CH: Preparation of heparin and its first clinical use. Circulation 19:79, 1959

145. Estes JW, Poulin PF: Pharmacokinetics of heparin: Distribution and elimination. Thromb Diath Haemorrh 33:26, 1974

146. Perry MO, Horton JA: Kinetics of heparin administration. Arch Surg 111:403, 1976

147. Cohen JA, Frederickson EL, Kaplan JA: Plasma heparin activity and antagonism during cardiopulmonary bypass with hypothermia. Anesth Analg 56:564, 1977

148. Hattersley PG: Activated coagulation time of whole blood. JAMA 196:436, 1966

149. Bull MH, Huse WM, Bull BS: Evaluation of tests used to monitor heparin therapy during extracorporeal circulation. Anesthesiology 43:346, 1975

150. Bull BS, Huse WM, Brauer FS, et al: Heparin therapy during extracorporeal circulation. II Use of a dose-response curve to individualize heparin and protamine dosage. J Thorac Cardiovasc Surg 69:785, 1975

151. Cargaff F, Olson KB: Studies in the chemistry of blood coagulation VI. Studies on the action of heparin and other anticoagulants. The influence of protamine on the anticoagulant effects in vivo. J Biol Chem 122:153, 1937-8

152. Ellison N, Ominsky AJ, Wollman H: Is protamine a clinically important anticoagulant? Anesthesiology 35:621, 1971

153. Eika C: On the mechanism of platelet aggregation induced by heparin, protamine, and polybrene. Scand J Haematol 9:248, 1972

Joel A. Kaplan, M.D.
Joseph M. Craver, M.D.

13
Assisted Circulation

MECHANICAL CIRCULATORY ASSIST DEVICES

Mechanical circulatory assist (MCA) devices have been used for 20 years to support the circulation in patients with cardiogenic shock. Initially, the cardiopulmonary bypass machine was used for circulatory assistance, since it was used during cardiac surgery, but with little success.[1] Since then, many devices have been developed to assist the failing circulation. These devices may be classified as shown in Table 13-1.[2,3] Total cardiopulmonary bypass has been used with femoral vein and femoral artery cannulation and either a bubble or membrane oxygenator. Prolonged perfusion has led to hemolysis and coagulation defects. Left heart bypass will also decrease preload. This has been accomplished by withdrawing blood from either the left atrium or ventricle and pumping it into the aorta or systemic arteries during diastole. The DeBakey pump has been employed in patients having difficulty coming off cardiopulmonary bypass.[4] In this system, blood is taken from the left atrium and pumped into the axillary artery. Recently, Litwak described a new left heart assist device that does not require another thoracotomy to remove it as the previous systems did.[5] Cannulae are placed in the left atrium and ascending aorta and brought out through the abdominal wall. Partial left heart bypass may be used for as long as necessary and then the cannulae closed off and left under the skin.

Clauss described the concept of counterpulsation in 1961, and this has been used since then to reduce afterload or arterial impedance.[6] His arterial counterpulsator withdrew blood from the aorta during systole and returned it during diastole. The idea was to reduce aortic and left ventricular systolic pressures, left ventricular wall tension, and thus myocardial oxygen consumption. At the same time, the increased aortic blood volume during diastole increased coronary perfusion.

Many techniques for counterpulsation have been developed, but the intra-aortic balloon pump (IABP) has become by far the most popular. Moulopoulus first produced diastolic augmentation in 1962 with a balloon catheter placed in the aorta.[7] His studies were later adapted by Kantrowitz, who perfected the technique in 1968 for clinical use in patients with cardiogenic shock.[8] The following advantages have led to the popularity of the IABP:[9]

1. Ease of insertion and removal without a thoracotomy
2. Ease of operation of the system
3. Effective diastolic augmentation with good clinical results, e.g., reversal of cardiogenic shock syndrome

Table 13-1

Classification of
Mechanical Circulatory
Assist Devices

I. Decreased preload
    1. Cardiopulmonary bypass
    2. Left heart bypass
II. Decreased afterload
    1. Arterioarterial pumping
    2. Aortic counterpulsation
III. Direct cardiac compression

---

4. Little patient discomfort
5. Acceptable complication rate

Noninvasive external counterpulsation over the legs has only been moderately effective in cardiogenic shock, and it does not appear that it will replace the IABP.[10] Direct cardiac compression has been tried clinically without success by compressing the entire heart with an inflated silastic membrane in a rigid cup.[11]

INTRA-AORTIC BALLOON PUMP

The IABP was first used in 1968 for patients in refractory cardiogenic shock. In 1970, Buckley showed that decreasing the arterial impedance was the main hemodynamic effect of the balloon and that improved coronary perfusion was a secondary effect.[12] In 1970, Mundth introduced the use of the IABP to stabilize patients with cardiogenic shock in preparation for surgery.[13] In 1973, Buckley reported the use of the IABP in patients who were unable to be weaned from cardiopulmonary bypass.[14] This was a great step in salvaging many cardiac surgical patients. Recently, the IABP has been used in an attempt to salvage ischemic myocardium and prevent further ischemic damage.[15] It has frequently been used as an interface between medical and surgical treatment modalities.

Physiological Principles

Left ventricular failure is characterized by decreased contractility in association with increased preload and afterload. This produces hypotension and a low cardiac output syndrome (cardiogenic shock) consisting of cold clammy skin, decreased urine output, decreased level of consciousness, and metabolic acidosis. These patients all require invasive monitoring with a Swan-Ganz catheter to determine their exact left ventricular function. Bolooki has classified these patients into hemodynamic subsets according to his "shock box" (Fig. 13-1).[9] Class A patients are relatively stable and do not require the IABP. Class B patients are hypovolemic and will improve with volume infusion.

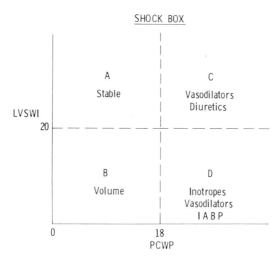

Fig. 13-1. Bolooki's "shock box" is demonstrated. (Reproduced from Bolooki H: Clinical Application of the Intra-Aortic Balloon Pump. Mt. Kisco, NY, Futura, 1977, with permission of author and publisher.)

Class C patients are in congestive heart failure and usually respond to afterload reduction therapy and diuretics. Some of these patients however, will require the IABP if they do not improve with vasodilators. Class D patients are the sickest and still have a high mortality associated with their cardiogenic shock. They have pulmonary congestion and poor peripheral perfusion. These patients have a cardiac index of less than 2.0 liters/min/m², a left ventricular stroke work index of less than 20 gm·m/m², and cardiac work (MAP × CI) of less than 150 units. Most of these patients require the IABP even after therapy with inotropes and vasodilators. The goals of IABP therapy in these patients are to unload the heart and allow it sufficient time for recovery while maintaining adequate peripheral perfusion.

The intra-aortic balloon is inserted into the descending thoracic aorta through a graft anastamosed end-to-side to the femoral artery. The tip of the polyurethane balloon catheter should be located just below the left subclavian artery (Fig. 13-2). The balloon is inflated with helium or carbon dioxide, usually at the same rate as the pulse (1:1 mode). It may also be used only on every other beat (1:2 mode) or 1:4 of 1:8. Either helium or carbon dioxide is used to inflate

the balloon because of their low viscosity which allows rapid movement of the gas in and out of the balloon.

The balloon is *inflated* during *diastole*, which is timed from either the T wave of the ECG or the dicrotic notch (aortic valve closure) on the arterial pressure tracing (Fig. 13-3). The adult balloon is inflated with either 30 or 40 cc of gas. As a result, a volume of blood in the aorta is displaced proximal and distal to the balloon, and the diastolic blood pressure is augmented. This produces an increase in coronary and cerebral blood flow. Since coronary blood flow occurs predominantly in diastole, an increase in the diastolic blood pressure should increase coronary blood flow. Mueller has demonstrated an increase in coronary flow with counterpulsation in patients with cardiogenic shock.[16] Timing of the inflation is critical and is best done from a central aortic pressure tracing. Early inflation will impede and prematurely terminate ventricular ejection. This can reduce stroke volume and cardiac output, increase end-systolic and end-diastolic volume, and increase instead of decrease left ventricular wall tension.[17]

The balloon is *deflated* just prior to the next *systole* during the phase of isometric contrac-

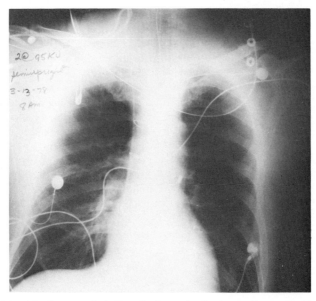

Fig. 13-2. The intra-aortic balloon is shown in the descending aorta. The tip is somewhat below the left subclavian artery.

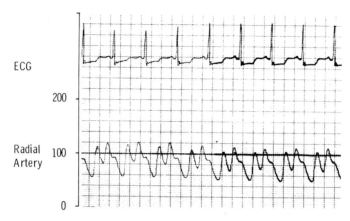

Fig. 13-3. The ECG and radial artery tracings of a patient undergoing balloon counterpulsation are demonstrated. The balloon is inflated on the dichrotic notch or the T wave of the electrocardiogram.

tion. It is timed to deflate just prior to the onset of the QRS complex of the ECG or just prior to the beginning of the arterial upstroke. The timing of deflation is also critical because prolonged inflation will decrease stroke volume and increase left ventricular wall tension. If the balloon is deflated too early, there is a large diastolic dip or "sink" that will pull blood out of the more peripheral arteries (e.g., carotid) back to the aorta and reduce cerebral and coronary blood flow. Deflation produces a negative intra-aortic pressure as a result of the rapid collapse of the balloon. The arterial impedance to ejection of blood from the left ventricle is thus decreased, and cardiac output is augmented. Weber has shown that the IABP can reduce mean ejection impedance by 21 percent,[17] while Mueller reported a 46 percent decrease.[16] Myocardial work and preload also fall as secondary features of the IABP unloading the heart.

The IABP favorably affects the delicate balance between the myocardial oxygen supply and the myocardial oxygen demand. This can best be seen by using the endocardial viability ratio (EVR) described by Buckberg and Hoffman[18] and modified by Philips.[19]

$$EVR = \frac{DPTI}{TTI}$$
$$= \frac{\text{diastolic pressure time index}}{\text{tension time index}}$$
$$= \frac{\text{supply}}{\text{demand}}$$

The DPTI is a measure of myocardial oxygen supply, while the TTI is a measure of myocardial oxygen demand or consumption (Fig. 13-4). The TTI is the area under the systolic portion of the arterial tracing, which is measured from the beginning of the upstroke to the dicrotic notch. The DPTI is the area under the diastolic part of the curve minus the left atrial pressure. The ratio of DPTI to TTI should normally be over 1.0. Ratios under 0.7 imply subendocardial ischemia. This ratio can be measured either by planimetry or by Phillip's formula (see Chapter 4). The IABP markedly increases the DPTI and decreases the TTI, thus improving the EVR and the myocardial oxygen balance. The IABP also decreases the LAP and frequently decreases the heart rate on a reflex basis as a result of improved perfusion. All of these factors tend to improve myocardial oxygenation.

By decreasing preload and afterload and by augmenting coronary blood flow and the myocardial oxygen balance, the IABP helps to improve left ventricular function. Patients tend to move from "shock box D" up toward "box A" (Fig. 13-5). In most cases, the move is gradual and needs to be supported by pharmacologic therapy with inotropes and vasodilators.

By displacing blood from the aorta, the IABP should also affect peripheral tissue perfusion. Results of studies in this area have been conflicting. Most studies have found a slight increase in carotid artery flow (5 percent) and unchanged renal artery blood flow.[20] Diastolic augmentation has been shown to increase aortic baroreceptor output and, in some studies, to

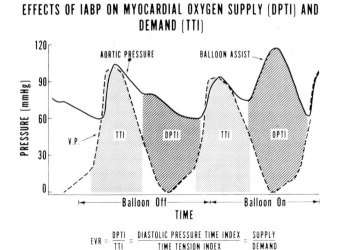

EFFECTS OF IABP ON MYOCARDIAL OXYGEN SUPPLY (DPTI) AND DEMAND (TTI)

$$EVR = \frac{DPTI}{TTI} = \frac{DIASTOLIC\ PRESSURE\ TIME\ INDEX}{TIME\ TENSION\ INDEX} = \frac{SUPPLY}{DEMAND}$$

Fig. 13-4. The effects of the IABP are shown on the endocardial viability ratio. (Reproduced from Bolooki H: Clinical Application of the Intra-Aortic Balloon Pump. Mt. Kisco, NY, Futura, 1977, with permission of author and publisher.)

decrease heart rate and vascular resistance by this mechanism.[21] The effects of the IABP are summarized in Figure 13-6 and Table 13-2.

Mechanics of the Intra-Aortic Balloon Pump

There are two types of balloons and pumping systems available at the present time: (1) the omnidirectional tricompartmental balloon used in the Avco-Roche* IABP, and (2) the unidirectional dual-chambered balloon used in the Datascope System 80† IABP. The two balloons are shown in Figure 13-7. The Avco-Roche omnidirectional balloon is trisegmented, with inflation beginning in the middle segment, followed by inflation of the two ends. This avoids entrapment of blood between the two ends of the balloon.[22] The Datascope unidirectional balloon has two chambers. The distal small balloon inflates first to occlude the aorta, and then the proximal balloon inflates. Bregman and Talpins have shown that this causes most of the augmented flow to travel proximal toward the coronary arteries.[23,24] In one study, Talpins found that the unidirectional balloon resulted in a 66 to 100

* Avco-Roche Medical Electronics, Cranbury, N.J.

† Datascope Corp., Paramus, N.J.

percent greater increment in coronary blood flow than the omnidirectional balloon. Both types of balloons are made of polyurethane, which, because of its surface properties, tends to be nonthrombogenic. The Avco-Roche balloon is inflated with helium, while the Datascope balloon is inflated with carbon dioxide.

We have had most of our experience with the IABP utilizing the two Avco-Roche systems shown in Figure 13-8. Therefore, we will discuss the mechanics and problems using these models. Most of the discussion, however, will apply to the Datascope system as well. The Avco-Roche Model 7 is the older system, while the Model 10 is the more recently introduced, updated version. New features of the Model 10 are a computerized color screen that identifies problems during use or setup of the balloon, automatic venting of the balloon, a built-in pacemaker to trigger the balloon at a fixed rate of 80 if desired on cardiopulmonary bypass (see section on pulsatile perfusion), an optional recorder for recording timing of the balloon, and an optional built-in cardiac output computer that can give frequent cardiac output readings on the computer screen.

While the surgeons are inserting the balloon catheter, which takes 15 to 30 minutes, the balloon console should be set up and checked out. The balloon is initially timed off an ECG trace.

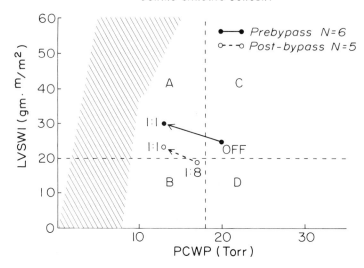

Fig. 13-5. The effects of the IABP on left ventricular function in 11 patients during cardiac surgery are demonstrated. Measurements were made from 6 patients in the prebypass period and 5 patients after cardiopulmonary bypass.

This ECG can be directly obtained from the patient by a second set of ECG electrodes, or it can be taken off the monitoring equipment and jacked into the back of the balloon console. We prefer to take it off the monitor and select the lead with the largest gain for the computer in the balloon console to read. The gain control is adjusted to give a peak-to-peak height of 2 cm. If the patient has no spontaneous heart beat or a very slow rhythm, then ventricular and atrial pacemaker wires are placed on the heart. The ventricular pacing spike will fire the balloon with good timing, but the benefit of atrial contraction is lost. Triggering the balloon off atrial pacing is much trickier. The atrial pacer spike must be made very small so that the console does not see it but instead triggers off the ensuing ventricular complex. If the balloon triggers off the atrial spike, it will not have proper timing. If the patient will not conduct an atrially paced beat, we prefer to use atrioventricular sequential pacing to trigger the balloon. This allows atrial contraction with a small pacer spike not seen by the console and correctly timed ventricular contraction with a larger pacer spike seen by the console and proper timing of the balloon off the ventricular complex. The assist interval switches are adjusted so that the balloon inflates on the peak of the T wave and deflates immediately before the QRS complex. When the balloon is inserted, the console end is handed off the sterile field by the surgeon and plugged into the back

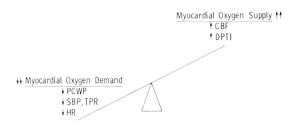

Fig. 13-6. The effects of the IABP on the myocardial oxygen balance are demonstrated.

Table 13-2
Hemodynamic Effects of IABP

Increased	Decreased
Diastolic aortic pressure	Systolic aortic pressure
Coronary blood flow	Left ventricular wall tension
Cerebral and renal blood flow	Preload-LVEDP, PCWP, LAP
Cardiac output	Afterload
Ejection fraction	Heart rate
	Tension time index

of the console. The balloon has to be flushed for 1 minute with helium to rid it of air. Pumping is then begun using half the volume of the balloon at first (e.g., 20cc in a 40cc balloon) to check for proper operation. The volume is then increased to its full amount by adjusting the large knob on the front of the console.

The initial timing is set using the ECG, but the final critical adjustment is made using the arterial pressure tracing. The balloon is set to inflate on the dicrotic notch and to deflate just before the beginning of the upstroke. This can be set using the radial artery trace as long as it is remembered that the radial artery tracing is delayed in its passage from the aorta by about

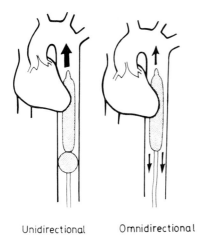

Unidirectional   Omnidirectional

Fig. 13-7. The unidirectional and omnidirectional intra-aortic balloons are demonstrated. (Reproduced from Bregman D: Dual-chambered intra-aortic balloon counterpulsation. *In* Ionesco M (ed): Current Techniques in Extracorporeal Circulation. London, Butterworth's, 1976, with permission of author and publisher.)

25–50 msec. Therefore, the balloon should inflate just slightly ahead of the dicrotic notch seen on the radial artery tracing. For ideal balloon timing, a needle may be placed in the aorta and a central aortic pressure tracing obtained and compared to the radial artery tracing.

The balloon should be set on 1:2 or 1:4 to adjust the timing properly. This allows both normal and balloon-augmented beats to be seen. After proper timing, the IABP is set on 1:1 for maximum benefit for the patient. Proper and improper balloon timing are shown in Figure 13-9. The balloon console may be triggered off the ECG or the arterial pressure tracing. In the operating room, the arterial pressure curve triggering is preferable, since it will not be interfered with by the electrocautery. The electrocautery will obliterate the ECG, and whenever it is used the IABP will misfire if it is being triggered off the ECG. This will not happen if the IABP is triggered off the arterial pressure tracing.

There is an elaborate system of alarms and warning lights built into the IABP console. On the new Model 10, the computer screen even indicates where the problem is located and how to correct it. Problems frequently encountered are helium leakage at the vent site or connection to the console, empty helium tanks, water vapor in the cable to the balloon, arrhythmias affecting the timing, poor ECG contact or tracings, and low battery power. These must all be attended to immediately to maintain good diastolic augmentation.

The Avco-Roche balloon pump should be operated on ac wall current whenever possible. It is also supplied with a dc battery pack for use during movement of the patient. It takes 18 hours to recharge an exhausted battery; therefore, the unit should remain plugged in and fully

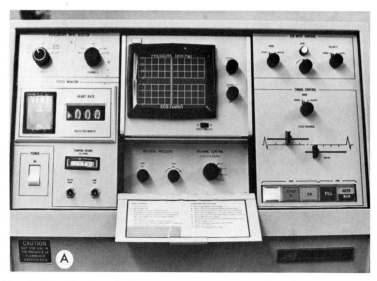

Fig. 13-8A. The Avco-Roche Model 7 intra-aortic balloon console is demonstrated

charged at all times. A fully charged battery is adequate for about 1 hour of transporting.[22] On the new model, a flashing light indicates a low battery, while on the older model, a voltmeter is located at the bottom. When this reads under 10 v, the battery is low and needs recharging.

Both models of the Avco-Roche IABP have a cardiac output computer that can be purchased as an option. In 1976, Herzlinger, from the Avco Everett Research Laboratory, described a new method of cardiac output determination using the radial artery tracing in patients receiving balloon pumping (Fig. 13-10).[25] The formula used by the computer for deriving the cardiac output is

$$CO = BV \times \frac{P_2 - P_0}{P_1 - P_0} \times HR$$

where   BV   = balloon pumping volume
            HR   = heart rate

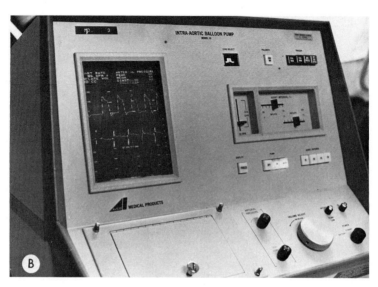

Fig. 13-8B. The Model 10 is demonstrated.

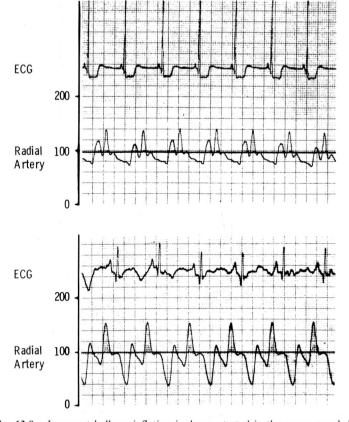

Fig. 13-9. Incorrect balloon inflation is demonstrated in the upper panel. The balloon is deflated too early. Correct balloon inflation and deflation is demonstrated in the lower panel.

$P_1 - P_0$ = balloon deflation pressure excursion

$P_2 - P_0$ = Ventricular ejection pressure excursion

P_1 = plateau-like region of the pressure tracing midway between peak diastolic pressure and end-diastolic pressure

P_2 = peak systolic pressure

P_0 = end-diastolic pressure

This formula can only be used when the patient is receiving diastolic augmentation with every heart beat (1:1 mode). The computer updates the cardiac output readout every 10 seconds to give continuous monitoring without additional equipment. Herzlinger compared this method with dye or thermal dilution techniques in 40 patients. The mean cardiac output was 4.84 liters/min using the formula as compared to 4.93 liters/min using thermal and dye dilution techniques. In 5 percent of the patients, this method could not be used because no plateau region could be identified. The overall correlation coefficient between this method and the standard methods was 0.928, while the standard deviation

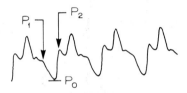

Fig. 13-10. Herzlinger's technique for measuring cardiac output off the radial artery tracing is demonstrated. The patient must be on the 1:1 mode of counterpulsation.

of the difference between the two methods was 12 percent. However, there are some problems with this technique:

1. It cannot be used during balloon weaning when it would be most useful; it can only be used on the 1:1 mode.
2. Occasional recalibration of the balloon pumping volume at various pressures is necessary.
3. To construct left ventricular function curves, a Swan-Ganz catheter to obtain the PCWP is still needed.

Clinical Use of the Intra-Aortic Balloon Pump

Indications for the IABP are shown in Table 13-3. The relative contraindications for the IABP are shown in Table 13-4.

CARDIOGENIC SHOCK

The IABP was first designed and used for patients with cardiogenic shock.[8] Since then, data have become available from a number of studies. Scheidt reported a cooperative multi-departmental trial of 87 patients with cardiogenic shock.[26] Mean heart rate decreased from 110 to 103 beats per minute, systolic pressure decreased from 76 to 57 mm Hg, diastolic pressure increased from 53 to 83 mm Hg, mean arterial pressure was unchanged, and cardiac output increased 0.5 liter/min. from 2.4 to 2.9 liter/min. About 70 percent of the patients had improved urine output, reduced acidosis, and decreased incidence of arrhythmias; 60 percent needed fewer pressor drugs, while showing improved peripheral perfusion; and about 40 percent showed improvement in their mental status and pulmonary congestion. However, 52 patients (60 percent) could not be weaned from the balloon, and only 15 of those taken off the balloon (17 percent) left the hospital. The author's

Table 13-3
Indications for the IABP

I. Ischemic heart disease
  A. Cardiogenic shock
  B. Acute myocardial infarction with mechanical complications
    1. Ventricular-septal rupture
    2. Acute mitral insufficiency
    3. Acute left ventricular aneurysm
  C. Refractory ventricular arrhythmias
  D. Progressive ischemia
  E. During cardiac catheterization
  F. Undergoing noncardiac surgery
II. Cardiac surgery
  A. Before cardiopulmonary bypass
  B. After cardiopulmonary bypass
  C. Postoperatively
III. Pulsatile cardiopulmonary bypass
IV. Pediatric congenital heart disease

attempts to predict survival ahead of time were totally unsuccessful. The mortality from cardiogenic shock is still over 50 percent even with the IABP. Ehrich defined hemodynamic changes with the IABP in the first 48 hours of its use and was able to distinguish survivors from nonsurvivors.[27] After 24 hours of balloon assist, those who were to become balloon-independent had significantly different hemodynamics than those who remained balloon-dependent. For example, the cardiac index rose 47 percent in the balloon-independent group, while it rose only 3 percent in the balloon-dependent patients. The two groups also had a different pattern on the "shock box" diagram (Fig. 13-11).

Surgical intervention in patients with cardiogenic shock has significantly improved the survival of certain types of patients with mechanical defects. Survival in patients with car-

Table 13-4
Relative Contraindications for the IABP

I. Moderate to severe aortic insufficiency
II. Severe disease of the aorta—e.g., aortic dissection
III. Severe lower extremity peripheral vascular disease—e.g., Leriche syndrome
IV. Severe extracardiac systemic disease

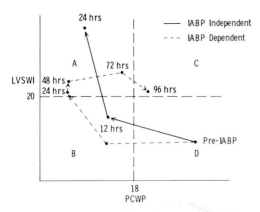

Fig. 13-11. The hemodynamic responses of two groups of patients to the IABP are demonstrated. One group of patients became independent of the balloon after 24 hours, while the others were dependent for 96 hours. (Modified from Ehrich DA: The hemodynamic response to intra-aortic counterpulsation in patients with cardiogenic shock complicating acute myocardial infarction. Am Heart J 93:274, 1977, with permission of author and publisher.)

diogenic shock and a mechanical lesion should be greater than 50 percent. Significant mechanical complications following infarction include:

1. Ventricular-septal rupture with a left-to-right shunt of greater than 2:1.
2. Acute mitral insufficiency with greater than 2+ mitral regurgitation.
3. Acute left ventricular aneurysm.

Bardet reported on the combined use of the IABP to stabilize the patients in shock and surgery to correct mechanical defects in 13 patients.[28] Twelve patients survived for more than 1 month, and 8 survived for more than a year. The results of mitral valve replacements performed up to 3 months after infarction have shown a 33 percent mortality, while mortality in the early postinfarction period ranged from 40 to 50 percent.[29] Many of the patients had associated coronary revascularization. Surgical mortality has been related to the extent of cardiac dysfunction, presence of shock, and time of onset of mitral regurgitation from the infarction. More than 300 cases of surgically corrected ventricular-septal rupture have been reported.[30] The operative mortality is highest when the operation is performed within 1 week of the infarction (70 percent), while it declines by about 10 percent for each week after the time of infarction. Mortality figures have consistently been about

50 percent for resection of an acute left ventricular aneurysm.

ISCHEMIC HEART DISEASE OTHER THAN CARDIOGENIC SHOCK

The IABP has been shown to be effective in reducing the severity of ischemic injury resulting from coronary artery occlusion.[31] It has been utilized clinically in the setting of:

1. Preinfarction angina[32]
2. Early acute infarction[33]
3. Acute infarction with extension[32]
4. Refractory ventricular arrhythmias[34]
5. Emergency coronary arteriography[35]

The IABP has been used in the medical management of these types of patients *after* initial therapy with inotropes, vasodilators, antiarrhythmics, and β-blockers has failed. In some situations the IABP is used to control the symptoms prior to surgery, while in other cases the IABP is not used, but the patient is taken immediately to surgery, where the maximum medical therapy is continued during anesthesia.

The IABP is used in preinfarction patients in an effort to improve coronary blood flow, especially coronary collateral blood flow, and to improve the myocardial oxygen supply/demand ratio. Saini has shown that the IABP can increase myocardial blood flow to ischemic areas of the heart.[36] Using a radioactive tracer technique, Saini showed that blood flow to the ligated ischemic area was reduced from a control value of 78 to 13 ml/min/100 gm myocardium. With institution of the IABP, the flow increased to 35 ml/min/100 gm myocardium. Powell showed that the IABP improved cardiac performance, oxygen consumption, and coronary blood flow in ischemic dogs.[37] Watson has shown a further improvement in coronary blood flow to the ischemic heart when the IABP is combined with an infusion of hypertonic 25 percent mannitol.[38] Combined therapy increased collateral flow 46 percent more than the use of mannitol alone and 27 percent more than the IABP alone. The markedly increased collateral flow resulted from the increased transmural pressure gradient produced by diastolic augmentation and the ability of mannitol to reduce coronary vascular resistance in the ischemic myocardium.

After an acute myocardial infarction, there

is an intermediate zone of tissue (twilight zone) between the necrotic area and the normal myocardium. The survival of this zone depends on the precise relationship between the oxygen supply and demand. It has been shown that this area can be preserved by drug intervention such as nitroglycerin and propranolol and also by use of the IABP.[39] Maroko showed that counterpulsation applied up to 3 hours after occlusion markedly reduced the extent and severity of myocardial ischemic injury in his dog model. He has also shown improvement in humans using the precordial mapping technique in which he demonstrated reversal of ST-segment abnormalities.[15] Gold reported on 11 patients who had recurrent chest pain 3 to 10 days after an acute myocardial infarction in spite of maximum medical therapy.[32] Use of the IABP eliminated ischemic pain in 9 patients and reduced the frequency of attacks in the other 2 patients. All the patients subsequently underwent cardiac catheterization and revascularization surgery.

There is still controversy concerning the role of combined pharmacologic therapy with counterpulsation in patients with acute myocardial infarction. Should the afterload, and thus the coronary filling pressure, be increased or decreased while using counterpulsation? Clayman recommended using a "hypertensive balloon"—adding an intravenous infusion of phenylephrine (Neo-Synephrine) along with the IABP.[40] Using epicardial mapping, he found that the combination of the IABP and phenylephrine led to smaller areas of damage than either the IABP alone or the IABP plus nitroprusside. Parmley, however, recommended combining nitroprusside with external counterpulsation for maximum improvement.[41] This controversy is still continuing at the present time.

Refractory ventricular arrhythmias indicate a poor prognosis when associated with an acute myocardial infarction. A small number of patients with recurrent ventricular arrhythmias cannot be controlled by conventional antiarrhythmic therapy, including propranolol. The new antiarrhythmic drugs such as bretylium may be a significant factor in the care of these patients. At the present time, however, recurrent episodes of ventricular tachycardia or fibrillation may require counterpulsation with the IABP to control them. Increased coronary blood flow to the ischemic irritable areas provided by

the IABP is frequently effective in decreasing the incidence of arrhythmias.[32]

In some institutions the IABP is frequently used prior to coronary arteriography. All the disease states mentioned above would be included in the group of patients needing the IABP before the arteriography. Our indications for the IABP during cardiac catheterization studies are very few. Because of the excellent care and skill provided by our cardiac radiology department, the IABP is rarely used during catheterization. Essentially, it is used only in those patients who required it previously in the coronary care unit for cardiogenic shock, severe heart failure with a probable mechanical defect, or an unstable acute myocardial infarction.

There is one other new indication for the IABP that we believe will increase its use in the future. That is the use of the IABP in patients with recent myocardial infarctions who are stable but who require emergency noncardiac surgery. The risk of an operation within 6 months of an acute infarction is considerably higher than for the general population with coronary artery disease. Tarhan showed that surgery within 3 months of an infarction will have an associated incidence of reinfarction of 37 percent and that the reinfarction carries over a 50 percent mortality.[42] That study was reported in 1972 but was recently updated with essentially the same results.[42A] Miller and Cohen reported on a patient who had an anteroseptal infarction and, on the thirteenth postinfarction day, required an emergency gastrectomy for massive gastrointestinal hemorrhage.[43,44] After receiving 26 units of blood, the patient arrived in the operating room with hypotension and pulmonary edema. The IABP was placed via the femoral artery using local anesthesia, and effective counterpulsation with a pressure of 110/140/60 mm Hg (systolic/augmented diastolic/diastolic) was obtained. The patient tolerated a morphine-based anesthetic and made an uneventful recovery without further infarction. The balloon was discontinued after 20 hours because of ischemia of the leg. Ideally, we believe, it should stay in place for 2 to 3 days, since Tarhan found that most of the reinfarctions occur within 2 to 3 days after surgery. We believe the use of the IABP to help high-risk cardiac patients through *noncardiac* surgery will increase with time as the anesthesiologist gains further experience with it.

USE OF THE INTRA-AORTIC BALLOON PUMP IN CARDIAC SURGERY

The use of the IABP in cardiac surgical patients was introduced by Buckley in 1973 and has become one of its most important applications.[14] There are four main periods when the IABP may be used in cardiac surgical patients (Table 13-5):[45]

1. Continued preoperative use
2. Intraoperative use before cardiopulmonary bypass
3. Intraoperatively in order to discontinue cardiopulmonary bypass
4. Postoperatively to treat the low-output syndrome

The exact role of the IABP in cardiac surgical patients is still unclear and is still evolving. Overall, the incidence of its use appears to be decreasing from the period of its peak use in 1976 and early 1977. We have recently looked at the role of the IABP in cardiac surgery and anesthesia at Emory University Hospital over the past 2 years (January 1976 to December 1977).[46] Overall, the IABP was used in 63 of 1738 (3.62 percent) of all adult surgical patients (Table 13-6). The most recent 6-month period showed a decrease in the use of the IABP to

Table 13-5
Perioperative Indications for the IABP

I. Preoperative
   A. Cardiogenic shock
   B. Acute myocardial infarction complicated by:
      1. Mechanical defects—ventricular-septal rupture, acute mitral insufficiency, or ventricular aneurysm
      2. Continued ischemic pain and extension
      3. Refractory ventricular tachyarrhythmias
   C. Catheterization laboratory problem
II. Intraoperative before cardiopulmonary bypass?
   A. Recent infarction with unstable angina
   B. Combined left main and right coronary artery disease, with poor left ventricular function and an unstable clinical condition
   C. Combined coronary artery disease and valvular heart disease
   D. Very poor left ventricular function
      1. Left ventricular end-diastolic pressure > 20 mm Hg
      2. Ejection fraction < 0.2
      3. Cardiac index < 1.8 liters/min/m^2
III. Intraoperative to discontinue cardiopulmonary bypass
   A. Unable to discontinue bypass within 30 minutes
   B. Inadequate hemodynamics *after* therapy with *both* an inotrope and a vasodilator
   C. Poor hemodynamics
      1. Cardiac index < 2.0 liters/min/m^2
      2. Left atrial pressure (PCWP) > 20 mm Hg
      3. Systolic blood pressure < 80 mm Hg
      4. Total peripheral resistance > 2500 dynes-sec/cm^{-5}
      5. Urine output < 0.5 ml/kg/hr
   D. Epinephrine dosage > 15 μg/min
   E. Persistent ventricular arrhythmias
IV. Postoperative
   A. Low-output syndrome
   B. Complicated intraoperative myocardial infarction

Table 13-6
A 24-Month Experience with the IABP

	Group*	January → June 1976	July → December 1976	January → June 1977	July → December 1977	Totals	% of Usage
IABP prior to operating room	I	1	1	6	—	8	12.70%
IABP prebypass	II-A	3	—	2	2	7	11.11%
	II-B	2	3	1	—	6	9.52%
IABP postbypass	III	13	13	9	7	42	66.67%
Total use IABP		19	17	18	9	63	
Total cardiac surgery		310	372	536	520	1738	
% of cases with IABP		6.13%	4.57%	3.36%	1.73%	3.62%	

* *Key:* Group I = IABP preoperatively; Group II-A = IABP placed in the operating room prior to the induction of general anesthesia using local anesthesia; Group II-B = IABP placed in the operating room after the induction of general anesthesia; group III = IABP placed after cardiopulmonary bypass

only 1.73 percent of cardiac surgical patients. The amount the IABP is used varies from institution to institution and depends on a number of factors:

1. Volume of cardiac surgery—probably is needed less in centers doing a large volume of surgery.
2. Skill and speed of surgical and anesthesia teams—this improves dramatically as the volume of cases increases to over 500 per year. The key factor is the shorter period of time on cardiopulmonary bypass.
3. Improved myocardial preservation techniques on cardiopulmonary bypass—hyperkalemic, hyperosmolar, cold solutions are being used in some institutions to arrest the heart on bypass and decrease the amount of ischemic damage.
4. Intelligent use of modern monitoring techniques, such as the Swan-Ganz catheter, and frequent cardiac output measurements during surgery (see Chapter 4).
5. Thorough understanding of anesthetic and cardiac drugs, anesthetic techniques, and cardiac pathophysiology, as pointed out in previous chapters.

PREOPERATIVE USE OF THE INTRA-AORTIC BALLOON PUMP

At our institution the balloon is used preoperatively for patients in cardiogenic shock, in severe heart failure with a mechanical defect, or with an acute unstable myocardial infarction. In the past 2 years, 8 patients had the IABP in place upon arrival in the operating room at Emory University Hospital. All the patients had been hypotensive and severely unstable when the IABP was placed. The IABP was used throughout the operative procedure in these patients to increase their coronary perfusion pressure and decrease the myocardial oxygen demand. A number of investigators have reported their experience with the use of the IABP to stabilize patients in shock before bringing them to the operating room. Sanders reported on criteria for patients with cardiogenic shock who needed emergency angiography and surgery:[47]

1. Failure to improve in 24 hours on the IABP and inotropes
2. Increased inotropic support needed while on the IABP
3. Dependence on the IABP after 24 hours

4. Recurrent deterioration after being weaned off the IABP

Fifteen of the 20 patients were operated upon, and 7 were long-term survivors. Bregman reported on 4 patients and Parker on 8 others who had the IABP in place to treat a low-output state before coming to the operating room.[48,49] Three of 4 survived in one series, and 4 of 8 in the other. In all cases, the authors thought that the IABP was an important factor in making the course of anesthesia and surgery safer. No episodes of severe hemodynamic deterioration were reported during the induction of anesthesia in these patients. Bolooki has even described a portable stretcher used for counterpulsation of patients in transit to the operating room.[50]

INTRA-AORTIC BALLOON PUMP USED IN THE OPERATING ROOM BEFORE CARDIOPULMONARY BYPASS

Use of the IABP prior to cardiopulmonary bypass is the most controversial and rapidly evolving area for the IABP. Many institutions have *widely differing indications* for the use of the IABP at this time in the surgical procedure. For this reason, a question mark has been placed after this section of Table 13-5. At Emory University Hospital, we tend to be very conservative in using the IABP prior to cardiopulmonary bypass, and we find that we are using it less and less at this time in the surgical procedures (Table 13-6). Twenty-one patients received the IABP before bypass (13 in the operating room and 8 preoperatively in the coronary care unit). Our overall incidence of using the IABP before bypass has decreased, and our indications have gradually changed. Our only use of the IABP in the prebypass period over the past year has been for patients with severe coronary artery disease combined with either valve replacement or repair of a mechanical defect, such as ventricular aneurysm. In the past year, 11 patients have had the IABP placed before bypass for these reasons. Some investigators have recommended the use of the IABP in the following cases:

1. All patients with lesions of the left main coronary artery
2. All patients with moderately depressed left ventricular function (LVF)
3. All patients with preinfarction or unstable angina

We do not believe these patients need the IABP if they receive good anesthetic and surgical care. In many cases, the IABP has been used instead of good monitoring and patient care.

Garcia and Cooper both recommend the use of the IABP before anesthesia in *all patients* with left main coronary artery (LMCA) disease.[51,52] Garcia reported on 18 patients who had LMCA or a left main equivalent (left anterior descending plus circumflex coronary artery disease) associated with right coronary artery disease. All the patients had excellent left ventricular function, with the lowest ejection fraction being 52 percent. In 2 of 5 patients who did not have the IABP before anesthesia, cardiac arrest occurred during or immediately after induction of anesthesia. The anesthetic technique and monitoring used are not described. Thirteen other patients had the IABP placed preoperatively using local anesthesia, and all had uneventful surgical and anesthetic courses. Cooper reported 28 patients with LMCA disease who received the IABP before surgery. Again, these patients had good left ventricular function, and the balloon was recommended because they had no problems in this ''high-risk'' group when the IABP was used before surgery.

In the past 30 months at Emory University Hospital, we have operated on 101 patients with LMCA disease. Many of these patients had had a prior myocardial infarction (33 percent) and poor left ventricular function (elevated left ventricular end-diastolic pressures in 16 percent and akinesia in 24 percent of the patients). The hospital mortality was 2 percent, and the perioperative infarct rate was only 3 percent. The IABP was used in only 1 patient before bypass and in 6 patients after bypass. Therefore, we believe the IABP is not routinely needed in *all* patients with LMCA disease. It may be needed in patients with combined LMCA and right coronary artery disease who have poor left ventricular function and who are clinically unstable. However, most patients with LMCA disease can be managed without the IABP as long as they receive:

1. Good preoperative preparation, including *continuation* of propranolol until surgery
2. Good myocardial preservation on bypass
3. Good anesthetic care which avoids both hypotension (very detrimental in patients with LMCA disease) and increases in myocardial oxygen demand (rate pressure product > 12,000).

The preoperative use of the IABP has also been recommended for all patients with preinfarction or unstable angia.[52] Also included in this group are patients who have had a recent infarction and who continue to have episodes of pain.[32,53,54] Cooper reported 27 patients with preinfarction or unstable angina who received the IABP before surgery. Two of these patients died, both of whom had had an infarction prior to surgery. We certainly do not agree that all patients with preinfarction or unstable angina require the IABP before anesthetic induction. This is the primary indication for coronary revascularization at Emory and would mean that most of our 1000 cases per year would need the IABP!

The situation of patients coming for revascularization surgery shortly after an acute infarction with impending extension (continued pain) is certainly different. Many investigators have recommended that all of these patients have the IABP placed before surgery to control the pain and stabilize the hemodynamics. Mundth and Gold reported two series of patients in whom the IABP was used prior to surgery.[32,54] The balloon reduced the ischemic attacks, which had been refractory to medical treatment. Six of 7 patients survived in one group, and 4 of 5 survived in the other series. Bardet reported on 17 patients who had postinfarction angina and required the IABP to stop the episodes of pain associated with the ECG changes.[53] The IABP relieved the patients of the pain, allowed safe coronary arteriography, and 16 of the 17 patients survived emergency revascularization.

In the past year, we have operated on 35 patients shortly after an acute infarction who continued to have pain.[55] Ten patients were revascularized within 24 hours of the infarct; 9 patients, within 2 to 7 days after infarction; and 16 patients within 8 to 30 days postinfarction. There was no hospital mortality. Left ventricular function rather than the interval between infarction and surgery was the most important prognosticator of hemodynamic stability. Four patients had the IABP inserted preoperatively, and 3 required it after bypass, while 14 percent of the patients required inotropic support after bypass. Therefore, we used the IABP only for those patients who had poor left ventricular function and revascularized the others without using the IABP.

Cooper and others have recommended the preoperative use of the IABP for all patients undergoing myocardial revascularization who have poor left ventricular function.[52,56–59] The problem occurs in defining poor left ventricular function (LVF)! Cooper reported on 6 patients who received the IABP preoperatively for poor LVF. This group of patients had ejection fractions that ranged from 0.41 to 0.56, with an average of 0.50. Understandably, all of these patients did well during surgery. Goldman used an ejection fraction of 0.4 as his indicator for the IABP, and Feola and Cleveland used 0.3.

Bolooki has defined his criteria for poor LVF requiring elective use of the IABP as follows:[57]

1. Severe left ventricular dysfunction: Cardiac index < 1.8 liters/min/m², ejection fraction < 30 percent, left ventricular end-diastolic pressure > 22 mm Hg.
2. Moderate left ventricular dysfunction: Cardiac index < 2.2 liters/min/m², ejection fraction < 40 percent, left ventricular end-diastolic pressure > 18 mm Hg.

He states that all patients with severe left ventricular dysfunction should have the IABP preoperatively. Patients with moderate left ventricular dysfunction need the IABP if they also have either (1) aortic stenosis (gradient > 80 mm Hg), (2) acute myocardial infarction, or (3) preinfarction angina. He also feels that patients need the IABP if their ejection fraction minus their left ventricular end-diastolic pressure is less than 5, e.g., EF 28 − LVEDP 25 = 3 = IABP.

We believe that left ventricular dysfunction must be severe before the IABP is indicated prior to anesthesia for elective coronary revascularization. We *may* use the IABP preoperatively if the cardiac index is less than 1.8 liters/min/m², together with an ejection fraction of less than 0.20 and a left ventricular end-diastolic pressure over 20 mm Hg, and the patient has signs and symptoms of congestive heart failure. This is now a rare indication for the IABP at Emory, since we believe these patients can be safely managed with good monitoring and anesthetic techniques utilizing the vasodilators to control hemodynamics. We studied 188 patients undergoing myocardial revascularization who had poor left ventricular function.[60] This group represented 16.7 percent of all coronary bypass procedures performed over 3 years. All patients who had other procedures (e.g., ventricular aneurysmectomy) were excluded. The patients were divided into three groups:

1. Ejection fraction < .35 (72 patients)
2. Total occlusion of left anterior descending and right coronary artery (57 patients)
3. Left ventricular end-diastolic pressure > 20 mm Hg (59 patients)

The IABP was not used before cardiopulmonary bypass in any of the patients. Inotropic drugs, vasodilators, and the intra-aortic balloon were used frequently after bypass (Fig. 13-12). Inotropes were needed in about 20 percent of these patients. Recently, with more liberal use of nitroprusside after bypass, we are using even less of the inotropic drugs. The IABP was used in 9 percent of the patients to discontinue bypass. The perioperative infarction rate was 11 percent,

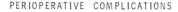

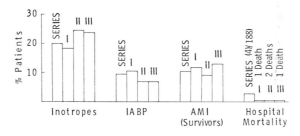

Fig. 13-12. Perioperative complications in 188 patients with poor left ventricular function.

and the hospital mortality was 2.1 percent (4 of 188).

The next problem is when to place the IABP in the patient if you are going to use it in the prebypass period of the operative procedure. Should it be put in under local anesthesia before the induction of general anesthesia, or should the balloon be placed after the patient is anesthetized but before surgery begins? We believe this has to be individualized for each particular patient. In some patients with a low-output syndrome, balloon insertion under local anesthesia is extremely well tolerated, while in some patients with preinfarction angina, the stress of surgery under local anesthesia is poorly tolerated and may even precipitate an ischemic episode. We have seen stable patients develop hypertension, tachycardia, and increases in wedge pressure in association with ST-segment depression during insertion of the balloon, which was being inserted in order to avoid these problems.

We then have induced anesthesia and given vasodilators to reverse the abnormal hemodynamics before the balloon was finally inserted (Fig. 13-13).

INTRA-AORTIC BALLOON PUMP AFTER CARDIOPULMONARY BYPASS OR POSTOPERATIVELY

The indications for the IABP are similar in the settings of both discontinuing cardiopulmonary bypass and the postoperative low-output syndrome. Improved anesthesia techniques, myocardial preservation, and vasodilator therapy appear to have decreased the need for the IABP in these situations. Included in this is the management of cardiopulmonary bypass, which is very important in determining the ease of discontinuing the extracorporeal circulation (see Chapter 9). During the past 2 years, we have used the IABP after bypass in 42 of 1738 patients (2.4 percent) (Table 13-6). However, 26 of these

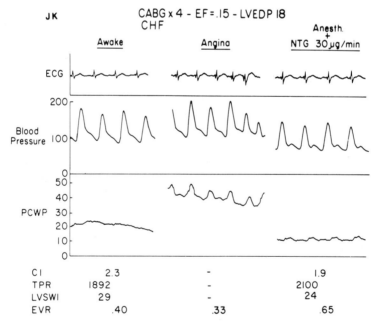

Fig. 13-13. With injection of local anesthesia by the surgeon, this patient became agitated, with increases in blood pressure and wedge pressure associated with premature ventricular contractions. Anesthesia was induced with morphine and diazepam, and nitroglycerin was administered, with a resultant decrease in blood pressure and wedge pressure. (Reproduced from Kaplan JA: Anesthesia and management of left ventricular failure. *In* Bolooki H (ed): Clinical Application of the Intra-Aortic Balloon Pump. Mt. Kisco, NY, Futura, 1977, with permission of author and publisher.)

were in 1976, when we did 682 cases (3.8 percent), while only 16 have been used in 1977, when we did over 1056 cases (1.5 percent). Our criteria for using the IABP after bypass are shown in Table 13-5 and agree almost entirely with Bolooki's recommendations.[57]

At the end of bypass, the pump flow is gradually reduced, and the heart is filled to a left atrial pressure (LAP) of 12–18 mm Hg. If bypass cannot be discontinued because of inadequate cardiac output and blood pressure, either an inotropic agent or a vasodilator is administered. If the patient is vasoconstricted and has a high afterload, a vasodilator is used. We use nitroprusside most often, or possibly nitroglycerin if the LAP is very high. If poor myocardial function appears to be the problem, an inotropic drug such as calcium, dopamine, isoproterenol, or epinephrine is used. Epinephrine is our preferred drug in the very sick patient, and nitroprusside is added to reduce the impedance to ejection from the left ventricle. Figure 13-14 shows a sick patient after bypass who is receiving epinephrine. He had a high preload and afterload and a low cardiac output. Nitroprusside, in small doses (0.5 µg/kg/min) corrected his hemodynamics and allowed him to come off bypass without the use of the IABP. We have seen many patients who have come off bypass with a *combination* of an inotrope and a vasodilator who would have otherwise required the IABP. In some patients, however, this pharmacologic combination does not work, and they then require the IABP. Once the IABP is inserted and counterpulsation is begun at 1:1, the inotropic and vasodilator drugs frequently may be reduced or discontinued. Occasionally, only the vasodilator may be continued to further decrease the patient's impedance to ejection.

In the past, too much use was made of vasoconstrictors alone in an effort to discontinue bypass, and the IABP was needed more often. Buckley and Craver first reported the use of the IABP to discontinue cardiopulmonary bypass in 1973.[14] They had 26 patients whose systolic blood pressure was less than 90 mm Hg

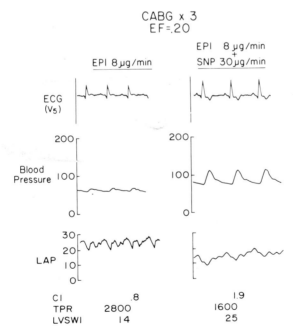

Fig. 13-14. At the end of bypass this patient was hypotensive, with an increased left atrial pressure (LAP) and elevated TPR. Nitroprusside (SNP) decreased the left ventricular wall tension, and blood pressure increased to a satisfactory level. (Reproduced from Kaplan JA: Anesthesia and management of left ventricular failure. *In* Bolooki H (ed): Clinical Application of the Intra-Aortic Balloon Pump. Mt. Kisco, NY, Futura, 1977, with permission of author and publisher.)

and whose LAP was over 25 mm Hg and who had inadequate circulation while receiving catecholamines. Four patients could not be brought off bypass even with the IABP, but 22 patients were brought off bypass, and 10 were long-term survivors. This was a very significant report and has led to other reports of successful use of the IABP after bypass.[61-63] Most recently, Stewart reported 15 patients requiring the IABP after bypass, with 13 surviving, and 8 patients who required the IABP in the postoperative period, with 5 survivors.[63] Wright has even reported the use of external counterpulsation to help discontinue bypass in 3 patients who otherwise could not be removed from extracorporeal circulation.[64]

Recently, other indices have been proposed to help manage extremely sick patients after cardiopulmonary bypass. Phillips and Bregman have recommended using the endocardial viability ratio (EVR) to determine when the IABP is needed.[19] They feel that this index will identify persistent unrecognized subendocardial ischemia and allow insertion of the IABP to prevent the development of necrotic areas. They reported the use of the EVR to determine the adequacy of subendocardial blood flow in 64 patients after bypass. The IABP was used in 14 patients who had a left atrial pressure over 25 mm Hg associated with an EVR below 0.7 for more than 30 minutes after cardiopulmonary bypass, even though the average blood pressure was 90/65 mm Hg. In 9 patients, there was hemodynamic improvement and they survived, while 5 patients died even with the IABP. The 50 patients with an EVR over 0.7 had a mean EVR of 0.87, and all survived. There was a statistically significant difference between the EVR of survivors and nonsurvivors.

Norman developed a scoring system to be able to predict the outcome of patients requiring the IABP.[65] This scoring system may be useful to follow the course of patients on the IABP (Table 13-7). Norman studied 46 patients using this scoring system and found significant differences between survivors and nonsurvivors. Patients with persistent scores of less than 6 were at greatest risk and usually died. In the surviving patients, the scores in the first 12 hours averaged 8.7 and rose to 10.9.

HEMODYNAMIC EFFECTS OF THE INTRA-AORTIC BALLOON PUMP DURING SURGERY

Most studies have shown that the effects of the IABP used during surgery are similar to those seen in patients in the preoperative period.[57,62] The systolic blood pressure decreases, and the augmented diastolic and mean arterial pressures increase. The left atrial pressure and left ventricular end-diastolic pressure decrease, cardiac output increases, and total peripheral resistance decreases. Coronary blood flow measured in saphenous vein grafts initially rises but then falls back almost to control values. Bolooki showed that the diastolic pressure increased by 100 percent, cardiac index increased by 30 percent, and end-diastolic pressure decreased by 20 percent. Results of studies we performed in the prebypass and postbypass period are shown in Tables 13-8 and 13-9 and in Figure 13-5. In general, the IABP decreased systolic blood pressure and total peripheral resistance. It increased diastolic and mean blood pressure, cardiac index, left ventricular stroke work index, and the endocardial viability ratio.[46]

Table 13-7
Norman's Circulatory Support Score

Parameter	Score				
	0	*1*	*2*	*3*	*4*
CI	< 1.5	1.5–2.0	2–2.5	2.5–3	> 3
PCWP	> 25	20–25	15–20	10–15	< 10
SVR	> 2500	2000–2500	1500–2000	1000–1500	< 1000
Urine output (ml/hr)	< 20	20–30	30–40	40–50	> 50

Table 13-8
Hemodynamics in 6 Patients with the IABP Before Cardiopulmonary Bypass

Patient	Surgery Indications, Cath Data	BP (torr) C	BP 1:1^A	CVP (torr) C	CVP 1:1	PCWP (torr) C	PCWP 1:1	CI (liters/min/m²) C	CI 1:1	LVSWI (gm·m/m²) C	LVSWI 1:1	TPR (dynes-sec/cm⁻⁵) C	TPR 1:1
1	CABG (3), MVR CHF, EF .41 LVEDP 14	90/68	75/90/55	6	5	27	20	2.4	2.5	23	23	869	812
2	CABG (4), VA CHF, EF .30 LVEDP 24	120/60	95/150/35	7	5	12	10	1.8	2.1	27	25	1985	1500
3	CABG (3), EF .25 LVEDP 35	128/75	115/120/68	11	11	14	12	2.1	2.3	25	30.	1790	1268
4	CABG (4), CHF EF .10 LVEDP 15	170/86	140/150/50	7	4	22	14	1.5	1.9	22	24	2100	1629
5	VA, CHF EF .05 LVEDP 35	110/70	110/150/30	10	6	22	16	1.7	1.8	14	19	1840	1683
6	CABG (3) EF .10 LVEDP 25	150/74	144/160/60	8	5	21	7	1.8	2.4	37	57	1899	1690
x̄	EF .20 / LVEDP 25	128/72	113/137/48*	8	6	20	13*	1.9	2.2*	25	30	1747	1430*
S̄E	.005 / 3.8	11.7/3.5	10.8/10.9/5.3	.8	1.0	2.3	1.9	.1	.1	3.1	5.7	181	140

* $P < .05$ by student's T test.

Key: C = Control baseline hemodynamics; 1:1 = IABP on 1:1 mode; CABG = Coronary artery bypass grafts; MVR = Mitral valve replacement; CHF = Congestive heart failure; VA = Ventricular aneurysm; A = systolic pressure/balloon-augmented diastolic pressure/diastolic pressure

461

Table 13-9
Hemodynamics in 5 Patients Who Required the IABP After Cardiopulmonary Bypass

Patient	Surgery Indications, Cath Data	BP (torr) 1:8	BP (torr) 1:1	PCWP (torr) 1:8	PCWP (torr) 1:1	CI (liters/min/m²) 1:8	CI (liters/min/m²) 1:1	LVSWI (gm · m/m²) 1:8	LVSWI (gm · m/m²) 1:1	TPR (dynes-sec/cm⁻⁵) 1:8	TPR (dynes-sec/cm⁻⁵) 1:1	EVR 1:8	EVR 1:1	Drugs
1	CABG (4), VA EF .30 LVEDP 24	112/64	90/115/40	12	10	1.8	2.3	14	18	1889	1148	.79	2.0	Dopamine, 3 μg/kg/min
2	CABG (3) EF .25 LVEDP 35	140/85	100/110/50	14	11	2.0	1.9	47	48	2022	1459	1.05	2.01	Nitroglycerin, 32 μg/min
3	CABG (4) EF .10 LVEDP 15	100/53	90/110/40	16	13	2.1	2.7	15	17	1205	853	.45	1.10	None
4	VA EF .05 LVEDP 25	105/60	90/120/40	25	20	2.0	3.0	10	22	2000	1866	.66	1.40	None
5	CABG (1) EF .21 LVEDP 25	70/60	60/80/40	19	13	.7	1.5	7	9	1700	1117	—	—	Epinephrine, 4 μg/min Xylocaine, 2 mg/min
$\bar{x}$	EF LVEDP .18 25	105/64	86/107/42*	17	13*	1.7	2.3*	19	23	1763	1289*	.74	1.63*	
S$\bar{\mathrm{E}}$	.05 3.2	11.2/5.5	6.8/7.0/2.0	2.3	1.8	.3	.3	7.2	6.6	151	173	.13	.23	

* $P < .05$ by student's T test.

Key: 1:8 = IABP on 1:8 mode; 1:1 = IABP on 1:1 mode; CABG = Coronary artery bypass grafts; VA = Ventricular aneurysm.

Complications of the Intra-Aortic Balloon Pump

The incidence and nature of complications resulting from use of the IABP vary with the indications for use, the duration of use, and the experience of the surgical team. The reported complications are shown in Table 13-10. Ischemia of the leg is the most frequent complication in our experience. Awareness of this complication and frequent checking of the peripheral pulses in the leg for signs of ischemia are extremely important. If severe ischemia develops, the IABP should be removed within 6 hours and a femoral embolectomy performed. If it is still needed, the IABP can be placed in the other leg. Lefemine recently reported on complications of the IABP in medical and surgical patients.[66] Serious arterial insufficiency developed in 7 of the 29 medical patients, and in the group with cardiogenic shock, the rate of this complication approached 50 percent. In the surgical group, 5 of 65 patients developed arterial insufficiency. Overall, there was a 17.4 percent incidence of complications and an 11.6 percent incidence of serious obstruction to the circulation of the leg. Alpert has suggested using a saphenous vein cross-graft from the opposite femoral artery distal to the balloon insertion.[67] We have not done this and would only suggest its possible use in patients in whom the opposite femoral artery cannot be used to insert the IABP.

Biddle reported a case of dissection of the aorta complicating the use of the IABP.[68] There was no intimal tear found in his case at autopsy, and it was suggested that lateral shearing forces were responsible for the dissection. Dunkman reported 2 cases of aortic dissection in his series.[69] In both cases, the IABP was passed into a false lumen and functioned fairly well, creating no problems. This complication occurs during insertion through an area of severe arteriosclerosis and can be prevented by careful surgical insertion.

Thrombus formation on the balloon catheter and peripheral embolization have been reported. Emboli have been reported in the testicular and renal vessels[69] and in the hepatic and renal arteries associated with multiple renal infarcts.[49] These can be prevented by anticoagulation of the patient or possibly by infusing low-molecular-weight dextran at the rate of 10 ml/hr.

Thrombocytopenia has been reported to occur after counterpulsation. In one series, approximately half of the patients dropped their platelet counts by 50 percent during 60 hours of IABP use.[69] The use of dextran has also been recommended to try to prevent this complication. Disseminated intravascular coagulation has also been seen in patients with cardiogenic shock who had the intra-aortic balloon in place. Red blood cell destruction and increased plasma hemoglobin may also be seen.

Wound infections after balloon insertion have also been observed.[62] The wound usually opens and is weeping by 4 to 7 days after insertion. Bolooki reported this complication in 4 percent of his patients and in up to 30 percent of obese patients.[9] These may require both topical and systemic antibiotics. Occasionally, it is necessary to open the incision and remove the graft material attached to the femoral artery in order to clear up the infection.

Gas embolization from the IABP into the aorta is rare owing to the precise construction of the balloon catheter. It has been reported to be a lethal complication, however.[70] If the Avco-Roche balloon ruptures, an automatic control allows only a small amount of helium to enter the aorta. If the console is in the manual mode of operation instead of the automatic mode, however, more helium can enter the aorta. If the Datascope balloon ruptures, 40 cc of carbon dioxide can enter the aorta. A leaking balloon should be removed immediately.

Lefemine lists the inability to pass the IABP as a complication.[66] He believes this is a serious limitation of the technique and reported it in 13 percent of his patients. This is a much higher figure than others report. He used aortic arch insertion in 5 percent of his surgical patients when it could not be passed up the femoral artery.

Table 13-10
Complications of the IABP

1. Ischemia of the leg
2. Dissection of the aorta
3. Thrombus formation and embolization
4. Thrombocytopenia
5. Infection
6. Gas embolization
7. Inability to place the IABP

Discontinuation of the Intra-Aortic Balloon Pump

When the patient appears to have improved satisfactorily, the IABP is weaned over a period of 18 to 24 hours. We try to discontinue inotropic infusions and sometimes vasodilators and the ventilator prior to weaning the balloon. This sequence is not fixed, and if the patient has severe respiratory insufficiency, the IABP may be discontinued while the patient is still on mechanical ventilation. Signs of hemodynamic improvement include the following:

1. Augmented diastolic blood pressure > 100 mm Hg
2. Pulmonary capillary wedge pressure decreased by 5 mm Hg
3. Cardiac output increased by 0.5 liter/min
4. Urine output > 50 ml/hr without diuretics
5. Decreased need for catecholamines
6. Systolic blood pressure increased to equal the augmented diastolic blood pressure by the pump

The balloon is weaned in steps from 1:1 to 1:2, then 1:4, and finally 1:8. Each of these steps can take from 1 to 24 hours, depending on the patient's hemodynamic response. Ideally, cardiac output and left ventricular function is checked at each step if the monitoring catheters are still functional. The balloon is removed after 6 to 8 hours of counterpulsation at 1:8 if the hemodynamics remain stable.

We do not remove the IABP in the operating room from any patient who required it during the operative procedure. All of these patients remain on counterpulsation in the postoperative intensive care unit for at least 12 to 24 hours. During this time, the inotropic infusion is decreased if possible, and the vasodilator infusion is frequently decreased. The IABP is weaned if the patient has good peripheral perfusion with a mean blood pressure over 70 mm Hg, LAP or PCWP less than 20 mm Hg, cardiac index over 2 liters/min/m², total peripheral resistance under 2000 dynes-sec/cm⁻⁵, and urinary output over 0.5 ml/kg/hr. The balloon is removed and the femoral artery repaired in the intensive care unit with continuous monitoring. We think it is an unnecessary risk to disconnect the monitoring and to move the patient back into the operating room for removal of the balloon.

PULSATILE ASSIST DEVICE

The pulsatile assist device (PAD) was introduced by Bregman in 1976.[71,72] The PAD has two major uses at present: (1) intraoperative counterpulsation, and (2) pulsatile cardiopulmonary bypass. The PAD was marketed by Datascope and originally powered by the Datascope System 80 Intra-Aortic Balloon Pump console. Recently, Datascope has developed a separate power source to control the PAD (Datascope System 42). In 1977, Kaplitt and Tamari introduced their version of the pulsatile assist device, which they called the Tamari-Kaplitt Pulsator (TKP).[73] This unit is powered by a separate power source. Early in 1978, the Avco-Roche Corporation introduced their version of the pulsatile assist device, which is powered by their Model 7 IABP console. For ease of discussion, we will refer to all of these types together as the PAD, since they all work on the same principle.

The PAD is applied *externally* in the cardiopulmonary bypass (CPB) circuit, to provide counterpulsation similar to the IABP.[74] The PAD is attached between the arterial roller pumps on the heart lung machine and the aortic cannula (Fig. 13-15). The device can be used with either aortic or femoral artery perfusion. As soon as the arterial perfusion cannula is inserted, synchronous arterioarterial counterpulsation can be begun. This may be useful in patients with severe left ventricular dysfunction or severe ischemia or where the prebypass period may be prolonged. If the proximal anastomoses of the coronary bypass grafts are done before instituting CPB, the prebypass phase of the operation can be quite long. In hospitals that do the proximal anastamoses before going on CPB, the PAD may be quite useful. In situations like ours, where all the anastamoses are done on CPB and, therefore, the prebypass period is brief, the PAD appears to have less application.

The PAD consists of a flexible, valveless, polyurethane balloon through which the arterial blood flows. The two ends have tubing that is compatible with the pump circuit. The TKP is molded from one continuous piece of PVC tubing. The balloon is contained in a rigid plastic tubing, which is connected via an air hose to the balloon console or power pack. The synchronous counterpulsation is timed by means of the ECG tracing in a manner similar to the IABP.

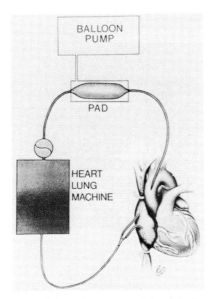

Fig. 13-15. Schematic diagram of the pulsatile assist device in the cardiopulmonary bypass circuit. (Reproduced from Bregman D: Hemodynamic effects of pulsatile blood flow. *In* Bolooki H. (ed): Clinical Application of the Intra-Aortic Balloon Pump. Mt. Kisco, NY, Futura, 1977, with permission of author and publisher.)

The PAD air hoses are kept sterile in the operative field for two reasons:

1. In the event of a mechanical problem, the surgeons can excise it from the circuit.
2. Counterpulsation is most effective when it is applied closest to the heart.

Bregman studied 125 patients undergoing cardiac surgery using the PAD in the CPB circuit.[71,72] A majority of these patients (92) had poor left ventricular function, with an ejection fraction less than 0.3, or a left ventricular end-diastolic pressure over 18 mm Hg. Counterpulsation was used before bypass in all patients, and the proximal anastomoses were performed at this time in the coronary bypass patients. All the patients were weaned successfully from CPB and the PAD. In 10 patients, the EVR was calculated off the PAD (1.06 ± .09) and on the PAD (1.38 ± .12) and was significantly improved on the PAD. One patient had an intraoperative myocardial infarction and required the IABP 2 hours after discontinuing CBP and the PAD. One other patient died of hemorrhage secondary to an iatrogenic intraoperative aortic injury.

The stated, though largely unproven, benefits of the PAD are as follows:

1. Improved postoperative left ventricular function
2. Decreased need for the IABP
3. Decreased need for inotropic drugs
4. Reduced incidence of myocardial infarctions
5. Improved perfusion on pulsatile CPB

Berger first called attention to the use of the IABP to create pulsatile CPB.[75] In a study using dogs, he showed improved urine output and creatinine clearance and less increase in peripheral resistance, fluid requirements, and lactate production with pulsatile perfusion. Pappas first used the IABP to produce clinical pulsatile CPB in 56 patients in 1975.[76] He compared these patients to others receiving the standard nonpulsatile perfusion and found pulsatile CPB to be superior. He suggested that pulsatile CPB improved myocardial metabolism, function, and peripheral perfusion and resulted in less heptocellular damage (lower SGOT). To sum up these earlier studies, pulsatile CPB had the following advantages:

1. Better myocardial perfusion
2. Better peripheral capillary perfusion
3. Less metabolic acidosis
4. Lower peripheral resistance
5. Better renal, cerebral, and hepatic perfusion

Bregman realized that insertion of the IABP was not justified to provide pulsatile CPB and thus developed the PAD to provide both pulsatile CPB and the possibility of intraoperative arterial counterpulsation. A tracing comparing the IABP to the PAD to provide pulsatile CPB is shown in Figure 13-16. A pulse pressure of 40–50 mm Hg is readily obtained while maintaining a mean perfusion pressure of 80–90 mm Hg. In both animal and patient studies, no significant hemolysis has been noted from the use of pulsatile CPB.

A number of patients develop acute right heart failure during surgery. The concept of using the IABP for right ventricular failure by pumping in the pulmonary artery is in its early stages of development. Bregman however, has proposed the use of the PAD inserted in the pulmonary artery as a means of providing temporary right heart counterpulsation timed off the

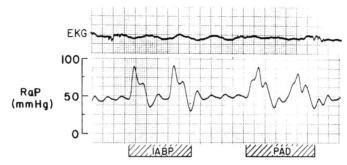

Fig. 13-16. Comparative effects of the PAD and IABP to create synchronous pulsatile cardiopulmonary bypass in a patient (Reproduced from Bregman D: Dual-chambered intraaortic balloon counterpulsation. *In* Ionescu M (ed): Current Techniques in Extracorporeal Circulation. London, Butterworth's, 1976, with permission of author and publisher.)

pulmonary artery tracing. This may also have application for pediatric patients who frequently die of right heart failure.

LEFT VENTRICULAR ASSIST DEVICES

Patients continue to die of left ventricular failure even with the use of the IABP and PAD. Therefore, investigators continue to look for other assist devices to temporarily support the sick left ventricle until it can recover its strength. Silvay reported on the use of the Litwak cannula and left heart assist device (LHAD) in 15 patients with a low-output syndrome after cardiac surgery.[77] A cannula was placed in the left atrium, with a second one in the ascending aorta. Both cannulae were brought out through the abdominal wall and attached to an external roller pump to assist the left ventricle. They employed their LHAD quite aggressively whenever the hemodynamics could not be stabilized with drug therapy and the IABP over 1 hour. The flow of the LHAD was adjusted to maintain a total cardiac index of 2.5 liters/min/m² and an LAP under 20 mm Hg. The period of support with the LHAD ranged from 6 to 501 hours. Using the LHAD, 14 of the 15 patients were weaned from CPB. Five patients could not be weaned off the LHAD, another 4 died after they were off the LHAD, and 2 others died 7 and 10

weeks postoperatively. There were 4 long-term survivors (27 percent).

Two other invasive devices are currently being developed. Norman is developing an abdominal left ventricular assist device (ALVAD) to be used in patients with severe cardiogenic shock unresponsive to therapy with drugs and the IABP.[78] The pumping chamber is placed in the abdominal cavity and powered by an IABP console. Blood is taken from the left ventricular apex and pumped into the abdominal or thoracic aorta. Norman is devising a scoring system to determine which patients will die with the IABP alone and thus will need the ALVAD. At the present time, patients on the IABP who have a cardiac index of less than 1.2 liters/min/m² or a cardiac index of less than 2.1 liters/min/m² together with a systemic vascular resistance over 2100 dynes-sec/cm⁻⁵ and a circulatory support score of less than 6, are candidates for the IABP-powered ALVAD. Peters has developed a transapical left ventricular bypass (TALVB) for use in both left- and right-sided heart failure.[79] This is a relatively simple system, using a transapical withdrawal system attached to an external roller pump that can be used to aid either ventricle. The blood can be pumped back into either femoral artery or the aorta. A removable left ventricular apical catheter is presently being developed which holds great hope for the future.

REFERENCES

1. Stuckey JH, Newman MM, Dennis C, et al: The use of the heart-lung machine in selected cases of acute myocardial infarction. Surg Forum 8:342-344, 1957

2. Sanders CA, Buckley MJ, Austen WG: Mechanical circulatory assistance: Current status. N Engl J Med 285:348-350, 1971

3. Kones RJ: Cardiogenic Shock: Mechanism and

Management. Mt. Kisco, NY, Futura, 1974, pp 327-381

4. DeBakey ME: Left ventricular bypass pump for cardiac assistance: Clinical experience. Am J Cardiol 27:3-11, 1971

5. Litwak RS, Koffsky RM, Jurado RA, et al: Use of a left heart assist device after intracardiac surgery: Technique and clinical experience. Ann Thorac Surg 21:191-202, 1976

6. Clauss RH, Birtwell WC, Albertal G, et al: Assisted circulation. I. The arterial counterpulsator. J Thorac Cardiovasc Surg 41:447-458, 1961

7. Moulopoulus SD, Topaz S, Kolff WJ: Diastolic balloon pumping (with carbon dioxide) in the aorta: Mechanical assistance to the failing circulation. Am Heart J 63:669-675, 1962

8. Kantrowitz A, Tjonnelarel S, Freed PS, et al: Initial clinical experience with intra-aortic balloon pumping in cardiogenic shock. JAMA 203:113-118, 1968

9. Bolooki H: Clinical Application of the Intraaortic Balloon Pump. Mt. Kisco, NY, Futura, 1977

10. Soroff HS, Giron F, Ruiz U, et al: Physiologic support of heart action. N Engl J Med 280:693-704, 1969

11. Skinner DB: Experimental and clinical evaluation of mechanic ventricular assistance. Am J Cardiol 27:146-154, 1971

12. Buckley MJ, Leinbach RC, Kastor JA, et al: Hemodynamic evaluation of intraaortic balloon pumping in man. Circulation 41 (suppl II):130-136, 1970

13. Mundth ED, Yurchak PM, Buckley MJ, et al: Circulatory assistance in emergency direct coronary artery surgery for shock complicating acute myocardial infarction. N Engl J Med 283:1382-1384, 1970

14. Buckley MJ, Craver JM, Gold HK, et al: Intraaortic balloon assist for cardiogenic shock after cardiopulmonary bypass. Circulation 47-48 (suppl III):90-94, 1973

15. Maroko PR, Bernstein EG, Libbey P, et al: Effects of intraaortic balloon counterpulsation on the severity of myocardial ischemic injury following acute coronary occlusion. Circulation 45:1150-1159, 1972

16. Mueller H, Ayres SM, Gianelli S, et al: Effect of isoproterenol, l-norepinephrine, and intraaortic counterpulsation on hemodynamics and myocardial metabolism in shock following acute myocardial infarction. Circulation 45:335-351, 1972

17. Weber KT, Janicki JS: Intraaortic balloon counterpulsation: A review of physiological principles, clinical results, and device safety. Ann Thorac Surg 17:602-636, 1974

18. Hoffman JIE, Buckberg GD: Pathophysiology of subendocardial ischemia. Br Med J 1:76-79, 1975

19. Philips PA, Bregman D: Intraoperative application of intra-aortic balloon counterpulsation determined by clinical monitoring of the endocardial viability ratio. Ann Thorac Surg 23:45-51, 1977

20. Chatterjee S, Rosensweig J: Evaluation of intraaortic counterpulsation. J Thorac Cardiovasc Surg 61:405-410, 1971

21. Feola M, Limet RR, Glick G: Direct and reflex vascular effects of intraaortic balloon counterpulsation in dogs at four levels of aortic pressure. Clin Res 19:313, 1971

22. Grover RR: The function of the Avco-Roche intraaortic balloon pump. In Bolooki H (ed.): Clinical Application of the Intraaortic Balloon Pump. Mt. Kisco, NY, Futura, 1977, pp 85-99

23. Bregman D: Dual-chambered intraaortic balloon counterpulsation. In Ionescu MI, Wooler GH (eds): Current Techniques in Extracorporeal Circulation. London, Butterworth, 1976, pp 407-516

24. Talpins NL, Kupke DC, Yellin E, et al: Hemodynamics and coronary blood flow during intraaortic balloon pumping. Surg Forum 19:122-126, 1968

25. Herzlinger GA: Absolute determination of cardiac output in intra-aortic balloon pumped patients using a radial arterial pressure trace. Circulation 53:417-421, 1976

26. Scheidt S, Wilner G, Mueller H, et al: Intraaortic balloon counterpulsation in cardiogenic shock. N Engl J Med 288:979-984, 1973

27. Ehrich DA, Biddle TL, Kronenberg MW, et al: The hemodynamic response to intraaortic counterpulsation in patients with cardiogenic shock complicating acute myocardial infarction. Am Heart J 93:274-279, 1977

28. Bardet J, Marquet C, Kahn JC, et al: Clinical and hemodynamic results of intraaortic balloon counterpulsation and surgery for cardiogenic shock. Am Heart J 93:280-288, 1977

29. Amsterdam EA, Hughes JL, Miller RL, et al: Early surgical intervention for complicated acute myocardial infarction: Initial and long-term results. Am J Cardiol 33:123, 1974

30. Schechter DC: Inventory of surgical operations for cardiac structural sequels of myocardial infarction. Part II. NY State J Med 75:1672-1680, 1975

31. Levine FH, Gold HK, Leinbach RC, et al: Management of acute myocardial ischemia with intraaortic balloon pumping and coronary bypass surgery. Circulation 58 (suppl I):70-72, 1978

32. Gold HK, Leinbach RC, Sanders CA, et al: Intraaortic balloon pumping for control of recurrent myocardial ischemia. Circulation 47:1197-1203, 1973

33. De Laria GA, Johansen KH, Sobel BE, et al: Delayed evaluation of myocardial ischemic in-

jury after intraaortic balloon counterpulsation. Circulation 49-50 (suppl II):242-248, 1974

34. Willerson JT, Curry GC, Watson JT, et al: Intraaortic balloon counterpulsation in patients with cardiogenic shock, medically refractory left ventricular failure and/or recurrent ventricular tachycardia. Am J Med 58:183-191, 1975

35. Guss SB, Zir LM, Garrison HB, et al: Coronary occlusion during coronary angiography. Circulation 52:1063-1068, 1975

36. Saini VK, Hood WB, Hechtman HB, et al: Nutrient myocardial blood flow in experimental myocardial ischemia. Circulation 52:1086-1090, 1975

37. Powell WJ, Daggett WM, Magro AE, et al: Effects of intra-aortic balloon counterpulsation on cardiac performance, oxygen consumption, and coronary blood flow in dogs. Circ Res 26:753-764, 1970

38. Watson JT, Fixler DE, Platt MR, et al: The influence of combined intraaortic balloon counterpulsation and hyperosmotic mannitol on regional myocardial blood flow in the ischemic myocardium in the dog. Circ Res 38:506-513, 1976

39. Maroko PR, Kjiekshus JK, Sobel BE, et al: Factors influencing infarct size following coronary artery occlusion. Circulation 43:171-174, 1971

40. Clayman R, Johansen KH, De Laria GA, et al: The hypertensive balloon: A beneficial synergism for the salvage of the ischemic myocardium. J Thorac Cardiovasc Surg 68:80-89, 1974

41. Parmley WW, Chatterjee K, Charuzi Y, et al: Hemodynamic effects of non-invasive systolic unloading (nitroprusside) and diastolic augmentation (external counterpulsation) in patients with acute myocardial infarctions. Am J Cardiol 33:819-825, 1974

42. Tarhan S, Moffitt EA, Taylor WF, et al: Myocardial infarction after general anesthesia. JAMA 220:1451-1455, 1972

42A. Steen PA, Tinker JH, Tarhan S: Myocardial reinfarction after anesthesia and surgery. JAMA 239:2566, 1978

43. Miller MG, Hall SV: Intraaortic balloon counterpulsation in a high risk cardiac patient undergoing emergency gastrectomy. Anesthesiology 42:103-105, 1975

44. Cohen SI, Weintraub RM: A new application for counterpulsation. Arch Surg 110:116-117, 1975

45. Kaplan JA: The role of anesthesia in surgical patients with left ventricular failure. In Bolooki H (ed): Clinical Application of the Intraaortic Balloon Pump. Mt. Kisco, NY, Futura, 1977, pp 263-276

46. Kaplan JA, Craver JM, Jones EL, et al: The role of the intraaortic balloon in cardiac anesthesia. Presented at the International Anesthesia Research Society annual meeting, 1978. In press

47. Sanders CA, Buckley MJ, Leinbach RC, et al: Mechanical circulatory assistance: Current status and experience with combining circulatory assistance, emergency coronary angiography, and acute myocardial revascularization. Circulation 45:1292-1313, 1972

48. Bregman D, Parodi EN, Edie RN, et al: Intraoperative unidirectional intraaortic balloon pumping in the management of left ventricular power failure. J Thorac Cardiovasc Surg 70:1010-1039, 1975

49. Parker FB, Neville JF, Hanson EL, et al: Intraaortic balloon counterpulsation and cardiac surgery. Ann Thorac Surg 17:144-151, 1974

50. Bolooki H: A portable radiolucent stretcher for intraaortic balloon counterpulsation. J Thorac Cardiovasc Surg 63:501-503, 1972

51. Garcia JM, Mispireth LA, Smyth NPD: Surgical management of life-threatening coronary artery disease. J Thorac Cardiovasc Surg 72:593-595, 1976

52. Cooper GN, Singh AK, Vargas LL, et al: Preoperative intraaortic balloon assist in high risk revascularization patients. Am J Surg 133:463-468, 1977

53. Bardet J, Rigaud M, Kahn JC, et al: Treatment of post-myocardial infarction angina by intraaortic balloon pumping and emergency revascularization. J Thorac Cardiovasc Surg 74:299-306, 1977

54. Mundth ED, Buckley MJ, Gold HK, et al: Intraaortic balloon pumping and emergency coronary artery revascularization for acute myocardial infarction with impending extension. Ann Thorac Surg 16:435-443, 1973

55. Jones EL, Douglas JS, Craver JM, et al: Results of coronary revascularization in patients with recent myocardial infarction. J Thorac Cardiovasc Surg 76:545-551, 1978

56. Goldman BS, Wlaker P, Gunstensen J, et al: Intraaortic balloon pump assist: Adjunct to surgery for left ventricular dysfunction. Can J Surg 19:128-134, 1976

57. Bolooki H, Williams W, Thurer RJ, et al: Clinical and hemodynamic criteria for use of the intraaortic balloon pump in patients requiring cardiac surgery. J Thorac Cardiovasc Surg 72:756-768, 1976

58. Feola M, Wiener L, Walinsky P, et al: Improved survival after coronary bypass surgery in patients with poor left ventricular function: Role of intraaortic balloon counterpulsation. Am J Cardiol 39:1021-1026, 1977

59. Cleveland JC, Lefemine AA, Madoff I, et al: The role of intraaortic balloon counterpulsation in patients undergoing cardiac operations. Ann Thorac Surg 20:652-660, 1975

60. Jones EL, Craver JM, Kaplan JA, et al: Criteria

for operability and reduction of surgical mortality in patients with severe left ventricular ischemia and dysfunction. Ann Thorac Surg 25:413, 1978

61. Housman LB, Bernstein EF, Braunwald NS, et al: Counterpulsation for intraoperative cardiogenic shock. JAMA 224:1131–1133, 1973

62. Berger RL, Saini VK, Ryan TJ, et al: Intraaortic balloon assist for postcardiotomy cardiogenic shock. J Thorac Surg 66:906–915, 1973

63. Stewart S, Biddle T, DeWesse J: Support of the myocardium with intraaortic balloon counterpulsation following cardiopulmonary bypass. J Thorac Cardiovasc Surg 72:109–114, 1976

64. Wright PW: External counterpulsation for cardiogenic shock following cardiopulmonary bypass. Am Heart J 90:231–235, 1975

65. Norman JC, Cooley DA, Igo S, et al: Prognostic indices for survival during postcardiotomy intraaortic balloon pumping. J Thorac Cardiovasc Surg 74:709–720, 1977

66. Lefemine AA, Kosowsky B, Madoff I, et al: Results and complications of intraaortic balloon pumping in surgical and medical patients. Am J Cardiol 40:416–420, 1977

67. Alpert J, Bhaktan EK, Gielchinsky I, et al: Vascular complications of intraaortic balloon pumping. Arch Surg 111:1190–1195, 1976

68. Biddle TL, Stewart S, Stuard ID: Dissection of the aorta complicating intraaortic balloon counterpulsation. Am Heart J 92:781–784, 1976

69. Dunkman WB, Leinbach RC, Buckley MK, et al: Clinical and hemodynamic results of intraaortic balloon pumping and surgery for cardiogenic shock. Circulation 46:465–477, 1972

70. Furman S, Vijaynayar R, Rosenbaum R, et al: Lethal sequalae of intraaortic balloon rupture. Surgery 69:121–129, 1971

71. Bregman D, Parodi EN, Bowman FO, et al: Clinical experience with a new cardiac assist device—the pulsatile assist device (PAD), abstracted. Clin Res 24:211-A, 1976

72. Bregman D, Bailin M, Bowman FO, et al: A pulsatile assist device (PAD) for use during cardiopulmonary bypass. Ann Thorac Surg 24:574–581, 1977

73. Kaplitt MJ, Tamari Y: Clinical experience with the Tamari-Kaplitt pulsator: A new device to create pulsatile flow or counterpulsation during open heart surgery. Am J Cardiol 39:260, 1977

74. Bregman D: Hemodynamic effects of pulsatile blood flow. In Bolooki H (ed): Clinical Application of the Intraaortic Balloon Pump. Mt. Kisco, NY, Futura, 1977, pp 29–39

75. Berger RL, Saini VK: Conversion of non-pulsatile cardiopulmonary bypass to pulsatile flow by intraaortic balloon pumping during myocardial revascularization for cardiogenic shock, abstracted. Circulation 45–46 (suppl II):130, 1972

76. Pappas G, Winter SD, Kopriva CJ, et al: Improvement of myocardial and other vital organ function and metabolism with a simple method of pulsatile flow (IABP) during clinical cardiopulmonary bypass. Surgery 77:34–44, 1975

77. Silvay G, Litwak RS, Lubkan SB, et al: Left heart assist device: Early clinical experiences with management of post-perfusion low cardiac output. Anesth Analg 56:402–408, 1977

78. Norman JC, Fuqua JM, Hibbs CU, et al: An intracorporeal (abdominal) left ventricular assist device. Arch Surg 112:1442–1451, 1977

79. Peters JL, McRea JC, Fukumasu H, et al: Transapical left ventricular bypass (TALVB) without an auxiliary ventricle. Trans Am Soc Artif Intern Organs 22:357–365, 1976

Postoperative Care of the Patient

Donald C. Finlayson, M.D.

14
Postoperative Intensive Care

TRANSPORT FROM THE OPERATING ROOM TO THE INTENSIVE CARE UNIT

At the end of a cardiac operation the patient has experienced many dynamic changes in the function of almost all organ systems. In the midst of these changes, he must be safely transported to an intensive care unit (ICU), which is frequently a long distance from the operating room. A fundamental prerequisite is the maintenance of stable cardiovascular and respiratory function. Implicit in this is adequate monitoring and ventilation.

Monitoring

Monitoring of cardiac function on a beat-to-beat basis is essential to the patient's safe transport. This is accomplished using a dual-channel portable oscilloscopic monitor. This unit is battery powered and has one channel for an electrocardiogram display and the second channel for an arterial blood pressure display. Lead II of the ECG is observed during transport, since the detection of arrhythmias is the primary purpose for the electrocardiogram. Many arrhythmias may occur during this part of the operative procedure. In order for treatment to be most effective, an accurate electrocardiographic diagnosis must be readily available. A portable

battery-powered defibrillator should also be part of the transport equipment for patients who are very unstable, with frequent ventricular arrhythmias.

A continuous display of the arterial pressure is also observed during transport. The display is observed for changes in arterial pulse contour, and a digital readout permits continuous observation of the systolic and diastolic blood pressures. This capability of observing blood pressure, heart rate, and rhythm simultaneously is invaluable in the management of very sick patients during transport to the intensive care unit. Indeed, the governing principle should be that those parameters considered essential for monitoring intraoperatively should be maintained and monitored during the transport of the patient to the intensive care unit.

If the transport monitor does not have a second channel for arterial pressure, an approximation of this information may be gained by leaving a long length of arterial pressure tubing attached to the arterial line. This tubing is left about one-third filled with air and closed at the distal end by a stopcock. Compression of the air bubble in the tubing will be proportional to the intra-arterial pressure. Significant changes in blood pressure and stroke volume are usually readily perceived. It is better, however, to place an aneroid blood pressure manometer dial on the end of the tubing to give a continuous reading of the mean arterial blood pressure.

Ventilation

Ventilation of the patient can normally be managed using a self-inflating resuscitation bag with supplemental oxygen. A length of breathing tubing should be placed on the air-input side of the self-inflating bag so that the entrained gases during the refilling cycle of the bag will be 100 percent oxygen.[1,2] The use of this length of tubing ensures that almost 100 percent oxygen will be delivered to the patient. If the breathing tubing is omitted, it will not be possible to give 100 percent oxygen, unless the oxygen flows into the system are greater than 20 liters/min. Flows of this rate are potentially dangerous and may jam the valving system of the bag, preventing exhalation. With lower flow rates, air will be entrained as the bag refills following compression so that the inspired oxygen concentration will be lowered. This air entrainment will lower the F_IO_2 in most bags to the range of 60 to 75 percent when using oxygen flows of 6–8 liters/min in adults with normal ventilatory patterns.

During transport, the patient should receive positive-end-expiratory pressure (PEEP) if it was required during surgery. Few valves to provide PEEP are readily available, but the Boeringer valve or other self-assembled valves may be used during transport.

Ventilation during transport may also be managed using a Bird or Bennett pressure-cycled ventilator mounted on the ICU bed. This can be equipped to provide PEEP, as well as a controlled F_IO_2 using an air-oxygen blender. The delivered tidal volume and inspired oxygen concentration should be checked with a portable oxygen analyzer and respirometer. This type of ventilator can also be used for the transport of patients from the intensive care unit to other areas in the hospital (e.g., x-ray).

The amount of oxygen in the tank and the necessary flow rates must be kept in mind by the anesthesiologist. A full E-cylinder of oxygen has a pressure of 1800 psi and contains 625 liters of oxygen. The amount of oxygen remaining in the cylinder can be estimated from the pressure on the dial and the duration of safe usage can be estimated from the rates of flow being used. A bird ventilator in an average patient may use 10 liters of oxygen per minute.

Admission Procedure to the Intensive Care Unit

Before disconnecting the patient from the ventilator and monitoring equipment in the operating room, a number of preparations should be made. Transfer from the operating room table should be directly to an ICU bed whenever possible rather than to a recovery room stretcher and then later to an ICU bed. This transfer should be made as smoothly as possible, keeping in mind the fact that protective autonomic reflexes may have been depressed by anesthetic drugs and the patient's underlying disease. Movement to the ICU should be carried out as expeditiously as possible. Elevators, when necessary, should be called for and waiting when the patient arrives. Immediately upon arrival in the ICU, all monitoring and ventilator systems should be connected and the chest tubes stripped as soon as possible and reconnected to active suction.

The large number of personnel at the ICU station at this time, those transporting and those receiving the patient, should not get in one another's way. The measures to admit the patient should be carried out in an organized fashion. The organizing involved should be the result of thoughtful planning and training and should have as its objective, assessment of the patient and a plan for his management.[3]

STEPS ROUTINELY INVOLVED IN
ADMITTING A PATIENT TO THE
ICU

1. Pressure monitoring: The patient is immediately connected to the transducer and oscilloscopic system, which has been previously leveled and zeroed. Automatic flushing systems are attached to all pressure lines.
2. ECG—MCL_1 or V_5 monitoring: Heart rate is continuously counted and displayed on a digital readout.
3. Pacemaker: Confirm adequate function.
4. Chest tubes: Active suction applied after initial stripping; note initial volume of blood.
5. Temperature.
6. Examination: CNS: level of consciousness, pupils; skin: color, temperature; chest: bilateral breath sounds, endotracheal tube position, cuff volume; heart: heart sounds, murmurs, gallops, and rubs.

7. Ventilator: Minute ventilation and $Paco_2$ 35–45. Large tidal volumes with an IMV circuit with slow ventilatory rates (8–10). Inspired oxygen: initial setting, 70 to 80 percent until first blood gas checked.
8. PEEP: As required.
9. Laboratory studies: Blood gases, hematocrit, electrolytes, and coagulation profile.

INTENSIVE CARE UNIT ORGANIZATION[4]

Contributing to the efficient delivery of care in the ICU are several features of its design and staffing. There is much agreement on the design criteria for the ideal ICU, and solutions have been suggested for the organizational problems that occur. Most ICUs, however, are far from the ideal and represent examples of the problems rather than the solutions. Nevertheless, consideration of some of the features of design and staffing is useful.

Design Features

Layout and Visibility. Ideally, all patients should be visible from the center of the unit.

Isolation. Partitions, walls, or curtains between patients should permit visual isolation. Under ordinary circumstances, a fixed wall is not required. Its omission permits more flexible use of the floor space in the event that additional support equipment is needed for the care of the patient. Isolation with respect to sound or bacteria requires a fixed wall system. Unlike the needs of patients in a coronary care unit, sound isolation is not necessary for the majority of surgical ICU patients. This type of isolation should be available to the occasional patient who is conscious and still needs the special facilities of the surgical intensive care unit. Bacterial isolation should be available for the management of severe infections and to provide reverse isolation precautions for the protection of susceptible individuals (e.g., patients receiving steroids and/or other immunologic suppressant drugs). These units require not only fixed walls but also special anterooms, scrub sinks, containers, disposals, and air-conditioning systems.

Monitoring. Bedside displays of all monitor information are necessary, reflecting the fact that most of the nursing care will be carried out at the bedside. Fewer data need to be transmitted to the central nursing station. In designing new facilities, attention should be given to the potential future use of computers, so that adequate space is available for terminals and conduits to the central station.[5,6] The display should include an electrocardiogram with a write-out, temperature, and at least three pressure channels. All of these monitored parameters should be able to be directly recorded. The monitoring in the intensive care unit is, in fact, very similar to that in the operating room. One major difference is that sampling and injection through monitored lines are carried out more frequently in the operating room setting than in the intensive care unit. In addition, the patient is heparinized throughout much of the procedure in the operating room, and therefore there is little risk of clotting of the monitoring lines and loss of these valuable tools. This risk of clotting is avoided in the intensive care unit by the use of automatic continuous flushing valves (e.g., Sorensen intraflo®) in the monitoring systems.

Other monitoring techniques may be used in the intensive care unit to supplement those in the operating room. One example is the transcutaneous oxygen electrode.[7] Transcutaneous values for oxygen parallel those of arterial blood and equilibrate rapidly enough to serve as useful trend monitors to detect changes occurring with events such as coughing, tracheal suction, and the removal of oxygen face masks.

Computers have been used for the recording of patient data, for the handling of laboratory tests, and for the control of intravenous fluid infusions, blood infusions, and even drug administration. Their value on a cost-effectiveness basis is not yet clear nor is their potential for the future. In combination with pressure and cardiac output monitoring, however, measurements obtained with the use of computers and mass spectrographs may add to our present capabilities and permit more appropriate therapy with a shorter response time.[8–11]

Lighting. Variable intensity, potentially bright lights should be available for the intensive care unit. These may be needed for minor or even major surgical procedures under emergency situations.

Services. Gases, suction, electrical power, and grounding and isolation transformers, are common services.

Staffing

For the acutely ill patient, one attendant per patient during each shift, or three per day, is the ideal. Attendants include a mixture of registered nurses, respiratory therapists, physical therapists, nurses and other paramedical personnel. The role of the registered nurse is one of the major factors governing the use of other personnel. The more specialized functions the nurse carries out (e.g., physical therapy, respiratory therapy), the fewer other personnel that will be needed; this also means, however, substantial changes in the traditional nursing roles will require extensive further training.

The specific staffing mixture to be found in any institution usually reflects tradition and is usually not readily susceptible to change. Indeed, change is usually not necessary. There would appear to be no absolute requirements for the proportions of personnel in this unit, only for their training.

Physicians involved in such a unit must contribute in a number of ways toward the training of the staff:

1. Administration
2. Provision of reasonably constant physician presence
3. Continuous postgraduate education

These contributions by the physician become more important as the case load becomes heavier. The rewards will be in the good results that follow rapid and appropriate responses by the unit personnel in urgent situations.

Charting

Although computer-assisted charting is possible to varying degrees, manual notation by the ICU personnel is the usual practice. Charts and flow sheets appear best adapted to the requirements of the situation in the ICU. These flow sheets facilitate sequential charting of information and assessment of the patient, especially of trends in hemodynamic and respiratory parameters. Charting like other aspects of patient care should be carried out mainly at the bedside.

RESPIRATORY CARE

Immediate Postoperative Changes

IMPAIRED OXYGENATION AND VENTILATION

Although the lungs are isolated and to some extent protected during cardiopulmonary bypass, a number of factors may contribute to the development of pulmonary problems in the postoperative period. These are:

1. Temperature—Shivering→increased oxygen demand and increased CO_2 production.
2. Cardiac output
3. Anesthetic agents and vasodilator drugs
4. Age
5. Lung changes
   a. Airway closure
   b. Lung volume—Reduced—PEEP
   c. Respiratory work increased
   d. Parenchymal damages
   e. Fluid shifts

Temperature. Hypothermia in the range of 35–36°C is usually seen in the immediate postoperative period. During anesthesia, this might be expected to reduce oxygen consumption by 6 to 7 percent per degree celsius. This must be balanced against the increased oxygen affinity seen with cardiopulmonary bypass in the presence of any degree of alkalosis. Shivering in response to hypothermia during emergence from anesthesia makes prediction of oxygen demand difficult. It may lead to increases in demand that are usually greatly in excess of any reduction as a result of the lower temperature. In one study, oxygen demand was increased 135 to 486 percent.[12] Increases in oxygen demand of this magnitude, coming at a time when the patient may still be severely hemodiluted, are undesirable and potentially dangerous. For example, a doubling of the oxygen demand in the face of a 50 percent reduction in oxygen-carrying capacity will necessitate a fourfold increase in cardiac output to maintain the same hemodynamic conditions. Since such an increase is not always possible, the results will be increased peripheral oxygen extraction with increased venous desaturation. Under these circumstances, the lung will be presented with blood that is grossly desaturated and that has a very short mean transit time. Both of these factors may operate to inhibit arterialization of the venous blood, thus contributing to hypoxemia.

Therefore, shivering should be minimized. In adults, chlorpromazine (0.5-2mg) in repeated intravenous doses is commonly used to reduce the amount of shivering. Rewarming should be gradual, paralleling the gradual improvement in cardiovascular function and oxygen-carrying capacity usually seen in the immediate postoperative period.

Cardiac Output. Cardiac output insufficient for ordinary demands may have a great effect on peripheral oxygen extraction.[13] In addition, with a low cardiac output, the relatively fixed volumes of anatomic shunts will become proportionately larger and add significantly to the already high levels of venous admixture that may be present. Finally, the inadequate cardiac output may lead to left ventricular failure and the development of pulmonary edema, compounding the problem. In addition, a low cardiac output may be associated with an increased V_D/V_T, making respiratory efforts less efficient and giving rise to further demands for respiratory and cardiac work.

Anesthetic Agents and Vasodilator Drugs.[14,15] Anesthetics and vasodilators may worsen hypoxemia and venous admixture by overcoming the reflex hypoxic pulmonary vasoconstriction that might ordinarily be expected to minimize this process.

Age.[16] Age correlates with the presence of postoperative hypoxemia and may be most closely related to airway closure.

Airway Closure and Reduced Lung Volume.[17-19] Respiratory function is further altered by the reduction in lung volume seen with anesthesia and surgery. Decline in the total lung capacity and the functional residual capacity does not appear to be matched by compensatory reduction in the closing capacity. Therefore, an increasing degree of airway closure and a worsening ventilation perfusion mismatch will be seen. Positive end-expiratory pressure may therefore be a useful adjunct to therapy under these circumstances, as well as when there is increased interstitial fluid.[20-22] The use of ventilation patterns with PEEP appears capable of preventing much of the reduction in functional residual capacity after open heart surgery and is unquestionably of value in minimizing the hypoxemia associated with pulmonary edema. Its use may be accompanied by improved oxygenation, and better respiratory mechanics and may permit the use of lower levels of inspired oxygen.

Initial ventilator adjustments may be difficult with respect to minute ventilation and alveolar CO_2 as a result of the presence of alterations in dead space, which may be associated with a low cardiac output state, and changes in carbon dioxide production, which may lead to levels markedly above or below normal. The use of nomograms with imposed corrections for temperature, height and weight, and body surface area, although satisfactory in the majority of patients, may occasionally lead to grossly abnormal values. The presence of either a low cardiac output or shivering or both should lead one to suspect an altered carbon dioxide production and the need to change the predicted ventilator settings.

Since there are many factors capable of compromising oxygenation, an initial F_IO_2 of 0.7 with an end-expiratory pressure of 0 is used for the initial ventilation of the average patient. This range is chosen in the hope of minimizing ventilation perfusion scatter while not increasing venous admixture, as is often the case with the use of 100 percent oxygen. PEEP is added, beginning with 5 cm of water and increased in 2½-cm increments until the initial arterial blood gases show an alveolar-to-arterial oxygen gradient of less than 250-300 torr.

Respiratory Work. Many patients, especially those undergoing aortocoronary bypass, have preexisting chronic obstructive pulmonary disease with significant alterations in their work of breathing. The normal levels of oxygen consumption for respiratory work are quite low, being approximately 2 percent of the total body oxygen consumption at rest. These levels rise after surgery, however. One group, studied by Peters, demonstrated more than a tenfold increase in work of breathing after median sternotomy, with the increase being most marked on the third postoperative day.[23] In these patients, any impairment in respiratory efficiency, necessitating an increase in ventilation, may give rise to insupportable levels of work with cardiac and respiratory decompensation.

Parenchymal damage to the lung as a result of insults that may be associated with open heart surgery may also be a problem, despite the relative isolation that the lungs enjoy from the bypass circuit during much of the cardiac surgical procedure. This may be a factor contributing to the prolonged need for respiratory care in many patients in the postoperative period.[24]

The increased work appears to be equally distributed into lung and chest wall components and can be expressed in terms of depression of lung and chest wall compliance. Among the factors contributing to the decreased lung compliance are the reductions in lung volumes, atelectasis, and increased abdominal visceral volume. The reduction in chest wall compliance is due almost entirely to the splinting associated with incisional pain.

These increases in work must be considered to be superimposed upon the ordinary basal requirements for oxygen and require proportionate increases in cardiac output. The terms "increased oxygen consumption," "respiratory work," and "cardiac output" may be thought of as being synonymous in these circumstances. The termination of ventilatory support must therefore be gradual enough so that additional requirements for oxygen delivery occasioned by spontaneous ventilation can be imposed progressively, under optimum circumstances, and assessed thoroughly before completion of the process.

The finding that respiratory work is markedly elevated and rises even further in the next several days after surgery suggests that extubation may be just as safely performed immediately after surgery as it is later, if carried out under reasonable conditions. Early extubation after surgery has become increasingly popular as surgical and anesthesia techniques, and understanding of the disordered physiology have improved. Since the work of breathing will apparently change very little in the initial postoperative period, early extubation may in some instances contribute positively to the patient care rather than detracting from it as was once thought to be the case. The cost and complexity of care is usually reduced with an increase in patient comfort. Presently, many patients undergoing coronary artery bypass surgery are extubated in the early postoperative hours (within 6 hours of surgery).[25] Most other cardiac surgical patients are ventilated at least overnight (12 to 18 hours postoperatively).

Criteria for extubation, either immediately after surgery or at a later time, are as follows:

1. Oxygen transport
   Adequate carrying capacity must be present
   Hematocrit value greater than 25 to 30 percent
   Hemoglobin affinity must be acceptable
   No severe alkalosis
2. Oxygen demand
   Stable
   No severe shivering
   Temperature greater than 36°C
   P_VO_2 greater than 35 torr
3. Myocardial function
   Good contractility, rhythm, cardiac output, and blood pressure must be maintained
4. Respiratory function
   Vital capacity greater than 10 ml/kg
   Inspiratory force greater than 20–25 cm H_2O
5. Hemostasis
   Less than 200 ml/hr of chest tube drainage
   Relatively normal coagulation studies
6. Metabolic state
   Normal electrolytes and blood sugar
7. Central nervous system
   Awake and alert patient

Respiratory Care After Extubation

OXYGEN THERAPY AFTER EXTUBATION

Although the majority of patients do not have impairment of lung function of major significance, all have changes that are usually reflected in an increased alveolar-to-arterial oxygen difference and in varying degrees of arterial desaturation. All require supplemental oxygen for several days and may demonstrate impaired oxygenation for as long as several weeks. Oxygen therapy must not be discontinued for meals or nursing procedures until adequate oxygenation has been demonstrated while breathing room air. Even in the best of circumstances, this usually takes several days.

Nasal prongs with flows of 5–6 liters/min of humidified oxygen should be used when it is necessary to remove a face mask. The maximal effective F_1O_2 from nasal cannulae in the usual patient under these postoperative circumstances will probably not exceed 30 percent. An ordinary, close-fitting oxygen face mask with a flow of 6–8 liters/min of humidified oxygen will be adequate for most patients and will give an effective F_1O_2 of approximately 40 percent. If this is not adequate, an increased amount of oxygen can be given in a controlled manner by the use of flows that exceed the patient's maximal mid-inspiratory flow rate and prevent the entrainment of room air in the inspired mixture. In the adult patient, oxygen flows of 20–25 liters/min through a double-flow meter assembly will suffice. The F_1O_2 can be set by adjustment of the air entrainment aperture on the humidifier bottle and confirmed by analysis.[26]

INTERMITTENT POSITIVE PRESSURE BREATHING (IPPB), BRONCHODILATOR THERAPY, AND CHEST PHYSIOTHERAPY

The exact place of IPPB after open heart surgery is unclear, and a clear demonstration of benefits is lacking. However, IPPB for the mobilization of secretions and delivery of bronchodilator drugs to the airway may be useful in some patients, particularly in patients with overt bronchospasm and a history of chronic obstructive lung disease. Drugs such as the β_2 stimulant isoethrane may be diluted in water and nebulized into the airway via face mask or mouthpiece. However, β_1 agonist activity is not entirely absent in these drugs and the frequent development of tachycardia and irritability is often a limiting factor to the use of these drugs in cardiac patients. Therefore, caution and careful ECG monitoring must be the rule for at least the initial use of these drugs and must continue until a pattern of safety is assured.

The use of IPPB to minimize atelectasis and other postoperative complications has, in most studies, been found to be about as effective as good nursing and physiotherapy. It should probably be regarded in most instances as simply another mode of therapy to encourage a degree of deep breathing and coughing, secretion mobilization, and an increase in the functional residual capacity. Some improvement may result if the target of IPPB is a breath of a measured volume, rather than one resulting from the application of a fixed pressure. These measures and others to increase lung function and reduce atelectasis (e.g., incentive spirometer) would appear to have a common objective, to be almost equal in value, and to be a fundamental component of postoperative chest care.[27]

Continued Postoperative Ventilation

The primary purpose for the continuation of tracheal intubation and artificial or mechanical ventilation has been the protection of the airway, the assumption of the work of breathing, and the assurance of adequate ventilation. The ventilatory equipment in the intensive care unit should have humidifiers, a safe design, a wide range of flexibility, and a range of ventilatory capabilities.

ENDOTRACHEAL INTUBATION

The oral rather than the nasal route of intubation would appear preferable in most cardiovascular patients, certainly in adults, during cardiac surgery. In children, the nares are approximately the same size as the diameter of the trachea, and therefore a tube of optimal size can be placed. In adults, however, the nares are much smaller than the trachea, and therefore this is not possible. Furthermore, nasotracheal intubation is more traumatic, with the hazard of turbinate injury, bleeding, and bacteremia. To risk injury, bleeding, and sepsis in a patient about to receive heparin and undergo cardiovascular surgery would seem unwarranted. Nasal hemorrhage, once experienced, is never forgotten and is thereafter carefully avoided. Similar considerations are operative should it prove necessary to reintubate the patient in the postoperative period.

The cuff on the endotracheal tube should be of the compliant, controlled, low-pressure variety.[28] The Lanz tube contains an inflating pressure bypass valve and a compliant pilot balloon inside a plastic envelope, as well as a low-pressure cuff. Air is injected into the inflating valve until the pilot balloon shows a moderate degree of inflation and occupies about one-third to one-half the space inside its envelope. This will give rise to a cuff pressure of 15–25 cm H_2O. In patients requiring very high inflation pressure for ventilation, this cuff pressure may be inadequate to effect a tracheal seal and prevent leakage of the ventilatory gases back around the cuff. If faced with this problem, air should be injected into the inflation valve until the pilot balloon expands to completely fill the envelope. Further injections of air will then be delivered to the cuff as in an ordinary tube, giving rise to higher cuff pressures and eventually sealing the trachea. The amount of air should then be carefully adjusted so that there is a seal up to the selected level of pressure and a leak thereafter.

Conventional low-pressure cuffs should have the amount of air in the cuff carefully adjusted at insertion and checked frequently thereafter. Initially, the seal should be up to, but not exceeding, 25 cm H_2O. A cuff leak should be apparent with ventilatory pressures significantly above this level. The threshold pressures used subsequently should be those indicated by the patient's condition.

Noncompliant high-pressure cuffs should not be used. Even very slight excesses of air above the levels required to seal the trachea to prevent gas leakage may give rise to catastrophically high lateral tracheal wall pressures. These pressures may totally prevent perfusion in the underlying trachea, leading to tissue necrosis and subsequent tracheal stenosis. If such a tube is used, the patient should be ventilated with a continuous leak at peak inspiratory pressure.

Tracheal stenosis is unlikely to be seen with the use of a controlled-pressure cuff tube and should not occur if an ordinary low-pressure cuff is in use and properly inflated. Its development should be suspected if the amount of air being put into the cuff increases with time and will be confirmed by serial x-rays showing the cuff to be increasing in size, finally becoming greater in diameter than the trachea. If the cuff is increasing its size, the patient should be ventilated with a leak at peak inspiratory pressure. The cuff, once inflated, should stay that way except for routine checking of its pressure and volume. Proper tubes may be left in place, with minimal risk, longer than was originally thought to be the case. The risk of damage to the trachea is minimal and while risk to the vocal apparatus is still real, it is perhaps reduced by the newer, less toxic materials used in endotracheal tube construction. Our experience would suggest that these tubes may be left in place, with minimal risk, for 5 to 6 days. If they are to be left in place for longer than this, withdrawal of the endotracheal tube from the trachea and inspec-

tion of the vocal apparatus may be indicated. The finding of relatively normal vocal cords will permit reinsertion of the tube. Significant damage will indicate the need for tracheostomy. This examination is performed using a fiberoptic bronchoscope passed down through the endotracheal tube.[29]

VENTILATORS

Many ventilators are available for use in the intensive care unit. The ideal ventilator should be:

1. Sturdy and reliable
2. Powerful–generate 85–100 cm of H_2O-air pressure
3. Safe—alarms, indicators, monitors
4. Easy to operate
5. Equipped with a proper humidifier[30,31]—Adequate and dependable
6. Flexible—assisted and/or controlled ventilation, intermittent mandatory ventilation (IMV), synchronized intermittent mandatory ventilation (SIMV), PEEP, continuous positive airway pressure (CPAP), and sighs.

The IMV mode is satisfactory for almost all patients and, at least at lower rates, gives some assurance that the patient's homeostatic mechanisms will contribute to the respiratory process, leading to more appropriate levels of $PaCO_2$ and pH. At the time of admission to the ICU the patient usually shows moderate to marked respiratory depression. Under these circumstances, there is usually no difference between IMV and controlled mechanical ventilation. The assist-control mode may be useful in the patient who, for reasons of agitation, pain, hypoventilation, or other causes, cannot smoothly adjust to IMV. Under these circumstances, one is often presented with a patient struggling to breathe. The use of manual or mechanically assisted respiration may tide one over until the situation can be more adequately assessed and, by providing more adequate ventilation, may stabilize the situation.

SIMV may prove more readily tolerated as respiratory support is being withdrawn, if for no other reason than the fact that it should be more comfortable than a nonsynchronized mode. Although this may not be true for patients on long-term ventilatory support at low IMV rates, it would appear to be the case for the cardiac patient being weaned from what is most commonly only short-term ventilation.

In most cardiac patients, very slow IMV rates (i.e., 1–2 per minute) may function only as a sigh and thus might be considered as part of the postoperative chest physiotherapy program. If this is the case, they should be given in large volumes. The sigh volume should be two to three times the usual tidal volume of 7.0 ml/kg.[32] The use of a sigh in a program of ventilatory support has fallen out of fashion in recent years. It has been considered only of equal value to a pattern of large tidal volumes and slow respiratory frequency. This may not be entirely true. Lung compliance may be improved by a sigh, even in patients being ventilated with slow rates, increased tidal volumes, and PEEP. Until the problem is clarified, a sigh at intervals of 5 minutes, with a volume of two to three times the tidal volume, should probably be part of the patient's ventilatory management.

PEEP is a well-established contribution to ventilatory support.[33] It gives rise to an increase in functional residual capacity, recruitment of increased numbers of alveoli, and, as would be expected, is effective in the management of diffuse reversible atelectasis and pulmonary edema. One or both of these are often present postoperatively. It must be kept in mind that in the emphysematous patient whose functional residual capacity is already greater than normal, PEEP is likely to be less useful and may even exacerbate the situation. To the extent that the pressure is transmitted through what is usually a stiff lung to the vascular compartment in the presence of a normal or reduced lung volume, there may be some inhibition of venous return, and decrease in cardiac output.

In assessing and managing incremental PEEP, the cardiac output should be evaluated whenever the PEEP level is altered.[34] If some depression in cardiac output is seen, a blood volume increase can be produced. This will usually overcome the cardiac output depression. Further increases in PEEP and blood volume will be contingent on improvement in oxygenation and may be continued until either a marked change in circulation is seen or until there is no further improvement in either lung compliance or arterial blood gases.

The physiological effects of ventilation with and without PEEP or superPEEP represent a spectrum of change involving the cardiovascular system, antidiuretic hormone, and fluid and electrolyte balance. Antidiuretic hormone secretion is increased under some circumstances of artificial ventilation at zero end-expiratory pressure and, in all likelihood, under all circumstances in which PEEP is used. The fluid retention thus engendered will ensure a more stable cardiovascular system but may pose problems in terms of lung and other organ-system functions as PEEP is withdrawn. Attention to fluid balance must be meticulous and accompanied by readiness to use diuretics. Water balance is also affected by the humidification systems of most ventilators in current use. They are very efficient, so much so as to largely eliminate insensible water loss, at least in the nonfebrile patient.

PROBLEMS DURING VENTILATORY CARE

The problems that stem from the use of artificial ventilation are related in part to its physiological consequences and in part to the potential for trauma inherent in the technique itself.

Cardiovascular function may be decreased by virtue of depression of venous return and cardiac output. The cardiovascular changes represent the balance between the effects resulting from the increased intrathoracic pressure, which tend to inhibit venous return and depress cardiac output, and those giving rise to increased autonomic system activation, which opposes the process. The increased intrathoracic pressure will be more marked if higher pressures are necessary for ventilation of the patient or if higher levels of PEEP are used. The level of increased intrathoracic pressure that will give rise to a decrease in cardiac output varies from patient to patient. The following factors are involved:

1. Blood volume
2. Degree of autonomic nervous system activity potentially available—drugs, disease
3. Ease of transmission of the intrathoracic pressure to the vascular compartment

In the emphysematous patient with diminished lung parenchyma, the pressure may be transmitted with little attenuation directly to the vascular compartment. In contrast, in the patient with edema, atelectasis, and a relatively normal lung, much of the pressure may be expended in maintaining expansion, with less available for transmission. Therefore, PEEP should be used with caution in the presence of hypovolemia, vasodepressive drugs, and emphysema. It should be started at 5 cm H_2O and increased by amounts as little as 2.5 cm H_2O with careful clinical assessment in regard to the cardiac output.

Marked cardiovascular stimulation in the absence of adequate sedation may result from the presence of a tube in the patient's trachea and/or an unsynchronized ventilatory pattern. It is only necessary to see a few patients agitated and coughing on an endotracheal tube to realize that the potential benefits of ventilation in terms of decreased work of breathing are being swept away by the inability to tolerate the tube and/or the ventilator. This often occurs in the patient after open heart surgery, particularly during the weaning process using unsynchronized intermittent mandatory ventilation breaths at slow rates. Thus the synchronized IMV mode (now becoming available) may be a better choice and less disturbing in some patients.

Pneumothorax and surgical emphysema may result from the application of positive pressure to the airway. The risk is magnified by preexisting disease and trauma to the lungs and is dependent upon the amounts of pressure being used. A pneumothorax should be suspected in the presence of the following:

1. Abrupt circulatory depression accompanied by the sudden development of marked increases in peak airway pressures, often setting off the pressure alarms on the ventilator.
2. Evidence of inadequate ventilation, such as tachypnea, accompanied by deterioration of arterial blood gases and cyanosis.
3. Diminished gas exchange on the affected side of the thorax which may be and often is obvious in terms of chest movement and auscultatory breath sounds.

The sudden appearance of any of the above should lead to the immediate examination of chest movement and breath sounds. Deterioration in the patient is often so rapid that diagnosis and treatment must be instituted immediately to avoid catastrophe. Chest-tube placement and underwater sealed drainage are required. X-rays should be used to confirm the diagnosis if time permits and must be taken after decompression. Emergency decompression of a tension-pneumo-

thorax may be necessary even while preparations for chest tube insertion are underway. This may be accomplished by insertion of a large-bore plastic intravenous cannula (14- or 16-gauge) attached to a syringe into the anterior third interspace in the mid-clavicular line. After detection of the pleural space by the loss of resistance, removal of the syringe will permit the air to escape. Continued positive pressure ventilation will prevent collapse of the underlying lung.

The appearance of a small asymptomatic pneumothorax as an incidental finding in the first postoperative x-ray is often a consequence of accidental and unappreciated damage to the pleura at operation, without damage to the lung.[35,36] In the absence of any clinical evidence of enlargement, continued surveillance both clinically and by x-ray is sufficient, and chest tube drainage is not required.

Prolonged intubation is mainly a hazard to the vocal apparatus and trachea, although occasional ulcerations involving the tongue and soft palate may be seen. In the early attempts to provide prolonged respiratory support, Lindholm and his co-workers noted that the risk to the vocal apparatus was time-dependent but approached 100 percent by about the fourth day.[37] The newer plastic materials are better tolerated than the original red rubber tubes, and the risk is therefore somewhat reduced. The degree to which the risk is decreased is not entirely clear, however, and the resultant ulceration, scarring, and granulation formation still occur. As noted earlier, if for any reason prolonged oral endotracheal intubation is desired, periodic withdrawal of the tube and laryngoscopy may be indicated. The appearance of significant damage to the vocal apparatus would then mandate a tracheostomy.

The risks of prolonged intubation must be balanced against those of tracheostomy in the early postoperative period. The worst complication of an early tracheostomy is probably infection of a median sternotomy. To avoid this, tracheostomies should be deferred until wound healing is well underway, a period generally thought to be between 5 and 8 days. The risks of endotracheal intubation for periods longer than this and the reversibility of the resulting lesion are not entirely clear. It is believed by many, however, that the risk is less than that of mediastinal infection.

Nasotracheal intubation is often used when prolonged intubation and ventilatory support are necessary in pediatric patients. The nares are approximately the same size as the trachea in children, while much less so in adults, making this route more suitable for children. Therefore, despite the risks of trauma and bacteremia, this method is considered the method of choice by some pediatric anesthesiologists. The advantages are thought to lie mainly in the potential for increased comfort for the patient. This factor is not often relevant in the adult ICU setting. Respiratory failure without diminution of consciousness is not common in adult patients in comparison with the situation found in younger patients with diseases such as poliomyelitis, Guillain-Barré, or myasthenia gravis.

Tracheostomy may be carried out in the intensive care unit if necessary using local anesthesia, sedation, and analgesia as appropriate to the patient's condition. After preparation, an incision is made into the upper tracheal rings, the endotracheal tube cuff is deflated, the tube withdrawn, and the tracheostomy tube inserted. There should be no blood in the surgical site to run into the trachea, the airway should be free of secretions, and the procedure should be carried out with dispatch.

Accidental dislodgement of the tube in the early postoperative period is a hazardous complication. The tissue planes at the site are mobile and poorly differentiated for several days until a moderate amount of granulation tissue develops. Therefore, the tract down to the trachea and stoma may not be obvious after accidental extubation. Intubation of the mediastinum under these circumstances is not uncommon. Therefore, if the tracheostomy tube cannot be easily and convincingly replaced in the trachea, the stoma should be occluded by an assistant's hand and bag and mask ventilation carried out until preparations can be made for orderly intubation and subsequent replacement of the tracheostomy tube under more controlled conditions.

If the cuff ruptures during this early period, the tube may be changed safely by removing it over a suction catheter inserted over its lumen into the trachea. A new tube is then inserted over the suction catheter.

The most feared late complication of tracheostomy is vessel erosion and hemorrhage, most commonly from the innominate artery. The hazards of such a complication in a patient who may be infected down to the eroded vessel are obvious.

Humidification of the inspired gases is necessary for the optimum maintenance of thermal and water balance and to minimize changes in tracheal mucous membranes. The Bennett/Cascade humidifier is the one most commonly used. It is effective, durable, and reliable. It can be set to deliver fully humidified gases to the airway at body temperature. Insensible water loss will be largely eliminated by the use of such equipment. This fact should be taken into account when making fluid balance calculations.

The x-ray examination of the chest is an essential part of the monitoring process in the ICU. The films should be taken upon admission, 6 to 8 hours later, after extubation or reintubation, and daily thereafter, as well as for other specific indications. Chest x-rays will represent a true monitoring method if they are taken as soon as needed and made available without delay. They should be kept for viewing in the intensive care unit or at least as close by as possible. The film should be taken in a standardized fashion using a fixed tube-to-film distance of 44–48 inches, with the patient in a 45° head-up tilt position, and using the same exposure from one film to another. When it is necessary, because of patient instability, to use the supine position, it should be noted on the film. This uniformity of technique will permit more adequate assessment of pulmonary congestion and edema, effusions, and intrapleural air as well as the evaluation of endotracheal tube and intravascular catheter position.

CARDIOVASCULAR CARE

The Cardiovascular Status in the Immediate Postoperative Period

RHYTHM

Many factors may be responsible for alterations in rhythm after open heart surgery. Among them are preexisting disease; the effects of operation including manipulation, cross-clamping, and ischemia; the use of myocardial preservation solutions; and metabolic changes in acid–base and electrolyte balance.[38]

The use of myocardial preservation solutions containing high concentrations of potassium (20–30 mEq/liter) may contribute to the development of varying degrees of heart block. This process may last for several hours and initially may be effectively managed from a hemodynamic standpoint by the use of a sequential atrioventricular pacemaker or by infusion of a glucose-insulin-potassium (GIK) solution. Simple ventricular pacing, although less effective, will suffice if the general level of myocardial function is adequate.

Ventricular irritability as manifested by premature ventricular contractions is probably the most common rhythm disturbance after open heart surgery. The rapid decreases in serum potassium that may be associated with prior and intraoperative use of diuretics along with alkalosis, and the humoral changes associated with operation, all may contribute to the development of myocardial irritability. Therefore, in the immediate postoperative period, sampling of serum potassium levels must be frequent and treatment must be aggressive, with the objective being the maintenance of the serum potassium level at the upper limits of normal. Potassium supplementation, if it is indicated in adults, is given by infusion from a metering intravenous set at the rate of 10 mEq/30–60 min. This may be repeated two to three times and then followed after 60 minutes by determination of the serum potassium level.

Lidocaine in a bolus of 1–1.5 mg/kg is commonly given for the treatment of premature ventricular contractions. If this results in significant improvement, it should be followed by a continuous infusion consisting of 1–4 mg/min in the average adult patient. Divided doses of propranolol may also be used (0.25–1 mg in the average 70-kg adult).

The acid-base status of the patient must also be evaluated. For reasons noted earlier, the new ventilation settings in the intensive care unit may cause inappropriate underventilation and elevation of the $PaCO_2$, which will be accompanied by increased levels of autonomic nervous system activity. Hypocarbia and respiratory alkalosis can result in rapid translocation of potassium from the blood into the cells and consequent hypokalemia and further arrhythmias.

Supraventricular tachyarrhythmias may also be seen. The approach to their treatment will depend on the cause, but usually consists of the use of propranolol, digitalis, and/or cardioversion (see Chapter 4).

CARDIAC TAMPONADE

Cardiac tamponade should be suspected when the central venous pressure is found to be rising while the cardiac output is falling. If actual measurements of cardiac output or left-sided pressures are available, evidence of reduced left-sided filling and output may assist in making the diagnosis. Other features are associated hemorrhage and chest x-ray evidence of mediastinal widening. In some patients, a pulsus paradoxus may also be present, but this finding is not very obvious in patients on controlled mechanical ventilation. Isoproterenol by infusion can be used to provide some degree of support while arrangements are being made for more definitive therapy. Once the diagnosis is suspected, however, failure to rule out tamponade should be followed by reexploration of the patient's chest (see Chapter 15).

CONTRACTILITY

Contractility may be altered in the immediate postoperative period. Moderate but reversible depression due to disease, manipulation, and ischemia is often seen. The appearance of problems of this sort for the first time, not at operation, but later in the patient's ICU course, is unusual, however, and should lead one to suspect a new event. In the absence of the above factors, the sudden occurrence of hypotension in the early postoperative period, especially after myocardial revascularization, must give rise to a provisional diagnosis of acute coronary insufficiency and impending or established myocardial infarction. Efforts must be made to exclude metabolic and respiratory disturbances, hypovolemia, hemorrhage, and tamponade as causes, and the ECG must be reviewed. New and localizing ischemic changes may raise the possibility of a return to the operating room. The vascular insufficiency may be due to correctable problems such as kinking or rotation of a graft or obstructive problems at either its origin or insertion. Return to the operating room, if contemplated, must be expeditious. In the normothermic patient, some degree of irreversible damage from absolute ischemia begins to appear after about 20 minutes and is probably not reversible after 60 to 120 minutes.

Cardiovascular Problems

RATE DISORDERS

Bradycardia. In bradycardia, the mechanism, degree of block, adequacy of cardiac output, and ventricular irritability must all be evaluated. Simple observation is permissible if the cardiac output seems adequate and PVCs are not present. Isoproterenol may be used in circumstances in which the adequacy of cardiac output is in question, the pulse rate low or normal, and PVCs absent. If PVCs are present, irrespective of the level of cardiac output, pacing may be carried out in the hope that raising the rate might reduce the level of ventricular irritability. Atropine may be given to these patients for diagnostic or therapeutic purposes (Fig. 14-1).

Tachycardia. In tachycardia, the mechanism and cardiac output must similarly be evaluated and the possibility of digoxin toxicity entertained. Carotid massage is frequently a useful maneuver. Slowing following the increase in vagal tones suggests that a paroxysmal atrial tachycardia may have been the problem. If a ventricular mechanism appears to be the problem, supplemental potassium in 10 mEq increments may be given even in the absence of laboratory assessment of pH and serum potassium measurements. This may also be accompanied by the use of lidocaine and preparations made

for cardioversion if the situation appears urgent (Fig. 14-2).

RHYTHM DISORDERS

Much of the rationale for the treatment of these problems will be obvious from the consideration of the algorithms below. The maintenance of normal sinus rhythm (i.e., the presence of atrial activity) can be expected to improve cardiac output by as much as 25 percent. This may be of critical importance in the very sick patient with an extremely low cardiac output. Propranolol, digoxin, or cardioversion may be used when the cardiac output is severely threatened and the mechanism is other than sinus or nodal. If the patient is awake, consciousness should be obtunded prior to cardioversion to the degree consistent with patient safety. If the patient is intubated or if there is reasonable assurance that his stomach is empty, this should not be a problem and, indeed, is true in most cases. Small amounts of diazepam are frequently used. If the patient has a full stomach and is alert, the problem becomes more difficult. The alternatives are either to administer little or no analgesia and hynotics or to give hypnotic drugs in combination with muscle relaxants to gain control over and protect the airway.

PRESSURE DISORDERS

Hypertension. Increased blood pressure is often an early event in the recovery period and is frequently severe with the return of autonomic

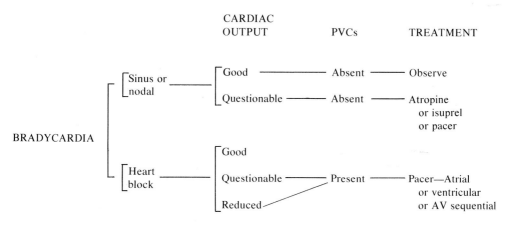

Fig. 14-1. Algorithm for diagnosis and treatment of bradycardia.

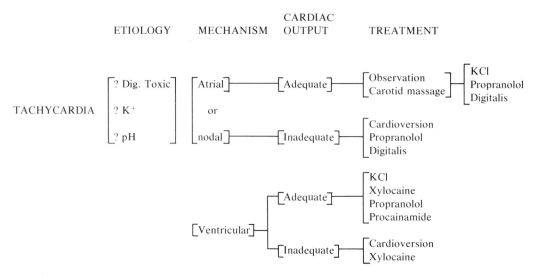

Fig. 14-2. Algorithm for diagnosis and treatment of tachycardia.

nervous system activity and consciousness.[39,40] At this time the patient is usually hypothermic, anemic, and to some degree in a low-output state. Since cardiac function and oxygen demand are dependent on afterload to a significant degree, control of this problem is quite important. Initial measures should include:

1. Supplemental analgesia—morphine in 2–5 intravenous aliquots
2. Chlorpromazine, 1–2 mg intravenous aliquots

If these two drugs are not effective, vasodilator therapy with nitroglycerin, nitroprusside, trimethaphan, or phentolamine may be indicated. A recent approach has been to manipulate the renin-angiotensin-aldosterone system with angiotensin-blocking drugs.

The nitroglycerin infusion used in the operating room should be taken to the intensive care unit with the patient and can be used for the initial treatment of this hypertension. In a recent study that we performed, doses between 32 and 120 μg/min of nitroglycerin were successful in controlling the hypertension in 80 percent of the patients.[41] In the remainder, the hypertension was not controlled by nitroglycerin, and the use of nitroprusside was required. Trimethaphan (1 mg/ml) or phentolamine (0.5–1 mg/ml) may also be given intravenously for the control of postoperative hypertension.

Nitroprusside is probably the most commonly used drug in this situation and is frequently made up in concentrations ranging from 100 to 400 μg/ml. It should be administered in the smallest amount capable of producing acceptable therapeutic results. Absence of vasodilatation with ordinary doses should suggest a search for evidence of possible cyanide toxicity. It should be discontinued immediately if there is any evidence of increasing metabolic acidosis.[42]

Hypotension—Low Cardiac Output State. The cardiac output and systemic vascular resistance are factors in the final production of any blood pressure. Hypotension for most patients after open heart surgery is usually associated with a low cardiac output and increased vascular resistance, rather than increased cardiac output and low peripheral resistance. Inherent in successful treatment of this problem is good diagnostic information; that is, cardiac output should be known. Therefore, any situation requiring other than modest levels of supportive care should dictate the placement of a thermal dilution pulmonary artery catheter.

Initial steps in therapy (Fig. 14-3) should include an assessment of cardiac efficiency in regard to rate and rhythm, blood volume, myocardial contractility, and oxygen delivery capacity. In addition, arterial blood gas studies should be carried out to assess the ventilatory and acid–base status.

Oxygenation should be made as complete as possible:

1. The F_IO_2 is set at 70 percent, since higher concentrations than this are potentially toxic and should be used for only short periods of time. Also, they are usually relatively ineffective in the face of degrees of venous admixture greater than 30 or 40 percent.
2. PEEP is most useful in the presence of reduced lung volumes and pulmonary edema.
3. $Paco_2$ should be adjusted to maintain the physiological level of pH.
4. Acid–base balance should be kept within the normal range to avoid cardiovascular depression often seen with acidosis and the effect on myocardial and cerebral blood flow which may follow marked alkalosis.

The blood volume status is usually assessed by inspection of the hemodynamic parameters for evidence of inadequate preload, i.e., right-sided (CVP) and left-sided (LAP or PCWP) pressures. A volume challenge may be given when this is not clear. Balanced salt solutions, such as Ringer's lactate or colloids such as dextran may be used.[43] The volume chosen for infusion should be approximately 5 percent of the patient's predicted blood volume. It should be administered fairly rapidly, given in four or five

equal parts a few minutes apart, preferably by injection using a syringe with inspection of the patient's clinical signs between aliquots.

Oxygen flux, i.e., oxygen delivery capacity, should also be assessed. Marked anemia is usually present immediately postoperatively and, to a lesser extent, is often seen later in the patient's postoperative course. The impairment of oxygen delivery, which is the underlying pathophysiological defect in the low-output state, can often be improved markedly by simply raising the hematocrit. Hematocrit levels much above the physiological range may, however, lead to impairment of tissue perfusion as a consequence of the impairment in flow properties of the blood under these circumstances, leading to eventual worsening of the problem. The target hematocrit value should therefore lie between 35 and 40 percent.

A low cardiac output state continuing from events in the operating room almost invariably represents impairment of contractility as well as other factors. Many of these are reversible with time, while others will require specific treatment.

General supportive therapy may include the use of glucose, insulin, and potassium infusions which appear to have a beneficial effect on the injured myocardium.[44,45] This solution is thought to provide its effect by presenting extra substrate for energy production in the myocardium. If this approach is to be used, the patient may be given an initial intravenous bolus dose of 25

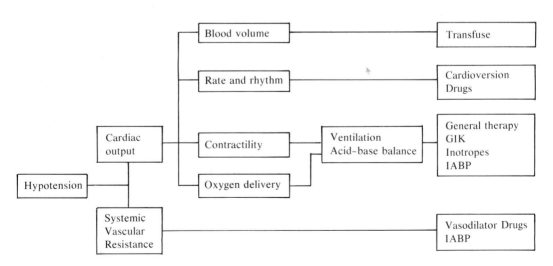

Fig. 14-3. Initial steps in therapy of hypotension.

gm of glucose (50 ml of 50 percent glucose) accompanied by 10 units of regular insulin. This can then be followed by an infusion containing 250 gm of glucose, 40 mEq of potassium, and 25 units of regular insulin. The infusion is given at the rate of 1.5 ml/kg/hr.

Specific drug therapy includes the use of calcium and other inotropic agents. If ionized calcium levels can be determined, such measurements should be carried out and calcium administered to bring the ionized calcium up to normal. If it is not possible to measure ionized calcium, a test dose of 250–500 mg can be administered. Usually the patients require 1–2 gm of calcium chloride to get the full hemodynamic response. This effect may then be supplemented with other inotropic agents, vasodilators, and the intra-aortic balloon pump as required (see Chapter 12 for the therapeutic algorithm).

CENTRAL NERVOUS SYSTEM STATUS

Anesthesia should be designed so that the patient will be reactive as soon as possible upon arrival in the ICU. This is especially true for those patients particularly at risk of complications involving the central nervous system, i.e., in whom the heart chambers were opened or in whom preexisting disease is present. The patient's hand grasp and ability to use all four limbs in sequence should be checked. If the patient is unresponsive, narcotic antagonists and physostigmine can be administered if narcotics and scopolamine have been used during the anesthetic procedure. The continued absence of neurological responsiveness should be followed by:

1. Discussion of the problem with all involved personnel
2. Guarded prognosis in any discussion with the family
3. Ventilatory readjustment so as to produce moderate hypocarbia—PaCO$_2$ 30–35 torr[46]
4. Decadron, 10 mg stat and 4 mg every 6 hours (four times a day)
5. Mannitol infusion, 20–40 gm
6. Repeated neurological examinations including fundoscopy

Air emboli are the most common central nervous system complication after open heart

surgery. The risk is greatest when the heart chambers have been opened. However, air may gain access to the left ventricle or the aortic root as a result of problems with the insertion or removal of the left ventricular vent or problems with cannulation or anastamosis of the aorta. Particulate emboli, including calcium, fibrous tissue, or atheromatous material, may be dislodged during valvular surgery or with placement of clamps on the ascending aorta. Air in the circulatory system shows axial streaming and gravitational effects. It tends to travel on the upper outermost stream of blood and thus flows preferentially in almost all circumstances to the head, more to the right side than to the left. In the circulation, air is widely distributed, breaking up into smaller and smaller bubbles and lodging finally in the distal arteriolar tree. If the bubbles contain only oxygen and are less than 0.1 mm in size, they should disappear after a few seconds. If they are even slightly larger and contain nitrogen they may persist for many hours.

The use of 100 percent oxygen has not proved very encouraging, since these bubbles are relatively inaccessible once they are in the distal cerebral vascular tree. One investigator observed that an increase in venous pressure and venous engorgement appeared to assist in bubble clearance through capillary beds.[47] This might suggest that nursing in the head-down position and higher levels of PEEP might also be worth exploring in the care of these patients. These techniques, however, would seem to be productive of more cerebral edema.

The data available in patients with preexisting cerebral vascular disease as manifested by carotid bruits, with or without signs and symptoms, would suggest that carotid lesions should be dealt with prior to or at the same time as the cardiac operation. If this has not been done, the weight of evidence would suggest that antiplatelet therapy be started as soon after surgery as possible.

RENAL STATUS

The renal status of the patient should be followed by a routine observation of the hourly urine output and specific gravity and by the daily determination of BUN and creatinine levels. Impairment of renal function may be produced by impaired perfusion and nephrotoxic substances, both of which may be present during cardiopulmonary bypass, and the risk of which increases with its duration.[48] Other risk factors are preexisting disease and the magnitude of the operation, expressed in terms of the manner of cross-clamping, total duration, and hemodynamic results.

The flow rates on bypass and the presence of hemoglobinuria appear to be related to later development of renal failure. The development of the more severe degrees of established renal failure, as might be expected, carries with it a very poor prognosis. A mortality of close to 100 percent is characteristic of cardiovascular patients sick enough to require frequent dialysis.

Attention should therefore be directed at prevention and avoidance rather than treatment of the disorder. General measures should be carried out to maintain a cardiac output with as little depression of renal blood flow as possible, principally by the avoidance of α-adrenergic vasopressors and by the use of vasodilator drugs and the intra-aortic balloon pump. An adequate rate of urine output should be maintained through the judicious administration of fluids and the use of diuretics. The urine should be alkalinized in the presence of large quantities of hemoglobin. Careful surveillance of the urinary electrolytes, osmolality and sediment microscopy in relation to the serum electrolytes, and the use of the urinary-to-serum creatinine ratio may permit more precise assessment of the degree of functional impairment.

Careful attention to fluid balance may reduce the need for dialysis.[49] The anuric patient with a normal water balance who is normothermic requires about 1 percent of body weight per day for insensible loss of water from the skin and airways. This is present to a normal degree while no other loss is present. This figure should be reduced about 50 percent for patients on a ventilator and must be adjusted to take into account the balance resulting from previous treatment. Although the peritoneal route can be used and is very effective for the exchange of water and electrolytes, hemodialysis is usually preferred. The prognosis, although gloomy overall, is, in individual cases, dependent upon the evidence of reversibility of other organ systems and renal dysfunction. The excellence of the general measures for supportive care that have been responsible for much of the recent improvement in the success of open heart surgery will also contribute to recovery in specific disorders such as renal failure.

REFERENCES

1. Priano LL, Ham J: A simple method to increase the inspired oxygen of resuscitator bags. Crit Care Med 6:48,1978
2. Carden E, Friedman D: Further studies of manually operated self-inflating resuscitation bags. Anesth Analg 56:202, 1976
3. Safar P, Grenvik A: Organization and physician education in critical care medicine. Anesthesiology 47:87,1977
4. Pontoppidan H, Wilson RS, Rie MA, et al: Respiratory intensive care. Anesthesiology 47:96, 1977
5. Endresen J. Hill DN: The present state of trend detection and prediction in patient monitoring. Intens Care Med 3:15, 1977
6. Ashcroft JM, Berry JL: The Wythenshawe hospital patient data display system. Intensive Care Med 1:49, 1975
7. Al-Diady W, Skeats SI, Hill DN, et al: The use of transcutaneous oxygen electrodes in intensive therapy. Intensive Care Med 3:35, 1977
8. Symposium: Mass-spectrometry at the bedside. Crit Care Med 4:219-264, 1976
9. Praicash O, Mei JS: Use of mass-spectrometry and infrared CO_2 analysis for bedside measurement of cardiopulmonary function during anesthesia and intensive care. Crit Care Med 5:180, 1977
10. Wilson RS: Monitoring the lung: Mechanics and volume. Anesthesiology 45:135-145, 1976
11. Osborn IJ: Monitoring respiratory function. Crit Care Med 2:217, 1974
12. Day J, Nunn JF, Prys-Roberts C: Factors influencing arterial PO_2 during recovery from anesthesia. Br J Anaesth 40:398, 1968
13. Kelman GR, Nunn JF, Prys-Roberts C, et al: The influence of cardiac output on arterial oxygenation: A theoretical study. Br J Anaesth 39:450, 1957
14. Sykes MK, Arnot RN, Jastrzebski J, et al: Reduction of hypoxic pulmonary vasoconstriction during Trilene anesthesia. J Appl Physiol 39:103, 1975
15. Wilson RS, Sullivan SF, Malm JR, et al: The oxygen cost of breathing following anesthesia in cardiac surgery. Anesthesiology 39:387, 1973

16. Nunn JF: Influence of age and other factors in hypoxemia in the postoperative period. Lancet 2:466, 1965

17. Rehder K. Marsh HM, Rodarte JR, et al: Airway closure. Anesthesiology 47:40, 1977

18. Meyers JR, Lembeck L, O'Kane H, et al: Changes in functional residual capacity of the lung after operation. Arch Surg 110:576, 1975

19. Hewlett AM, Branthwaite MA: Postoperative pulmonary function. Br J Anaesth 47:102, 1975

20. Downs JB, Mitchell LA: Pulmonary effects of ventilatory patterns following cardiopulmonary bypass. Crit Care Med 4:295, 1976

21. Stokke DB: Review: Artificial ventilation with positive end-expiratory pressure (PEEP). Historical background, terminology, and pathophysiology. Intensive Care Med 2:77, 1976

22. Douglas FG, Finlayson DC: Effect of positive end-expiratory pressure on lung mechanics during anesthesia in dogs. Can Anaesth Soc J 24:425, 1977

23. Peters RN, Wellons HA, Howe TM: Total compliance in work of breathing after thoracotomy. J Thorac Cardiovasc Surg 57:348, 1969

24. Kaison KE, Seltzer V, Lee S, et al: Influence of thoracotomy on pulmonary mechanics. Association of increased work of breathing during anesthesia and postoperative pulmonary complications. Ann Surg 162:973, 1965

25. Klineberg PL, Geer RT, Hirsh RA, et al: Early extubation after coronary bypass graft surgery Crit Care Med 5:272, 1977

26. Welch BE, Morgan TE, Clamman HB: Time concentration effects in relationship to oxygen toxicity in man. Fed Proc 22:1053, 1963

27. Pfenninger J, Roth F: Intermittent positive pressure breathing (IPPB) versus incentive spirometry (IS) therapy in the postoperative period. Intensive Care Med 3:279, 1977

28. McGinnis GE, Shively JG, Patterson RL, et al: Engineering analysis of intratracheal tube cuffs. Anesth Analg 50:557, 1971

29. Holley HS, Gilvea JE: Vocal cord paralysis after tracheal intubation. JAMA 215:281, 1971

30. Steward DJ: A disposable condenser-humidifier for use during anesthesia. Canad Anaesth Soc J 23:191, 1976

31. Chamney AR: Humidification requirements and techniques including a review of the performance of the equipment in current use. Anaesthesia 24:602, 1969

32. Bendixen MHH, Egbert LD, Hedley -Whyte J, et al: Respiratory Care. St. Louis, CV Mosby, 1965

33. Pontoppidan H, Geffin B, Lowenstein E: Acute respiratory failure in the adult. Boston, Little, Brown, 1973

34. Zarins CK, Virgilio RW, Smith DE, et al: The effects of vascular volume on positive end-expiratory pressure-induced cardiac output depression and wedge-left atrial pressure discrepancy. J Surg Res 23:348, 1977

35. Pennock JL, Pierce WS, Waldhausen JA: The management of the lungs during cardiopulmonary bypass. Surg Gynecol Obstet 145:917, 1977

36. Modry DL, Chiu CJ, Hinchey EJ: The roles of the ventilation and perfusion in lung metabolism. J Thorac Cardiovasc Surg 74:275, 1977

37. Lindhold CE: Prolonged endotracheal intubation. Acta Anaesthesiol Scand [Suppl] 13: 33, 1969

38. Sanchez MG, Finlayson DC: Dynamics of serum potassium with hyperventilation. Can Anaesth Soc J (in press)

39. Taylor KM, Morton IJ, Brown JJ, et al: Hypertension and the renin-angiotensin system following open-heart surgery. J. Thorac Cardiovasc Surg 74:840, 1977

40. Roberts AJ, Niarchos AP, Subramanian VA, et al: Systemic hypertension associated with coronary artery bypass surgery. J Thorac Cardiovasc Surg 74:846, 1977

41. Kaplan JA, Woodward S, Finlayson DC: Vasodilator therapy after cardiac surgery: A comparison of the efficacy and toxicity of nitroprusside and nitroglycerin. Abstract presented at the American Society of Anesthesiology annual meeting, 1977

42. Gross L, Trembley NA, Davies DW: The toxicity of sodium nitroprusside. Can Anaesth Soc J 23:480, 1976

43. Virgilio RW, Rice CL, Smith DE, et al: Crystalloid versus colloid resuscitation: Is one better? Intensive Care Med 3:113,1977

44. Kones RJ, Phillips JH: Reduction in myocardial infarction size: Prevention of heart cell death. South Med J 69:442, 1976

45. Kones RJ, Phillips JH: Glucose-insulin-potassium (GIK) therapy for ischemic heart disease. Crit Care Med 3:143, 1975

46. Siesjo BK: The influence of respiratory disturbances on acid-base and energy metabolism of the brain. Intensive Care Med 3:245, 1977

47. Use of compression chambers for therapy. Department of the Air Force, 1972

48. Abel RM, Buckley MJ, Austen WL: Etiology, incidence and prognosis of renal failure following cardiac operations. J Thorac Cardiovasc Surg 71:323, 1976

49. Lee HA: The management of acute renal failure following trauma. Br J. Anesth 49:697, 1977

Joel A. Kaplan, M.D.

15
Pericardial Diseases

CARDIAC TAMPONADE

Cardiac tamponade (commonly called pericardial tamponade) can be a true medical emergency when associated with profound cardiovascular collapse. By definition, it is the low-output syndrome caused by *impairment of diastolic filling* of the heart resulting from an unchecked rise in intrapericardial pressure.[1] Fluid accumulates in the closed pericardial space, producing the elevated intrapericardial pressure. The fluid in the pericardial space may be due to chest trauma,[2] postoperative bleeding,[3] perforation of the ventricle by pacemakers[4] or venous pressure catheters,[5] malignant diseases, infections, or chronic renal failure.[6] The incidence of tamponade following cardiac surgery ranges from 3 to 6 percent.

Hemodynamic alterations depend on the *amount of fluid* in the pericardium or mediastinum and the *rapidity* of its accumulation. A liter of fluid may be tolerated if it gradually accumulates, while a few hundred milliliters may produce tamponade if it is rapidly accumulated. Because of the low compliance of the pericardium, the fluid raises intrapericardial pressure, raises ventricular end-diastolic pressure, and impairs diastolic filling of the ventricles. The high ventricular end-diastolic pressure produces early closure of the atrioventricular valves and further reduces ventricular filling volume.[7] The ventricular end-diastolic *volume* is reduced, but ventricular end-systolic volume tends to be normal.[8] This leads to reduced stroke volume, ejection fraction, and cardiac output. Myocardial function is depressed as a result of the decreased preload (end-diastolic volume) and coronary blood flow, which is decreased as a result of arterial hypotension, tachycardia, and high ventricular wall tension.[9] The decreased stroke volume leads to a compensatory tachycardia, vasoconstriction, and increased venous return in an effort by the autonomic nervous system to maintain an adequate cardiac output. These compensatory mechanisms fail when, in the face of a mounting left ventricular end-diastolic pressure, stroke volume falls so greatly that the tachycardia cannot maintain adequate blood pressure and cardiac output. The patient then passes from a period of autonomic compensation to a state of profound cardiovascular collapse.[10] Wechsler showed that there may be three stages of compensation:[11]

1. Compensated hemodynamic obstructive phase—with augmented sympathetic tone and somewhat decreased cardiac output.
2. Intermediate phase—with subendocardial ischemia (as a result of decreased coronary perfusion pressure and a reduced endocar-

dial to epicardial blood flow ratio), and arterial hypotension.

3. Hemodynamic and myocardial decompensation phase—with severe myocardial ischemia, decreased myocardial contractility, and cardiogenic shock.

Diagnosis

Beside suspicion is vital for the accurate diagnosis of cardiac tamponade. The patient may be dyspneic, anxious, diaphoretic, ashen colored or cyanotic, and complaining of chest pain. Beck's triad[12] is frequently present, consisting of (1) neck vein distention, which increases with inspiration (Kussmaul's sign); (2) hypotension with a decreased pulse pressure; and (3) distant muffled heart tones. In addition, a pericardial friction rub may be heard.

The presence of a pulsus paradoxus is an important diagnostic sign of cardiac tamponade. This is an *abnormal* inspiratory fall in the systolic blood pressure. The term is misleading, however, since it is not paradoxical but only an *exaggeration* of a normal physiological phenomenon. Normally, the blood pressure during inspiration is less than 5 mm Hg lower than in expiration. This is due to transmission of intrathoracic pressure and transit time delay of increased right-sided blood volume through the pulmonary circulation to the left side of the heart.[13] Any inspiratory decline of the systolic blood pressure by more than 10 mm Hg is abnormal, and it is frequently over 20 mm Hg in cardiac tamponade. Guntheroth showed that the exaggerated pulsus paradoxus in cardiac tamponade reflects the normal respiratory effects on right ventricular stroke volume delayed by transit through the pulmonary circulation and *exaggerated* by the small *left* ventricular stroke volume in a *vasoconstricted* state.[14] A paradoxical pulse may also occur in patients with chronic obstructive pulmonary disease, obesity, and right-sided heart failure.[15] Massumi recently reported a *paradoxical* pulsus paradoxus that is the reverse of the usual situation—a rise of the blood pressure on inspiration. This may be seen with idiopathic hypertrophic subaortic stenosis, left-sided heart failure with positive pressure ventilation, and isorhythmic ventricular rhythms.[16]

When a blood pressure cuff is used to diagnose a pulsus paradoxus, attention to detail is important. The patient must breathe as normally as possible, since deep breathing will exaggerate the decline. The cuff pressure is gradually decreased while listening for the Korotkoff sounds, which will first be heard only during expiration, and then further decreased until all beats are heard. The difference between where the intermittent sounds and the regular sounds are heard is the paradoxical pulse. Direct arterial pressure monitoring allows this to be determined more easily and accurately. As seen in Figure 15-1, the paradoxical pulse is 24 mm Hg, while by cuff it was heard as only 10–15 mm Hg.

A progressive increase of the central venous pressure (CVP) to a level of over 15 mm Hg may be indicative of tamponade. Weeks demonstrated that a "pressure plateau" may occur with tamponade, in which the right atrial pressure (CVP), pulmonary artery diastolic pressure, and pulmonary capillary wedge pressure (left atrial pressure) all equalize near 20 mm Hg.[17] Other authors feel, however, that the CVP may be a more sensitive monitor to detect tamponade than the Swan-Ganz catheter. Field pointed out that with the development of tamponade, the CVP will increase relatively more from its baseline level than the pulmonary capillary wedge pressure, which starts at a higher level.[18] Occasionally, in the postoperative patient, we have seen tamponade of only the right side of the heart as a result of blood clots over the right ventricle. This has presented as a very high CVP with a normal PCWP. Rittenhouse has demonstrated that jugular venous flow velocity can be measured by a Doppler flowmeter and that it decreased early during cardiac tamponade in dogs.[19] This technique has not yet been reported in patients, but this might be a simple and useful diagnostic tool in the future. The jugular venous waveform also changes in cardiac tamponade (see Chapter 4). The y descent is absent or even transformed into an abnormal positive wave of venous pressure, and no forward flow occurs after the v wave. The a wave also becomes more prominent than the v wave.

The electrocardiogram is usually not very helpful in diagnosing tamponade. It may show reduced QRS and T-wave voltage or elevated ST segments. Simultaneous electrical alternation of atrial and ventricular complexes is rare but, if present, is diagnostic of tamponade. Ven-

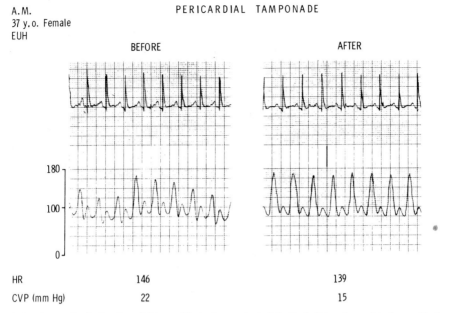

A.M.
37 y.o. Female
EUH

PERICARDIAL TAMPONADE

BEFORE   AFTER

	HR	CVP (mm Hg)
BEFORE	146	22
AFTER	139	15

Fig. 15-1. A paradoxical pulse of 24 mm Hg is demonstrated in the left-hand panel before relieving the pericardial tamponade. In the right-hand panel, after removal of the fluid, the paradoxical pulse has essentially disappeared.

tricular electrical alternans is much more common and less specific, but if marked and persistant, it is strong evidence for tamponade.[20]

The routine chest x-ray usually shows clear lung fields and a normal or enlarged cardiopericardial silhouette in patients with tamponade. Contrast angiocardiography or radioisotope scanning of the chest can be used to confirm the presence of a pericardial effusion.

Echocardiography represents one of the most reliable and clinically useful methods of diagnosing an effusion in the pericardium. This is because the fluid media reflects little or no ultrasonic energy as compared to the solid structures such as the pericardium and heart walls. Diagnosis rests on demonstrating an echo-free space between the pericardium and moving heart (Fig. 15-2).[21]

Treatment

Most patients with tamponade are treated outside the operating room by pericardiocentesis. A small percentage of patients, however, will be rushed to the operating room with a very unstable circulatory system. Intraoperatively,

these patients should be extensively monitored. A 20-gauge Teflon catheter is placed in the radial artery, while a 16-gauge intracath is placed in the internal jugular vein for continuous measurement of blood pressure, pulsus paradoxus, and central venous pressure. In addition, the electrocardiogram, urine output, and blood gases are monitored. These can all be put in place in less than 10 minutes in the operating room. The treatment of cardiac tamponade is divided into two phases: (1) temporary measures and (2) definitive treatment.[22,23]

TEMPORARY MEASURES

Blood Volume Expansion. The blood volume may be expanded by a rapid infusion of a colloid or crystalloid solution in an effort to raise the central venous pressure above 15–20 mm Hg. This will increase the effective filling pressure of the heart and help to oppose the elevated intrapericardial pressure. As the gradient of blood flow between the large veins and atrium is restored, stroke volume and cardiac output should increase. In dogs studied with an induced tamponade, volume expansion has been a very

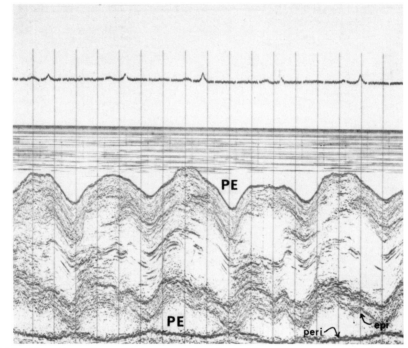

Fig. 15-2. The echocardiogram demonstrates a patient with a severe pericardial effusion (PE) between the epicardium and pericardium. Later, 750 ml of bloody fluid was tapped from this patient's pericardium.

effective method of increasing stroke volume. In one study, 20 ml/kg of whole blood was administered and led to elevations in the central venous pressure, pulmonary artery pressure, left atrial pressure, arterial blood pressure, stroke volume, and cardiac output.[24] Subsequent phlebotomy of the same volume of blood totally reversed the hemodynamic benefit. In another study, smaller volume infusions consisting of 10 ml/kg also effectively increased stroke volume, cardiac output, and blood pressure, and decreased total peripheral resistance.[25]

Inotropic Infusion. Isoproterenol appears to be the most effective temporizing measure until the pericardial fluid is removed. Infusion rates of 0.25–0.5 μg/kg have been used in dogs with tamponade to markedly increase stroke volume, heart rate, and cardiac output while decreasing total peripheral resistance. Fowler compared isoproterenol (0.5 μg/kg) to norepinephrine (0.5 μg/kg) in dogs with cardiac tamponade.[26] Norepinephrine increased peripheral resistance and blood pressure by 20 mm Hg but

had little effect on heart rate, stroke volume, or cardiac output. Isoproterenol increased the heart rate, doubled the stroke volume, and tripled the cardiac output while dropping the total peripheral resistance by 50 percent with an unchanged blood pressure. Triester compared treatment with isoproterenol, volume expansion, and acetylstrophanthanin, a rapid-acting digitalis preparation.[25] Digitalis was the least effective therapy, even though it undoubtedly exerted a positive inotropic effect. This effect was counterbalanced by a large increase in peripheral vascular resistance, and thus in a manner similar to norepinephrine, the stroke volume and cardiac output were not elevated. Isoproterenol was the most effective therapy, elevating cardiac output by 240 percent, while volume expansion increased output by 170 percent. The new inotropic drugs dopamine and dobutamine have not been studied in cardiac tamponade. However, both dopamine at low doses (less than 5 μg/kg/min), and dobutamine, which is primarily a β-adrenergic stimulator, should be effective in increasing cardiac output and decreasing total peripheral resistance in a manner similar to isoproterenol.

Correction of Metabolic Acidosis. Sodium bicarbonate ($NaHCO_3$) is a very useful drug in this situation, since the patients are frequently acidotic secondary to poor peripheral perfusion with a low cardiac output. An arterial blood gas should be checked when the patient is first seen, and any base deficit greater than -5 mEq/liter should be totally corrected. It has been shown that catecholamines (especially epinephrine) are less active in acidotic states, and acidosis may itself depress myocardial function.[27] Fortunately, isoproterenol was the catecholamine least affected by severe acidosis in a study in dogs in which acidosis was induced by hydrochloric acid.[28] Sodium bicarbonate may also have useful hemodynamic effects in patients with tamponade. In volunteers anesthetized with halothane, $NaHCO_3$ increased stroke volume and cardiac output and decreased total peripheral resistance.[29] Oxygen should also be administered to these patients, who frequently have hypoxemia secondary to their low cardiac output. If not absolutely required, positive pressure ventilation is best avoided, however, since it will further decrease venous return and the venoatrial gradient.

DEFINITIVE TREATMENT

The ultimate therapy for cardiac tamponade is drainage of the fluid. Pericardiocentesis is the treatment of choice for the routine management of a patient with nontraumatic tamponade. The preferred technique is via the subxyphoid approach, aiming toward the left shoulder at a 30° angle.[10] The needle position can be monitored electrocardiographically by attaching a V lead with an alligator clip to the needle.[30] Marked ST elevation or premature ventricular contractions indicate contact with the epicardium and mean the needle should be withdrawn a few millimeters. Removal of as little as 25 ml of fluid may lead to dramatic hemodynamic improvement with increased blood pressure and cardiac output and reduced pulsus paradoxus. It is important to remember, however, that failure to obtain fluid by pericardiocentesis does not rule out a pericardial effusion or tamponade.

Surgical intervention (pericardiotomy) is the therapy of choice for tamponade:

1. As a result of trauma, especially for penetrating wounds of the heart and great vessels
2. After cardiac surgery
3. When fluid reaccumulates or cannot be removed by pericardiocentesis.

In many cases, the pericardiocentesis may serve only as a temporizing measure until the surgical procedure can be performed. Skillful surgical exploration entails less risk to the patients than does repeated pericardiocentesis.[31] The surgical approach may be through either the fourth left interspace in an anterolateral thoracotomy, through a subxyphoid window, or through a midline sternotomy in which the lower third is reopened in the postcardiac surgery patient.

Anesthesia for Patients with Cardiac Tamponade

It should be obvious that these patients are at high risk during general anesthesia. Severe hypotension and cardiac arrests have been reported when many types of general anesthesia were administered to patients with tamponade who had impaired cardiac filling and reduced cardiac outputs. All the inhalational anesthetics are known myocardial depressants, and most of them are peripheral vasodilators as well. Administration of these drugs may lead to hypotension, bradycardia, and cardiac arrest in patients with an unrelieved cardiac tamponade. Murray reported 2 patients with cardiac tamponade who were anesthetized with thiopental, nitrous oxide, and halothane, 0.5 percent, in whom severe hypotension occurred.[32] The hypotension was unresponsive to fluids or vasopressors and was only corrected by relieving the tamponade. In both of these patients, positive pressure ventilation also appeared to play a role in producing hypotension. Guntheroth and Morgan have shown that positive pressure ventilation further decreases the venous return to the heart and the subsequent cardiac output.[14,33]

The preferred form of anesthesia for these patients is *local anesthesia* until the tamponade is removed and *then* a general endotracheal anesthesia for exploration of the mediastinum if this is necessary.[34] In most patients, a subxyphoid pericardial window can be created or the lower end of the sternum reopened, using less than 30 ml of 1 percent lidocaine. Through this

incision, the fluid can be partially or totally removed and the hemodynamic situation markedly
improved. If required, a mild degree of sedation
can be provided with fentanyl or ketamine in
subdissociative doses (0.25 mg/kg). Fentanyl appears to be a venoconstrictor and does not reduce venous return, while morphine is a venodilator and will markedly reduce the venoatrial
gradient. We have had excellent results using
ketamine to sedate a number of these patients.
The blood pressure and heart rate usually rise,
and peripheral perfusion appears to improve.
Recently, Mathrubhutham reported a study of
ketamine anesthesia in dogs with cardiac tamponade.[35] Ketamine, administered intravenously
in a dose of 5 mg/kg, increased cardiac output
in dogs with cardiac tamponade who were either
normovolemic, hypervolemic, or hypovolemic.
Cardiac index increased from 1.42 to 2.35 liters/
min/m², while no significant changes occurred
in heart rate, mean arterial pressure, central
venous pressure, pulmonary artery pressure, or
pulmonary capillary wedge pressure.

After the tamponade has been relieved, a
safe induction of anesthesia, including positive
pressure ventilation, can be undertaken if an
exploration of the mediastinum or great vessels
is necessary. We have usually used fentanyl and
diazepam for induction and nitrous oxide, oxygen, pancuronium, and fentanyl for maintenance. Fentanyl and diazepam have been reported to have minimal hemodynamic effects in
patients with pericardial effusion.[36] In chronically ill patients, we have continued with ketamine, nitrous oxide, oxygen, and muscle relaxants.

CHRONIC CONSTRICTIVE PERICARDITIS

Current medical management of acute pericarditis is successful in most cases. There are
a number of patients, however, who develop
recurrent constrictive pericarditis. Causes of
chronic constrictive pericarditis include radiation therapy, neoplasms, uremia, rheumatoid
arthritis, and tuberculosis.[37] This disease is similar to cardiac tamponade in that both impede
diastolic filling and expansion of the ventricles
and equally affect both sides of the heart. Thus,
equalization of the atrial, ventricular diastolic,
and pulmonary artery diastolic pressures occurs
in both disease states. The venous pressure trac-

ing characteristically shows a deep y trough in
constrictive pericarditis. Pulses paradoxus only
occurs in one-third of the patients with constriction, however, while atrial fibrillation and Kussmaul's sign occur commonly in these patients.
The patients frequently present with recurrent
chest pain and/or symptoms of right-sided heart
failure with venous congestion, hepatomegaly,
ascites, and edema. The electrocardiogram is
usually not diagnostic. Low voltage of the QRS
complexes and inversion of the T waves may
occur. Atrial fibrillation or flutter is present in
one-fourth of the patients. The heart on chest x-
ray may be small or large. Calcium in the pericardium is seen in over 50 percent of the cases.

At Emory University Hospital, over 50 peri-
cardectomies have been performed for chronic
pericarditis in recent years. These have been
performed through either a median sternotomy
or a thoracotomy incision. Cardiopulmonary bypass has not been used routinely, but only when
necessary to be able to dissect the pericardium
from the heart. We have been impressed by how
much manipulation these hearts in a "peel" can
stand and still maintain reasonable hemodynamics. Occasionally, it has been necessary to
support the circulation with isoproterenol during
the dissection or to treat ventricular arrhythmias
with lidocaine, but only rarely has bypass been
needed. Atrial arrhythmias are also fairly common, since the sinoatrial node is superficial and
may be affected by the disease process. All peri-
cardectomies have been performed with a
"pump standby" in case difficulties were encountered during the dissection, and the patients
were monitored with direct arterial and venous
pressures. The anesthetic used most often has
been fentanyl and diazepam with nitrous oxide,
oxygen, and pancuronium. Any anesthetic technique that does not markedly decrease venous
return or depress the myocardium can be used,
however.

Hatcher reported 24 of these procedures
done for recurrent pericarditis at Emory.[38]
There were no operative complications, no use
of cardiopulmonary bypass, and no mortality in
this series. Relief of pericardial pain was complete in 84 percent of the patients. The surgical
group from Stanford University has reported a
series of 11 cases of surgical treatment of constrictive pericarditis using cardiopulmonary bypass.[39] They feel that their ability to dissect the
relatively empty heart is improved while on car-

diopulmonary bypass, which facilitates removal of the constricting tissue and shortens the operation. Their operations were performed through a median sternotomy, with cannulation of the right atrium and ascending aorta for bypass. The medium duration of bypass was 60 minutes, and 7 of the 11 patients required inotropic support after bypass. In addition, their median postoperative blood loss was 1201 ml, with a range of 526 to 6780 ml, and 1 patient had to be brought back to the operating room because of bleeding. We believe the use of cardiopulmonary bypass makes this operation more complicated and, therefore, have elected not to use it whenever possible. In the past, the mortality for this operation was stated to be 25 percent and was only recommended when patients were severely disabled. At the present time, with modern monitoring, anesthetic, and surgical techniques, patients can have the operation performed safely at earlier stages of the disease process.

POSTOPERATIVE PERICARDITIS

Postoperative pericarditis frequently begins within 2 to 3 days of a cardiac surgical procedure. It has been reported to occur in 13.7 percent of postoperative patients,[40] but at our hospital it appears to be much more common than this figure. Engle has shown that patients with this syndrome have circulating antiheart antibodies, and thus the disease is thought to have an autoimmune basis.[41]

Typically, in the postoperative period, the patient complains of fever and chills and frequent episodes of chest pain, which are very different from previous anginal attacks. The pain is commonly referred to the neck and sometimes to the back, abdomen, or either arm. It is frequently aggravated by deep breathing and rotation of the chest, while relieved by sitting up and leaning forward. Pericardial friction rubs are present in most of the patients. The postoperative ECG may show ST-segment elevation without reciprocal depression. This is distinguished from acute infarction by the lack of developing Q waves. Many of the patients develop rapid supraventricular tachyarrhythmias, most often atrial fibrillation or flutter. These arrhythmias are frequently difficult to control and poorly tolerated by the patients. Large doses of digoxin and propranolol are administered until the ventricular rate slows to under 100 beats per minute. Rarely has cardioversion been required in the immediate postoperative period. Other medical treatments for pericarditis include aspirin (15 grains q.i.d.), indomethacin (25 mg q.i.d.), and prednisone (20 mg daily for 4 to 6 weeks).

As reported by Berger, some of the patients may develop a delayed postcardiotomy tamponade syndrome.[42] The onset of tamponade is insidious and develops about the fifth or sixth postoperative day. By this time, the patients are out of the intensive care unit and all the monitoring devices have been removed. Berger reported 6 patients who developed this syndrome after valve replacements. The initial complaints were weakness and generalized malaise, gastrointestinal symptoms, and finally, cardiovascular symptoms that progressed to a low-output syndrome and shock before the diagnosis was made. All the patients were taking anticoagulants because of the artificial valve replacements, and this may have contributed to the disease process. Pericardiocentesis was the only necessary treatment and yielded 500–700 ml of bloody fluid, while surgical intervention was not required in any of the 6 patients. Brown has recently reported a syndrome of pericardial tamponade and constriction after coronary revascularization,[43] while Douglas reported cardiac tamponade within 6 to 31 days of surgery in 2.6 percent of patients.[44] Both of these studies emphasize that a mediastinal and pericardial collection of blood is common after cardiac surgery. This can organize and finally fibrose and produce cardiac constriction and tamponade.

REFERENCES

1. Fowler NO: The recognition and management of pericardial disease and its complications. *In* Hurst JW, Logue RB (eds); The Heart (ed 4). New York, McGraw-Hill, 1978, pp 1640–1659

2. Jones EW, Holmsworth J: Penetrating wounds of the heart; Thirty years experience. Arch Surg 96:671–682, 1968

3. Fraser DG, Ullyot DJ: Mediastinal tamponade

after open-heart surgery. J Thorac Cardiovasc Surg 66:629–631, 1973

4. Kalloor GJ: Cardiac tamponade: Report of a case after insertion of a transvenous endocardial electrode. Am Heart J 88:88–89, 1974

5. Lawton RL, Rossy NP, Funk DC: Intracardiac perforation. Arch Surg 98:213–216, 1969

6. Singh S, Newmark K, Ishikawa I, et al: Pericardectomy in uremia: The treatment of choice for cardiac tamponade in chronic renal failure. JAMA 228:1132–1135, 1974.

7. Shabetai R, Fowler NO, Guntheroth WG: The hemodynamics of cardiac tamponade in constrictive pericarditis. Am J Cardiol 26:480–489, 1970

8. Craig RJ, Whalen RE, Behar VS, et al: Pressure and volume changes of the left ventricle in acute pericardial tamponade. Am J Cardiol 22:65–74, 1968

9. O'Rouke RA, Fischer DP, Escobar EE, et al: Effect of acute pericardial tamponade on coronary blood flow. Am J Physiol 213:549–552, 1967

10. Spodick DH: Acute pericardial tamponade, pathologic physiology, diagnosis and management. Prog Cardiovasc Dis 10:64–96, 1967

11. Wechsler AS, Awerbach BJ, Graham TC, et al: Distribution of intramyocardial blood flow during pericardial tamponade. J Thorac Cardiovasc Surg 68:847–856, 1974

12. Beck CA: Two cardiac compression triads. JAMA 104:715, 1935

13. Shabetai R, Fowler NO, Gueron M: The effects of respiration on aortic pressure and flow. Am Heart J 65:525–533, 1963

14. Guntheroth WG, Morgan BC, Mullin S: Effect of respiration on venous return and stroke volume in cardiac tamponade: Mechanism of pulsus paradoxus. Circ Res 20:381–390, 1967

15. Rebuck AS, Pengelly CD: Pulsus paradoxus in the presence of airways obstruction. N Engl J Med 288:66–69, 1973

16. Massumi RA, Mason DT, Vera Z, et al: Reverse pulsus paradoxus. N Engl J Med 289:1272–1275, 1973

17. Weeks KR, Chatterjee K, Block S, et al: Bedside hemodynamic monitoring: Its value in the diagnosis of tamponade complicating cardiac surgery. J Thorac Cardiovas Surg 71:250–252, 1976

18. Field J, Shiroff RA, Zelis RF, et al: Limitations in the use of the pulmonary capillary wedge pressure. Chest 70:451–453, 1976

19. Rittenhouse EA, Barnes RW: Doppler jugular flow velocity to differentiate cardiac tamponade from failure. Arch Surg 11:67–70, 1976

20. Spodick DH: Electrical alternation of the heart: Its relation to the kinetics and physiology of the heart during cardiac tamponade. Am J Cardiol 10:155–165, 1962

21. Gramiak R: Echocardiography. JAMA 229:1099–1101, 1974

22. Stein L, Shubin H, Weil MH: Recognition and management of pericardial tamponade. JAMA 225:503–506, 1973

23. Kaplan JA, Bland JW, Dunbar RW: The perioperative management of pericardial tamponade. South Med J 69:417–419, 1976

24. DeCristofaro D, Liu CK: The hemodynamics of cardiac tamponade and blood volume overload in dogs. Cardiovasc Res 3:292–298, 1969

25. Treister B, Gianelly RE, Cohn KE, et al: The circulatory effects of isoproterenol, acetylstrophanthanin, and volume loading in acute pericardial tamponade. Cardiovasc Res 3:299–305, 1969

26. Fowler NO, Holmes JC: Hemodynamic effects of isoproterenol and norepinephrine in acute cardiac tamponade. J Clin Invest 48:502–507, 1969

27. Darby H: Effects of metabolic acidosis on ventricular function and response to epinephrine and norepinephrine. Circ Res 8:1242–1250, 1960

28. Kaplan JA: Hemodynamic effects of metabolic acidosis and alkalosis on positive inotropic agents. Abstract presented at the American Society of Anesthesiologists annual meeting, 1977

29. Kaplan JA, Bush GL, Lecky JH, et al: Effects of sodium bicarbonate on systemic hemodynamics on halothane anesthetized volunteers. Anesthesiology 42:550–559, 1975

30. Bishop LH, Estes EH, McIntosh HD: The electrocardiogram as a safeguard in pericardiocentesis. JAMA 162:264–265, 1956

31. Boyd TF, Strieder JW: Immediate surgery for traumatic heart disease. J Thorac Cardiovasc Surg 50:305–315, 1965

32. Murray BRP, Robertson DS: Anaesthesia for mitral valvotomy complicated by hypotension due to pericardial effusion. Br J Anaesth 36:256–258, 1964

33. Morgan BC, Guntheroth WG, Dillard DH: Relationship of pericardial to pleural pressure during quiet respiration and cardiac tamponade. Circ Res 16:493–498, 1965

34. Stanley TH, Weidaur HE: Anesthesia for the patient with cardiac tamponade. Anesth Analg 52:110–114, 1973

35. Mathrubhutham M, Rao TLK, Shanmugham M, et al: Hemodynamic effects of ketamine in cardiac tamponade dog model with normovolemia, hypervolemia, and hypovolemia. Abstract presented at the American Society of Anesthesiologists annual meeting, 1977

36. Konchigeri HN, Levitsky S: Anesthetic considerations for pericardiectomy in uremic pericardial effusion. Anesth Analg 55:378–382, 1976

37. Hancock EW: Constrictive pericarditis: Clinical clues to diagnosis. JAMA 232:176–177, 1975

38. Hatcher CR, Logue RB, Logan WD, et al: Peri-cardiectomy for recurrent pericarditis. J Thorac Cardiovasc Surg 62:371–378, 1971

39. Copeland JG, Stinson, EB, Griepp RB, et al: Surgical treatment of chronic constrictive peri-carditis using cardiopulmonary bypass. J Thorac Cardiovasc Surg 69:235–238, 1975

40. Keith TA, Fowler NO, Helmsworth JA, et al: The course of surgically modified mitral stenosis. Am J Med 34:308–319, 1963

41. Engle MA, Zabrickie JS, Senterfit ZB, et al: Postpericardiotomy syndrome. A new look at an old condition. Mod Concepts Cardiovasc Dis 44:59–64, 1975

42. Berger RL, Loveless G, Warner O: Delayed and latent postcardiotomy tamponade. Ann Thorac Surg 12:22–28, 1971

43. Brown DF, Older T: Pericardial constriction as a late complication of coronary bypass surgery. J Thorac Cardiovasc Surg 74:61–64, 1977

44. Douglas JS, King SB, Hatcher CR, et al: Late cardiac tamponade after open heart surgery: A problem of differential diagnosis, abstract ed. Am J Cardiol 35:132, 1975

John T. Bonner, M.D.

16
Cardiopulmonary Resuscitation

Competence in the skills and knowledge of resuscitation is demanded in the practice of anesthesia for cardiovascular surgery. Although modern methods of gathering data pertinent to physiological variables allow early detection of deterioration, the situation still arises in which circulation cannot be maintained by pharmacologic or other techniques, and then the therapy known as cardiopulmonary resuscitation (CPR) is used.

CPR has been described in a form currently taught to physicians and nonphysicians.[1] It includes techniques of artificial ventilation, artificial circulation, and drug therapy that are the result of national conferences featuring participation from several medical disciplines. Further training, supported by the American Heart Association and other organizations, has taken the form of advanced life support described by Carveth, Burnap, and others.[2] Some of the material in this chapter is borrowed, with permission, from this program.

In the situation of circulatory collapse, immediate measures must be taken to restore circulation of oxygenated blood to vital organs. Irreversible central nervous system damage probably occurs after 4 minutes of total cessation of circulation at normal body temperature. The therapeutic goals of *basic life support* are establishment of a patent airway (A: Airway); artificial ventilation of the apneic victim (B: Breathing); and provision of artificial circulation (C: Circulation) by external cardiac compression (and possibly internal cardiac compression).

The ABCs of basic life support are taught to the public by community organizations using mannequin simulation. Such an approach deals effectively with mouth-to-mouth (or mouth-to-nose-and-mouth) artificial ventilation, sternal compression, and immediate problem solving, but it cannot deal entirely with the hospital setting of cardiac arrest. The victim may be intubated, in bed, and connected to many wires and tubes. Performance of proper sternal compression, for example, is entirely different in a patient who is lying in a soft bed than in a mannequin lying on a floor. The essentials of basic life support must be satisfied, however, and will be reviewed in this chapter. Also, limitations and commonly encountered deviations from the accepted standards will be discussed.

In the approach to a victim of an *unwitnessed* cardiac arrest, the diagnosis of unresponsiveness is made by a "shake and shout" maneuver. This would not be appropriate for an anesthetized patient in whom the diagnosis of cardiac arrest would be made by loss of palpable pulse, change in audible cardiac sounds, arterial pressure, or skin color. Therefore, consideration of the unwitnessed cardiac arrest would not be indicated for the properly monitored cardiac surgery patient. Another questionable maneuver taught in mannequin practice of basic life support is the chest thump applied to the unresponsive victim of a witnessed cardiac arrest. In our opinion, the chest thump should *not* be included in resuscitative measures in postoperative patients unless ventricular tachycardia is likely. The usefulness of the chest thump seems to be limited to the well-oxygenated heart with ventricular tachycardia.[3] It should be emphasized that the chest thump does not circulate blood but creates a small electrical current that may cardiovert a relatively healthy heart from ventricular tachycardia.[4] We have observed a similar phenomenon when the surgeon physically taps the exposed heart in ventricular tachycardia.

BASIC LIFE SUPPORT

Airway Establishment

It is not appropriate in this discussion to consider in detail a skill so essential and commonly practiced in anesthesiology. Several points might be mentioned, however, which should be considered in airway management in the setting of cardiac arrest.

Initially, backwards (posterior) head tilt is employed to open a victim's airway. This maneuver must often be combined with a jaw lift maneuver if the nonintubated patient has central nervous system depression sufficient to cause loss of tone in the temporalis muscle, with a relaxed lower jaw.[5]

Frequently, an endotracheal tube will have already been placed if circulatory collapse has occurred in the setting of cardiac anesthesia. Patency and proper positioning of the tube cannot be assumed, particularly in the pediatric patient. "Sudden" obstruction of the small endotracheal tube can occur if blood within its lumen becomes clotted or if secretions dry. Unintentional extubation, endobronchial intubation, and kinking of the endotracheal tube are all airway accidents to be excluded by physical examination of the chest or inspection of the upper airway. Blind palpation for the presence of the endotracheal tube cuff in the oropharynx can quickly diagnose accidental extubation. Assurance of a patent airway remains the *initial* ob-

ligation of resuscitation. This obligation can usually be fulfilled within seconds but should not be excluded or assumed to have been satisfied by simple presence of an endotracheal tube protruding from the patient's mouth or nose.

Breathing

Attention is paid to adequate ventilation before any attempt is made to diagnose the absence of a pulse in a victim who has collapsed or suffered some change in consciousness.

This sequence is appropriate in providing basic cardiac life support, since so many airway accidents with impairment of ventilation can eventually result in cardiac arrest. Soft tissue airway obstruction in the unconscious victim without airway support is common and results in inadequate ventilation, even in the presence of the victim's spontaneous ventilatory efforts.[6] Proper airway management, including the use of an endotracheal tube, should minimize the problem of soft tissue airway obstruction in the setting of cardiac anesthesia.

The presence of adequate ventilation is a more difficult diagnosis to make. The American Heart Association's recommended method of listening, looking, and feeling for exhaled gas to establish apnea may not be appropriate in the morphinized patient, who may be breathing three to four times a minute, with a 15-second pause between each breath. The monitored surgical patient who has circulatory collapse demands attention to support of circulation that does not allow the luxury of a 15-second pause in resuscitative efforts to diagnose presence or absence of ventilation. Therefore, ventilation should be guaranteed by artificial positive pressure methods while listening to breath sounds and observing the chest wall for symmetrical and definite movement. Four or five breaths with as close to 100 percent oxygen as possible should satisfy the second requirement of resuscitation, that of adequate ventilation.

Hyperventilation during the initial phases of resuscitation is appropriate. A respiratory alkalosis can partially compensate for a metabolic acidosis, but chronic hyperventilation and alkalemia should be avoided. Circulatory depression associated with controlled ventilation, shift of the oxyhemoglobin dissociation curve, decreases in cerebral blood flow, decreases in ionized calcium, increased oxygen consumption, and blunted ventilatory drive are consequences of alkalosis that should be avoided after initial resuscitation is accomplished.[7,8]

Circulation

Artificial circulation is provided to the pulseless victim by either closed or open chest cardiac compression. The potential damage of closed chest cardiac compression in the patient who has recently undergone thoracotomy or sternotomy is probably greater than in the patient who has not been subject to cardiac surgical intervention. We know of no data to indicate that properly performed sternal compression after a recent sternotomy gives a cardiac output that compares favorably with compression of the intact sternum. However, the time required to reopen a sternotomy wound must be balanced against the immediate restoration of some circulation by artificial means and avoiding further deterioration in the pulseless patient.

The diagnosis of absent circulation, then, is critical. The common error of the too-rapid pulse check is to be avoided. At least 5 and preferably 10 seconds should be spent palpating a proximal, easily accessible pulse. The carotid artery at its bifurcation immediately in front of the sternocleidomastoid muscle at the level of the thyroid cartilage is a satisfactory pulse to seek, as is the femoral artery at the inguinal ligament. The diagnosis of an absent pulse is made *after* the airway is established and after several large-volume breaths are provided the victim of cardiovascular collapse.

Closed chest cardiac compression is accomplished by pressure from the heel of the hand in the midline, two fingerbreadths cephalad to the xiphoid process. In the adult, enough force is exerted on this point to depress the sternum 1½ to 2 inches, with the victim supine. Compression is done at 80 per minute (one rescuer) and 60 per minute (two rescuers). A firm support or board should be placed behind the victim. The ratio of downstroke to upstroke should be approximately equal. Studies in animals and humans suggest that rapid thrusting is to be avoided and that a downstroke time of about 50 percent of the compression cycle is desirable. [9–11] The optimum technique of cardiac compression, as we currently understand it, provides only a fraction of the normal cardiac output. The mechanism by which circulation is supported by ster-

nal compression may not be as simple as it seems, since other maneuvers such as coughing have seemed to aid in circulatory support.[12] Until further data become available, however, attention should be paid to the proper performance of cardiac compression as taught in currently accepted standards. The standards dictate proper hand placement, force of compression, downstroke-to-upstroke ratio, rate, and avoidance of pauses in compression longer than 5 seconds in the pulseless victim.

Open chest cardiac compression is probably indicated if properly performed closed chest massage results in inadequate circulation with no evidence of pulses, and deterioration of the acid–base status.

Again, the inclusion of the chest thump in resuscitative measures is controversial. The chest thump has proved effective in the patient with documented ventricular tachycardia whose myocardium is oxygenated and not acidotic.[3,4] We feel that it has no place in prolonged resuscitation efforts and detracts from more appropriate support of circulation in the pulseless victim.

ADVANCED LIFE SUPPORT

After the ABCs of basic life support have been satisfied, attention is then turned to specific pharmacologic intervention for the treatment of acidemia and arrhythmias.

Drugs

Of the drugs available for use in cardiac arrest, three are almost always used and constitute the mainstay of therapy. These are oxygen, sodium bicarbonate, and epinephrine. Other essential drugs are atropine, lidocaine, morphine, and calcium chloride. This group of agents is classified as "essential drugs" in the American Heart Association's Advanced Life Support Course (Table 16–1).[13] Other useful treatments during CPR are shown in Table 16–2.

OXYGEN

Ventilation of the victim of cardiovascular collapse should be accomplished using as close to 100 percent oxygen as possible. No danger of oxygen toxicity exists for the minutes to hours required to resuscitate and stablize the adult

Table 16-1
Summary of Essential Drugs

	Indication	Dose (I.V.)		Remarks
		Adult	Child	
Oxygen	Cardiac arrest	100%	100%	Modify self-inflating bag to give highest percentage oxygen.
Epinephrine	Absent pulse	0.5–1 mg	10 µg/kg	Give I.V. or intratracheal, not intracardiac.
Sodium bicarbonate	1–2 min after absent pulse	1 mEq/kg initial dose	1 mEq/kg initial dose	Repeat one-half initial dose in 10 min or get blood gas. Do not mix epinephrine or calcium. Give I.V. only.
Atropine	Bradycardia and hypotension	0.5–1 mg	0.03 mg/kg	Reassess ventilation and oxygenation, since hypoxia causes bradycardia.
Lidocaine	Myocardial ectopy and ischemia	1 mg/kg	0.5 mg/kg	Follow bolus with continuous infusion. Watch for CNS toxicity. Lower dose if liver dysfunction or CHF.
Morphine	Pain or pulmonary edema	1–5 mg titrated	Titrate up to 0.15 mg/kg	Do not give I.M.
Calcium chloride	Electromechanical dissociation or asystole	250–500 mg bolus	10–20 mg/kg	Watch Q-T interval. Watch for bradycardia.

Table 16-2
Summary of Useful Modalities

Drug or Therapy	Action	Adult Dose	Remarks
Levarterenol (norepinephrine)	Vasoconstriction Positive inotropic	Drip 4–16 μg/min (8 mg/500 ml = 16 μg/ml)	Causes renal and mesenteric vasoconstriction.
Isoproterenol (Isuprel)	Positive inotropic and chronotropic (β-adrenergic agonist)	Drip 2–10 μg/min (2 mg/500 ml = 4 μg/ml)	May increase myocardial oxygen consumption disproportionate to supply.
Dopamine (Intropin)	α- and β-adrenergic Dopaminergic	Low: 1–5 μg/kg/min Medium: 5–20 μg/kg/min High: more than 20 μg/kg/min	Does not compromise renal circulation at low doses. High doses cause more vasoconstriction.
Propranolol (Inderal)	β-adrenergic blocker (competitive for agonist)	0.25–1 mg I.V. increments	May potentiate bronchial smooth muscle constriction and myocardial depression.
Methylprednisolone (Solumedrol) or Dexamethasone (Decadron)	Questionable	Up to 30 mg/kg Up to12–20 mg q. 6 hr or 60–100 mg I.V.	May stabilize subcellular membranes. Used in cerebral edema (dexamethasone) and pulmonary dysfunction (methylprednisolone).
Defibrillation (Countershock)	Myocardial depolarization	3.5–6 w/sec/kg (400 w/sec in average-sized adult)	Useful for ventricular tachycardia, fibrillation. Synchronized cardioversion for symptomatic atrial tachyarrhythmias
Intra-aortic balloon counterpulsation	Augment coronary filling and aortic flow; while decreasing preload and afterload	1:1 mode	Used in cardiogenic shock.

505

victim. Decreased cardiac output, even when cardiac compression is properly performed, results in mixed venous and arterial blood desaturation. The resulting hypoxemia is augmented by abnormalities in ventilation-perfusion relationships within the lung. High inspired concentrations of oxygen can minimize shunting as a result of ventilation-perfusion imbalance. A change in the inspired concentration of oxygen can itself affect the ventilation-perfusion relationship within the lung, but it should be emphasized that in an arrest situation, as close to 100 percent inspired concentration of oxygen as possible should be used for ventilation.[14] Concern for altering ventilatory drive or oxygen toxicity is appropriate only for long-term ventilatory support and not for the acute resuscitation.

Self-inflating bags must be modified to give more than 40 to 60 percent oxygen. A reservoir should be added to the oxygen inlet to increase the oxygen percentage of a self-inflating bag.

SODIUM BICARBONATE (NaHCO$_3$)

After effective ventilation with oxygen is accomplished, chemical buffering of the acidemia present in an arrest situation should then be considered. An empirical dose of about 1 mEq/kg of sodium bicarbonate can be given to any patient who has had circulatory collapse. Subsequent doses of buffer may be given intravenously either on the basis of "base deficit" calculated from arterial Pco$_2$ and pH, or on a time basis of 44 mEq in adults every 10 minutes of artificial circulatory support. The cardiac responsiveness to catecholamines is diminished in the presence of acidemia.[13] Potential hazards of buffer administration are volume overload, sodium overload, and severe metabolic alkalosis. Increased osmolarity and arterial Pco$_2$ have been noted in dogs and in patients in whom empirical buffering with sodium bicarbonate was used.[15,16] Inactivation or precipitation of catecholamines or calcium salts will result if they are added to sodium bicarbonate. The relatively large volume of drug administered prevents the use of any but the intravenous route of administration. In our experience, the intratracheal route of bicarbonate administration finds little use except perhaps in the setting of massive, acid pulmonary aspiration.

Tromethamine (THAM) has potential advantages for the buffering of acidemia, since no sodium load is given with the drug. In practice,

however, NaHCO$_3$ remains the agent that is the most useful.[17]

EPINEPHRINE

The cardiovascular effects of epinephrine are dose-related and include the following: increased myocardial contractility, increased heart rate, increased arterial blood pressure and systemic peripheral resistance, increased myocardial oxygen consumption, and increased automaticity.[13,18] Both α- and β-adrenergic receptors are stimulated by this sympathomimetic-amine. Small doses produce primarily a β effect, which may result in a lower blood pressure. In the large doses used during resuscitation, epinephrine elevates the perfusion pressure of the coronary circulation and redistributes blood centrally, away from muscle and skin. Long-term use results in a detrimental effect on the renal circulation. Epinephrine may also be used in asystole (to stimulate spontaneous contraction) and in "fine," low-amplitude ventricular fibrillation in an attempt to convert the fibrillation to a coarse pattern that is more favorable to electrical cardioversion. The doses and volumes of epinephrine given make it feasible to administer it intratracheally (down an endotracheal tube) as well as in a peripheral or centrally placed venous line. The old practice of percutaneous intracardiac injection of epinephrine is to be *strongly discouraged* because of the consequences of complications from this technique. These complications include myocardial and coronary vascular laceration and intramyocardial injection, which may produce intractable fibrillation, an especially hazardous complication.

Epinephrine is frequently diluted from a 1:1000 solution (1 mg/ml) to a 1:10,000 concentration. In adults, 0.5–1 mg is a reasonable dose to be employed intravenously during a resuscitation; this dose may be repeated in 5 to 10 minutes.

In patients with an intact circulation, 2–4 μg (2/1000 or 4/1000 the dose used in resuscitation) will produce a noticeable response of heart rate and contractility if given intravenously. Continuous infusions of epinephrine are employed in a concentration of 8 μg/ml, and the infusion rate (2–16 μg/min) is adjusted according to response of blood pressure, heart rate, and contractility. For resuscitation from complete circulatory collapse in infants and children, a 1:10,000 solution is prepared (0.10 mg/ml), and 0.10 ml (10μg) per kilogram of body weight given intravenously.[1,19]

OTHER ESSENTIAL DRUGS

Atropine. The parasympatholytic actions of atropine block vagal effects on the sinoatrial node and other portions of the conduction system, increasing heart rate.[13]

As with epinephrine, the cardiovascular effects of atropine are dose-related. Very small doses of atropine may enhance vagal effects and result in bradycardia. Heart rate (as well as blood pressure) must be balanced against myocardial oxygen consumption in treatment of bradycardias. Atropine is useful in the patient with hypotension associated with bradycardia. Escape ectopy in the setting of bradycardia is another indication for the use of atropine. Doses used in resuscitation of the adult are 0.5-2 mg, given intravenously. Ventricular arrhythmias have been noted to occur after the intravenous administration of atropine.[13,20]

The bradycardia that occurs in resuscitation frequently responds to effective ventilation and oxygenation of the patient. One axiom pertinent to the pharmacology of resuscitation should be remembered: "Think of oxygen if you think of atropine."[21] Atropine may be used in a dose of 0.03 mg/kg in children and infants, supplied as 0.4 mg/ml.[19] This would be about 0.10 ml/kg body weight.

Lidocaine. Lidocaine is an amide local anesthetic used to suppress ventricular dysrhythmias. Ectopic activity in the setting of myocardial ischemia has the potential to deteriorate into ventricular tachycardia or ventricular fibrillation. Lidocaine tends to prevent this deterioration by affecting the rate of phase 4 spontaneous depolarization, affecting excitability of Purkinje fibers, and elevating the fibrillation threshold.[13,22]

Therapeutic blood levels of lidocaine for suppression of ectopic activity are about 2-5 μg/ml. Higher doses approach the blood level associated with CNS stimulation, including generalized seizures. A bolus dose of 1 mg/kg should be followed by a continuous infusion of 20-50 μg/kg/min, or about 1-4 mg/min in the adult. Early CNS toxicity is manifested by slurring of speech, dysphoria, tinnitus, and tremulousness. In doses therapeutic for arrhythmias, ventricular contractility is not significantly af-

fected. Alone, in moderate doses, lidocaine may slightly increase blood pressure. Total intravenous bolus doses should not exceed 200 mg in the adult in the absence of drugs suppressing seizure activity such as diazepam or a barbiturate. Circulatory depression with prolonged QRS complexes and decreased contractility results after excessive doses.[13] Since lidocaine biodegradation is accomplished in the liver, reduced doses should be given if liver dysfunction is present. Liver dysfunction may be associated with congestive heart failure.

Morphine. The indications for the use of morphine in a cardiac emergency are pain and pulmonary edema. Its favorable effects on total body oxygen consumption in the anxious patient, peripheral pooling of blood in dilated venous capacitance vessels, and other poorly defined effects on the pulmonary circulation effect an improvement in the patient who is in overt congestive failure with pulmonary edema. The potential for bronchoconstriction mediated by histamine release is probably more theoretical than real in humans.[23]

No reduction in myocardial contractility occurs with therapeutic doses, and any blood pressure drop associated with small doses is due to arterial and venous dilation.

Bolus doses should always be given intravenously, since absorption from muscle and skin is erratic in the patient with compromised circulation. From 1 to 5 mg is given intravenously to the patient with pain or pulmonary edema. Drops in blood pressure and respiratory rate should be the limiting factors to dosage. Expiratory abdominal muscle rigidity is often associated with the slow ventilatory rate resulting from the administration of morphine.

Calcium Chloride. The complex cardiovascular effects of calcium may be summarized by considering the calcium ion as having positive inotropic activity. The calcium ion is necessary for normal cardiac muscle contraction, and potentiates contractility in a dose-related manner.

Electrical activity can theoretically be restored in cases of true electrical standstill.[1] Calcium enhances ventricular excitability and may potentiate digitalis toxicity, as well as producing bradycardia after rapid administration. When used to increase myocardial contractility, calcium chloride is the preferred preparation, having more ionized calcium than the gluconate or gluceptate forms. Calcium chloride is given intravenously in 250–500 mg bolus doses of the 10 percent solution (100 mg/ml). A maximum dose has been suggested of 100 mg/5 kg, or about 1.5 gm in the adult.[1] In our experience, this dose has been successfully exceeded when withdrawing patients from extracorporeal circulation. Shortening of the Q-T interval and increasing

direct arterial pressure upstroke are noticeable manifestations of the cardiovascular effects of calcium.

Useful Modalities

The indications, actions, and doses of the other useful therapeutic interventions during a cardiopulmonary resuscitation are summarized in Table 16-2.

REFERENCES

1. Gordon AS: Standards for cardiopulmonary resuscitation (CPR) and emergency cardiac care (ECC). JAMA [Suppl.] 227:833–868, 1974
2. Carveth SW, Burnap TK, Bechtel J, et al: Training in advanced cardiac life support. JAMA 235:2311–2315, 1976
3. Yakaitis RW, Redding JS: Precordial thumping during cardiac resuscitation. Crit Care Med 1:22–26, 1973
4. Pennington JE, Taylor J, Lown B: Chest thump for reverting ventricular tachycardia. N Engl J Med 283:1192–1195, 1970
5. Guildner CW: Resuscitation—opening the airway. J Am Coll Emerg Physicians 5:558–590, 1976
6. Safar P, Escarraga LA, Chang F: Upper airway obstruction in the unconscious patient. J Appl Physiol 14:760–764, 1959
7. Stone DJ: Respiration in man during metabolic alkalosis. J Appl Physiol 17:33–37, 1962
8. Khambatta JH, Sullivan S: Effects of respiratory alkalosis on oxygen consumption and oxygenation. Anesthesiology 38:53–57, 1973
9. Birch LH, Kener LJ, Doornbos F, et al: A study of external cardiac compression. J Mich Med Soc 61:1346–1352, 1962
10. Taylor GJ, Tucker WM, Green HL, et al: Importance of prolonged compression during cardiopulmonary resuscitation in man. N Engl J Med 296:1515–1517, 1977
11. Del Guercio LRM, Coomaraswamy RP, State D: Cardiac output and other hemodynamic variables during external cardiac massage in man. N Engl J Med 269:1398–1403, 1963
12. Criley JM, Blaufuss AH, Kissel GL: Cough induced cardiac compression. JAMA 236:1246–1249, 1976
13. Advanced Cardiac Life Support. American Heart Association, 1975
14. West JB: Ventilation-perfusion relationship. Am Rev Respir Dis 116:919–943, 1977
15. Bishop RL. Weisfeldt ML: Sodium bicarbonate administration during cardiac arrest. JAMA 235:506–515, 1976
16. Mattar JA, Weil MH, Shubin H, et al: Cardiac arrest in the critically ill. (II) Hyperosmolar states following cardiac arrest. Am J Med 56:162–168, 1974
17. Bleich HL, Schwartz WB: Tris buffer (THAM). An appraisal of its physiologic effects and clinical usefulness. N Engl J Med 274:782–786, 1966
18. Lappas D, Powell WM, Daggett WM: Cardiac dysfunction in the perioperative period: pathophysiology, diagnosis, and treatment. Anesthesiology 47:117–137, 1977
19. Gregory G: Resuscitation of the newborn. Anesthesiology 43:225–237, 1975
20. Massumi RA, Mason DT, Amsterdam EA: Ventricular fibrillation and tachycardia after intravenous atropine for treatment of bradycardia. N Engl J Med 287:336–338, 1972
21. Stone JG: Personal communication, 1976
22. Collingsworth KR, Kalman SM, Harrison DC: The clinical pharmacology of lidocaine as an antiarrhythmic drug. Circulation 50:1217–1230, 1974
23. Goodman LS, Gilman A: The Pharmacological Basis of Therapeutics (ed 4). Toronto, Macmillan, 1970, p 247

Index

Abdominal left ventricular assist device (ALVAD), 466
Acetaminophen, 190, 317
Acetylcholine, 27, 211
Acetylsalicylic acid (ASA), 428, 430
Acetylstrophanthanin, 494
Acid-citrate-dextrose (ACD), 416
Acidemia, 506
  with CPR, 503
Acidosis, 41, 212, 286, 288, 324, 332, 334, 384
  and CPB, 310, 423
  and hypothermia, 302
  and IABP, 442, 450, 465
  metabolic, correction of, 60
  and perfusion, 304
  postoperative, 317, 318
  and renal disease, 188
  and tamponade, 495
Aciduria, 416
Acrocyanosis, 286. See also Cyanosis
Activated clotting time (ACT) 305–306, 307, 315, 319
  and CPB, 422, 427
  and heparin, 428, 429
  monitoring of, 334, 335
Acute tubular necrosis (ATN), 189
Acyanotic shunt, 330
Adenosine diphosphate (ADP) release, 416
Adenosine 3',5'-cyclic monophosphate. See Cyclic AMP
Adrenal medulla, 8
  and halothane, 10
  output increase, 13
Adrenalin, adrenaline. See Epinephrine
Adrenergic blocking drugs, 11

Adrenergic nerve endings, 10, 13, 25
Adrenergic receptors, 22, 39
  alpha, 12, 18, 43, 44, 46, 47, 51, 134, 178, 201, 212, 220, 262, 271, 423
  beta, 11, 41, 42, 43, 46, 47, 60, 62, 178, 182, 201
  and halothane, 8
  primary groups of, 40
Adrenergic stimulation, 104
Adult-onset diabetes mellitus (AODM). See Diabetes mellitus
Afterload, 101, 256, 317, 486. See also Impedence
  and congenital heart disease, 380
  and counterpulsation, 441
  and CPB, 270, 432
  defined, 199
  and IABP, 442, 459
  and pacemakers, 352
  reduction of, 267, 328
  in ventricular function, 99
A-H interval and heart block, 145, 147
Air embolism
  and CVP monitoring, 85
  enlargement of, 7
Akinesia
  and catheterization, 176
  and stenosis, mitral 209
Albumin, 104, 192
  and CPB, 410, 411, 423
  and liver disease, 191
Aldosterone, 177, 412
Alkalosis, 59, 108, 184, 506
  and CPB, 384, 405, 424, 425, 430, 476, 484
  and extubation, 478

and hypotension, 487
and hypothermia, 413
Allen's test, 72, 77, 258, 290
Alpha, adrenergic receptors. See Adrenergic receptors
Alpha, adrenergic vasopressors, 404, 423
Alpha, methyldopa, 12
Alphaprodine, 20
American Heart Association, 145, 248, 501, 502
  Advance Life Support Course, 503
American Pacemaker Bifocal Pacer, 362
American Society of Anesthesiologists, Physical Status Scoring System, 381
Aminoglycocides, 188
Aminophylline, 10, 47, 182
Amnesia, 5
  and anticholinergics, 53
  and diazepam, 144
  and drugs, 383, 385
  and ketamine, 25
  and lorazepam, 18
  and narcotics, 19
  and nitrous oxide, 266
Analgesia
  as anesthetic objective, 3
  and drugs, 385
  and ketamine, 25
Anectine, 27. See also Succinylcholine
Anemia, 486
  and hypotension, 487
  intraoperative, 108
  and ischemia, 275
  and oxygen, 243
  and stenosis, mitral, 207

Anesthesia Consultation Form, items
        on, 333
Anesthesia protocol, checklist,
        335–336
Anesthetizing barbiturate
        concentration (ABC), 261
Aneurysm, 369, 376
    aortic, 226
    thoracic
        classification, 370
        dissection types, 370–372
        etiology-pathogenesis, 369
        and IABP, 451
        management principles, 372–374
        surgical technique, 370
    ventricular, 173, 174
Aneurysmectomy, ventricular, 457
angina, 6, 46, 132, 170–171, 206,
        214, 224, 227, 233, 243–245,
        253, 274, 377, 380, 383
    and beta-blocking drugs, 11
    decubitis, 245
    drug treatment, 253–254
    and IABP, 455, 456
    management of, 51
    and MVO₂, 108
    nocturnal, 381
    and oxygen, 251
    preinfarction, 451, 457
    and RPP, 246
    stable/unstable, 244, 246
    and stenosis, aortic, 222, 225
    types of, 244
    unstable, 252, 253
Angina pectoris. See Angina
Angiography, 6, 101, 178, 370, 455,
        493
Angiotensin, 44–45, 229
    and blood pressure, 177, 178
    effects of, 212
    formation of, 192
    and MR, 217
    and stenosis, mitral, 210
Anileridine (Leritine), 20
antiarrhythmic drugs, 61–64, 142
    choice of 62–64
    mechanisms of, 62
Anticholinergics, 9, 52–54
Anticoagulation, 171, 305-307, 315,
        319, 334-335, 422, 427-429
    and bypass, 307
    reversal of, 315
Anticonvulsants, 317
Antidiabetic drugs, metabolism of,
        186
Antidiuretic hormone (ADH), 189
Antihistamines and hypotension, 21,
        26

Antihypertensives, 12, 169, 171, 179
Anuria, 303
Anxiety, 243
    and catecholamines, 171
    and drugs, 18
    and embolism, 388
    and heart failure in children, 285
    and myocardial stimulation, 17
    and premature ventricular beats,
        381, 383
    preoperative, 192–193, 242
    and stenosis, valvular, 202
Aorta, 118, 374, 375. See also Aortic
        valve
    anastomosis of, 483
    and aneurysms, 369, 370
    cannulation of, 481, 488
    coarctation of, 281, 284, 294, 328,
        394
    in CPB, 311, 399, 419, 420, 424
    cross-clamping of, 372
    dissection, 463
    IABP in, 443, 444, 452, 463
    and vascular disease, 379
Aortic cannula, 268
Aortic pressure, 72, 74, 76, 101, 103,
        105, 107, 197, 198, 202, 203
Aortic pulse contour analysis, 98
Aortic regurgitation (AR), 205, 222,
        226–232
    acute, 227–228
    anesthetic considerations, 231–232
    and AVR, 235
    chronic, 204, 228–229
    and LV, 208
    and MR, 220
    pathophysiology of, 227–231
Aortic stenosis (AS), 200, 202–204,
        206, 210, 211, 214, 220–226,
        229, 284, 324, 328
Aortic valve. See also Aorta; Aortic
        pressure; Aortic regurgitation
    area of (AVA), 221, 222, 227
    artificial, 283
    and bypass, 311, 314
    and catheterization, 176
    disease of, 21, 85, 273, 328, 380
    insufficiency, 22
    replacement of (AVR), 225,
        230–231
Aorticopulmonary window, 283, 284,
        310
Aortocoronary bypass surgery, 42,
        206, 241–242, 393-440
Aortography, 252
Aramine, 44, 45. See also
        Metarminol
Arfonad, 46. See also Trimethaphan

Arrhythmias. See Cardiac arrhythmia
Arterial blood gases (ABG), 174
Arterial occlusive disease, 65
Arterial pressure, 44
    and bypass, 88
    measurement of, 72, 104
    monitoring of, 277–299
Arteriograms, 176, 241, 248–249,
        379, 451, 452, 456
Arteriosclerosis. See also
        Atherosclerosis
    and aneurysm, 369
    and CPB, 400, 422
    and surgery, 37
Aspiration, precautions against, 25
Aspirin, 171, 188, 410, 416, 497
Asthma, 10, 182
Asymmetric septal hypertrophy
        (ASH), 232–235
    nonobstructive, 232–233
    obstructive, 233–235
Asynchronous pacemakers, 350–351.
        See also Pacemakers
Asystole, 53, 292, 313, 314, 421. See
        also Cardioplegia
Atelectasis, 319, 379, 478, 481
Atherosclerosis, 17, 23, 64, 149, 186,
        205, 206, 214, 215, 246
    and CAD, 273
    generalized, 186
    and oxygen, 243
    risk factors in, 242
Atherosclerotic heart disease, 42, 224,
        225
Ativan, 18. See also Lorazepam
Atresia, pulmonary, 285
Atrial fibrillation, 55, 57, 64, 78,
        141, 174, 496. See also Atrial
        flutter
    conversion of, 143
    and coronary artery disease, 386
    and digitalis, 381
    and ECG, 134, 135
    and pacemakers, 349
    and stenosis, mitral, 209–210, 211,
        212, 213, 216
Atrial flutter, 57, 60, 63, 64, 133,
        134, 174. See also Atrial
        fibrillation
    conversion of, 143
    and ECG, 127, 135
    treatment of, 141
Atrial kick, 219, 220, 233
Atrial pacemakers, 351. See also
        Pacemakers
Atrial pacing wires, 297
Atrial septal defects, detection of, 284
Atrioventricular canal, 286

Atrioventricular (AV) node, 58, 60,
        61, 63, 64, 117, 118, 120, 138
    and arrhythmias, 128, 129
    and cholinergics, 53
    and conduction, 12, 13, 121, 161,
        174
    function of, 248
    and heart block, 64, 147–149, 248,
        348
    and pacing, 431
    tissue in, 55, 56
    and valve stenosis, 301
Atrium, 265
    and aneurysm, 370
    cannulation of, 441, 497
    and cholinergics, 53
    contraction and heart rate, 352
    and CPB, 314, 418, 419, 431
    enlarged, 325–326
    giant, 143
    and pacemakers, 347
    pressure, postoperative, 319
    and ventricles, 173
Atropine, 12, 21, 44, 103, 131, 231,
        267, 333
    action of, 53–54
    and bradycardia, 10
    and cardiac arrest, 503
    for children, 291, 317
    and CPB, 314
    and CPR, 507
    and ECG, 136, 137
    effects of, 386, 485
    and heart block, 148, 149
    and hypotension, 9
    and vagal tone, 63
Automaticity in cells, 61
Autonomic nervous system, 423
    and blockade, 25
    and heart rate, 93
    receptors, 40
Avco-Roche IABP, 445, 447, 448,
        463, 464
a Wave, 173, 223, 226
Axillary artery, 77
Axis of heart and ECG, 122
Azotemia prerenal, 187, 189, 192.
        See also Hypoperfusion

B-44-3 pump tubing, 396
Bacteremia, 328, 329, 483
Ballistocardiogram (BCG), 8, 103
Balloon rupture, in catheterization,
        92–93. See also Intra-aortic
        balloon pump
Barbiturates, 6, 383
    and liver disease, 191

    ultrashort-acting, 14–15
Baroreceptors, 44
    activation of, 42
    and blood pressure, 55, 63
    cardiac functions, 6
    and ketamine, 25
Barostatic reflexes and barbiturates,
        15
Basilic vein, cannulation of, 84–85
Beck's triad, 492
Bennett ventilator, 474
Bennett Cascade humidifier, 483
Bentley, 399, 402
Benzodiazepine, 261
    derivatives, 16, 17–18
Beta-adrenergic effects, 220, 231,
        385, 506
Beta-adrenergic receptors, 11, 41, 42,
        43, 46, 47, 60, 62, 178, 182,
        201. See also Beta-blocking
        drugs
Beta-blocking drugs, 14, 47, 104,
        253–254, 263, 264. See also
        Beta-adrenergic receptors
    and CABG, 275, 383
    for children, 292, 293, 294
    and IABP, 451
    and MR, 217
Beta stimulation of heart, 200, 201,
        226
Bicarbonate, 48, 356. See also
        Sodium bicarbonate
Bicuspid valve, 220, 328
Bifascicular block, 350
Bigeminy, 9, 58, 174
Bird ventilator, 474
Blalock-Hanlon atrial septectomy, 286
Blalock-Taussig shunt, 292, 299, 333
Blood pressure (BP), 72, 99, 199
    arterial, 71, 86
    and baroreceptors, 63
    and cardiac output reduction, 52
    and CPB, 422, 423, 432
    and digoxin, 55
    direct measurement of, 72–78
    and dobutamine, 43
    and droperidol, 19
    and ECG, 246
    and enflurane, 13
    and epinephrine, 41, 42
    and halothane, 8
    and humoral substances, 177
    and IABP, 452, 453, 464, 473
    indirect measurement of, 72
    and ketamine, 25, 26
    and muscle relaxants, 27
    and nitrous oxide, 6–7
    and renal disease, 187

    and revascularization, 272
    and tamponade, 492
    venous, 78
Blood pressure cuff, 71, 74, 474, 479,
        480, 492. See also Blood
        pressure
    for children, 293
    and monitoring, 295
Blood urea nitrogen (BUN), 252, 488
    and creatinine, 169, 178, 184, 186,
        187
    of infant, 290
Body temperature, infants and
        children, monitoring of, 301–
        302
Boeringer valve, 474
Bohr effect, 188
Brachial artery, 77, 176, 258
Brachial plexus, injury of, 85
Bradyarrhythmia
    in children, 292
    and pacemakers, 350
Bradycardia, 23, 64, 227, 231, 254,
        255, 267
    and anticholinergics, 53, 54
    atropine-reversible, 10
    and bypass, 314
    and calcium, 59
    and CPR, 507
    and drugs, 386
    and ECG, 160
    effects of, 63
    and hypotension, 9, 21
    and muscle relaxants, 27
    and pacemakers, 349, 352, 353
    postoperative, 317, 484
    and pulmonary blood flow, 293
    reflex, 307
    and tamponade, 495
Bradytachyarrhythmia, 131
Bretylium, 62, 64, 138, 140, 452
Bronchiectasis, 182
Bronchitis, 251, 379
Bronchoconstriction, 46, 47, 182,
        507. See also Bronchospasm
Bronchodilators, 182, 251, 379, 479
Bronchoscopy, 328, 480
Bronchospasm, 10, 479
    and epinephrine, 41
    and heart failure, 285
    and ketamine, 25
Brown-Harrison heat exchanger, 398
Bruits, 379
Bundle branch block, 381
Bundle of His, 117, 118, 145, 347,
        348, 349, 350, 354
Bundle of Kent, 133, 134
Butyrophenone, 8, 43, 262

CABG. *See* Cardiac artery bypass grafting
Cachexia, 205
Caffeine, 182
Calcium, 47, 59–60, 268, 502
  and ACT, 190
  and AR, 231
  and blood pressure, 177
  and cardiac contraction, 318
  and CNS, 488
  and CPB, 412, 421, 422, 425, 431
  and CVP, 299
  and digitalis, 255
  and digoxin, 54, 56
  and ECG, 160, 161
  and halothane, 11
  and hypotension, 9
  and IABP, 459
  levels, postoperative, 317
  monitoring of, 304
  and oxygen, 105
  and oxygenator, 410
  and pericardium, 496
  and renal disease, 188
Calcium chloride, 141, 161, 255, 267, 333
  and ASH, 234
  and cardiac arrest, 503, 507–508
  and CPB, 60, 270, 271, 341
  and hypotension, 488
  monitoring of, 304
  and potassium, 319
  precautions, 335
Calcium gluceptate, 60
"Camel hump" wave, 161
Cannon wave, 173. *See also* "a" wave
Cannulae, removal of, 315
Cannulation, 78, 334. *See also* Catheterization
  and aneurysm, 370, 371
  of artery, 73, 76–78, 258, 297
  and CPB, 143, 311, 418, 419
  of IJV, 84
  and ischemic symptoms, 77
  and monitoring, 299
  percutaneous, 33
  rhythm disturbances during, 268
  and thrombosis, 75
Capillary wedge pressure, 52, 219
Carbon dioxide tension
  for balloon inflation, 92, 463
  and bypass surgery, 4, 308, 309, 379, 401, 404, 405, 407, 408, 409
  and coronary blood flow, 108
  and respiration, 477
  retention of, 183

and venoconstriction, 21
Carcinoid syndrome, 235
Cardiac arrest and halothane, 8.
Cardiac arrhythmia, 40, 130–135, 138–141, 213, 233, 275, 378, 379, 380, 496, 497
  and AR, 231
  and catheters, 90, 92, 127
  in children, 293
  and congestive heart failure, 286, 328
  and coronary blood flow, 431
  diagnosis of, 149
  and digitalis, 54, 452
  and drugs, 160–163, 385, 386
  and ECG, 119, 296
  and embolism, 388
  factors causing, 128
  fatal, 173
  and IABP, 447, 450, 451, 452
  in infant, 291
  and infarction, 387
  and LCOS, 317
  and lung disease, 182
  monitoring of, 473
  perioperative, 128
  physiologic basis of, 128–129
  postoperative, 318
  and stenosis, aortic, 226
  symptoms of, 171
  treatment of, 46, 61 64, 141–145, 383
Cardiac cycle, 198
Cardiac drugs, 39
  antiarrhythmic, 61–64
  cardiovascular, preparations/ dosages, 337, 338
  cholinergic/anticholinergic, 52–54
  diuretics, 64–65
  glucagon, 60–61
  glycosides, 54–59
  sympathetic blocking, 45–47
  sympathomimetic, 39–45
  vasodilator, 47–52
Cardiac index, 26, 42, 93, 99, 100, 265, 331, 381–382, 443, 457, 466, 496
Cardiac massage, 9
Cardiac output, 44, 421, 432, 491
  and cardiac index, 331
  and catheters, 301
  and CPB, 431
  curve, 97
  data for, 329
  and dopamine, 43
  and enflurane, 13
  factors determining, 317
  formulas, 93, 97, 98

and glucagon, 60
and glycosides, 55
and halothane, 8
and hypotension, 487
and heparin, 25
maintenance of, 485
measurement of, 93–98, 247, 267
monitoring of, 304–305
and muscle relaxants, 27
and narcotic analgesics, 23
and nitrous oxide, 7
postoperative, 316, 317, 318, 319, 321
and respiration, 477, 482
and tamponade, 494
and ventilation, 481
and ventricular function, 99, 100
Cardiac pacing, 141
Cardiac Slide Rule, 95, 96
Cardiac stroke volume, 59
Cardiogenic shock (CS), 42, 52, 272
Cardiomyopathies, obstructive, 46, 284, 349, 383
Cardioplegia, 60, 313, 431. *See also* Asystole
  potassium induced, 270
  and CPB, 313, 425
Cardiopulmonary bypass (CPB) 85, 86, 99, 101, 181, 186, 189, 191, 231, 269–271, 393, 455, 458, 460, 464, 496–497
  algorithm for, 433–435
  and aneurysm, 370, 372
  and blood pressure, 72
  and calcium, 60
  checklist for, 430
  circuit, 395, 396
  coming off of, 430–436
  complications after, 254
  conduct of, 418
  and core-cooling, 283
  and CVP, 289
  development of, 281
  and digoxin, 58
  and ECG, 127, 135, 296
  equipment for, 393–396
  and flutter, 127
  and hypothermia, 323, 324
  initiation of, 419
  institution of, 311–312
  and intraoperative fluids, 306–307
  and kidney, 188
  maintenance, 289
  monitoring for, 307–315
  myocardium in, 312–314
  perfusion, 44
  physiology of, 410–418
  precautions in, 334–335

and respiration, 250
termination of, 314–315
therapeutic decisions in, 100
and urine output, 303
and vasodilators, 47, 52
and ventricular failure, 330
Cardiopulmonary resuscitation (CPR),
    2, 501, 504, 505
life support
    advanced 503–508
    basic, 502–503
Cardiovascular depression
    and barbiturates, 15
    and diazepam, 16
    and halothane, 8, 9, 11
    and methoxyflurane, 14
    and narcotic analgesics, 20
    and nitrous oxide, 7
    and propranolol, 46, 47
Cardioversion, 141–145
    complications of, 144
    internal/external, 143
Carlen's tube, 372, 374
Carotid artery, 84, 85, 379
    arteriogram of, 181–182, 252
    bruits, 170, 273, 488
    disease of, 178–181
    endarterectomy of, 149, 274
    massage of, 133, 134, 485
    pulse, 201
    tracings of, 103
Carotid sinus, pressure, 57
Catecholamines, 212, 243, 245, 385.
        See also Dopamine,
        Epinephrine, Isoproterenol,
        Norepinephrine, Dobutamine
    and arrhythmia, 128
    and blood pressure, 177
    and CPB, 430
    and CPR, 506
    depression, 382
    and diabetes, 185
    and digitalis, 255
    effects of, 171
    and enflurane, 13
    and halothane, 10, 11
    heart sensitization to, 22
    and hypothermia, 302
    inactivation of, 25
    infusion, 60
    and LV, 261
    and methoxyflurane, 14
    and myocardium, 10
    and nitrous oxide, 6
    and oxygen, 105
    potencies of, 44
    production of, 263
    release, 295, 386

and PBF, 293
and stress, 192
and sweating, 284
and sympathomimetics, 39
and tamponade, 495
and vasoconstriction, 262, 473
Catheterization, 6, 176, 201, 236,
    246–247, 330. See also
    Cannulation
and arrhythmia, 127
and ASH, 234
and bladder, 302
and blood pressure, 72
central venous, 334
for congenital problems, 288
and CPB, 308, 393
in CVP, 266
data for, 329
diagnostic, 26
and diazepam, 17
and heart failure, 249
and IABP, 452
and LV, 155
of pulmonary artery, 234, 388
and PVCs, 174
of radial artery, 74, 75, 304, 384
and regurgitation, 203
of right atrium, 301
and stenosis, valvular, 202, 211
and tamponade, 491
transthoracic, monitoring of, 300–
    301
urethral, 328
and ventricular dysfunction, 245,
    249
Celite, 190
Central nervous system (CNS)
    and anticholinergics, 53
    depression of, 20, 21
    and diazepam, 16
    and droperidol, 18
    and lidocaine, 63
    and morphine, 21
    postoperative care of, 488
    seizures in, 58
Central venous pressure (CVP), 173,
    191, 192, 219, 220, 236, 266,
    384, 432, 487, 492, 493, 496
    and catheterization, 78–85, 86, 87,
        89, 120
    monitoring of, 258, 299–300
    in prebypass, 307
    and preload, 99
    postoperative, 318
Centripetal noncompressing pump,
    394
Cephalic vein, cannulation of, 84–85
Cephalosporin, 333, 334

Cerebral blood flow (CBF), 181
Cerebral perfusion, 42
Cerebral steal syndrome, 181
Cerebrospinal fluid (CSF), 183
Cerebrovascular accidents (CVA), 252
Cerebrovascular disease, 178–181
Chaotic atrial mechanism (CAM),
    133, 134
Chest thump, developed, 145
Chlordiazepoxide (Librium) 17–18
Cholinergic/anticholinergic drugs,
    52–54
Cholinergic receptors, 26, 40
Cholinesterase inhibition, 27
Chloroform, 19
Chordae tendineae, 206, 209, 214,
    216, 230, 236
Chlorpropamide, 186
Chlorpromazine, 43, 48, 269, 486
    blocking effects of, 46
    and bypass, 271, 423
    compared, 18
    and temperature, 302
Chronic obstructive pulmonary disease
    (COPB), 182, 250
Chronotropic/inotropic drug effects,
    40
Chylothorax, 287
Cineangiography, 176, 201, 204, 205,
    206, 209, 247, 329
Circulation, assisted, 441
    IABP, 442
    mechanical devices for, 441–442
Citrate-phosphate-dextrose (CPD),
    416, 417
Clonidine, 12, 178
CM_5 lead, 150
Coagulation
    disorders, 190–191, 251, 441
    and heparin, 427
    and platelets, 417
Cocaine and arrhythmia, 128
Commisurotomy, 225
Computers
    and cardiac output, 98
    for patient data, 475
Congenital heart defects
    anesthesia for, 281
    cardiopulmonary bypass, 307–315
    diagnostic techniques for, 282
    hemodynamic data in, 327–330
    historical background, 281–282
    intracardiac shunt flows, 330–332
    pathophysiologic aspects, 283–288
    postoperative care, 315–321
    and RVH, 124
    special problems, 321
    surgical management, 282

Congenital heart defects *(continued)*
  vascular resistance, calculation of,
    332
Congestive heart failure, 4, 171–173,
    249, 283, 285, 286, 377, 378,
    380–381, 387
  and arrhythmia, 328
  and CABG, 275
  causes of, 57, 284
  and CPB, 404, 411
  diuretics, 255
  and dobutamine, 43
  and halothane, 9, 12
  and IABP, 443, 457
  in infants and children, 285, 325,
    326, 327
  medical management of, 291
  postoperative, 317, 318
Consumptive coagulopathy, 191
Continuous positive airway pressure
    (CPAP), 319, 480
Coronary arteriovenous fistulae, 284
Coronary arterioles, vasodilation of,
    43
Coronary artery bypass grafting
    (CABG), 271–274
Coronary artery bypass surgery
    (CABS), 106, 252, 264, 270,
    275, 328. *See also* Coronary
    artery disease
Coronary artery disease (CAD), 6, 86,
    104–110, 133, 149, 178, 186,
    241–245, 261, 353, 377–380,
    381, 384, 386, 388. *See also*
    Coronary artery bypass
    grafting
  complications in, 378
  detection of, 246
  and diazepam, 17
  and diuretics, 255
  lesions, 169
  occlusive disease, 4, 8, 9, 19, 26,
    156
  other related problems, 242,
    273–275
  patients, grouped, 250
  prevalence of, 149
  stenosis, artery, 249
  surgery, 22, 109, 155, 193, 242,
    250
  treatment of, 52
Coronary blood flow (CBF), 256,
    261, 265, 460, 487
  and CABG, 275
  and fentanyl, 24
  formula for, 105–106
  and IABP, 451, 452
  and ischemia, 274

and oxygen consumption, 229
  total, measurement, 106
Coronary circulation, status of, 206
Coronary perfusion pressure (CPP),
    13, 42, 51, 107, 225, 260, 275
Coronary sinus thermodilution, 106
Corticosteroids
  and bypass, 310
  and glucose metabolism, 306
  and myocardium, 275
Cor triatriatum, 284
Counterpulsation, 159, 441, 443, 452,
    455, 463, 464, 465
Countershock. *See* Cardioversion
CPK enzyme, 153–154
CPK-MB levels, 174
CPAP, 326
Creatinine, 153, 154, 155, 290, 465
  clearance of, 187, 188, 189, 465
  and hypertension, 178
  levels, 488
Cross-clamping and aorta surgery, 87,
    269, 270
CS₅ lead, 150
Curare, 26, 386
c Waves, 173
Cyanide release, 49
Cyanide toxicity, 486
Cyanotic heart disease, 283, 286, 330,
    380
  in adults, 327
  and air bubbles, 334
  and bypass, 309, 311
  and catheters, 300
  causes of, 285, 287
  and embolism, 388
  and hypotension, 293
  intravenous induction for, 294–295
  and prebypass, 307
  and respiration, 482
  and TAPVD, 288
Cyclic AMP (adenosine 3′,5′-
    monophosphate), 60
Cyclopropane, 19, 27, 128

Dacron fabric, 283, 370
Datascope system, 80
  and IABP, 445, 464
Datascope balloon, 463
DeBakey pump, 441
Debubbling in CPB, 406
Decadron, 488
Decannulation, 75
Defibrillation and electric shock, 144
Delirium
  and ketamine, 25
  and side effects, 25

Delta waves, 421
Demerol, 20. *See also* Meperidine
Desmethyldiazepam and diazepam, 16
Dextran, 410, 411, 463, 487
Dextrose 306, 323
  and CPB, 417
  and diabetes, 186, 187, 274
  and nitroglycerin, 51
  precautions with, 335
Diabetes mellitus, 78, 81, 184–187,
    353, 379, 380
  adult onset, 184, 185–187
  and electrolytes, 184
  juvenile, 184–185
Dialysis, 189, 320
Diastolic filling time, 105
Diastolic pressure (DP), 72, 107
  and CPP, 107
  and diazepam, 17
  failure in, 491
  and heart rate, 227
  mean, 107, 110
  and PVP, 380
  and regurgitation, 226
  and revascularization, 241
  and stenosis, aortic, 224–226
  time index (DPTI), formula, 107,
    444
Diastolic pulmonary arterial pressure,
    (PA_D) 86, 87, 89
Diazepam, 63, 191, 193, 265, 274,
    383, 485, 496
  and aneurysm, 371, 372
  and anticholinergics, 53
  and barbiturates, 15
  and bypass, 269, 423
  cardiovascular effects of, 17
  for cardioversion, 144
  for children, 292
  and coronary blood flow, 181
  and CPR, 507
  and LV function, 261, 266
  and morphine, 385
  as premedication, 383
  properties of, 16–18
  and seizure, 58
  and tamponade, 496
Diazoxide and bypass, 271, 382
Diffuse intravascular coagulation,
    (DIC), 191
Digitalis, 54, 55, 169, 171, 173, 174,
    184, 188, 199, 216, 222, 245,
    268, 484, 494
  for arrhythmia, 318
  and ASH, 234
  and beta-blockade, 255
  and cardiac output, 381
  and contractility, 205

and CPB, 412, 431
and ECG, 123, 125, 128, 131, 134, 135, 147, 148, 159–160
and edema, 387
and infants/children, 285, 291, 317, 327
and liver, 192
and myocardium, 275
and oxygen, 105
and stenosis, valvular, 209, 226
and ST-segments, 152
until surgery, 383
toxicity, 12
Digitalization. *See also* Digitalis
and calcium, 59, 60
and dysrrhythmia, 64
and glucagon, 60
prophylactic, 58
and ventricle failure, 57
Digitoxin, 191, 255
Digoxin, 47, 54–60, 61, 63, 64, 191, 211, 222, 255, 383, 430
and conduction/heart rate, 55–56
and dysrhythmia, 56
and heart disease, 245
inotropic effect, 53–54
and pacemakers, 355
prophylactic use of, 57–59
therapeutic indications for, 56–59
toxicity, 485
Dilaudid, 200. *See also* Hydromorphine
Dimethyl tubocurarine, 26, 27, 386
Diphenylhydantoin, 61, 64, 129, 160. *See also* Phenytoin
Dipyrridamole, 410, 416
Diuresis postoperative, 310
Diuretics, 64–65, 169, 171, 245, 266, 387, 489
and aneurysm, 371, 372
characteristics of, 180
and CPB, 412, 421, 424
and ECG, 160
and hypertension, 178
and IABP, 443
and infants, 285, 291, 327
and liver, 192
and pacemakers, 355
and ST-segments, 152
thiazide-related, 12
uses of, 255
and ventricles, 484
Dizziness and arrhythmia, 171
Dobutamine, 43, 494
Dopamine, 10, 39, 43, 267, 268, 333, 494
and cardiac output, 318
and cardiogenic shock, 52

and CPB, 271, 314, 432
and heart failure, 99
and IABP, 459
and prebypass, 307
Doppler flowmeter, 72, 77, 78, 492
Doppler principle devices, 258, 293
Doppler transducer, 73
Dorsalis pedis artery, 77–78, 258
Dose-response relationship, 5
Double-roller head pump, 394
Dow Corning Medical Antifoam A, 406
Dreams, as side effect, 25
Drug therapy, preoperative, 253
Droperidol, 18–19, 25, 181, 262
cardiovascular effects of, 18–19
properties of, 18
for unconsciousness, 261
Ductus arteriosus, 324, 325, 326
patent in infants, closure of, 284
Dye dilution curve, 97, 247
Dyskinesia, 173, 176
Dysphagia, 18
Dyspnea, 222, 233
and embolism, 388
on exertion (DOE), 183
and heart failure, 171, 173
and lung disease, 182
and operative risk, 380
paroxysmal nocturnal, 208, 245, 249
and stenosis, mitral, 207, 210
symptoms of, 202, 205
Dysrhythmias, cardiac, 179, 244, 268. *See also* Arrhythmia
and calcium, 60
and catecholamines, 10
and diazepam, 16
digitalis-induced, 64
and digoxin, 54, 56, 57, 58, 59
and dopamine, 43
drug use, 62–63
and enflurane, 13
and epinephrine, 19, 41
and glucagon, 60
and halothane, 9–11
and hypotension, 9
and isoproterenol, 42
and ketamine, 26
and norepinephrine, 46
pressure-sensitive, 4

Ebstein's anomaly, 235, 285
Ecchymosis, 76
Echocardiography, 104–105, 201, 203, 205, 228, 232, 493, 494
described, 247

for congenital problems, 289
Ectopic activity ventricular, 54
Ectopic beats, 63
Ectopic impulses, 56
Ectopic pulsations, precordial, 173
Edecrin, 64. *See also* Ethacrynic acid
Edema
arteriolar, 178
cerebral, 181
fluid, mobilization of, 64
interstitial, 176, 183, 210
and lung disease, 182
periorbital, 285
peripheral, 170, 244
pulmonary, 23, 80, 350, 352, 380, 381, 387, 408, 419, 423, 496
acute, 215
alveolar, 173
care for, 477
and CNS, 488
and IABP, 452
and morphine, 22
and respiration, 481
Edrophonium (Tensilon), 53, 64, 133, 134
Einthoven's triangle, 119, 120, 122
Eisenmenger's syndrome, 380
Ejection fraction, 215, 247, 491
and contractility, 216
depressed, 266
and dysfunction, 208–209
factors in, 205
formula for, 198
and IABP, 456, 457
increased, 200
and infarction, 272
levels of, 269
and LV, 209
and regurgitation, 229, 230
ventricular, 329
Ejection phase indices, 205
Electrical conduction through heart, 118
Electrocautery, 127
and pacemakers, 356
Electrocardiogram (ECG), 71, 102, 104, 169, 201, 206, 242, 244, 262
and atrial pressure, 88
and calcium, 59, 304
and cardiac risk, 383, 384
and CPB, 88, 270, 314, 394, 421, 425, 431
as data, 328
electrodes, 333
and electrolytes, 125, 139, 160–161
and emphysema, 123

Electrocardiogram *(continued)*
  and extubation, 479
  for heart enlargement, 326
  and IABP, 443–447, 456
  and intensive care, 316, 475
  ischemic changes, 108, 110
  and monitoring, 117, 257, 260,
      295, 296–297, 335, 473
    and arrhythmia, 119
    and drugs, 159–160
    and electrolytes, 160–161
    electrophysiology, basic,
        117–119
    and heart blocks, 145–149
    and hypothermia, 161–162
    and infarction, 149–156
    lead systems, 119–121, 145,
        146, 150, 159
    in operating room, 125–127
    surgical, 385, 386, 388
    systematic approach to, 121–125
    uses of, 119
  and pacemakers, 347–353, 355,
      357
  postoperative, 319, 484, 497
  and RPP, 109
  uses of, 119, 122
Electrocardioversion, 268
Electroencephalogram (EEG)
  and CPB, 420, 421
  and monitoring, 306
  patterns, 12
Electrolytes, 169, 475, 489
  and blood pressure, 177
  and CPB, 421, 425, 430
  and diabetes, 184
  and digitalis, 255
  and ECG, 125, 139, 160–161
  in infants, 290, 327
  and LCOS, 317
  monitoring of, 297
  and oxygenator, 410
  and pacemakers, 351, 354, 355
  and respiration, 481
  therapy, 306
Embolectomy
  catheter, No. 3 French, 76
  femoral, 463
Embolism
  and countershock, 143
  and CPB, 312, 397, 421
  pulmonary, 387–388
Emphysema, 182, 482
  and ECG, 123
  and RVH, 124
Endocardial viability ratio (EVR),
      107, 110, 259–260
  and IABP, 110, 444, 445, 460, 465

Endocarditis, 214
  acute, 218
  infective, 226
    prevention of, 328, 329
Endo/epi ratio, 110
Endomyocardium and bypass, 313
Endotracheal cuff, 479–480.
Endotracheal tube, 242, 263, 474,
      479, 502, 506
  intubation, 45, 128, 262, 293, 316,
      385
  and respiration, 481, 482
Enflurane (Ethrane), 12, 24, 48, 136,
      188, 219, 220, 233, 235, 261,
      262, 263, 269, 330, 383
  anesthetic effects of, 12, 265
  and aneurysm, 371
  and bypass, 269, 270, 312
  cardiovascular effects of, 12–13
  and CBF, 181
  for children, 294, 295
  drug interactions of, 13
  and epinephrine, 13
  and LV function, 266
  and myocardium, 385
  and neuromuscular blockade, 304
  and pacemakers, 354
  in prebypass, 307
  and stenosis, mitral, 212
  and temperature, 302
Enterocolitis necrotizing, 327
Ephedrine, 9, 10, 43, 44, 45, 136,
      267, 268
Epicardium, 241
Epinephrine (Adrenalin, Adrenaline),
      10, 39, 40, 41, 44, 45, 141,
      268, 495
  and bypass, 271, 335, 430, 432
  and cardiac arrest, 503
  and cardiac output, 318
  in cardiac surgery, 102
  and CPR, 506–507
  dose-response relationship, 41
  and droperidol, 19
  and dysrhythmia, 19
  effects of, 41
  and enflurane, 13
  functions of, 41
  and halothane, 10
  and IABP, 459
  and prebypass, 307
  uses of, 41–42
  and vasodilation, 52
Erytherityl tetranitrate, 253
Erythromycin, 329
Erythrophoresis, 291
Ethacrynic acid (Edecrin), 64, 424
Ethrane. *See* Enflurane

Ethylenediaminetetracetate (EDTA),
      59
Excitability, of cell, 61
Exercise
  and heart function, 208
  testing, 171, 245–246
  tolerance test (ETT), 171
Expectorants, 379
Experimental design and
      pharmacology, 5
External jugular vein, cannulation of,
      84
Extracellular fluid (ECF), 411, 412
Extubation
  accidental, 483
  care after, 478–479
  criteria for, 478

Femoral artery, 379
  and aneurysm, 370, 372
  cannulation of, 369, 371
  catheterization of, 77, 176
  and CPB, 441
  and CPR, 503
  and IABP, 443, 463, 552
  monitoring of, 258, 299
  perfusion, 464
Femoral vein
  and aneurysm, 370
  and CPB, 441
  and IABP, 452, 463
Fenn effect, 105
Fentanyl (Sublimaze) 20, 261, 496
  and blood pressure, 267
  and CBF, 181
  properties of, 24
Fetal circulation, persistance of
      (PFC), 287–288
Fever
  and embolism, 388
  postoperative, 317
Fibrillation
  and catheters, 92
  myocardial, 58
Fibrillators, ac/dc, 144
Fibrin
  and ACT, 422
  clot, 189
Fibrinolysis, 324
Fibroelastosis, 206, 212, 216
  intimal, 210
Fibrosis
  interstitial, 183
  and LV, 200
  and MR, 225
  postoperative, 327
Fick
  method, 93, 247

and dye dilution, 96–97
principle, 106, 331
Filtration in CPB, 397–398
Fistula, arteriovenous, 76
and CVP monitoring, 85
Flaxadyl, 26. *See also* Gallamine
Flexer retinaculum, 73
Fluoride ions
and enflurane, 12
release of, 14
Fluotec Mark II vaporizer, 407
Fluothane, 70. *See also* Halothane
Foley catheter, 303, 334, 355
Foramen ovale, 314
and catheter, 286
closure of, 284
and TAPVD, 288
Forced Expiratory time (FET) and
lung disease, 182, 183
Force-velocity curve and heart, 101
Frank-Starling
compensation, 221, 222
mechanism, 26, 99, 210
preload, 223
principle, 201, 204, 207
relationship, 55, 228, 301
reserve, 214, 230
Franz XYZ leads, 159
Fresh-frozen plasma (FFP), 417, 418
Furosemide, (Lasix), 64, 303, 306,
319, 333
and aneurysm, 371, 372
and bypass, 309, 424
and edema, 387
postoperative use, 319

Gallamine (Flaxadyl), 26–27, 188,
212, 231, 304, 386
Gamma globulin production, 191
Ganglia, sympathetic autonomic, 8
Gangrene, 72
Gentamycin, 188, 329
Globulin/albumin ratio, 191
Glucagon, 11, 47, 60–61, 185, 255
and ischemia, 275
Glucocorticoids, 185, 412
and pacemakers, 354
Glycogenolysis, 41
Glucose, 48, 161
blood, monitoring of, 306
and bypass, 310, 312, 425
and conduction, electrical, 270
and congestive heart failure, 266
and glycogen, 191
and hypotension, 487, 488
and infants, 327
infusion, and ST-segment, 152
levels

in diabetes, 184–187
and renal disease, 188
and myocardium, 295
and pacemakers, 354, 356
and potassium, 319
Glucose-insulin-potassium (GIK) 422,
484
Glucuronic acid, 18
Glycopyrolate, action of, 53
Glycosides, 171. *See also* Digoxin
cardiac, 12, 54–59, 255
preparations, 172
and stenosis, mitral, 212
Gott, E. V., 372, 397, 436
Gott external shunt, 77
Green dye, 318
dilution, 305
Guanethidine, 12, 382
Guillain-Barré, 483

Haloperidol, 43
Halothane, 6, 19, 23, 24, 26, 48, 101,
128, 136, 219, 220, 233, 235,
261, 262, 263, 269, 330, 383
anesthetic effects of 7–8
and aneurysm, 371
and arrhythmia, 128
and bypass, 269, 270, 312
cardiovascular actions of, 8–9
and CBF, 181
for children/infants, 294, 297, 327
compared, 12–14
drug interactions of, 11–12
and dysrhythmia, 9–11
and heart disease, 4
and hypertension, 9, 21, 22
and hypotension, 9
and LV function, 266
and myocardium, 385
and neuromuscular blockade, 304
and pacemakers, 354
in prebypass, 307
and ST elevation, 156
and stenosis, 212
and tamponade, 495
and temperature, 302
and TR, 236
for ventricular fibrillation, 324
Hamilton cardiac output method, 98
Haptoglobin, 416
Harvey oxygenator, 403
Heart. *See also entries beginning with*
cardiac
and autonomic receptors, 40
block, 4, 63
and bypass, 270
and cardiac output, 317
and countershock, 143

degrees of, 147–149
development of, 484
diagnosis/treatment of, 145–149
and ECG, 78, 119, 123, 125,
131, 147, 148, 297
localization of, 121
and pacemakers, 348–350, 352,
381
third degree, 92, 248
disease
congenital, 85
operable, 332
electrical conduction, 118
axis of, and ECG, 122
electrophysiology of, 61–62, 64
failure
afterload reduction, 52
congestive, 266
murmurs in infants, detection of,
284
rate, 46, 95, 108, 110, 243, 261,
265
and block, 147, 148
and bypass, 314, 317
and calcium, 59
and cardiac output, 93, 99, 100,
102, 353
and catecholamines, 171
and ECG, 121–122
and ectopic beats, 63
and epinephrine, 41, 42
and EVR, 110
and ketamine, 26
and LA contraction, 200
and LV, 261
and muscle relaxants, 27
and nitrous oxide, 7
and oxygen, 105, 108
and propranolol, 46
and renal disease, 187
and stenosis, valvular, 207, 221
and TI, 109
and vasodilation, 48, 52
Heart-lung machine, 394, 396, 398,
404. *See also*
Cardiopulmonary bypass
development of, 281
and platelets, 416
priming of, 410–411
and venous return, 419
Heat exchangers in CPB, 398
Heat transfer coefficient, 398
Helium
and CBF, 106
and IABP, 443, 464
Hematocrit, 304, 306
and bypass, 310, 421
and hypotension, 487

Hematocrit *(continued)*
  monitoring of, 297, 334, 478
  values, 108, 326, 327
Hematoma
  and CVP monitoring, 85
  formation, 76
Hemiblocks, 146–147
Hemochron device, 305
Hemodilution, 250
  and bypass, 4, 319, 410–415, 419,
    422, 423
  and calcium, 60
  techniques, 306, 309
Hemodynamic monitoring, 71, 260
  arterial blood pressure, 71–
    78, 86–93
  ischemia, 104–110
  venous pressure, 78
  ventricular function, 98–104
Hemodynamics of surgery, 102
Hemoglobin, 188, 489
  in arterial blood, 105
  and bypass, 310, 397, 405, 406,
    411–413, 416, 423, 424
  and extubation, 478
  of fetus, 327
  and heart defects, 286
  monitoring of, 295, 297, 304, 306,
    334
  and oxygen, 256, 317, 326
    dissociation curve, 108, 266
  unsaturation in infants/children, 287
Hemoglobinuria, 64, 421
Hemolysis, 304, 441
  postoperative, 319
Hemoptysis, 93, 287
Heparin, 75, 77, 190, 333, 334
  and ACT, 305, 315, 428, 429
  and aneurysm, 372
  and embolism, 387
  infusion, 86
  and lidocaine, solution of, 299
    and bypass, 315
    half-life of, 306
  loss of, 426
  in prebypass, 307
Heparinization, 371, 372
Hepatic encephalopathy, 191, 192
Hepatitis
  and blood transfusions, 416, 418
  and bypass, risk, 309
  postanesthetic, 12
Hepatomegaly, 285, 311, 496
Herzlinger technique, 449
Hexafluorenium, 27
Hexamethonium, 25
Hill's contraction model, 101
His bundle, 147

electrograph, (HBE), 145
His-Purkinje. *See also* Purkinje
  fibers, 13
  system, 148
Histamine, 262
  H$_1$/H$_2$ receptors, 21
  and hypotension, 20, 21, 23, 24
  and muscle relaxants, 26
Horner's syndrome, 85
H-R interval
  in ECG, 121
  and heart block, 145
H-V interval and heart block, 145
Hyaluronidase, 156
  and myocardial infarction, 159
Hydralazine, 12
  and vasodilators, 48, 51
Hydromorphone (Dilaudid), 30
Hydrothorax, and CVP monitoring, 85
Hydroxyzine (Vistaril), for children,
  292
Hyperalimentation, 327
Hypercalcemia, 200
  and ECG, 160–161
Hypercarbia, 13, 20, 22, 58, 171,
    183, 212
  and arrhythmia, 128
  in children, 295
  and drugs, 8, 19, 62
  and dysrhythmia, 10
  and halothane, 8
  and narcotics, 19
  postoperative, 379, 386
Hyperglycemia, 306, 307
Hyperkalemia, 161, 188, 272, 431
  and aneurysms, 371
  and ECG, 125
  and pacemakers, 356
Hyperosmolarity, 185
  coma, nonketotic, 306
Hypertension, 45, 58, 176–178, 184,
    210, 223, 263, 379, 382, 386
  and anesthetics, 4
  and aneurysm, 371, 379
  and arrhythmia, 63
  arterial, 249
  and bypass, 269, 271, 311, 423
  and droperidol, 19
  and halothane, 8
  and IABP, 458
  and LV function, 266
  and morphine, 22
  and muscle relaxants, 27
  and oxygen, 170, 241
  and pacemakers, 353
  postoperative, 380
  preoperative control of, 12
  and propranolol, 11, 12, 46

pulmonary, 223
  chronic, 184
  venous, 210, 284
  and regurgitation, aortic, 226
  and surgery, 100, 385
  treatment, 485–486
Hyperthermia
  in children, 302
  in infants, 325
Hyperthyroidism, 132
  and propranolol, 46
  and stenosis, mitral, 207
Hypertrophy, 205, 206
  atrial, 215, 216, 221
  and regurgitation, aortic, 227
  and stenosis, aortic, 224, 225
  ventricular, 173, 177, 178,
    228–229
Hyperventilation, 9, 412
  and CPR, 502
  and EEG patterns, 12
Hypervolemia, 301, 386, 424
Hypocalcemia, 60, 161, 412
  and ECG, 125
Hypocarbia, 108, 484, 488
  and arrhythmia, 128
Hypoglycemia, 186, 187, 191, 306,
    307
  and diabetes, 184–186
  and insulin, 60
  and ischemia, 275
Hypokalemia, 58, 59, 60, 64, 124,
    178, 184, 188
  and bypass, 310
  and infants, 291
  and pacemakers, 356
  and ST-segment, 152
  and U wave, 124
Hypokinesia
  and catheterization, 176
  and stenosis, mitral, 209
Hypomagnesemia, 161
Hyponatremia, dilutional, 192, 285
Hypoperfusion, 189, 191
Hypoplastic left heart syndrome, 284
Hypotension, 6, 263, 378, 379, 382,
    491
  and aneurysm, 370
  and arrhythmia, 63, 64
  arterial, systemic, 9
  and arterial pressure, 297
  and bypass, 269, 310, 311, 313,
    315, 398, 421, 422
  deliberate, 72
  development of, 12–14
  and drugs, 254–255, 383, 386
    barbiturates, 15
    diazepam, 16, 17

droperidol, 18
epinephrine, 41
glycosides, 55
halothane, 9, 21, 22
meperidine, 23
morphine, 21, 23
muscle relaxants, 26, 27
norepinephrine, 42
vasodilators, 47, 49, 52, 385
and ECG, 134, 136
and histamine release, 24
and IABP, 452
and ischemia, 275
and oxygen, 243, 261
and pacemakers, 350
postoperative, 317–319, 484
prebypass, 307
and surgery, 387
and tamponade, 492, 495
treatment for, 46, 267–268,
    486–488
and vasodilation, 385
and ventricular failure, 57
Hypothermia, 18, 212, 250, 272, 406
and ACT, 305
and aneurysm, 371
and blood pressure, 72
and bypass, 4, 269, 270, 308,
    310–313, 405, 410–415,
    420–425
corrected, 281
deliberate, 72
and ECG, 127–129, 139, 161–162
and EEG, 306, 314
effects of, 302
and oxygen, 386
postoperative, 319
profound, 321–324
surface-induced, 283
treatment, 476–477, 486
and urine output, 303
Hypoventilation, 171
and drugs, 383
and IMV, 480
Hypovolemia, 26, 44, 80, 132, 192,
    213, 234, 255, 265, 266, 268,
    297, 299, 303, 317, 386, 482,
    484, 496
circulatory, 4
and hypertension, 12
hypotension from, 43
Hypoxemia, 212, 225, 286, 414
and bypass, 312
in children, 290, 293, 294, 302
and CPR, 506
noncardiac causes of, 287
and oxygen, 231, 243
postoperative, 317, 319

reduction of, 58
Hypoxia, 22, 108, 171, 183, 286,
    288, 321, 330
and arrhythmia, 128, 139
defined, 243
and dysrhythmia, 10
and epinephrine, 41
and heart failure, 57, 62, 63
and ischemia, 275
and monitoring, 295
myocardial, 356, 421, 476–477
postoperative, 379, 380, 386
and vascular resistance, 332

Idiopathic hypertrophic subaortic
    stenosis (IHSS), 57, 89,
    233–235, 294
Idiopathic respiratory distress
    syndrome (IRDS), 324
IJ wave, 8, 103
Iliac artery, 370, 379
Imipramine HCl and ECG, 160
Impedance, 101, 256, 317, 486
Impulse conduction pathways, 348
Inapsine, 18. See also Droperidol
Inderal, 46. See also Propranolol
Indomethacin, 327, 497
Infarction. See also Myocardial
    infarction
  acute, 103
    with IABP, 451
    and drugs, 178
    ischemia, 174, 176
    subendocardial, 173
Infection
    and catheters, 93
    and CVP monitoring, 85
Inferior vena cava, 288
    and bypass, 311, 313, 418, 419
    and oxygen saturation, 330, 331
    and urinary output, 303
Infundibular stenosis, 285
Inhalational anesthetics, 5, 58. See
    also Enflurane, Halothane,
    Nitrous oxide
Inotrex, 43, 45. See also Dobutamine
Inotropes, 9, 11, 104, 494–495. See
    also Dobutamine, Dopamine,
    Epinephrine, Isoproterenol,
    Norepinephrine
    and IABP, 443, 444, 451
    and oxygen, 105
Inotropy, 99. See also Contractility
Insulin, 161, 184–185, 333
    and bypass, 425
    and conduction, electrical, 270
    and diabetes, 184–186

and hypoglycemia, 60
and myocardium, 275
and pacemakers, 354, 356
and potassium, 319
preparations of, 185
Intensive care unit (ICU)
    admission procedure, 474–475
    charting in, 476
    for children, 316
    clinical observation, 320
    flow sheets for, 320–323
    organization of, 475–476
    staffing of, 476
    ventilation, 321
Intermediate coronary syndrome, 244
Intermittent mandatory ventilation
    (IMV), 319, 480–482
Intermittent positive pressure
    breathing (IPPB), 479
Internal defibrillator paddles, 268
Internal jugular vein. See Jugular
    vein, CVP
Intra-aortic balloon pump (IABP),
    110, 156, 220, 252, 258, 267,
    269, 297, 329, 384, 394, 397,
    441–443, 454, 489
    and blood pressure, 458, 459
    and bypass, 271, 394, 432
    clinical use of, 450
    complications of, 463
    discontinuation of, 464
    effects of, 446, 447
    hemodynamic responses, 451,
        460–462
    and hypotension, 488
    indications for, 450
    and infarction, 272–273
    and inotropes, 443
    and left main coronary artery
        disease, 271, 272
    and other LV-assist devices, 466
    and oxygen, 107
    and PAD, 464–466
    perioperative indications for, 453
    postoperative use, 458–460
    and surgery, 453–458
    therapy with, 99–100
    types of, 447
Intravenous drugs
    anesthetic, 4
    barbiturates, ultrashort-acting,
        14–15
    diazepam, 16–18
    droperidol, 18–19
    ketamine, 24–26
    muscle relaxants, 26–27
    narcotic analgesics, 19–24
Intravenous fluids and hypotension, 9

Intropin, 43, 45, 333. *See also*
    Dopamine
Intubation, 260
    endotracheal, 212, 262, 479–480,
        483
    and muscle relaxants, 27
    nasotracheal, 483
Ischemia, 65, 92, 108, 119, 120, 122,
        124-126, 227, 233, 252, 256,
        492
    and bypass, 270, 309
    and CAD, 273
    causes, 284
    and coronary blood flow, 181,
        274–275
    cerebral, 140
    and congestive heart failure, 286
    and drugs, 178
    and ECG, 244, 246, 296
    extension of, 42
    and infarction, 92, 174, 176
    and left main coronary artery
        disease, 271
    and monitoring, 257–261
    myocardial, 9, 47, 54, 57, 133,
        139, 214, 215, 218, 219, 225,
        243
        and aneurysm, 371
        anterior, 159
        and bypass, 421, 424, 425, 432,
            442, 450, 455
        defined, 243
        and ECG, 149–152, 155
        hemodynamic measurements of,
            104–110
        and IABP, 451–452, 456, 460,
            463, 464
        incidence of, 377–379, 386, 387
        onset of, 156
        and oxygenation, 410
        and pacemakers, 351, 354–356
        protection in, 274–275
        and transmural/subendocardial,
            151
    and overdistension, 266
    and oxygen, 326
    and RPP, 264
    subendocardial, 106–108, 110, 234
        measurement of, 110
    and surgery, 302
    symptoms of, 77
    and ventricular hypertrophy, 328
Isoflurane, 235
Isoproterenol (Isuprel), 10, 11,
        42–45, 47, 48, 63, 110, 136,
        141, 156, 158, 182, 213, 255,
        484
    and asymmetrical hypertrophy
        (ASH), 234

    for bronchospasm, 10
    and cardiac output, 318
    and heart block, 148, 149
    and heart rate, 317
    and IABP, 459
    infusion of, 131, 356
    and ischemia, 158, 275
    and LV dysfunction, 209
    and tamponade, 484, 494, 495
Isosorbide dinitrate (Isordil), 230, 253
Isovolumic contraction phase, 227
Isovolumic phase indices, 205
Isovolumic pressure, 101
Isovolumic relaxation, 215
Isuprel. *See* Isoproterenol

J point (ECG), 124, 151
J wire, 258
    in catheterization, 84
Jugular vein, 92, 173, 300, 371, 417
    external, 170
    internal, 81–83, 89, 90, 93
        cannulation of, 80–84, 89

Kerley B lines, 284
Ketaject. *See* Ketamine
Ketalar. *See* Ketamine
Ketamine, 19, 24–26, 212
    and arrhythmia, 128
    cardiovascular effects of, 25–26
    and cerebral blood flow, 181
    for children, 294–295, 380
    and LV outflow, 330
    and pacemakers, 355
    properties of, 24–25
    and tamponade, 496
Ketoacidosis, 184, 185
Kidneys
    and aneurysms, 372
    artificial, 407
    and autonomic receptors, 40
    and blood flow, 43
    and bypass, 395, 416
    dysfunction, 192
    preservation of, 319, 321
    and renal disease, 187–189
Korotkoff sounds, 72, 74, 297, 492
Krypton, and coronary blood flow,
        106
Kussmaul's sign, 492, 496

Lactic
    acidosis, and diabetes, 185
    dehydrogenase (LDH),153,154, 155
Laplace relationship, 215
Laryngoscopy, 262, 263, 295

Lasix, 64, 333, 387. *See also*
    Furosemide
Lateral plantar artery, 77
Lanz tube, 479
LDH isoenzymes, 174
Lee-White clotting time, 190
Lead
    intracardiac electrocardiographic,
        145
    systems
        for ECG, 119–121, 125, 126
        for ischemia, 149, 151
Left anterior hemiblock (LAH), 146,
        147
Left anterior oblique, view, of LV,
        247
Left atrial
    catheter, 219, 301
    contraction, with mitral stenosis,
        209
    hypertrophy, 123
    pressure (LAP), 71, 80, 110, 197,
        200, 201, 204, 208, 487
        and AR, 230
        catheter, 226
        and contractility, 26
        and CPB, 432, 436
        and DPTI, 107
        and IABP, 459, 460, 464
        mean, 332
        and monitoring, 85, 86, 87, 89
        and MR, 215, 217, 218, 219,
            220
        and regurgitation, 203, 229
        and stenosis, valvular, 207–211,
            222–223
Left atrium, 230
    contraction, 201
        and MR, 215, 216, 218
        and stenosis, aortic, 223
    and LAP, 85
    role of, 209–210
Left bundle branch, 118
    block (LBBB), 122, 145–146, 147,
        152
    and pacemakers, 347
Left main coronary artery (LMCA),
        456
    disease, 271–272
Left posterior hemiblock (LPH), 146
Left-to-right shunting, 293, 305, 324,
        326, 330, 382
Left ventricle
    and aneurysms, 371–372
    and AR, 230–231
    catheter at, 176
    and catheterization, 176
    contractility, 215–216, 222
    diastolic unloading, 206

dysfunction, 171, 208
dyssynergy, 200
and ECG, 120
ejection, 204
enlarged, 202, 325–326
failure in, 326, 327, 442
function, 385, 457
and hypertrophy, 232–236
impaired, 6, 52
and LA, 223
and regurgitation, 227, 228
and stenosis, valvular, 208–210, 213, 222–226
stroke work index, 460
and TR, 235
and vasodilation, 48
wall movement 155
Left ventricular
assist devices (LVAD), 466
contractility, 4, 229
ejection time (LVET), 102, 103, 104
end-diastolic pressure (LVEDP), 59, 89, 100, 105, 108, 109, 247, 249, 256, 261, 266, 269, 436, 457, 460
and barbiturates, 15
and catheterization, 176
and contractility, 205, 216
and CPP, 107
decrease, 49, 51
and diazepam, 17
and hypertrophy, 232–234
increased, 200, 202, 204
and lesions, 207
and MR, 215, 218
normal, 197–199, 201
and preload, 98
and regurgitation, 228–231
and stenosis, valvular, 207, 209, 210, 212, 222, 225, 227
end-diastolic volume (LVEDV), 171, 173, 199, 204
and contractility, 205
increased, 202
and LA, 223
and MR, 201, 213–218, 221
normal, 197, 198, 200
and regurgitation, 227–230
and stenosis, valvular, 207–209, 213, 224, 226
end systolic volume (LVESV), 198, 200, 201, 204, 215, 227
filling pressure (LVFP), 98, 266
function, 4, 89, 99, 104, 247, 249
and CVP, 80
and epinephine, 102
overextended, 107
and ventricle function, 99, 101

function group, 261–269
hypertrophy (LVH), 123, 124, 146, 192, 232, 233
pressure (LVP)
drop in, 215
and MR, 218
normal, 197, 198
volume loop, 207, 228
sinus rhythm, normal, 198
systolic pressure (LVSP)
and aortic pressure, 197
overloading of, 220–222
and regurgitation, 214
and stenosis, aortic, 224–226
Lenegre's disease, 349
Leritine, 20. See also Anileridine
Leukopenia, with CPB, 406
Levarterenol, 42, 45. See also Norepinephrine
Lev's syndrome, 349
Librium, 17. See also Chlordiazepoxide
Lidocaine, 10, 16, 58, 59, 62, 63, 82, 129, 262, 263, 333, 381, 385, 485, 495
and cardiac arrest, 503
for children, 295, 317
and contractions, 484
and CPR, 507
for dysrhythmias, 41
and ECG, 134, 135, 138, 140, 160
and monitoring, 301
and pacemakers, 354, 358
Lipids, 12
Lipolysis, 41
Lithium
for pacemakers, 353
Liver
enlargement of, 184
and halothane, 8
and prebypass, 307
sinusoids, 2
Lorazepam (Ativan), 18, 383
Low cardiac output syndrome (LCOS), 317, 319
Lown-Ganong-Levine Syndrome, 123
Lungs
and autonomic receptors, 40
compliance with mitral stenosis, 212
cysts on, congenital, 287
diseases, 182–184
and heart block, 146
functions, with nitrous oxide, 5
and heart disease, in infants, 326
intraoperative management of, 184
obstructive, 182, 183
restrictive, 183
and stenosis, mitral, 210

and surgery, 250
volume, with respiration, 477
Luxury Perfusion Syndrome, 181
LVSWI, 95
formula, 95
and ventricular work, 99
Lyosomes, with CPB, 396

MAC levels, 5, 354
Magnesium
and digitalis, 54, 255
and ECG, 160, 161
and hemodilution, 412
and oxygenator, 410
sulfate, for arrhythmias, 58–59
Malnutrition, postoperative, 317
Mammary artery, internal, and revascularization, 272
Mannitol, 48, 411, 488, 489
and bypass, 309, 312, 424, 425
and myocardium, 275
and urine output, 303, 319
MAO inhibitors, 382
Marfan's syndrome, 369, 370
Maroko dog model, 156, 157
Massage
of carotid sinus, 53
MCL$_1$ lead, 120, 121, 474
Mean arterial pressure (MAP) 95, 181, 220, 318, 496
and afterload, 99
and CPB, 432
formula, 421
Mean cardiac index, 215
Mean cardiac output, 449
Mean perfusion pressure (MPP), 181
Mean pulmonary arterial pressure ($\overline{PAP}$), 86, 87, 89
Mean systemic arterial pressure ($\overline{SP}$), 259, 260
Mean systemic diastolic pressure ($\overline{DP}$), 259
Mechanical circulatory assist devices (MCA), 441–442
Medtronic pacemakers, 359–361, 363–365
Mellaril, 160. See also Thioridazine
Meperidine (Demerol), 20
properties of, 23–24
Mephentermine (Wyamine), 10, 43
Mercury-zinc pacemakers, 353
Metaraminol (Aramine), 44, 45
Methoxamine (Vasoxyl), 9, 44, 45, 234
and AR, 229
and MR, 217
and vasodilation, 51
Methoxyflurane (Penthane), 12, 14, 188, 263

Methoxyflurane (Penthane) *(continued)*
  analgesia, 144
  and counter shock, 143
Methyldopa, 382. *See also* Alpha-
    methyldopa, Aldomet
Methylprednisolone, 48, 333, 334
Metocurine, 212, 262. *See also* d-
    Tubocarine, Dimethyl-
    tubocurine
Metubine, 26. *See also*
    d-Tubocurarine,
    Dimethyl-tubocurine
Mineralocorticoids, 177, 354, 412
Minimal alveolar concentration
    (MAC), 5, 261, 354
Mitral regurgitation (MR), 200, 201,
    204, 210–211, 212–213,
    272–273, 328
  acute, 214–215
  anesthetic considerations, 219–220
  chronic, 215
  pathophysiology of, 213–218
  and stenosis, 218
Mitral stenosis, 57, 124, 201, 203,
    205, 206–213, 222, 230, 284
  pathophysiology of, 206
  and regurgitation, 218
  sinus rhythm, 208
Mitral valve, 197, 201, 202, 228, 425
  area (MVA)
    disorder in, 206–207
  and catheterization, 176
  disease, 55, 85, 183, 184, 206,
    328, 380
  and hypertrophy, 233
  and LV, 209
  prosthesis, 211, 220
  replacement (MVR), 52, 211–214,
    216, 218–220, 222, 451
Mobitz blocks, 147, 160, 174, 348,
    350
Modified chest lead one (MCL1),
    129–130
Modulung, 395. *See also* Travenol
Monitoring, 256–258
  hemodynamic, principles of,
    295–306
Morphine, 5, 17, 20, 100, 131, 193,
    212, 213, 226, 265, 269, 274,
    486
  and bypass, 269–271
  and cardiac arrest, 503, 507
  and CBF, 181
  and IABP, 452
  for children and infants, 297, 317,
    327
  in intensive care, 21
  and LV, 261, 266, 267
Morphine sulfate, 226, 333, 383

Mouth-to-mouth resuscitation, 501
Murmurs, systolic, in infants, 325,
    326
Muscle relaxants, 26–27
Myasthenia gravis, 483
Myocardial blood flow, with oxygen
    demand, 13
Myocardial cells, 61–63
Myocardial contractility, 9, 219, 261,
    317, 318, 492, 506
  and ASH, 235
  and barbiturates, 15
  and cardiac cycle, 204, 205
  defined, 199
  and diazepam, 17
  and enflurane, 13
  and epinephrine, 42
  and halothane, 8
  and heart rate, 93, 352
  increased, 200
  and oxygen, 108, 243, 257
  postoperative, 484
  and ventricular function, 99, 215–
    216
Myocardial depression, 23, 100, 263,
    284, 330
  and anesthesia, 330
  and drugs, 193, 386
  and hypothermia, 302
  and morphine, 385
  and oxygen, 302
Myocardial infarction, 152–156
  acute, 98, 246
  and anticholinergics, 54
  and dobutamine, 43
  and CABG, 275
  and drugs, 253–255
  and ECG, 119, 153
  and epinephrine, 42
  and IABP, 451, 452, 457, 465
  incidence of, 378–380, 387
  inferior wall, 122
  and LV, 200
  management, summarized,
    272–273
  mapping for, 120
  and MR, 218
  and PBF, 293
  posterior, 349, 350, 377
  and vasodilators, 47
Myocardial ischemia, 170, 200
Myocardial oxygen consumption
    (MVO2), 105-109, 156, 202,
    253, 254, 255, 256, 260, 270
  determinants of, 253
  measurement of, 258–260
Myocardial preservation, 328, 371
Myocardial oxygen supply, 262
Myocarditis, and ECG, 125

Myocardium
  and bypass, 269, 312–314
  and catecholamines, 10, 11
  and CPB, 419
  dysrhythmias of, 19
  functional status of, 204–205
  and hypotension, 487
  and IABP, 451, 452, 458
  and oxygen debt, 410
  and pacemakers, 357–358
  preserved, 318, 324, 424–426,
    458, 484
Myomectomy, 234
Myxedema, 252, 274
  and ECG, 123

NaHCO3, 327
Narcotic analgesics, 7, 19–24
  anesthetic effects of, 19–20
  and anticholinergics, 52
  cardiovascular effects of, 20–23
  and droperidol, 18, 19
  and halothane, 11
Narcotics, 269, 283
  and AR, 231
  and children, 291
  compared, 20
  and CPB, 423
  and liver disease, 191
  for prebypass, 307
Nasopharyngeal temperature, 302
National Transfusion Hepatitis Study,
    418
Nausea
  and blood toxicity, 49
  and drugs, 171
Necrosis
  and CPK-MB, 156
  and cystic, 369
  hepatocellular, 192
  of tissues, 335
Neo-Synephrine, 44, 333, 452. *See
    also* Phenylephrine
Neostigmine, 131, 386
Nephron functioning, 189
Nernst equation, 354
Neuroleptic state, 18
Neuromuscular blockade,
    monitoring for, 304
Neuromuscular blocking drugs, 24
New York Heart Association
    (NYHA), 169, 204, 205, 210,
    245, 246, 380
  classification of, 245
Nipride, 49, 301, 333. *See also*
    Nitroprusside, Sodium
    nitroprusside
Nisentil, 20. *See also* Alphaprodine
Nitrate therapy, 215

Nitrates, 48, 253, 383
   and vasodilators, 51
Nitroglycerin, 22, 156, 220, 233,
      247, 253, 264–265, 272, 318
   and aneurysm, 371
   and angina, 170, 271
   and ASH, 234
   and bypass, 269, 271, 423, 432
   and CVP, 266
   for hypertension, 486
   and IABP, 452
   intraoperative use, 382
   and MR, 218
   and myocardium, 275
   patient response to, 267, 268
   and ST-segment, 159
   and stenosis, valvular, 210, 224,
      225
   and vasoconstriction, 46
   and vasodilation, 49, 50, 51–52
Nitroprusside, 22, 48, 156, 231, 264,
      265, 267, 273, 318, 319
   and aneurysm, 371
   and bypass, 269, 271, 432
   for hypertension, 486
   and IABP, 452, 459
   and ischemia, 275
   and TPR, 99
   and vasodilation, 46, 49, 51–52
Nitrous oxide (N_2O), 8, 63, 262, 265,
      267, 269, 274, 372, 383, 385,
      496
   for amnesia, 266
   as anesthesia, 3
   anesthetic effects of, 5–6
   and aneurysm, 371
   and bypass, 270
   cardiac effects of, 212
   cardiovascular actions of, 6–7
   cardiovascular changes, 7
   and CBF, 106
   for children/infants, 294, 295, 327
   and CPB, 406
   dose-effect relationship, 5
   and enflurane, 13
   and morphine, 23
   and MR, 219
   and narcotic analgesics, 20
   and neuromuscular blockade, 304
   in prebypass, 307
   and tamponade, 495, 496
   and seizures, 58
   and surgery, 100
Nocturnal angina, 249
Nomograms, 422
Norepinephrine, 10, 39, 44, 45, 128,
      494
   and AR, 229
   and ketamine, 25

   and MR, 217
   and muscle relaxants, 26–27
   and nitrous oxide, 6
   and oxygen, 105
   release of, 43, 46
   uses of, 42
Nodal bigeminy, in ECG, 136, 137
Nodal rhythms, 9
Noncardiac surgery, anesthesia, 377
   anesthetic techniques, 384–386
   congenital heart disease, 380
   congestive heart failure, 380–381
   coronary artery disease, 377–380
   monitoring in, 383–384
   perioperative complications,
      386–388
   postoperative care, 386
   preoperative measures, 381–383
   valvular heart disease, 380
Norman's Circulatory Support Score,
      460
Normocarbia, 8, 13
Numorphan, 20. See also
      Oxymorphone

Obesity, 379
   and blood pressure, 72, 73
   and hyperglycemia, 185
Obtundation, mental, 317, 318
Ohm's law of electricity, 72
Oliguria, 205, 213, 288, 303
   and CPB, 423
   postoperative, 317, 318
Open heart surgery, 43
   anesthesia protocol for, 333–336
Optiflo I, Cobe, 399, 402
Oropharyngeal airway, 263
Osborn wave, 161, 162
Orthopnea, 249
   and LVD, 171
Oscilloscope,
   and ECG, 126
Oscillotonometer, 72
Ostium secundum atrial septal defect,
      294
Overload ventricular, 201
Oxacillin, 333, 334
Oxazepam (Serax), 18
Oxyhemoglobin
   and CPB, 405
   and CPR, 502
   dissociation curve, 254, 413
Oxygen
   and aneurysms, 371, 372, 374
   and angina, 206, 224
   and AR, 231
   balance, myocardial, 105, 107, 244
   and body temperature, 302, 414

   and bypass, 308, 309, 311, 312
   and cardiac arrest, 503, 504–506
   and cardiac output, 97
   and cardiac risk, 384
   cerebral demand for, 181
   for children, 292
   consumption, 212, 214
      and digoxin, 55, 57
      and droperidol, 18
      ketamine, 26
      limiting, 41
      myocardial, 254, 255, 256
         and barbiturates, 15
         and vasodilators, 48, 49, 51
   in CPB, 395, 398, 399, 401–410,
      422, 423, 424, 425
   in CPR, 506, 507
   demand
      blood flow, 13
      and diazepam, 17
   and hypotensive patient, 170
   myocardial, 4, 108, 110, 243, 245
   and narcotic analgesics, 23
   of fetus, 327
   and hemodilution, 412
   and hypertension, 486
   and hypotension, 487
   and hypothermia, 413
   and IABP, 444, 451, 452
   and ICU, 475
   and ischemia, 275
   maintenance of, 388
   and monitoring, 295
   and myocardium, 352
   and nitrous oxide, 5, 7
   in prebypass, 307
   and pulmonary disease, 326
   pressures, as data, 329
   and regurgitation, 227, 229, 230
   and respiration, 476
   saturations, 330, 331
   and stenosis, aortic, 225
   and ST-segment, 159
   supply
      and angina, 243
      and halothane, 8–9
      myocardial
         consumption, 105
         and coronary circulation, 107
         factors in, 104–105
         and IABP, 107
         maximization of, 108
         measurement of, 105–108
   and surgery, 379, 385
   and tamponade, 495
   tension, 317
      arterial, 138
   therapy, 386
   and ventilation, 474

Oxygenation
   bubble, 441
   and chest thump, 145
Oxygenator
   blood flow requirements, 409
   bubble size, 404–406
   and CPB, 400, 401–410, 430
   critical volumes for, 403
   and hypothermia, 413
   membrane, 408
   and platelets, 415, 416
   and venous return, 419, 420
Oxymorphone (Numorphan), 20
Ouabain, 54, 432
   toxicity, 19
   ventricular fibrillation, 12

Pacemakers, 347
   anesthetic considerations, 353–358
   and arrhythmias, 128, 145
   atrial, 131–132
   benefits of, 350–351
   clinical use of, 358
   complications in, 358
   conduction block, types of,
      347–349
   conduction system, anatomy, 347
   and ECG, 119, 136
   examples of, 359–365
   and halothane, 10
   and heart block, 148, 381
   and IABP, 446
   lead wire, break in, 357
   monitoring of, 474
   permanent, indications for, 349
   and tamponade, 491
   temporary, indications, 147,
      349–350
   transvenous, 80, 141
   types of, 350, 351
   wandering atrial, 136
Pacing wires, epicardial, 58
$PaCO_2$, 107, 128, 181, 183, 184,
   266, 274, 421, 424
Pancuronium (Pavulon), 17, 25–27,
   53, 188, 191, 212, 231, 262,
   274, 295, 304, 327, 333, 371,
   372, 386, 496
Papillary muscle, 218
   dysfunction, 273
   of LV, 248
   and MR, 214
PA_D pressure, 93. See also Diastolic
      pulmonary arterial pressure
   and preload, 98
Parasympathetic nervous system
   blockade of, 46
Parasympathomimetic drugs, 128

Parasystole, in ECG, 138
Paroxysmal atrial tachycardia (PAT),
   133–135, 160
Paroxysmal nocturnal dyspnea (PND),
   171
Partial bypass, 44
   left heart, 373
Patent ductus arteriosus, 283, 284,
   286, 288, 291, 294, 302,
   326–329
Patent foramen ovale, 285, 286, 300
Patient evaluation, preoperative,
   290–291
Pavulon, 27. See also Parcuronium
P cells and pacemaker, 347
PCO_2, 286, 309, 326
Penicillin, aqueous-procaine, 329
Pentaerythritol tetranitrate (Peritrate),
   253
Penthane, 14. See also
      Methoxyflurane
Pentobarbital
   for children, 292
Pentolinium, 48
Pentothal, 14, 261, 354–355. See
      also Thiopental
PEP
   and contractility, 103
   LVET ratio, 103, 104
Perfusion
   coronary, 424
   and CPB, 422, 424
   and IABP, 443
   isolated organ, 394
   rate, and bypass, 309–312, 314,
      327
   subendocardial, 270
   and tamponade, 496
   and urine output, 421
Pericardial diseases, 119, 491–497
   cardiac tamponade, 491–496
   constrictive pericarditis, 496–497
   and ECG, 119
Pericardial effusions, and ECG, 123
Pericardial tamponade and CVP
      monitoring, 85
Pericardiocentesis, 495
Pericardiotomy, 495
Pericarditis, 173, 327, 496, 497
   constrictive, 57
Pericardium, 241
   and bypass, 313
   and heparin, 334
Peripheral circulation
   and AR, 229, 230
   and stenosis, mitral, 210–211
Peripheral resistance, 460
   and blood pressure, 72

and calcium, 59
   and catecholamines, 171
   and drugs, 385
   and tamponade, 494
Peripheral vascular disease, 379
Petechiae, 300
pH balance, and pacemakers, 356
Phenformin, and glucose, 185
Phenobarbital, 16
Phenothiazines, 18
   and dopamine, 43
Phenoxybenzamine, and CPB, 423
Phentolamine (Regitine), 46, 48, 212,
   220, 226, 267
   and bypass, 269, 271, 312, 423
   for hypertension, 486
   intraoperative use of, 382
   and vasodilators, 49–51
Phenylephrine (Neo-Synephrine), 9,
   44–46, 134, 233-235
   and bypass, 269
   and CPB, 423
   and IABP, 452
   for hypotension, 268
Phenytoin (Diphenylhydantoin), 64
Pheochromocytoma, 10, 60, 63, 178 ,383
Phlebitis, and diazepam, 16
Phlebotomy, 494
Phonocardiogram, 102, 103
   chest, 102
   and microphone, 103
   venous tracing on, 78
Phosphokinase, (CPK) levels,
   and vasodilators, 51
Physical therapy, pulmonary, 319
Platelets
   and ACT, 306, 319, 422, 428
   and clotting, 189–190
   count, 417
      and coagulation, 251
   and CPB, 397, 416
   and heparin, 427
Plethysmographs, 72
   photoelectric, 72, 73
Pleural effusions, 174
P-mitrale, 123
Pneumothorax, 7, 84, 182, 184, 287,
   482
   and CVP monitoring, 85
PaO_2, 181, 421
   and CPB, 416
   and edema, 387
   levels, postoperative, 316
Polypropylene, 407
Polyurethane, for IABP, 445
Polyuria, 306
Polyvinylpyrrolidone, (PVP), 288,
   410, 411

Positive end expiratory pressure (PEEP), 87, 374, 420, 474–477, 481, 482, 487, 488
Positive pressure ventilation, 20, 182
Postoperative care, 315–321, 373
  cardiovascular care, 483–488
  central nervous system, 488
  ICU, 315, 473–476
  problems in, 316–321
  renal status, 488–489
  respiratory, 476–483
  transport, patient, 473–475
Potassium, 128, 174, 183, 383, 423, 485
  and cardioplegia, 270
  and CBF, 106
  and children, 293
  and CPB, 412, 421, 422, 431
  and diabetes, 186, 274
  and digoxin, 54, 56–58, 255
  and ECG, 160–161
  and hypertension, 178
  and hypotension, 487, 488
  ions, and calcium, 59
  levels, 182, 184, 311
    postoperative, 317, 319
  monitoring of, 304, 306, 334
  and muscle relaxants, 27
  and myocardium, 275, 425
  and pacemakers, 354–356
  and renal problems, 188
  and ST-segments, 152, 156
Potts' shunt, 311, 327
P-pulmonale, 24
Practolol, 263
Prazosin, 48, 218
Prebypass
  checklist, 419
  period, anesthesia maintenance in, 307
  procedures, 418
Prednisone, 497
Preejection period (PEP), 102, 103
  and LVET, 205
Pregnancy and stenosis, mitral, 202, 207
Preinfarction angina, 244
Preinfarction syndrome, 244
Preload, 101, 256, 262, 317
  defined, 198–200
  and IABP, 442
  and pacemakers, 352
  reduction of, 267
  and tamponade, 491
  in ventricular function, 98
Premature atrial contractions, (PACs), 130–131, 174
Premature infants, 324-327

Premature nodal contractions (PNCs), 137
Premature ventricular contractions, (PVCs) 89, 131, 138, 173–174, 485
  and catheters, 90, 92
  and bigeminy, 160
Premedication
  for adults, 185–187
  for children, 291–292
Preoperative management, 169
  coronary artery disease, 170–176
  diseases, associated, 176
  ECG, 173–174
  essential data for, 169–170
Pressure transducers, 77
P-R interval, 161, 209, 297, 317, 431, 432
  in ECG, 56, 119, 123, 135, 147, 148, 160
  and heart block, 348, 353
  and LA, 223
  and LV contraction, 200
  prolonged, 381
  normal, 351, 352
  and stenosis, mitral, 209
  subdivision of, 121
Prinzmetal's angina (Varient angina), 151–152, 170, 173, 265, 271
Priscoline, 301. See also Tolazoline hydrochloride
Procainamide, 57, 61, 62, 64, 129, 134, 138, 354, 381
  and ECG, 125, 160
Procaine, 425
Propranolol (Inderal), 46–47, 61, 62, 64, 129, 138, 156, 174, 222, 226, 234, 235, 253–255, 263, 268, 272, 274, 484, 485, 497
  and aneurysms, 371
  for angina, 271
  arrhythmias, 131
  and bradycardia, 127
  for children, 292, 293, 394, 317–318
  and CPB, 430, 431
  and ECG, 134, 135, 137, 140, 160
  and enflurane, 13
  and glucagon, 60
  and halothane, 11–12
  and hypertension, 178
  and IABP, 452
  indications for, 265
  and ketamine, 25
  and LV dysfunction, 209
  and methoxyflurane, 14
  and myocardium, 275
  and pacemakers, 354

and ST-segment, 159
  and sympathetic stimulation, 58
  for tachycardia, 10–11
  uses of, 383
  and vasoconstriction, 47
Protamine, 48, 190
  and ACT, 305, 306, 430
  and anticoagulation, 315
  and CPB, 42, 393
  effects of, 429
  sulfate, 333, 334
Proteins
  and CPB, 410–411, 422
Prothrombin time (PT), 190–192, 251, 319, 417
  and ACT, 306
Psychosis, postoperative, 192
Pulmonary artery catheterization, 87, 219, 226, 267
  surgical indications for, 87
Pulmonary artery pressure (PAP), 86–93, 206, 208, 219, 236, 326, 332, 496
  and AR, 231
  catheterization, 89, 91, 92
  increased, 206
  and MR, 219, 220
  and PCWP, 93, 95
  and stenosis, valvular, 209, 210, 212, 213, 222
  systolic/diastolic, 86–87
  tracings of, 102
Pulmonary atresia, 281, 293, 319
Pulmonary blood flow, 332
  in children
    adaptation to, 287
    and cyanosis, 283
    and heart failure, 284–286
    and lesions, 293
    and prebypass, 307
    postoperative, 316, 319
    and pulmonary artery, 324
  and congenital heart defect, 328, 330
  and systemic blood flow, 330–331
Pulmonary capillary wedge pressure (PCWP), 86–90, 95, 191, 203, 204, 206, 208, 212, 259–261, 265, 267, 272, 273, 371, 372, 421, 423, 436, 450, 487, 492, 496
  and afterload, 99
  and AR, 229, 231
  and catheter malfunction, 93
  and contractility, 103
  and IABP, 264, 464
  and MR, 215, 216, 218, 219, 220
  and preload, 98, 99

Pulmonary *(continued)*
  and stenosis, valvular, 207, 209,
    210, 211, 212, 222, 226
  and TI, 109
  traces, 110
  and ventricular function, 100
Pulmonary circulation, and RV, 206
Pulmonary extravascular water
  (PEVW), 210
Pulmonary fibrosis, 182
Pulmonary function
  and age, 176
  tests (PFTs), 174, 182
Pulmonary infarction, 92–93, 94
Pulmonary rupture, 93
Pulmonary stenosis, 285, 324, 328
Pulmonary vascular disease, 183–
  184, 223
Pulmonary vascular resistance,
  (PVR), 208, 210–213, 220,
  222, 231, 288, 328–330
  formula for, 95, 332
  and infant, 284
Pulmonary venous congestion
  and cyanosis, 283
  and heart failure, 284
Pulmonary venous pressure, 380
Pulsatile assist device (PAD), 252,
  465
  and IABP, 464–466
Pulsus paradoxus, 319
Purkinje
  cells, 61–63, 347, 348
  fibers, 507
  system, 350, 354
    and arrythmias, 129
    ventricular, 117–118
P waves, 117–126, 130, 133–135,
  138, 160, 174, 388
  and conduction blocks, 174
  and heart block, 145, 148
  and pacemakers, 344, 351

QRS
  complex, 78, 102, 173, 174, 304,
    496
  and ECG, 160
  and IABP, 444, 446
  mapping, epicardial, 156
  and pacemakers, 348–351
  waves, 118–124, 127, 130, 132,
    134, 147, 148, 156, 492
Q-T$_c$ interval, 160
  in ECG, 125
Q-T interval, on ECG, 56, 119, 121,
  125, 128, 160–161, 508
  and calcium, 59
  prolonged, 304

Q-U interval, 161
Quinidine, 57, 61, 62, 64, 129, 134,
  138, 143, 174
  and ECG, 60, 125
  and pacemakers, 354
  sulfate, 381
Q-wave, 145, 146, 153, 155, 383,
  497
  and arrhythmias, 128
  and infarction, 173
  and QRS complex, 124, 125, 157

Radial artery
  and aneuryms, 372
  and blood pressure monitoring,
    73–78
  cannulation, 258
  catheter in, 304, 384, 493
  and IABP, 447
  monitoring of, 299
Radioisotopic
  methods, 205
  techniques, 104
Radionuclide
  described, 247
  scans, 201
Rashkind balloon atrioseptostomy
  catheter, 286
Rate pressure product (RPP), 108–
  110, 246, 258–261, 264, 265
  meter, 259
Reentry excitation, 129
Regitine, 46. *See also* Phentolamine
Regurgitation, 202
  aortic, 227
  tricuspid, 206
  valvular severity, quantitative,
    203–204
Regurgitant Fraction (RF), 204, 213,
  216, 218, 227
Reinfarction, and mortality, 378
Renal
  arterioles, vasodilation of, 43
  artery, 379, 463
  blood flow, 44
  disease
    and blood pressure, 177, 178
    vascular, 252
  dysfunction, 252
  failure, 274, 372
    and digoxin, 58
    postoperative, 316, 319
    and tamponade, 491
  function and glycosides, 54
  perfusion, 171, 465
  status, postoperative, 488–489
  toxicity, 14
  vein, and urine output, 303

Renin
  activity, and CPB, 395
  angiotensin-aldosterone system, 22,
    486
  blockage of, 46
  and blood pressure, 177
  production, 263
  release, 192
Reserpine, 12, 152, 382
Respiratory failure, postoperative,
  316, 319
Reticuloendothelial system (RES),
  189, 191, 251
Retina, arteriolar changes in, 178
  and diabetes, 185
Return-to-flow method, 74
Revascularization, 457, 484
  coronary, anesthesia for, 241
    anesthetic management, 255
    cardiopulmonary bypass
      management 269–271
    ischemic myocardium protection
      of, 274–275
    preoperative drug therapy,
      253–255
    preoperative evaluation,
      242–252
    special problems, 271–274
Rheumatic disease, 220, 226
  heart, 349
  of valves, 230
Rheumatic fever prophylaxis,
  328–329
Rhodonase enzymes, 49
Rhythm, in ECG, 121–122
Right anterior oblique (RAO) view, of
  LV, 247
Right atrial hypertrophy, 122, 123
Right atrial pressure, 78, 86, 88
  mean, 332
Right atrium, 80, 88, 92
  and bypass, 135
  and catheter, 96
  contraction, 78
  pressure, 266
Right bundle branch block (RBBB),
  118, 122, 124, 146, 147
Right-to-left shunt, 294, 305, 317,
  330, 380
Right ventricle, 89, 99, 330, 371
  and bypass, 330
  and cardiac output, 301
  catheter in, 90–91, 92, 93
  hypertrophy (RVH), 122–126
  pressure, 173, 206
Riva-Rocci occlusive cuff, 72
Robertshaw tube, 372
Robin Hood Syndrome, 181

RPP, 272
R-R interval, 174
  in ECG, 119, 125
Rubidium, and CBF, 106
RVEDP, 235, 236
RVSWI, formula, for, 95
  and ventricular function, 99
R-waves, 104
  and countershock, 141
  in ECG, 123, 124, 156
  and heart block, 145, 146
  and infarction, 153
  voltage, 173

S₃/S₄ gallops, 170, 173, 178
SA node, 130, 132, 133
  and ECG, 136
Saphenous vein
  bypass grafts, 138
  grafts, aortocoronary, 17
Saralasin, 48
Sarcoplasmic reticulum, 200
Sarns heat exchanger, 398, 399
Scopolamine, 17, 53, 183, 193, 211, 269
  action of, 53
  and bypass, 269
  for children and infants, 291, 292
  and CPB, 423
  and morphine, 385
  and premedication, 383
Secobarbitol, for children, 292
Sedation, and anticholinergics, 53
Seizures, postoperative, 317
Seldinger technique, 77, 87
Sentorr system, for blood gas
  analysis, 77
Sepsis, 287, 301
  gram-negative, 303
  postoperative, 191, 316, 317, 321
    and infants, 326
Septum
  hypertrophied, 232
  interatrial, 248
Sequential pacemakers, 351
Serax, 18. See also Oxazepam
SGOT, 153–154, 465
  and liver, 192
Shock
  and blood pressure, 72, 80
  and body temperature, 302
  cardiogenic, 441–443, 492
  and catheterization, 87
  and IABP, 450–452, 463
Sick sinus syndrome, 131, 349
SI, formula, 95
Sinoatrial node (SA), 60, 61, 117, 118, 233

and cholinergics, 53
and pacemaker, 347
Sinus bradycardia, 131
Sinus node artery, 248, 347
Sinus rhythm, ECG, 126, 127
Sinus tachycardia, 132, 133
Sinus venosus, closure of, 284
Sodium (NA⁺)
  and CPB, 411, 421
  and diabetes, 186, 187, 274
  and digoxin, 54
  and hemodilution, 412
  ions, 56
  and liver, 192
  reabsorption of, 65
  and renal problems, 188, 189
Sodium bicarbonate, 161, 333, 384
  and bypass, 310
  and cardiac arrest, 503
  and CPR, 506
  and dehydration, 188
  for PFC, 288
  and potassium, 319
  and tamponade, 495
Sodium nitroprusside
  (Nipride), 41, 49, 52, 129, 210, 212, 218, 220, 226, 229–230, 264, 301, 318, 333. See also
  Nitroprusside
  for bypass, 312, 324, 423
  intraoperative use, 382
Solumedrol, 333, 334
Sorensen intraflow, 475
Spirometer
  incentive, 479
  interpretation of, 175
Starling
  curve, 95, 98–100, 267, 384, 388, 432
  equation, 411
  forces, 423
  law, 201
Stenosis, 423
  aortic, 219, 380, 457
  idiopathic hypertrophic subaortic, 232
  isolated, 181
  pulmonary, 283, 285
  tricuspid/pulmonary, 78
  valvular, aortic, 233
Sternotomy, 220, 260, 262, 264, 319, 327, 496
  and aneuryms, 371
Steroids, 274, 425
  and pacemakers, 354
Stethoscope

precordial, 333, 335
  for children, 293
  esophageal, 334
  for children, 307
Stewart-Hamilton equation, 305
STIs, and contractility, 103
Stokes-Adams
  attacks, 349
  syndrome, 149
Stroke, 181
Stroke index, 265
Stroke volume (SV), 93, 95, 491
  and AR, 230
  and cardiac output, 24
  determinants of, 200, 233
  and dysfunction, 208
  formula, 93, 95
  forward, 204
  and heart block, 352, 353
  monitoring of, 473
  and MR, 215, 216, 218, 220
  and oxygen, 256, 261
  and regurgitation, aortic, 227–229
  and stenosis, aortic, 221, 222, 224
  and tamponade, 494
  and ventricular function, 99
ST-segment, 152–155, 173, 257, 262, 272, 296, 314, 384, 452, 492, 497
  changes, 151–154, 157, 246, 260
  depression, 56, 171, 173
    therapy for, 264
  in ECG, 121, 123–126, 128, 132, 134, 138, 160, 161
  and IABP, 458
  and ischemia, 149–152, 158
  and left main coronary artery
    disease, 271
  mapping techniques, 156–159
  stenosis, aortic, 226
ST-T-waves, 244, 383
  changes, 133
  and heart blocks, 146, 147
Subclavian artery, 370
  puncture of, 85
Subclavian vein, cannulation of, 85
Subendocardium, and stenosis, aortic, 224
Sublimaze, 20. See also Fentanyl
Succinylcholine (Anectine), 20, 26, 27, 136, 262, 333, 354, 355
  for children, 294, 295
  side effects, 386
Superior vena cava, 90, 118, 120, 258, 266, 288, 299, 300
  and bypass, 311, 313
  catheter in, 90
  and CPB, 418, 419, 421

Superior vena cava *(continued)*
  and oxygen saturation, 330, 331
  and pacemakers, 347
Supraventricular arrhythmias, 130, 131
Swan-Ganz catheters, 71, 80, 84–86,
    88, 89, 90–96, 127, 211, 260,
    267, 305, 384, 388, 411, 492
  and aneurysms, 370–371
  and IABP, 442, 450, 455
  indications for, 267
  and infarction, 273
  sizes of, 87
  value of, 379
Sympathetic nervous system
  blockage of, 46
  and cardiac output, 201
  and catecholamines, 10
  and disrhythmias, 10
  and glycosides, 55, 58
  and halothane, 8, 10, 11
  and lidocaine, 63
  and methoxyflurane, 14
  and muscle relaxants, 26–27
  and narcotic analgesics, 21, 22
  and nitrous oxide, 6, 13
Sympathomimetics, 11, 18, 39–44,
    45, 63
  for bradycardia, 10
  compared, 60
  dobutamine, 43
  dopamine, 43
  effects of cardiovascular, 40
  epinephrine, 42
  noncatecholamines, 43–45
  norepinephrine, 42
  and pacemakers, 354
Synchronized intermittent mandatory
    ventilation (SIMV), 480
Synchronous pacemakers, 351, 353,
    356
Syncope, 181, 222, 380
  and embolism, 388
  unexplained, 387
Systematic arterial hemoglobin
    unsaturation, 302. *See*
    Cyanosis
Systematic blood flow, and pulmonary
    blood flow, 331, 332
Systemic shunts, 327
Systemic vascular resistance (SVR)
    199, 201, 210, 212, 213, 216,
    217, 219, 220, 223, 226, 227,
    229, 231, 284, 329, 330
  formula for, 332
Systole
  and arterial vasodilation, 48
  and counterpulsation, 441
  and IABP, 443
  and ventricular function, 199

Systolic blood pressure, 72, 74, 243
Systolic time intervals (STI),
    102–103, 205
  influencing factors, 104

Tachyarrhythmias, 129, 131, 318,
    350, 380, 430, 432, 484, 497
  AV nodal, 137
  and diastolic filling, 205
  and pacing, 141
  supraventricular, 57, 174, 262
Tachycardia, 8, 10–11, 45, 56, 63,
    64
  and atropine, 54
  and catecholamines, 171
  and catheter, 90, 92
  and CBF, 107
  and chest thump, 145
  in children, 292, 317
  in CPR, 502, 507
  diagnosis, 486
  and drugs, 386
  ECG, 132, 133
  and edrophonium, 53
  and epinephrine, 41
  and glucagon, 60
  and halothane, 9
  and hypertension, 23
  and IABP, 452, 458
  and IPPB, 479
  and ischemia, 233, 275
  and isoproterenol, 42
  and LAP, 86, 104
  and LV, 202
  and morphine, 22
  and MR, 214
  and muscle relaxants, 26
  and oxygen, 15, 243, 258, 261–
    263
  pacing induced, 201
  and propranolol, 46
  reflex, 265
  and regurgitation, 227, 228
  retardation of, 268
  and stenosis, 209, 211–212, 224
  supraventricular, 226
    and pacemakers, 350, 381
  and tamponade, 491
  treatment of, 10–12, 485
  types of, 57–58
  ventricular, 138–139, 143, 381,
    430
Tachypnea, 182, 284, 286
Tamari-Kaplitt Pulsator (TKP), 464
Tamponade
  cardiac, 484, 491–496
    anesthesia for, 495–496
    diagnosis of, 492–493
    and pericarditis, 497

  postoperative, 317, 318–319
    signs and symptoms of, 319
    treatment of, 493–495
  pericardial, 57
Ta wave, 152
  of ECG, 118, 125
Tc interval, 159
T-connector, 297, 298, 334, 424
Tc pyrophosphate scan, 156
Technicium, with CBF, 106
Teflon catheters, 75, 76, 77, 78, 85,
    89, 90, 372, 493
Tensilon, 53, 133. *See also*
    Edrophoniun
Tension time index (TTI), 109, 110,
    259, 260, 261, 265, 444
Terbutaline, 42
Tetralogy of Fallot, 281, 285, 292,
    293, 294, 301, 302, 319, 324,
    330, 380, 419
Thallium, and CBF, 106
Theophylline, 182
Thermal dye dilution, 384, 449
Thermistor probes, 334
Thermodilution, 247, 318
  cardiac output curve, 97
  for cardiac output, monitoring of,
    305
Theta rhythm, 421
Thiamylal, and morphine, 23
Thiazide, 255
Thiocyanate, 189
  and cyanide, 49
Thiopental (Pentothal), 14, 23, 24,
    63, 261, 262, 274, 495
  cardiovascular effects of, 15–16
  and CBF, 181
  for children, 291, 294
  and countershock, 143
  and pacemakers, 354–355
Thioridazine (Mellaril), and ECG, 160
Thiosulfate, and cyanide, 49
Thoracic aorta
  aneurysms of, 369
  and bypass, 311
Thoracic duct, and CVP monitoring,
    85
Thoracotomy, 374, 496, 503
Thrombectomy, catheter, 76
Thrombin-antithrombin complex, 425
Thrombocytopenia, 189, 463
Thrombocytosis, 189
Thrombophlebitis, 387
  and CVP monitoring, 85
Thromboplastin time (PTT), 251, 319
Thrombo-resistance, with CPB, 397
Thrombosis, 75
  intravascular, 287, 295
  and monitoring, 301

Thrombus function, 463
Thyroid
  cartilage, 84
  disorders, 252–253
Thyrotoxicosis, treated, 383
Thyroxine, 274
Titration, with drug effects, 330
Tolazoline
  for PFC, 288
  and stenosis, mitral, 211
Tolazoline hydrochloride (Priscoline), 301
Total anomalous pulmonary venous drainage (TAPVD), 288
Total electromechanical systole (QS₂), 102, 103
Total peripheral resistance (TPR), 95, 99, 421
  and afterload, 99, 100
TP segment, 124
TQ segment depression, 156
TQ-ST- segment mapping, 156, 159
Trachea, 263
  anesthetized, 295
Tracheal intubation, 26, 127
Tracheoesophageal fistula, 287
Tracheostomy, 480, 483
Tranquilizers, 6, 11, 18, 269
  for children, 292
Transapical left ventricular bypass (TALVB), 466
Transitional cells
  and pacemakers, 347
Travenol, 395
  microporous lung, 408, 409
Trendelenberg position, 15, 80, 81, 262
Triaxial reference system, for ECG, 122, 123
Trichlorethylene, 263
Tricuspid atresia, 281, 285, 293, 319
Tricuspid endocarditis, 235
Tricuspid regurgitation (TR), 210, 211
  isolated, 235
  and other lesions, 235–236
Tricuspid valve, 78, 220
Tridodecylmethylammonium chloride (TDMAC), 372
Trigemony, 58
Trimethapan (Arfonad), 17, 46, 48, 51, 371, 382
Triple index (TI)
  formula, 259
  and RPP, 109, 260, 265
Thromboplastin time, partial (PTT), 190–192, 417
  and ACT, 306
Tromethamine (THAM), 410, 424, 425, 506

Tropin, with calcium, 59
Truncus arteriosus, 283, 288, 291
Tubing, in CPB, 396, 398
d-Tubucurarine, 26, 27, 53, 262, 294, 295, 304, 338. See also Dimethyl tubucurarine
T waves, 120–122, 124–127, 130, 132–134, 138, 151–153, 155, 159, 161, 388, 443, 446, 492, 496
  and ECG, 161
  and pacemakers, 351, 355, 356
T-wave inversion, 173, 174
Tygon 5-50-HL pump, 396
Tympanic membrane thermisters, 302

Ulnar artery, 76–77, 258
UMI Intro-set, 87
Unconsciousness, as anesthetics, 3, 5, 8
Uremia, 496
Urethral catheter, 263
Urine
  and diabetes, 187
  flow, and bypass, 309–311, 334–335
  output, 266, 421, 493
    and aneurysm, 371
    and CPB, 423, 424
    and IABP, 450, 464, 465
    monitoring of, 303–304, 306
    and morphine, 21
    and pacemakers, 352
    and ventricular failure, 57
Urine-to-plasma (U/P) urea, 189
U wave, of ECG, 118, 121, 124, 159, 160
  and arrhythmias, 128

Vagal
  activity, and blood pressure, 55
  activation, 57, 59
  nerves, 9, 26
    and cholinergics, 53
    increased activity of, 21
  nervous activity
    and halothane, 10
  stimulation
    baroreceptor-induced, 10
    of heart, 200
  tone, reduction of, 63
Valium, 16, 261. See also Diazepam
Valsalva, 300
  and CPB, 420
  maneuver, 82, 234, 300, 352
Valvotomy, aortic/pulmonary, 282
Valvular disease, 197
  heart disease, 89, 103, 267, 272, 274, 380, 388, 420

aortic regurgitation, 226–232
aortic stenosis, 220–226
  chronic, 4
  evaluation of, 201–206
  hypertrophy, 232–235
  lesions, specific, 206
  and normal functioning, 197–201
  tricuspid regurgitation, 235–236
stenosis, 202, 330
severity, quantitative, 202–203
Valvulotomy, closed, 211
Variant angina, 244, 271. See also Prinzmetal's angina
Vasoactive drugs, dosages, 339, 340
Vascular
  disease, peripheral, 251–252
  resistance, 330
Vasoconstriction, 235, 262
  and angiotensin-induced, 223
  and blood flow, 41
  and body temperature, 302
  and bypass, 311, 312
  and CBF, 181
  and CPB, 424
  and dopamine, 43
  and drugs, 477
  and IABP, 459
  in infants, 324
  and adrenergic receptors, 46, 47
  and norepinephrine, 42
  and PBF, 293
  peripheral, 212, 213
  postoperative, 318
  results of, 44
  and tamponade, 491
  and TAPVD, 288
  and vascular resistance, 332
Vasodilation, 330
  and afterload, 328
  arterial/venous therapy for, 48
  and bypass, 312
  coronary, 23
  and glucagon, 60
  halothane-induced, 12
  and hypotension, 268
  monitoring of, 301, 302
Vasodilators, 22, 47–52, 263–265, 267, 384
  actions of, 51
  and afterload, 380
  and aneurysm, 370, 371, 373
  cardiac indications for, 47
  and CPB, 432
  and IABP, 451, 458
  indications for, 47
  mechanics of, 48
  and MR, 220
  and PCWP, 273

Vasodilators *(continued)*
  and peripheral demand, 381
  preparation and dosage, 50
  sites and mechanisms, 48
  and stenosis, mitral, 210
  and surgery, 385
  therapy, 388
Vasopressin, and blood pressure, 177
Vasopressors, 43, 301, 383, 422, 482
  drugs, 263
    and hypotension, 21
Vasoxyl, 44, 45. *See also*
    Methoxamine
Vectorcardiogram, 159
V electrodes, 129–130
Vena cava, 235
  superior, 80, 82
    and catheterization, 83
Venodilation, 64, 385
  and CPB, 432
    and IABP, 443, 444, 457, 459,
      464
  and hypotension, 488
  and hypoxemia, 477
  therapy, 486
Ventilation, 479–483
  and ketamine, 25
  monitoring of, 474, 475
  and perfusion, 566
  in surgery, control of, 20
Ventilatory depression
  and diazepam, 16
  and fentanyl, 24
Ventricular
  arrhythmias, 138-141
  asystole, 140–141
  contractions, 484
    premature, 56
  end-diastolic volume, 109
  failure, 57
  fibrillation, 12, 64, 139, 141, 161,
    269, 270

and bypass, 312
  countershock for, 59, 143, 144
  and CPB, 420, 421, 425, 430
  danger of, 174
  and digoxin, 54, 56–59
  and epinephrine, 42
  and halothane, 9
  induction of, 63
  and narcotic analgesics, 22
  and pacemaker, 351, 354, 355
  risk of, 380
  treated, 324
function
  contractility measurements, 101–
    104
  measurements of, 98–104
  noninvasive techniques, 102–104
  and patients, treatment of, 99
hypertrophy, 120, 124, 201
inhibition pacemakers, 351, 353–
  354
muscle
  arrhythmias in, 127
myofibrils, 63
performance and disease, 17
pressure, 78
  and blood flow, 107
  and contractility measurement,
    101
  and epinephrine, 102
  and preload, 98
  rise in, 59
relaxation, 200
septal detect (VSD), 272, 273, 283,
  284, 291
Ventricular-triggered pacemakers,
  351, 353–354
Ventriculogram, 176, 177
Ventriculography, 234
  left, 246
Vineberg's procedure, 241
Vistaril, 292. *See also* Hydroxyzine

Vitamin K (Aquamephyton) 190, 191,
  319
V_5 lead, 125, 126, 149-151, 153, 154
  225, 226, 231, 257, 260, 272,
  296, 355, 384, 474
Volume ventilators, 319
VSD, 328, 330
V/Q ratio, 206
V wave, 173, 203, 216, 492
  pressure, 215, 218, 219

Walton-Brodie strain gauge arch, 101
Warfarin factors and coagulation, 190,
  191
Waterston shunt, 292, 310
Wenckebach block, 147–148, 174,
  348, 350
Wheatstone bridge, 96
Wolff-Parkinson-White (WPW)
    syndrome, 57, 123, 133, 134,
    152
Wyamine, 43. *See also*
    Mephentermine

Xanthine drugs, 49, 182
Xenon, and CBF, 106
X-rays, 201
  and cannulation, 84
  and catheters, 91, 92, 93
  and coronary disease, 169, 174,
    178, 184
  and edema, 381
  and embolism, 388
  of infant, 290
  for lung disease, 182
  and pacemakers, 355, 356
  and pneumonia, 284
  for premature infants, 325–326
  and respiration, 482, 483
  and tamponade, 493
Xylocaine, and CPB, 430